The Founders of Child Neurology

CHILD NEUROLOGY SOCIETY

The Founders of Child Neurology

EDITED BY STEPHEN ASHWAL, M.D.

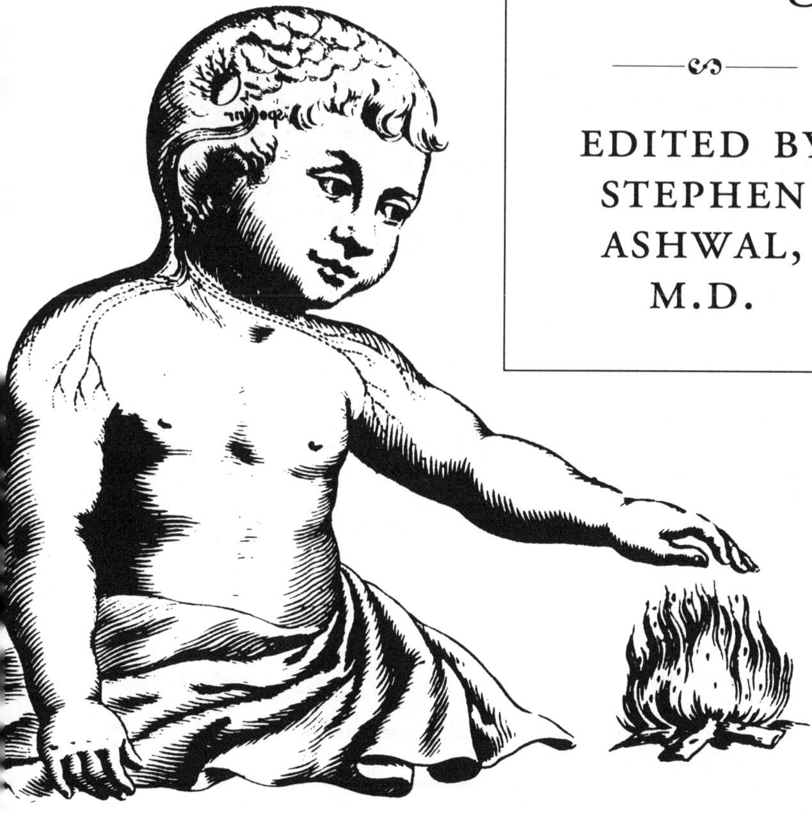

NORMAN PUBLISHING
in association with the Child Neurology Society

SAN FRANCISCO 1990

Published by Norman Publishing
in association with the Child Neurology Society.
Norman Publishing
720 Market Street
San Francisco, California 94102

Library of Congress Cataloging-in-Publication Data

The Founders of Child Neurology / edited by Stephen Ashwal.
p. cm.
Includes bibliographical references.
Includes index.
ISBN 0–930405–26–9
1. Pediatric neurology—History. 2. Neurologists—Biography.
I. Ashwal, Stephen, 1945–
[DNLM: 1. Nervous System Diseases—in infancy & childhood.
2. Neurology—biography. WZ 112.5.N4 F771]
RJ486.F65 1990
618.92'8'0922—dc20
[B]
DNLM/DLC 90–1827
for Library of Congress CIP

This book is printed on acid-free paper, and its binding materials have been chosen for strength and durability.

Norman Neurosciences Series, No. 1

Manufactured in the United States of America.

CONTENTS

ACKNOWLEDGMENTS

As 1990 ushers in the "Decade of the Brain," it is with delight and satisfaction that THE FOUNDERS OF CHILD NEUROLOGY is published. The development and publication of this book required the interest and efforts of many people. I would first like to thank Dr. Marvin Fishman, past president, and Dr. Darryl DeVivo, current president, of the Child Neurology Society, in particular, and the members of the Society for their encouragement and support. Drs. Kenneth Swaiman and Isabelle Rapin appropriately directed my inquiries so that I was able to contact colleagues in England, Europe, and Japan to enlist their interest and participation in this book. Dr. Lawrence Longo from Loma Linda not only kindled my interest in the history of medicine but also helped improve the scholarship of this work. I was also fortunate to have been introduced to Dr. Elizabeth Lomax at the University of California, Los Angeles, and Dr. Robert Aird at the University of California, San Francisco. Their knowledge of the history of medicine, particularly in the fields of pediatrics and neurology, and their willingness to review and comment on the introductory material was of inestimable value. The thoughtful suggestions of Dr. Enrique Chaves-Carballo, who served on the Archives Committee of the Child Neurology Society, Dr. Philippe Evrard from the University of Louvain, Belgium, Dr. Francis Schiller from the University of California in San Francisco, and Dr. Philip Dodge from Washington University in St. Louis, were greatly appreciated as were the comments and support of my colleagues, Drs. Sanford Schneider and Lawrence Tomasi.

A special expression of thanks to those who kindly listened to this proposal and then volunteered to write one or more of the biographical sketches. This book contains 124 biographical sketches written by more than 100 different authors from all over the world. My secretary, Ann Elliott, was responsible for all the initial manuscript typing and preparation. Jill Lustig and Martha Nicholson Steele from Norman Publishing were always available to answer questions that arose during all stages of preparation. This book would not have been possible without the special expertise of many librarians who were both willing and interested in pursuing requests for books, obscure pieces of information, and the majority of photographs and portraits. This included Gudrun Williams, Gilbert Abella, Leslie Hassett, and Carroll Westermeyer from the Del Webb Memorial Library and Paul Kittle and Laura Brown from the Medical Library Information Center at Loma Linda University; Margaret Kaiser, Jan Lazarus, Madeline Crisci and Lucinda Keister at the History of Medicine Division of the National Library of Medicine, Bethesda, Maryland; Cynthia Becht and Kathy Donahue of the History and Special Collections Division, Louise M. Darling Biomedical Library, University of California, Los Angeles; and Caroline Peck and Mr. William Schupbach, Curator, of the Wellcome Institute for the History of Medicine, London. Finally, a special thanks to my wife Eileen and children Alexander and Susannah who left me alone when I needed to be left alone and humored me when I needed to be humored.

Stephen Ashwal, M.D.

INTRODUCTION

THE DEVELOPMENT OF CHILD NEUROLOGY as an integrated field of medicine had its beginnings in the early 1800's, but it was not until a century later that this specialty began to flourish. With a rich heritage derived from traditional neurology and pediatrics, child neurology over the ensuing fifty years moved in many directions, reflecting the numerous social, technical, and medical trends occurring throughout the world. In the 1950s and 1960s, child neurology evolved into a very complex, distinct discipline. Formal training programs were initiated in many countries under the tutelage of those who had either trained themselves or received basic guidance from the early founders of child neurology. For example, in the United States, the National Institute of Neurological Diseases and Blindness began funding pediatric neurology training in 1957. The following year, a National Institute of Health ad hoc committee, consisting of Doctors Philip Dodge, Sidney Carter and David Clark, with the assistance of representatives from pediatrics and neurology, outlined guidelines for child neurology training. Ten years later the American Board of Psychiatry and Neurology began certification in neurology and psychiatry with special competence in child neurology. Child neurology societies or their namesakes were established in several countries: Japan (1961), Scandinavia (1962), England (1971), the United States (1972), and Belgium (1978). Out of the Oxford Club meeting, sponsored by Ronald MacKeith in 1970, and attended by thirty pediatric neurologists, the European Federation of Child Neurology Societies was organized. The EFCNS created regional societies based in large part on language preferences and an affiliation primarily with pediatric organizations. These societies included Dutch, Eastern European, French, German, Scandinavian, United Kingdom, and Eastern Mediterranean groups. In 1973, primarily because of the efforts of Sabine Pelc, the International Child Neurology Society was founded with a truly international membership and an orientation and allegiance closer to adult neurology. Certainly, as world communication and transportation technologies minimize distances, child neurology will continue to evolve and mature as it benefits from the international exchange of people and their ideas.

Child neurology is a "new" specialty, and its roots for most of us remain somewhat mysterious and uncertain. It is inevitable that the constant advances in medicine to which we are all exposed change the character and destiny of a specialty, like child neurology, almost on a daily basis. Yet it is certain that over generations the organization of our ideas and attitudes towards the patient, our conceptual frameworks about disease, research proposals, and our day-to-day bedside contacts are based on a heritage derived from the efforts of many previous clinicians and scientists.

Members of the Child Neurology Society expressed interest and supported an effort to compile a recorded history of this discipline. Excellent models of well-recognized related works in neurology include, *Garrison's History of Neurology* by Lawrence McHenry (1969), and in pediatrics, *Abt-Garrison History of Pediatrics* (1965). In McHenry's 552–page book the following is the only paragraph that considers the field of child neurology:

The neurological diseases of childhood and the development of the field of pediatric neurology (Levinson, 1949; Peterman, 1957) began in the early Nineteenth Century with the work of North (1826), Gerhard (1833), C. L. Klohss (1837), Copeman (1873), and others. Little (1853, 1861–62), gave the first report on cerebral diplegia, while Sturges (1881), Osler (1889, 1894) and others wrote on chorea and cerebral palsy in childhood. The first separate textbook of pediatric neurology was the classic work of Bernard Sachs (1895). Hydrocephalus was described by Cheyne (1808) and Brachet (1818), and a good example is shown in Bright's (1831) atlas. Porencephaly was described by Kundrat (1882). Other late Nineteenth Century neurology texts, such as Gowers' Manual *and Oppenheim's* Lehrbuch, *contain sections on neurological disorders occurring in childhood. Freud (1897) also prepared a review of pediatric neurology. In the early part of the Twentieth Century, the most notable work was that by Bruns, Cramer and Ziehen (1912).* (McHenry, 1969, 444)

McHenry cited articles by Abraham Levinson (1949) and Mynie G. Peterman (1957) that gave brief biographical overviews of several well-recognized physicians, such as Hippocrates, Thomas Sydenham, John Clarke, and Friedrich von Recklinghausen, who, among their many contributions to medicine, made relevant and important observations on childhood neurologic diseases.

In Arthur F. Abt's more concise *Abt-Garrison History of*

Pediatrics, there are but two paragraphs in 316 pages devoted to child neurology:

Of treatises on nervous disease in children, perhaps the earliest was L. W. Mauthner's Diseases of the Brain and Spinal Cord *(1844). A number of monographs on special subjects preceded and followed this, but apart from the Lumelian* [sic] *lectures of Charles West (1871), perhaps the earliest systematic treatises of importance were those of C. Pavone (Milan, 1892), B. Sachs (1895), B. K. Rachford (1905), M. Thiemich and J. Zappert (1910) and G. Peritz (1912).*

Of original descriptions of nervous diseases, those of cerebrospinal meningitis by Gaspard Vieusseux (1805), tetany by John Clarke (1815), S. L. Steinheim (1830), and J. B. K. Dance (1832), softening of the brain by Rostan (1820), poliomyelitis by M. Underwood (1786) [sic], *John Badham (1835), Jacob Heine (1840) and Duchenne of Bologne (1865), with the subsequent work of O. Medin (1890), Simon Flexner (1910–1916), Peabody, Draper, Dochez and the report of the Swedish Medical Institute (1912), the various forms of progressive muscular atrophy by Duchenne and Aran (1847–1868), Charcot and Joffroy (1869), Charcot and Marie (1886), Erb (1884–91), Guido Werdnig (1890–94) and Johann Hoffmann (1894), congenital spastic paraplegia by William John Little (1861), hereditary ataxia by Nikolaus Friedreich (1863–76), amaurotic family idiocy by Bernard Sachs (1887), hereditary cerebellar ataxia by Pierre Marie (1893), progressive interstitial hypertrophic neuritis by Jules Dejerine and Jules Sottas (1893) called erythema infectiosum by Salomon Stricker (1899) and amyotonia congenita by Hermann Oppenheim (1900) may be noted.* (Abt, 1965, 113)

From another perspective, medical history is also biographical. The lives of physicians, their contributions, the period in which they lived and their influence on medicine in general and their specialty in particular have formed the majority of such writings. Pediatrics and neurology are indeed fortunate to have several valuable sources that are fascinating, educational, and inspirational. George Frederic Still's *The History of Paediatrics* (1931), John Ruhräh's *Pediatrics of the Past* (1925) and *Pediatric Biographies* (1932), Abraham Levinson's *Pioneers of Pediatrics* (1943), and Borden Veeder's *Pediatric Profiles* (1957) are illustrative. In neurology, Webb Haymaker's and Francis Schiller's *The Founders of Neurology*

(1953, 1970) is exceptional and served as the model for the current volume.

This book consists of a series of biographical sketches of individuals who, from the seventeenth century to the present, have in some way made notable contributions to the understanding or care of children with neurological disorders. It is certainly not complete; those included are representative of many others who also deserve similar recognition. The biographical section of this book has been chronologically divided into five major time periods that reflect major trends occurring in pediatrics, neurology and child neurology. These sketches have been written by over one hundred authors from many different backgrounds in medicine and from many countries. Each sketch is not just a biography, but will also provide a better understanding of what was happening in child neurology or the related fields of pediatrics or neurology at the time the particular founder was caring for children. In some instances, quotations from the original principal contribution have been included to illustrate the attentiveness to clinical detail that is characteristic of the field. Each sketch also includes a portrait style photograph (if available) and in many instances reproductions from the original work, including pictures of children with specific neurologic disorders, drawings, handwriting samples, and an occasional informal photograph of the founder. Finally, each sketch is referenced with the major and some of the minor works of each founder as well as other historically important cited texts or papers.

As an introductory overview, a brief history of the field of child neurology has also been included. Its purpose is to give the reader a general idea of what comprises the field of child neurology and to furnish several chronological reference points, so that one can indeed appreciate the contributions made by the physicians included in this book.

There are essentially four ways to trace the development of child neurology aside from delving into the lives of the founders of this field. The first would be to examine the separate national histories of pediatrics and neurology and to search for the beginnings of interest in childhood neurologic disorders. For many reasons, this is a complex and unsettling task and justifies a volume of its own. The second approach would be to catalogue the important discoveries and contributions, and create a work similar to that of Leslie T. Morton's *A Medical Bibliography* (1983). A third alternative would be to assemble an annotated catalogue of the works in the field with perhaps some biographical information about both the book and the author. Finally, a brief subject-by-subject historical review could be considered. This last approach seemed to be the most sensible way to provide an overview of child neurology. I have chosen to do this before presenting the biographies of those physicians from many disciplines who had both a scientific interest and a very personal concern for children with neurologic disorders.

EPILEPSY

Generalized Seizures

Because seizures are so dramatic in their character, observations of their occurrence date back to the beginnings of recorded medical history. Hippocrates (460–370 B.C.) is credited with one of the earliest descriptions of seizures in children:

> *Now in children convulsions occur if there has been acute fever, and if the bowel has not been open, and if they have been sleepless, and if frightened, and if they have been screaming, and if they have changed colour acquiring a greenish or pale or livid or red colour. Convulsions occur most readily in children from just after birth up to the seventh year. But older children and men are no longer liable to convulsions in fevers, unless some complication with violent and very grave symptoms has arisen, as, for instance, happens with acute delirium.* (Still, 1931, 9)

Hippocrates wrote much about convulsions in children; he believed that they were due to diseases in the brain, proposing that epileptic attacks were caused by phlegm obstructing air in the cerebral veins. The Hippocratic writings also suggested that genetic factors were of importance in the etiology of epilepsy, as were prenatal and perinatal events (Wallace, 1984, 80). Seizures were noted to occur most commonly during the eruptions of the canines, which is at about twelve months of age. This coincides with the onset of febrile seizures that were further recognized by the writers of that time to occur in children under age seven years.

Many of the early writers also addressed the issue of treatment.

Paul of Aegina (625–690 A.D.) recommended baths for children suffering from convulsions, a remedy still used today in infants seen in emergency rooms with suspected febrile seizures (Levinson, 1949, 225). Rhazes (869–962), the famed Arabian physician, in his treatise on children, gave accurate descriptions of nocturnal seizures, febrile seizures, and night terrors. Paulus Bagerlardus (1472) favored treating childhood convulsions with the oil of white lilies or wet hyssop, while also stating that "convulsions are relieved and cured by the favor of the Lord" (Ruhräh, 1925, 40). In the fifteenth century Bartholomaeus Metlinger (1497) attributed convulsions to immoral conduct on the part of the mother during pregnancy or to imbecility "in the head of the fetus due to the influence of the stars." His ideas were, obviously, influenced by the prevailing theologies and philosophies of the Middle Ages. For treatment and prevention, he recommended nursing women to conduct themselves properly and "to refrain from eating apples" (Ruhräh, 1925, 86).

In the Middle Ages, epilepsy and seizures were described by almost all writers on pediatrics, yet to the modern day reader it is evident that the difference between these two topics was not very clear. However, many interesting and accurate observations were communicated. Cornelius Roelants (1450–1525), who had studied at the University of Louvain and written the most recognized pediatric treatise of the sixteenth century, included chapters on epilepsy. Thomas Phayre (1510–60) in *The Boke of Chyldren* (1545), the first treatise on pediatric diseases in the English language, and Hieronymus Mercuriali (1530–1606) in his pediatric treatise (1583), were the principal contributors to this subject after Roelants. Phayre recognized that age was a factor in the prognosis of epilepsy. A century later both Robert Pemell in *The Diseases of Children* (1653) and J. Starsmare in *Children's Diseases* (1664), observed that a common reason for seizures was that "the Child is born of Parents that have this Falling Sickness" (Still, 1931, 258). With the description of chorea by Thomas Sydenham (1686) as a "sort of convulsion," one suspects that the term "convulsion" was more descriptive of different types of involuntary movements, in contrast to the term "epilepsy," which was reserved for use as it still is today.

Thomas Willis (1621–1675) described in 1667 post-mortem

findings of "a considerable quantity of grummous blood" in the brain in the fourth child of a family who died from convulsions, but Willis was uncertain as to whether this was an effect rather than cause of the seizures (Levinson, 1943, 39). Willis also stated that epilepsy could be inherited or acquired, "Primary or Sympathetick," and also thought that age was a critical factor. Franciscus de le Boë or Sylvius (1614–1672), after whom the Sylvian fissure is named, also described a fatal convulsive episode lasting for several hours in his own eight-month-old daughter in *De morbis infantum et aliis quibusdam memoratu dignis affectibus* (1682) (Wallace, 1984, 85).

Although the concept of reflex activity of the nervous system originated in the eighteenth century, convulsions were thought to be due to the sudden rush of blood or nervous fluid to the peripherally affected part. In *Lexicon Physico-Medicum* (1726), John Quincy observed that epilepsy differed from convulsions in that in epilepsy "sensation suddenly ceases with an immediate prostration of the body" (Wallace, 1984, 88). In 1754 Petrus Sundius from Uppsala, Sweden, published a dissertation entitled *Epilepsia infantili*. This work represents one of the first treatises to appear on this subject. Sundius listed nine different causes of epilepsy, but it is his mention of "*meconio retento*," "*Febribus exanthematicis*," and "*Febre intermittente*" that is of note. It was William Heberden (1767–1845) in his *Commentaries* (1802) who observed that, although children were more susceptible to epilepsy, they were also more likely to recover completely. He also cautioned that one must separate true epilepsy from the occasional convulsion of childhood.

With the beginning of the nineteenth century, interest in infantile and childhood convulsive disorders became more apparent and complete monographs solely discussing these disorders were published. Jean Baptiste Timothée Baumes's *Des convulsions dans l'enfance, de leurs causes, et de leur traitement* (1797) was revised and a second edition published in 1805. John Clarke in his *Diseases of Children* (1815) provided the first description of infantile tetany and seizures that we now accept as secondary to hypocalcemia. Jean Louis Brachet's *Mémoire sur les causes des convulsions chez les enfans et sur les moyens d'y remédier* (1824) was an elaborate presentation of the many forms of childhood seizures. Brachet included many personal observations and those of other writers of the period. John North, a surgeon, wrote an extensive monograph entitled *Practical Observations on the Convulsions of Infants* (1826). The pediatric treatises of this time all had very extensive sections on generalized convulsions in children. Among these were those of Charles Michel Billard (1828), François Valleix (1838), and Frederic Rilliet and Antoine Barthez (1838–43). Charles West's *On Some Disorders of the Nervous System in Childhood* (1871) also gave a good overview of the understanding of this problem. Probably the first systematic approaches to the clinical analysis of epilepsy were those of John Hughlings Jackson (1863) and William Gowers. Gowers's monograph *Epilepsy and Other Chronic Convulsive Diseases* (1881a) contains several sections devoted primarily to children. In the early part of the twentieth century, the majority of writings on epilepsy appeared as book chapters in pediatric texts or separately as journal articles. Independent monographs on pediatric epilepsy included those by Heinrich Vogt (1910), Edward Bridge (1949), and Samuel Livingston (1954), and the exhaustive, though more general, works of Wilder Penfield and Herbert Jaspar (1954), and William and Margaret Lennox (1960). Owsei Temkin's *The Falling Sickness: A History of Epilepsy from the Greeks to the Beginnings of Modern Neurology* (1945) continues to remain an eloquent reference for those wishing to read in depth about the history of epilepsy.

There are many important dates recorded in the treatment of epilepsy (Temkin, 1945; Lennox and Lennox, 1960). A few of the most notable include the introduction of: potassium bromide by Sir Charles Locock (1857); phenobarbital by Alfred Hauptmann (1912); the ketogenic diet (1924); diphenylhydantoin by H. Houston Merritt and Tracy Putnam (1938); ethosuximide (1958); carbamazepine (1950s); valproic acid (1964); and diazepam (1966). Henry Ashby of Manchester, England, established the first residential school for epileptic children in 1900. One of the first multidisciplinary epilepsy clinics for children was established at Johns Hopkins in 1927 by Edwards A. Park and Adolph Meyer.

Petit Mal Epilepsy

The first case report of this disorder in a child was by the Swiss neurologist Simon André Tissot in 1772 who described a fourteen-year-old girl with abnormal eyelid movements and momentary loss of consciousness. Her symptoms began at age seven (Lennox and Lennox, 1960, 69). These episodes were originally thought to be tics, but were then recognized as convulsive attacks. Four months later she began to have generalized seizures. Jean Esquirol in 1815 is credited with first describing brief seizures but he did not use the term *petit mal* until later in 1838 in a chapter of the book *Des Maladies mentales* (Lennox and Lennox, 1960, 68). Esquirol noted that it was common to differentiate between "*le grand et le petit mal*" seizures. Louis Calmeil used the term *l'absence* for a seizure that represented an abortive vertiginous attack (1824), actually a form of seizure that we now consider a type of partial complex epilepsy. According to Temkin (1945), the term *absence* was used to express a period of passing mental confusion without other symptoms, whereas *petit mal* described a wider variety of attacks with loss of consciousness.

In 1854 Louis Delasiauve, in his *Traité de l'épilepsie*, separated seizures into four types: *vertiges*, or dizzy episodes; *accès complets* for generalized seizures; *chutes* for drop attacks; and *absences* for petit mal. William Gowers also mentioned petit mal under "minor attacks" in the second edition of his well-known book on epilepsy (1901), but did not provide a specific description of these attacks. Almost thirty years later Hans Berger made the first EEG recording of a somewhat atypical petit mal disorder in an eighteen-year-old girl with a five-year history of both generalized and absence seizures. This was reported in 1933 (Lennox and Lennox, 1960, 95). Two years later, Frederic Gibbs, Hallowell Davis, and William Lennox reported a more typical petit mal episode taken from one of their night sessions in the physiology laboratories at Harvard Medical School. The patient, who had been originally evaluated by William Lennox, continued to be followed by Lennox for many years thereafter, both clinically and with serial EEG tracings. Lennox later also demonstrated that medications such as phenobarbital or bromides were capable of temporarily eliminating paroxysmal EEG abnormalities in children (1936). Trimethadione was reported in 1945 to be an effective treatment by Lennox and by Meyer Perlstein (1946). Later ethosuximide and valproic acid became the mainstays of treatment.

Myoclonic Epilepsy

Although Galen may have described a case suggestive of myoclonic epilepsy, Tissot clearly recognized this type of seizure in an eleven-year-old boy with the intelligence and language function of a two-year-old. His head-nodding seizures began at eighteen months of age, presumably after being frightened by the sound of a pistol shot fired close to his ears by someone who had been drinking. The physician, W. J. West (an earlier West than the famous Great Ormond Street pediatrician, Charles West, who wrote on neurological diseases), published a detailed account of these head-nodding seizures in his own child. This type of seizure is still frequently referred to as West syndrome. West (1841) mentions that he had taken his son to see Dr. Charles Clarke in London, who had previously seen four children with similar seizures and termed them a "salaam convulsion." Newman reported four cases and referred to these as "*epilepsia nutans*" (1849) and Barnes in 1873 described successful treatment with bromides in one child in a paper entitled "Epilepsia nutans, or the Nodding Convulsions of Infancy."

Later in the nineteenth century, brief mention of myoclonic seizures was made by physicians such as William Heberden, Jr., and William Gowers (Lennox and Lennox, 1960, 125). However, it was the clinical and pathological studies of Heinrich Unverricht (1891), Herman Lundborg (1903), and Gonzalo Lafora (1911), who delineated several of the different clinical syndromes associated with this seizure type. James Ramsay Hunt also described true drop attacks, which he called "astatic epilepsy" after having observed ten cases at the Craig Colony. This was soon followed by the pioneering experimental and clinical work of the Dutch physician L. J. J. Muskens (1928) and that of Henri Gastaut (1947) which resulted in the foundations of our current understanding of myoclonic epilepsy. Since then this type of seizure has undergone numerous reclassifications as our understanding of the underlying causes has changed. The studies of P. M. Jeavons and B. D. Bowers, Peter Kellaway, and Jean Aicardi are amongst many that have helped redefine these disorders in modern child neurology (see Lennox and Lennox, 1960; and Aicardi, 1986, for uncited references).

Focal Motor Seizures

Hippocrates and Erastus were among the ancient medical writers who wrote on motor seizures involving one side of the body.

And, for the most part, convulsions seize the other side of the body, for if the wound is situated on the left side, the convulsions will seize the right side of the body, or if the wound be on the right side of the head, the convulsion attacks the left side of the body. (Hippocrates, in Lennox and Lennox, 1960, 200)

It was not, however, until the nineteenth century that more astute clinical observations recognized the true nature and cause of focal seizures. This realization commenced with the description of partial epilepsy and even post-ictal paralysis by James Cowles Prichard in *A Treatise on Diseases of the Nervous System* (1822), a forerunner of the later and more definitive studies by Robert Todd (1856). The clinical studies of Louis François Bravais (1827) on hemiplegic epilepsy and the clinicopathological studies of Richard Bright (1831, 1835) provided evidence for the cortical origins of focal seizures and formed the basis of the early clinical and anatomical classifications prior to the monumental studies of John Hughlings Jackson. The latter were published in a series of papers *On the Scientific and Empirical Investigation of the Epilepsies* (1874–76), which were later collected and edited by James Taylor (Jackson, 1931). These formed the foundation of our current understanding of focal (Jacksonian) and other types of seizure disorders and established the concept that epilepsy was an expression of an excessively discharging neuronal lesion.

Focal Sensory Seizures

Focal sensory seizures were first described by Galen (131–201 A.D.):

This I first saw in a boy of some 13 years of age when I was myself a young fellow, in company with our leading physicians, who had met to consider the treatment. I heard the boy relate that the condition began in his leg, and rose straight up through his thigh, flanks, side and neck, right to his head, and that as soon as it reached this, he could no longer follow it. Asked, however, by the doctors what sort of thing it was that rose to his head, the boy was unable to say. Another young lad, however, older than he, not unintelligent, able to appreciate fairly well what had happened, and better able to explain than the other boy, said that what rose up was like a cold current of air (aura). . . . (Lennox and Lennox, 1960, 215).

It was from this description that the word *aura* (in Latin, "wind") was derived. Temkin further traces the history of these types of seizures (1945). The studies of Gowers, Hughlings Jackson, and Penfield and Theodore C. Erickson (1941) stand out as major contributions both descriptively and in regard to pathogenesis.

Benign Rolandic Seizures

Martinus Rulandus in 1597 described a ten-year-old boy whose seizures involved the left eye, mouth, and left hand, with loss of speech and paralysis of the left arm (van Huffelen, 1989). This type of seizure was rediscovered in 1952 with the reports of Y. Gastaut and were called seizures with prerolandic spikes without focal significance. Following the work of Frederick and Erna Gibbs (1959) and later Cesare Lombroso (1967), the disorder is now termed benign focal epilepsy of childhood (van Huffelen, 1989).

HYDROCEPHALUS AND DEVELOPMENTAL ANOMALIES

Hydrocephalus

Hydrocephalus was known to Hippocrates and other early medical writers. However, the concept at that time related to any fluid collection in the head rather than our current understanding. Thus, three forms of hydrocephalus were recognized by Oribasius (325–403 A.D.): an accumulation of fluid between the skin and the pericranium; between the pericranium and bone; and between the dura mater and the bone (Fisher, 1951). In the seventh century, Paul of Aegina (625–690) described the same forms of hydrocephalus but did not agree with the treatments that Oribasius had proposed. It was not until the time of Andreas

Vesalius (1514–1564) that internal hydrocephalus was recognized with the description of a young girl whose ventricular system contained about nine pounds of water. Two centuries later, Giovanni Morgagni (1682–1771) commented that hydrocephalus in infants and children was associated with a large head in contrast to adults where the head size could be normal. Cornelius Roelants, in his pediatric work that appeared in the late fifteenth century, gave a comprehensive review of "water gathered in the head of children" based on his review of the writings of Avicenna, Rhazes and others (Ruhräh, 1925, 99). Treatment by attempting to dehydrate the young infant with dried foods of low-water content and cathartics followed by the use of "sneeze provocatives" was beneficial according to Rhazes (869–962):

And let the head be measured with a thread from the first day of the waning of the moon and seek the first day of its newness and it will be found diminished from its inflation. (Ruhräh, 1925, 115)

In the Middle Ages, many pediatric illnesses were thought to cause hydrocephalus, the most common being rickets, later made known through the works of Francis Glisson (1597–1677). It was Robert Whytt (1714–1766), however, who described *hydrocephalus internus* far more accurately than ever before. His *Observations on the Dropsy in the Brain*, published two years after his death (1768), is regarded as the first and perhaps most influential of many important monographs written over the next century. These included works of varying length and complexity by Monro (1803), Cheyne (1814), Smyth (1814), Göelis (1821), Bricheteau (1829), Charpentier (1829), Abercrombie (1836), Davis (1840), Bennett (1843), Smith (1845), Cooke (1850), and D'Astros (1898) (see Fisher, 1951; McHenry, 1969; Ring-Mrozik and Angerpointer, 1986, for uncited references).

Our modern understanding of the pathogenesis of hydrocephalus dates from the studies of François Magendie (1783–1855) who demonstrated the presence and free communication of cerebrospinal fluid in the ventricular system. This actually had been described earlier by Domenico Cotugno and Albrecht von Haller. Hubert von Luschka confirmed the presence of the foramen of Magendie and also described the lateral foramen of the fourth ventricle that now bears his name. The origins of cerebrospinal fluid production were first considered by Ernest Faivre, who in 1853 showed that the choroid plexus produced cerebrospinal fluid. The modern era of our understanding of the pathogenesis of hydrocephalus began with the studies of two of the most eminent early pediatric neurosurgeons: Harvey Cushing (1869–1939), who observed "sweating" on the choroid plexus and Walter Dandy (1886–1946) and his pediatric colleague Kenneth Blackfan (1883–1941), who found that obstruction of the foramen of Monro did not result in hydrocephalus if the choroid plexus was obliterated. Understanding the cause of hydrocephalus also required knowledge of the mechanisms of cerebrospinal fluid reabsorbtion. Axel Key and Gustaf Retzius showed that the Pacchionian bodies were important, but the absence of these structures in infants suggested an alternative resorptive pathway (1875–76). Lewis Weed proposed that the arachnoid villi served this purpose (1920). Dandy and Blackfan had also concluded that cerebrospinal fluid was absorbed through veins in the subarachnoid space (1914). It was, again, the classical studies of Dandy and Blackfan that proved that hydrocephalus could be produced by third ventricular obstruction. They also defined both the obstructive and communicating forms of hydrocephalus, the latter being due to impaired reabsorbtion of cerebrospinal fluid from the subarachnoid space over the brain convexities. Numerous pathological conditions, especially congenital or developmental malformations, were shown to cause hydrocephalus and these were concisely reviewed and further delineated by Dorothy Russell in her 1949 monograph on this subject.

Early attempts to treat hydrocephalus in infants using trephining and drainage were reported by the ancient Greeks. Fabricius Hildanus reported that such methods were sporadically attempted again in the eighteenth century (Fisher, 1951). Remmet of Plymouth, England, in 1778 removed eighty ounces of fluid from a patient. Alexander Monro advised that the opening be made away from large arteries or sinuses and advocated use of compressive bandages to minimize bleeding. Frequently, ventricular tapping was combined with the instillation of astringents as exemplified in the 1856 report of Boinet, who injected tincture of iodine into the ventricles of an infant with congenital hydrocephalus. In the early nineteenth century, C. W. Quinn recommended keeping the hydrocephalic infant in an upright position as well as applying external pressure to the cranium. Satisfactory results using compressive adhesive plasters or rubber bands were reported as early as 1821 by G. Blane, and later by T. Girdlestone and C. Costerton (1822). The history of the later nineteenth century and modern era of neurosurgical treatment is reviewed by Robert Fisher, in his chapter entitled "Surgery of the Congenital Anomalies," which appeared in A. E. Walker's *A History of Neurological Surgery* in 1951.

Spina Bifida

Although Greek, Roman, and Arab physicians alluded to defects of the spinal cord, the first definite mention of a spinal malformation was that made by Peter van Forest who, in 1610, described a two-month-old girl with a neck malformation that was probably a form of spina bifida; Casper Bauhin, Professor of Anatomy at Basel, gave an accurate description of this lesion (Fisher, 1951, 352). However, it was Nicolaas Tulp, made famous by Rembrandt in his *Anatomy Lesson of Dr. Tulp* (1632), who, in his *Medical Observations* (1641), gave the first complete description and name of the malformation spina bifida. It was soon appreciated that varying degrees of paralysis occurred in children with spina bifida, as noted in the account of ten cases by the Dutch anatomist, Frederick Ruysch (1691). Morgagni recognized that spina bifida occurred with and without hydrocephalus and believed that it was the local pressure from a hydromyelic spinal cord that created this malformation. In contrast, Jean Cruveilhier believed that spina bifida was due to an abnormality of development rather than a hydrostatic phenomenon. Further descriptions of this condition were made by Rudolf Virchow, who coined the term *spina bifida occulta* (1875), and by Friedrich von Recklinghausen (1866), who developed a classification of the different types of dysraphic states that is still in use today. Julius Arnold in 1894 and Hans Chiari in 1895 described the posterior fossa malformations seen in many children with this disorder. In 1892 C. Bayer reported the first surgical repair of an open meningomyelocele defect, but it was not until the advent of satisfactory ventriculoperitoneal shunting procedures almost sixty years later that the neurosurgical treatment of such patients became satisfactory (Ring-Mrozik and Angerpointer, 1986).

Porencephaly

Jean Baptiste Cazauvielh in *Recherches sur l'agenesie cérébrale* (1827), one of the first scientific works on paralysis in children, noted that congenital hemiplegia was associated with cerebral atrophy and he differentiated those due to *l'agenese cérébrale* (congenital cerebral agenesis) from *l'atrophie consecutif* (acquired cerebral atrophy). Perhaps one of the most outstanding early descriptions of the many different types of cerebral atrophy in children is found in the atlas of Jean Cruveilhier (1835–42). Descriptions of microcephaly, hemiatrophy, porencephaly, hydrocephaly, and cerebral dysgenesis are among the many stunning color illustrations, with accompanying histories of the patients, contained in this work. Descriptions since then have focused both on further characterizations of these malformations and the pathogenesis of cerebral atrophy. For example, fetal encephalitis and meningitis were considered a likely factor as early as 1834 (Breschet, 1834; von Lallemand, 1834; Henoch, 1842). Duges suggested that atrophy could be due to subarachnoid or subdural fluid collections (1826). Jean Louis Cotard felt it was difficult to determine etiology from the type of atrophy and believed that about one-fifth of atrophic cases might be due to birth injury. Cotard also noted that the cranium was smaller on the affected side, that aphasia was relatively uncommon, and that intelligence could be normal (Cotard, 1868). Adolf Strümpell believed that many cases were due to intrauterine encephalitis (1884, 1889) and R. Heschl coined the term *porencephaly* (1859).

The importance of fetal or perinatal vascular disease as a cause of porencephaly or atrophy was also promoted at this time. Hans Kundrat (1882) believed that focal cerebral ischemia in the fetal or perinatal period was the most common cause. Jules Parrott (1873) and V. Hutinel (1877) believed that venous congestion and thrombosis could cause cerebral injury. William Little's earlier clinical reports supported these ideas (1843); he also believed that hypoxia rather than trauma was a major factor. However, the works of Parrott and Hutinel were not well known in the English-speaking countries (see Ingram, 1964, for uncited references).

Craniosynostosis

Although Hippocrates realized that the cranial sutures in part determined the future shape of the infant's head, it was the great German pathologist Rudolf Virchow who coined the term *craniostenosis* and classified abnormalities of the size and shape of the head into macrocephalus, microcephalus, dolichocephalus (elongated head), and brachycephalus (shortened or square shaped-head). Virchow also differentiated between microcephaly and craniosynostosis, the term currently in use. The first craniectomy for craniosynostosis was performed by Odilon Marc Lannelongue (1890), who removed strips of bone adjacent to the closed suture. Because many of the early patients either had microcephaly or died from operative complications, surgical treatment was criticized by many, including Abraham Jacobi (1894). More careful selection of cases and a variety of new technical approaches, including subtemporal decompression by R. Dorfman and Anton von Eiselsberg (1908); orbital decompression by Hermann Schloffer (1913); subtotal craniectomy by K. H. Bauer (1932); a morcellation procedure by J. E. J. King (1938); creation of a temporoparietal flap by Dandy (1943); bilateral craniotomy by David Fairman and Gilbert Horrax; and the use of fibrin, tantalum foil, and polyethylene interposed along the site of the suture lines by Franc Ingraham and his colleagues, initiated the modern era of extensive craniofacial surgery (see Fisher, 1951, for all uncited references).

MENTAL RETARDATION

From the earliest times, children and adults with mental retardation were for the most part ridiculed, perceived as possessed by demons, exploited, ostracized from society, or simply eliminated by infanticide and other deliberate practices (Deutsch, 1946). Concern about the treatment of the mentally retarded began in the early nineteenth century, by those who later advocated and promoted social changes (Kanner, 1964). Care of the disadvantaged was, in part, a reflection of the political and economic changes sweeping Europe, England, and the United States that were associated with the American and French revolutions, the philosophical and intellectual movements expressed as the Age of Reason and the Age of Enlightenment, and the changes brought about by the Industrial Revolution. In general, the history of mental retardation can be separated into several overlapping conceptual and chronological periods that can only briefly be stated here.

Differentiation Between Mental Retardation and Mental Illness

Until the nineteenth century there was little differentiation between the mentally ill and mentally defective. Jean Etienne Dominique Esquirol (1722–1840), renowned psychiatrist at the Salpêtrière and the Bicêtre, was the first to clearly separate the mentally retarded from the emotionally disturbed in his work *Maladies mentales* (1828). It was not until 1886 in England that a distinction between psychosis and mental subnormality was legally defined (Balthazar and Stevens, 1975).

Individual Efforts to Improve the Conditions of the Mentally Retarded

Many individuals were responsible for the early development of the care, education, and training of the developmentally disabled. Some are particularly representative of specific ideas or trends that first appeared in the nineteenth century and include:

Treatment of the Mentally Retarded and Insane as Patients rather than Prisoners or Criminals Philippe Pinel (1745–1826), superintendent of the Bicêtre, was responsible for radically changing and humanizing the care of institutionalized insane and retarded patients. He is credited with developing the ideas that led to the unshackling the chains of the inmates and providing moral treatment.

Sensory Deprivation and its Relation to Mental Retardation Jean Marc Gaspard Itard (1774–1838) took in Victor, the "Wild boy of Aveyron," to educate. Although he believed that he had failed in his goals, he clearly demonstrated that even profoundly delayed children could be improved.

The Role of Special Education in the Care of the Mentally Retarded
Jacob Rodrigues Pereire (1715–1780) taught deaf-mutes a simplified form of sign language and served as the model for teaching the blind and feebleminded. Itard used Pereire's techniques as a basis for his educational training program.

Johann Jacob Guggenbuhl (1816–1863), who opened a treatment center especially for cretins called the Abendberg in the mountains of Switzerland, developed the concepts of physical and occupational therapy still in use today, and served as a model for many visiting physicians and others concerned with social welfare.

Edouard Séguin (1812–1880), who worked at the Hospice des Incurables and at the Bicêtre, developed methods of educational training for the mentally retarded that are summarized in his book *Traitement moral, hygiène, et éducation des idiots et des autres enfants arrières* (1846). He emigrated to the United States where he disseminated his educational philosophy and opened several institutions.

The Rise of Institutional Care of the Mentally Retarded

In the middle of the nineteenth century, private and public institutions were founded to care for the mentally retarded throughout Europe, England, and the United States. The history tracing the rapid formation of these facilities is reviewed in Leo Kanner's *A History of the Care and Study of the Mentally Retarded* (1964) and in Albrecht Deutsch's *The Mentally Ill in America* (1946).

The Development of Standardized Psychological Testing

The work of Alfred Binet (1857–1911) and Theodore Simon (1873–1961) at the beginning of the twentieth century was of fundamental importance in developing objective methods for the assessment of intelligence. Their work was translated and adapted for American use by Henry Goddard in 1910 and by O. Bobertag in Germany in 1914. The implications of their work were far-reaching because it was now possible to more accurately classify the mentally retarded and to develop similar scoring systems for vocational testing, personality and adaptive behavior, and sensorimotor development. The historical aspect of the development of psychological testing has been well reviewed (see Schultz, 1981; Caudle, 1984; Benner, 1985, for all uncited references).

Early Genetic Studies, the Eugenics Movement, and the Mentally Retarded

Richard Dugdale's *The Jukes; A Study in Crime, Pauperism, Disease and Heredity* (1877) and Henry Goddard's *The Kallikak Family; A Study in the Heredity of Feeblemindedness* (1912) reflected opinions raised by many on the hereditary nature of immorality and criminality and the fact that these problems were more prevalent among the mentally retarded (Deutsch, 1946; Balthazar and Stevens, 1975). Coupled with the rise of the eugenics movement, which was based on the work of Sir Francis Galton, much was written about the threat of the mentally retarded and the need to exert some form of control on their reproduction. Kanner rightly termed this period "the Eugenics Scare," and he pointed out that the world had more to fear from intelligent people busily planning war than from the feebleminded (Kanner, 1964, 128).

The Recognition of Individual Causes of Mental Retardation

The recognition, first of endemic cretinism (Kanner, 1964, 88) and later mongolism, served as the beginning of the extraordinary developments that have occurred over the past century in the pathological and biochemical understanding of mental retardation. These are briefly covered in sections on the neurometabolic and degenerative diseases of this Introduction.

CEREBRAL PALSY

The first scientific paper on paralysis in children was published in 1827 by Jean Baptiste Cazauvielh, who wrote on cerebral agenesis and congenital paralysis, dividing the disorders into congenital and acquired forms. He also observed the disorder to be more common in boys and to involve the right side of the body. Charles Michel Billard (1800–1832) was one of the first to correlate neurological symptoms and pathology in the newborn. In his

Traité des maladies des enfans nouveau-nés et à la mamelle (Treatise on the Newborn and the Nursing Infant) (1828), Billard recognized the relation between prolonged labor and intracranial hemorrhage:

The length of the labor, the necessary tractions in certain manoeuvres, the difficulty with which respiration is established, the changes which the circulation undergoes, explains how this apparatus is often the seat of sanguinous congestions, varying from simple injection of the meninges to true apoplexy. (Levinson, 1943, 54)

It was less than twenty years later that William John Little reported his well-known observations on orthopedic deformities, which he attributed in large part to birth injury (1843–44). In his later papers, Little classified these forms of birth paralyses into three types: hemiplegic rigidity, paraplegia, and generalized rigidity (1861–62). He also mentioned a fourth type of paralysis with "disordered movement." According to James Collier there had been earlier reports of cerebral diplegia by Nicholas André in 1741 and Jacques Delpech in 1828 (Collier, 1899). Little also recognized that intellectual impairment and, to a lesser extent, epilepsy, commonly accompanied this disorder. Little's paraplegia and generalized rigidity subsequently became known as diplegia or "Little's disease." The fourth category later was recognized as a form of *athetosis*, a term that William Hammond had used in his description of involuntary movements in several adult patients (1871); William Gowers later differentiated the choreoid from dystonic types of cerebral palsy (1876). Gowers also objected to the term *obstetrical paralyses* and preferred the term *birth palsy*, as he believed that one could not attribute obstetrical mishap as a cause in all cases. He also separated birth palsies into two classes: the peripheral and the cerebral and alludes to a third spinal form (1888). His use of the word *cerebral* in this context may be the first published record of its use for this descriptive purpose, although D. Burgess in the same year published a case report entitled *A Case of Cerebral Birth Palsy* (Wolf, 1969, 7). It is likely, however, that the term *cerebral palsy* was in common usage, because the following year William Osler published his monograph *The Cerebral Palsies of Children: A Clinical Study from the Infirmary of Nervous Diseases* (1889).

The first attempt at clinical categorization of the subgroups of cerebral palsy was that of Bernard Sachs and Frederick Peterson (1890), who suggested a classification based on etiology (prenatal, natal, and acquired), as well as according to the pattern of body involvement (diplegia, paraplegia, hemiplegia, ataxia, choreic, and athetoid). Several years later in 1897 Sigmund Freud introduced the term *cerebral diplegia* when bilateral motor involvement was present and compared this to hemiplegia, generalized rigidity, paraplegic rigidity, bilateral hemiplegia, generalized chorea, and double athetosis. He also used the term *ataxic cerebral palsy*, which ten years later Frederick Batten designated as congenital cerebellar diplegia to describe those children who had cerebellar involvement with some degree of spasticity (Ingram, 1964).

At the end of the last century, just as today, there was much controversy about the cause of cerebral palsy (Ingram, 1964). Rudolf Virchow in 1865 described what he called congenital encephalitis, consisting of yellowish masses in the white matter that he felt represented an inflammatory process. Adolf Strümpell also suggested that an intrauterine infection could cause such a problem (1885). However, more efforts were continuing to be focussed on brain damage as the mechanism of injury. Sarah McNutt considered that subdural and meningeal hemorrhages were the most common cause of cerebral palsy. Gowers (1888), Osler (1889), Robert Lovett (1888), and Sachs and Peterson (1890) all commented on the relation between birth trauma and cerebral palsy, although Sachs and Louis Hausman later expressed the opinion that it was hypoxia associated with prolonged delivery that was important (1926). In Germany, a broader view was held that hereditary or other factors were of importance (see Ingram, 1964). In England, Batten also expressed the view (1913) that intrauterine vascular occlusion or arrests of cerebral development were more important than birth trauma. The works of Hugo Ehrenfest (1922), an obstetrician, and Frank Ford, Bronson Crothers and Marian Putnam (1927) also carefully examined the issues of the relation between birth injury and cerebral palsy.

Over the next fifty years numerous approaches to the classification of such children were entertained. The early work of Bronson Crothers, especially his book *Disorders of the Nervous System in Childhood* (1926), created much medical interest in this problem. Winthrop Phelps (1950), who is credited with popularizing the term *cerebral palsy* in the United States, and Meyer Perlstein (1952), who suggested the term *dyskinesia*, viewed these patients according to the nature of the functional impairment of how different forms of cerebral palsy affected their posture and movement. Crothers and Richmond Paine (1959) examined the extrapyramidal types of cerebral palsy and the various forms of "mixed involvement." Thomas Ingram, in his well-researched book entitled *Paediatric Aspects of Cerebral Palsy* (1964), provides both a fascinating historical review of the development of the different forms of cerebral palsy as well as the results of many years of careful study of nosology, etiology, and treatment. The Spastic Society of Great Britain in the 1950's founded a medical advisory board known as the Little Club (in memory of William John Little) and arranged annual meetings at Oxford that were attended by child neurologists invited from many countries. Numerous highly regarded publications have originated from these efforts.

Ataxic Cerebral Palsy

In 1903 Frederick Batten described eight children with congenital ataxia, or *cerebellar diplegia*. Batten observed that the majority of these children improved and he suggested that congenital ataxia could be due to cerebellar damage at birth, but that in other cases it was likely the result of a brain developmental malformation. This in part had already been demonstrated by André-Thomas, who had published a large series of reports on children with agenesis or hypoplasia of the cerebellum (1897). Batten also realized that childhood ataxia could be acquired secondary to infections or tumors and in 1905 he distinguished acute post-infectious ataxia (*encephalitis cerebelli*) from the congenital and progressive forms of ataxia, such as Friedreich's disease. Batten's observations, on congenital and acquired non-progressive forms, established ataxia as a category of cerebral palsy (Ingram, 1964, 246).

At the same time, it was realized that hypotonia could be a prominent feature in infants with cerebral palsy. Ataxic children who had prominent hypotonia were reported by Otfrid Foerster (1909–10) and then by L. Pierce Clark (1918), who employed the term *Infantile cerebro-cerebellar diplegia of the flaccid ataxic astasic type.*

Since then, further cases have been reported by James Ramsay Hunt (1918), Winthrop Phelps (1940), Meyer Perlstein (1952), Frank Ford (1952), and Herman Yannett and Frank Horton (1952), who commented on the different forms and causes of "atonic cerebral palsy." The studies of R. C. Baker and G. O. Groves (1931), B. Brouwer and A. Biemond (1938), and Thomas Ingram (1964) helped clarify that either developmental abnormalities, in part on a genetic basis, or birth injuries could explain the cause of non-progressive ataxia in most children (see Ingram, 1964, and Wolf, 1969 for all uncited references).

Choreoathetotic Cerebral Palsy

Involuntary movements in children with hemiplegia were recognized by Jean Baptiste Cazauvielh (1827), Jean Martin Charcot (1853), Jakob von Heine (1860), and Jean Louis Cotard (1868). Jacques Delpech described a microcephalic child with continuous movements of his arms (1828) and several of Little's patients (1861) also had involuntary movements (Ingram, 1964). However, it is William Hammond who is credited with the first systematic observations of involuntary movements. In his paper "On Athetosis" (1871), he described two adults with hemiplegic athetosis due to post-natal cerebral injury, possibly involving the corpus striatum. Two years later, seven patients were reported by C. Shaw in a paper entitled "On Athetosis or Imbecility with Ataxia" in whom the abnormal movements had always been present. Fulgence Raymond, who followed Charcot as Professor of Neurology at the Salpêtrière, emphasized the frequent association of abnormal movements with hemiplegia and also distinguished two types: hemichorea and hemiathetosis (1876). He did not, however, recognize bilateral athetosis or chorea as forms of cerebral palsy.

Gowers (1876) further categorized the post-hemiplegic movement disorders and stated that athetosis was in reality a symptom of numerous neurologic disorders. Paul Oulmont described two forms of hemiathetosis: *hemiathetose symptomatique*, which was associated with obvious hemiplegia or other signs of cerebral injury; and *hemiathetose primitive*, in which there were no other neurological manifestations (1878). Oulmont presumed that this was due to a small focal cerebral lesion, as had been earlier suggested by

Charcot (1886). Others observed that, in some children, the involuntary movements worsened as the hemiplegia improved (see Ingram, 1964, for all uncited references).

Athetose double (*athetose générale*) was the term Oulmont used to describe similar involuntary movements seen in hemiathetosis, except that they were bilateral and usually seen in profoundly delayed children (see Ingram, 1964). Numerous case reports followed, including several by Osler, among which was the first observation of jaundice as a possible etiology (1894). In contrast to athetosis, Huét described a series of children who appeared to have chronic chorea on a congenital basis (1889). One of the most extensive clinicopathologic investigations was that of J. Audry, who reviewed ninety-three patients with chorea and athetosis, and observed significant basal ganglia and cerebral atrophy (1892). Freud considered both congenital chorea and athetosis to be closely related with many of his patients demonstrating spasticity and a history of perinatal distress (1893, 1897). Thus, by the beginning of this century, the definition of a form of cerebral palsy in which involuntary movements were the predominant feature was well established. Studies by Cécile and Oskar Vogt during the next twenty years delineated *status marmoratus* as a specific pathological entity of prenatal onset (1919, 1920). However, Crothers (1921) disagreed with the Vogt's concept of a prenatal developmental etiology and stressed the likelihood of birth injury as being a significant contributing factor. Further studies by Phillip Schwartz (1921), Ford (1927), Otto Marburg (1936), Randolph Byers (1942), Clemens Benda (1945), Ronald Norman (1947), Cyril Courville (1950), Meyer Perlstein (1952), Bronson Crothers and Richmond Paine (1959), and many others, subsequently delineated the importance of perinatal asphyxia as an important mechanism producing this lesion (see Ingram, 1964, and Wolf, 1969, for all uncited references).

Kernicterus Johannes Orth in *Über das Vorkommen von Bilirubinkingstalten bei neugebornen Kindern* (1875) first reported an infant with basal ganglia pigmentation in association with icterus gravis. Similar findings were later reported by Georg Schmorl in six infants dying from icterus gravis (1903). Intermittent rigidity and opisthotonus with hyperbilirubinemia were noted by Cornelia de

Lange (1924–25) and H. Gruenwald and W. Messer (1927), as were many other symptoms by several investigators (Ingram, 1964, 294). Initially it was believed that infection and hepatic immaturity were the precipitating factors causing hyperbilirubinemia and kernicterus, but it was not until the studies of A. Hoffman and L. Hausmann (1926) that a hemolytic factor was suggested. Philip Levine and Rufus Stetson stressed the importance of the Rh factor (1939) and for some time erythroblastosis was considered the sole cause of brain involvement. However, subsequent studies, especially those of Wolf Zuelzer and Roxie Mudgett (1950), clearly proved the importance of other factors. That same year R. Aiden and colleagues reported on twenty-four kernicteric preterm infants who had no blood group incompatibility. Considerable controversy remains about the importance of various causative factors (see Ingram, 1964, and Ford, 1966, for all uncited references).

Acquired Hemiplegia

Descriptions of hemiplegia occurring after infections can be found in the works of Cazauvielh (1827), C. von Lallemand (1830–34) and Eduard Henoch (1842). The first comprehensive clinical account was that of Jakob von Heine (1860), who reported two patients who became hemiplegic after scarlet fever and vaccination. Over the next forty years, a variety of reports described the clinical presentations of acquired hemiplegia in children. H. Richardière characterized the evolution from flaccid to spastic hemiparesis (1885). Post-hemiplegic involuntary movements were noted by Gowers (1876) and B. Greidenberg (1886). Théodore Wuillamier considered that focal or grand mal seizures frequently accompanied acute infantile hemiplegia (1882), and Martin Bernhardt (1885) and Freud (1891) noted the presence of aphasia. Bernhardt, (1885) and later Achille Souques (1894), described writing difficulties in hemiplegic children, and hemianopia was observed by Freud (1889). By the turn of the century, three large studies described most of the features of acquired hemiplegia (Osler, 1889; Sachs and Peterson, 1890; Freud and Rie, 1891) and a comprehensive understanding of what we now call the acute infantile hemiplegia syndrome was developed. Cases purporting cerebral emboli as the cause of this syndrome were first reported by James Taylor (1880), Johann Otto Heubner (1883), and John Abercrombie (1888). Osler found emboli in only a small number of his cases (1889) and thrombosis was felt to be more prevalent (Ross, 1882; Marie, 1885; Gowers, 1888). Hemorrhage was rarely considered a contributing factor (Sachs and Peterson, 1890). In contrast, non-pyogenic infection (Vizioli, 1880) or polioencephalitis (Strümpell,1889) were also raised as potential etiologies of acquired hemiplegia. This concept was strenuously criticized by Freud, but it was ultimately shown to be important (Ingram, 1964, 31–34). Adolf Wallenberg stressed that multiple etiologies were responsible (1886). Eventually, numerous viral agents were shown to be associated with acquired hemiplegia and the role of venous thrombosis was also recognized (Brett, 1983) (see Ingram, 1964, for all uncited references).

NEUROMUSCULAR DISEASES

One of the major areas of emphasis in child neurology is the evaluation of weakness in children. Until the nineteenth century, differentiation of neuromuscular disorders from other "wasting" diseases due to malnutrition, infection, rickets, and other conditions, was not possible. Likewise, the separation of disorders due to atrophy on a neurogenic basis from primary muscle diseases was principally on a clinical basis and often erroneous. It was the development of neuropathology that ultimately led, over a relatively short period of forty or fifty years, to the accurate differentiation of a group of diseases which now are beginning to be understood at the cellular, biochemical, and genetic level. A historical overview of these disorders has recently been written by Victor Dubowitz (1980).

Muscular Dystrophy

Amand Duchenne first reported a patient in 1861 and in a series of papers by 1868 had published thirteen cases of the disorder that bears his name. He suggested the name *paralysie musculaire pseudohypertrophique* because of the unusual combination of muscle enlargement with progressive weakness. In later works, he published a series of papers on muscle histopathology, which he obtained by muscle biopsy using his *harpon du Middledorph* (1872). Paul Broca may have mentioned this disease in 1851 (see Duchenne essay). In 1852 Edward Meryon described this disease in his paper entitled "On Fatty and Granular Degeneration of the Muscles" described four affected boys from the same family and included pathology material similar to that of Duchenne dystrophy. Sir William Gowers, in 1879, presented 21 cases of his own and reviewed 139 published cases in his clinical lectures *Pseudo-Hypertrophic Muscular Paralysis*. He also described the proximal muscle weakness of the lower extremities noted in the Duchenne patients as they tried to stand (Gowers' maneuver), and popularized the term *pseudo-hypertrophic* coined by Duchenne (Dubowitz, 1980).

Louis Théophile Joseph Landouzy and Joseph Jules Dejerine (1884) are credited with delineating the facioscapulohumeral form of muscular dystrophy but, in fact, Duchenne had described nine patients with this disorder in 1872 in the third edition of *De l'Electrisation localisée* (Dubowitz, 1980). The limb-girdle form of dystrophy was separately described by Ernst von Leyden (1877) and Paul Möbius (1879). Many of these forms of muscular dystrophy were summarized by Wilhelm Erb in *Dystrophia muscularis progressiva* (1891). To add confusion to the nomenclature of these disorders, Erb's name at that time was associated with the juvenile, or scapulohumeral, form of muscular dystrophy. Gowers described a distal form of muscular dystrophy (1902), but the existence of this disorder was in doubt until the 1951 description by L. Welander from Sweden. P. E. Becker and F. Keiner (1955) are credited with describing the milder X-linked recessive form of muscular dystrophy. The history of the evolving concepts of the pathogenesis of the muscular dystrophies, gene linkage studies of the X chromosome, and discovery of dystrophin have also been recently reviewed (Walton, 1981; Dubowitz, 1989).

Myotonic Disorders

Myotonia Congenita In 1876, Julius Thomsen described myotonia congenita. Although afflicted himself with this disorder, he did not publish his observations until his son, who was similarly affected, was refused medical release from the military. Thomsen described the disease in his article "Tonische Krämpfe in willkürlich beweglichen Muskeln in Folge von ererbter psychischer Disposition (Ataxia muscularis?)" ("Tonic Cramps in the Voluntary Muscles as a Consequence of an Inherited Psychical Disposition. [Ataxia muscularis?]").

In 1881 Adolf Strümpell reported a patient with this disorder and classified the disease as a primary myopathy. Later, Wilhelm Erb wrote an extensive monograph on myotonia congenita (*Die Thomsen'sche Krankheit*, 1886) and demonstrated both the characteristic histopathology of the disorder and the production of myotonia by electrical stimulation. Dejerine and Jules Sottas disagreed with Erb and believed that the pathologic changes he observed were the result rather than the cause of the disease (1895). Sergio Pansini (1908) and then K. Nissen, a grand-nephew of Thomsen, wrote further extensive papers on this disorder (1923). Nissen's studies are interesting as he completed the genealogical investigations of the original Thomsen family through seven generations, demonstrating an autosomal dominant inheritance. P. E. Becker, more recently, described a variant of myotonia congenita with recessive inheritance (1961). Some of the historical aspects are reviewed in Eivind Thomasen's *Myotonia* (1948).

Myotonic Dystrophy The first case report of myotonic dystrophy, made by Johann Hoffmann (1896), was followed by several other isolated reports before the well-recognized descriptions of Hans Steinert, and separately, Frederick Batten and H. P. Gibb, in 1909 (Thomasen, 1948). Batten and Gibb recognized the unusual degree of facial and sternocleidomastoid muscle atrophy and felt that this suggested a unique myopathic disease. Steinert further stressed the speech and swallowing difficulties and multisystem organ involvement. For the next forty years it was generally believed that myotonic dystrophy did not begin in childhood. Maas and Peterson in their 1948 study briefly mention a three-year-old child. Eivind Thomasen stated that he had records on eight children under fifteen years of age with the youngest child being two-years old and, in several of the remaining children, symptoms began around age six years (1948). Nevertheless, it was not until the more recent reports of T. M. Vanier (1960) and Phillip Dodge, Ingrid Gamstorp, Randolph Byers and Patricia Russell (1965), that the onset of this disorder in infancy and more common prevalence in children were recognized. Other forms of myotonic disorders such as myotonic chondrodystrophy are also of recent description (see Thomasen, 1948, for all uncited references).

Mitochondrial and Congenital Myopathies

The concept of mitochondrial myopathies was introduced by Rolf Luft in 1962 when he described a woman with severe hypermetabolism of non-thyroidal origin with skeletal muscle mitochondrial ultrastructural abnormalities and a defect of mitochondrial respiratory control. Soon thereafter, Milton Shy and his colleagues defined several subtypes affecting both the structure and function of muscle mitochondria (1964, 1966). Some of these patients were later shown on biopsy by Olson and others to have ragged red fibers (1972). In the past two decades, with the realization that mitochondrial dysfunction could also result in a variety of encephalopathies, as well as other organ involvement, these disorders have undergone numerous reclassifications as the genetic, metabolic, and structural abnormalities have been identified.

At the same time, another category of muscle disease, congenital myopathies, was also being delineated, based principally on ultrastructural abnormalities. Milton Shy and several coinvestigators were also instrumental in the original descriptions of some of these disorders, such as central core disease (1956), nemaline myopathy (1963), and myotubular myopathy (1966). Other forms have been and continue to be described, although there has been little advance in understanding how specific structural abnormalities are translated into muscle dysfunction. This is in contrast to the rapid gains that have been made in the past fifteen years in several of the metabolic myopathies, pioneered by the studies of Andrew Engel and Salvatore DiMauro, as well as other investigators in this field.

Spinal Muscular Atrophy

The original observations of the weak hypotonic infant by Guido Werdnig (1891, 1894) and Johann Hoffmann (1893, 1897, 1900), in a series of papers in the late nineteenth century, clearly indicated a genetically determined anterior horn cell disorder that is now recognized as infantile progressive spinal muscular atrophy. Hermann Oppenheim (1900) proposed the term *myatonia congenita* for a condition that was associated with early hypotonia but without deterioration. Because of the similarity to the terminology of Thomsen disease (*myotonia congenita*), James Collier and Kinnier Wilson (1908) suggested the term *amyotonia congenita* as a less confusing alternative. This was accepted with reservations by most pediatricians and neurologists until the work of Sven Brandt (1950) who studied infants with spinal muscular atrophy, and John Walton (1956), who reviewed the large experience at both the National Hospital for Nervous Disease at Queen's Square and the Hospital for Sick Children, Great Ormond Street, London. Based on the relatively favorable prognosis, Walton suggested that benign congenital hypotonia would characterize those infants better than the confusing array of names formerly employed (see McHenry, 1969; Dubowitz, 1980; and Brett, 1983; for all uncited references).

Peripheral Neuropathy

The first physician known to recognize that diseases could effect the peripheral nerves was Robert Graves, who was also known for his description of hyperthyroidism. Graves had cared for patients during a Paris epidemic of neuritis in 1828 and in 1848 published his observations (McHenry, 1969, 433). Other forms of alcoholic and infectious neuritis were described in the middle part of the nineteenth century. It was not until the concurrent well-known reports of Jean Charcot and Pierre Marie from Paris and Howard H. Tooth from Cambridge, England (1886), that genetically determined neuropathies of childhood were first recognized. The history of several of the genetically determined neuropathies that are first seen in children, such as Charcot-Marie-Tooth or Dejerine-Sottas disease, are well summarized by Peter James Dyck (Dyck, 1975).

METABOLIC DISORDERS

The concept of inborn errors of metabolism originated with the studies of Archibald Garrod, as published in his Croonian Lecture of 1908. Garrod designated four disorders as meeting his criteria: alkaptonuria, albinism, cystinuria, and pentosuria, and later published his book *Inborn Errors of Metabolism* in 1909. Garrod implied that the transmission of a single character was probably governed by a single enzyme. The later studies of George Beadle and Edward Tatum (1945) introduced the concept of one gene being responsible for one enzyme. The ensuing revolution in molecular genetics has become inordinately complex and certainly too extensive to elaborate upon in this context. However, it was not long after Garrod's publications that the transition from the use of neuropathology to neurochemistry in understanding childhood nervous system diseases began to unfold. This occurred in several principal areas although many other neurometabolic diseases have been described (see Watson and Tooze, 1981, and Scrivner et al., 1989, for all uncited references).

Amino Acid Disorders

The first disorder that presented primarily with neurological symptoms was phenylketonuria, described by Asbjörn Fölling in 1934. George A. Jervis in 1939 showed that large amounts of phenylalanine accumulated in the body, that the disorder was inherited, and that there was an inability to oxidize phenylalinine to tyrosine. Following this, diets low in phenylalanine were developed and shown by H. Bickel and coinvestigators in 1954 to be effective in improving neurological outcome. Later, newborn screening programs were implemented.

The second well-recognized disorder with catastrophic neurologic symptoms was maple syrup urine disease, described by John Menkes and coworkers in 1954 and demonstrated to be caused by a block in oxidative decarboxylation by Joseph Dancis and colleagues in 1963. More recent studies have defined several subgroups of this disorder and further elucidated the metabolic defects.

Homocystinuria, another of the classic amino-acid disorders, was described independently by two groups of investigators: Nina Carson and D.W. Neil (1962), and Theo Gerritsen and coinvestigators in 1962. Demonstration of the deficient enzyme in most patients (cystathione beta-synthetase) was published two years later by S. Harvey Mudd and collaborators. Numerous investigators since then have continued to amplify upon the clinical and biochemical presentation of this disorder.

Mention of the above three amino-acid disorders serves simply as a brief historical reminder of the complexities of this field whose history is less than a century old and whose impact on the understanding of nervous system function and pathology is not yet fully appreciated (see Scriver et al, 1989, for all uncited references).

Lysosomal Diseases

It is interesting to recall that when Bernard Sachs first described Tay-Sachs disease (1887), he considered it to be a disorder of arrested cerebral development rather than a neurometabolic disease. As is well known, his description of amaurotic familial idiocy was the beginning of an era of unitarian confusion, as has been presented in Wolfgang Zeman's exceptional review, *Historical Development of the Nosological Concept of Amaurotic Familial Idiocy* (Zeman, 1970). Zeman acknowledged the influence of Emil Kraepelin (1856–1926), the well-known psychiatrist, who insisted on the importance of neuropathology in elucidating the structural causes of mental retardation (1909). This was followed by the observations of Karoly Schaffer and Walther Spielmeyer, who demonstrated neuronal swelling in patients with amaurotic idiocy, the presence of the so-called Schaffer-Spielmeyer cell process, which was believed characteristic for these disorders (see Zeman, 1970). By 1923, when Spielmeyer critically reviewed this unitarian concept, there appeared to be general agreement as to its validity, although many different forms of these disorders were described. As emphasized by Zeman:

Obviously, neuropathology played the leading role in the delineation of amaurotic familial idiocy and its age dependent variants; however, the unfounded confidence in the anatomical approach did not only preclude a better understanding of the basic disease process but actually imparted a backward thrust upon clinical and genetic efforts to delineate the nosology of other heritable nervous disorders, for example Niemann-Pick disease and gargoylism. (Zeman, 1970, 228)

The origins of our current understanding of the lysosomal diseases, which include the sphingolipidoses, mucopolysaccharidoses, glycogen storage diseases, and glycoproteinoses, was the work of E. Klenk, who in 1939, demonstrated a twelve-fold increase of gangliosides (then known as substance X) in the brains of two patients with Tay-Sachs disease. Lars Svennerholm showed this to be GM2 ganglioside in 1967 and two years later Shintaro Okada and John S. O'Brien demonstrated the deficiency of two isoenzymes of hexosaminidase. Subsequently, screening programs for Tay-Sachs disease were developed. Almost simultaneous to these advances were the fundamental studies of Christian de Duvé and his colleagues (1958), which elucidated the structure and function of the lysosome, and the investigations of H. G. Hers and F. Van Hoof (1973), who introduced the concept of lysosomal diseases. The historical evolution of the scientific advances of the lysosomal disorders is very complex and has been reviewed to some degree in some of the standard works on inherited neurometabolic disorders (see Scriver et al, 1989, for all uncited references).

Peroxisomal Disorders

Nineteenth century neurologists had used the terms *diffuse* or *disseminated* sclerosis to separate a group of adult neurological disorders from multiple sclerosis as delineated by Charcot and others. The beginning of our understanding of these disorders in children is attributed to Paul Schilder, who in 1912 reported a patient with encephalitis periaxialis diffusa, felt by later writers to be similar to multiple sclerosis. The following year, Schilder reported another child whose disorder was familial and later considered to be the prototype for the genetically determined leukodystrophies associated with lyosomal dysfunction. This was followed by the report of Ernest Siemerling and Hans Creutzfeldt on a cerebral demyelinating disease in association with adrenal insufficiency (1923) and a year later by yet another report by Schilder of a patient with an encephalitic type of demyelinating process. In 1928 Max Bielschowsky and Richard Henneberg proposed the term *leukodystrophy*, dividing the entities with diffuse sclerosis into either an exogenous inflammatory type or an endogenous, familial, progressive type. The studies of Ludo van Bogaert and Ivan Bertrand (1933), L. Einarson and A. V. Neel (1938), Ronald Norman (1947), and J. Godwin Greenfield (1952), all contributed to the reclassification of these disorders proposed by Charles M. Poser and Ludo van Bogaert in 1956. In this classification, the diffuse scleroses were divided into three groups: Schilder's cerebral sclerosis, Leukodystrophies, and Subacute encephalitis. Over the past three decades our understanding of these disorders has changed dramatically. Initially, Hugo Moser and others recognized that the majority of patients with "Schilder's disease" had X-linked adrenoleukodystrophy. The discovery of the peroxisome by Christian de Duvé and the later recognition of abnormalities of peroxisomal structure and function in patients with X-linked adrenoleukodystrophy by Moser and others have very recently defined an entirely new group of neurometabolic diseases. At least ten different metabolic disorders are now reported as defects of peroxisomal metabolism (Lazarow and Moser, 1989). The majority of other forms of diffuse sclerosis categorized as leukodystrophies, such as metachromatic leukodystrophy and Krabbe's disease, are now also clearly recognized as lysosomal disorders.

Neuronal Ceroid Lipofuscinoses

The concept of progressive neurological disorders in children associated with loss of mental, motor, and visual function (amaurotic idiocy) as described at the turn of the century, was given further credence by the reports over the next twenty to thirty years of a distinct group of disorders now collectively known as the neuronal ceroid lipofuscinoses. Frederick Batten, in 1903, described two sisters, aged four and six years in whom a striking macular degeneration of the retina was associated with progressive cerebral impairment. Marmaduke Mayou, a London ophthalmologist, described a similar disorder the following year in three of seven children that he examined and this was followed in 1914 by Batten's description in his article entitled "Family Cerebral Degeneration with Macular Changes (So-called Juvenile Form of Family Amaurotic Idiocy)." (Batten, 1914) Although clearly describing a different disorder from Tay-Sachs disease, the subtitle of Batten's paper created some confusion. This was compounded by the already existing reports from 1905 of Heinrich Vogt, who discussed eight children; and Walther Spielmeyer, who reported on four siblings with similar symptoms to Batten's patients, including retinal degeneration; and by the reports of Jan Jansky (1908) and Max Bielschowsky (1913) of somewhat younger children with similar symptoms but without retinal changes, the so-called late-infantile form of neuronal ceroid lipofuscinoses (NCL). In 1931 Tage Sjögren reported 115 patients with the juvenile amaurotic idiocy with most developing blindness in middle childhood and eponymically this variant of NCL is called the Spielmeyer-Vogt-Sjögren syndrome. The biochemical nature of this disorder is uncertain, but early contributions toward understanding this disorder were those of E. Klenk (1939), Svennerholm (1962), Zeman and Alpert (1963), among others (see Zeman, 1970). More recently, the contributions of P. Santavuori and J. Haltia have defined a form of this disorder beginning in infancy. Currently several major types of neuronal ceroid lipofuscinoses are recognized clinically but nosology awaits further biochemical definition (see Zeman 1970, and Zeman, et al, 1970, for all uncited references).

ACQUIRED AND DEGENERATIVE DISORDERS

Disorders of the Gray Matter

Description of this little-understood group of disorders, currently classified as progressive infantile poliodystrophy, is credited to Bernard Alpers in his paper "Diffuse Progressive Degeneration of the Gray Matter of the Cerebrum" (1931), although earlier case reports by Moore (1879) and William Norton Bullard (1890) were published (Dreifuss and Netzky, 1964). Over the past sixty years, other disorders considered to be gray matter degenerative diseases have been delineated, such as the neuronal ceroid lipofuscinoses, the progressive myoclonic epilepsies, Rett syndrome, and some of the peroxisomal disorders. These for the most part, have already been considered in this Introduction.

Disorders of the White Matter

As previously mentioned, the classification and evolution of our understanding of diseases of the white matter began a little over one hundred years ago with the differentiation of multiple from diffuse scleroses, and more recently with the realization that many forms of white matter diseases, classified as leukodystrophies or Schilder's diffuse sclerosis, were caused by specific lysosomal or peroxisomal metabolic abnormalities. White-matter diseases associated with subacute encephalitis still remain an enigma, although the early investigations of subacute sclerosing panencephalitis by James Dawson (1933), H. Pette and G. Döring (1939), and Ludo van Bogaert (1945), as well as that of Carleton Gajdusek on the relation between slow virus infections and chronic neurologic disorders (1957) continue to unfold. The history of these disorders is that of neurology for the past thirty years (Dyken, 1989).

Multiple Sclerosis Hodemaker, working in Erb's clinic, reported a seven-year-old boy who died of this disorder at age fourteen (1879). Charcot, who is credited with defining the disease of multiple sclerosis (1868), initially did not believe that it could occur in children but changed his mind, as is evident in some of his later *Tuesday Lessons* (1872–1893). John Keating in his *Cyclopaedia of the Diseases of Children* (1891) records that more than fifty cases had been reported in children. By 1959, a total of 178 children with multiple sclerosis had been reported and soon thereafter the relation between optic neuritis and the development of multiple sclerosis in children was further examined by Charles Kennedy and Sidney Carter (1961) (Ford, 1966, 216).

Rare Disorders of the White Matter Three primary disorders, well known to child neurologists in spite of both their rarity and almost complete lack of understanding of etiology, are those described by Friedrich Pelizaeus (1885) and Ludwig Merzbacher (1910), Myrtelle Canavan (1931), and W. Stewart Alexander (1949). All represent reports of patients with severe neurological disorders, unique neuropathology, and except for the recent studies showing an aspartoacylase deficiency in Canavan's disease (Matalon, Michals, and Sebesta, 1988), essentially no metabolically known cause is evident (Myrianthopoulos, 1981).

Ataxia

Spinocerebellar Degenerative Disorders Interest in ataxic disorders of childhood was recorded in the mid nineteenth century when several French pathologists reported patients with abnormalities of cerebellar development (Combettes, 1830; Lallement, 1832). However, clinical interest in these problems began when Nikolaus Friedreich published his first paper on these disorders in 1863, "Über degenerative Atrophie der spinalen Hinterstrange," and continued to add further descriptions up to 1877. Friedreich's ideas were initially discounted by most neurologists, including Charcot and others of the French school, because it was believed that his patients had multiple sclerosis or amyotrophic lateral sclerosis but with onset in childhood. However, as others such as Gowers (1880) and Sachs (1895) recognized other children with "Friedreich's disease," it became accepted as a distinct neurological disorder. Freud (1893, 1897) described several children in whom ataxia presented either at birth or within the first year or two of life and thought that they could represent either a congenital form of Friedreich's disease or possibly a form of ataxic cerebral palsy.

The forms of hereditary cerebellar ataxia described by Pierre Marie (1893) and Gordon Holmes (1907) were of the type that began in mid to late life, as did most of the reported forms of olivopontocerebellar atrophy. The works of Joseph Jules Dejerine and André-Thomas (1902) and J. Godwin Greenfield (1954) summarize much of the historical development of this complex area (see Konigsmark and Weiner, 1970, for all uncited references).

Acquired Ataxia Acute or persistent ataxia as a complication of common childhood infections was well recognized in the late nineteenth century. Scarlet fever (Shepherd, 1868; Voelcker, 1905), measles (Clapton, 1871; Batten, 1905, Guthrie, 1905), pertussis (Hammarburg, 1892; Gordon, 1924), typhoid fever (Lenhartz, 1833; Feith, 1873; Marie and Joltrain, 1910), diphtheria (Serog, 1916; Wilson, 1919), influenza (Bastian, 1898; Taylor, 1904; Batten, 1907), chicken pox (Dagnelie and Dubois, 1932; Grenet and Georges, 1938), rubella (Margolis et al, 1943) and mumps (Miller et al, 1956) have all been reported. Both Gowers (1899) and Sachs (1926) were among the first to recognize that purulent intracranial infections that most often complicated middle ear disease could progress to abscess formation or sinus thrombosis with permanent ataxia (see Ingram, 1964, and Ford, 1966, for all uncited references).

Movement Disorders

Chorea The original descriptions of chorea date from the Middle Ages when many epidemics of both infectious and hysterical chorea occurred, including one in Strasbourg. To "protect" the inhabitants of Strasbourg, the chief magistrate ordered those afflicted with the "dancing mania" to stay at the chapel of Saint Vitus in Zabern, a small village in Alsace; thus the origin of the eponym St. Vitus' Dance to describe the form of chorea that was described by Thomas Sydenham in 1686. Sydenham's characterization remains accurate, succinct, and worth reading today. Little else was written until the work of P. Brouzet (1754), in which he devoted a chapter entitled "Of the Kind of Convulsion called Chorea St. Viti, or Vitus's Dance," stating that earlier writers since Sydenham had confused this disorder with "Tarantism," the convulsive movements caused by the bite of a tarantula (Still, 1931, 395). Later writers, including Etienne Michel Bouteille (1810), Richard Bright (1831), German See (1850), Henri Roger (1886), and Gowers (1886–88), felt that there was a relation between chorea and rheumatism. Others, such as Hermann Eichhorst, Adolf Strümpell, Moritz Romberg, and Bernard Sachs were uncertain that a relation did indeed exist; for example, Bernard Sachs observed that rheumatic heart disease activated chorea in only about one-tenth of children that he examined with this condition (1891, 1895). Octavius Sturges wrote an excellent and comprehensive monograph on childhood chorea entitled *On Chorea and Other Allied Movement Disorders of Early Life* in 1881, in which he also confirmed the connection between chorea and rheumatic diseases. This preceded William Osler's *On Chorea and Choreiform Affections*, which was published in 1894 (see McHenry, 1969, for all uncited references).

Early pathologic studies of chorea found numerous nonspecific findings. German See considered tuberculosis (1850); Theodor Meynert found degeneration in the basal ganglia (1868); others, such as William Dickinson (1876), found hyperemia; and Hughlings Jackson, thrombosis secondary to emboli (1864). Meynert (1875) and Harald Hirschsprung (1881) reported on the presence of subcutaneous nodules, and the association with heart disease was reviewed in many papers, including the *British Medical Association Collective Investigation Committee Report* (1887). It was not until the studies of Angelo Taranta and Gene Stollerman (1956) that a firm relation between streptococcal infection, rheumatic fever, and Sydenham chorea was established. At the turn of the century, arsenic was the remedy preferred by many physicians, although others strongly urged the use of bromides and chloral hydrate (see Sachs, 1891 and 1895, for all uncited references).

The history of Huntington chorea, described in 1872, is well known (McHenry, 1969). More recently the studies of Randolph Byers and Phillip Dodge have reviewed the juvenile form of this disorder, associated with rigidity, ataxia, and seizures (1967).

Dystonia Musculorum Deformans The term *dystonia musculorum deformans* was first used by Hermann Oppenheim in 1911 in a paper entitled "Über eine eigenartige Krampfkrankheit des kindlichen and jugendlichen Alters (Dysbasia lordotica progressiva, Dystonia musculorum deformans)." He presented his own observations and also included those from the earlier 1908 dissertation of Marcus W. Schwalbe (Herz, 1944). Credit is also given to Edward Flateau, the father of Polish neurology, and his student, William Sterling, for their description of this disorder, which also appeared in 1911. Over the past half century, the genetic and kindred studies of Wolfgang Zeman (1959) and Roswell Eldridge (1970) have added much to the understanding of these disorders in children (Eldridge, 1970).

Juvenile Parkinson's Disease The first description of this extremely rare disorder is credited to James Ramsay Hunt, who described four sporadic cases in which the onset ranged between thirteen and thirty years (1917). Hunt's description came one hundred years after the original description of this disorder in adults by James Parkinson (1817). Since then, isolated case reports have been published, but little information has been added since the original clinical description (Neophytides, 1981).

INFECTIONS OF THE NERVOUS SYSTEM

Poliomyelitis

The first definitive description of poliomyelitis is credited to Michael Underwood in the second edition of his *Treatise on the Diseases of Children*, (1789) in a section entitled "Debility of the Lower Extremities." Jakob von Heine, in his book *Beobachtungun über Lahmungszustande der unteren Extremitaten und deren Behandlung* (1840), called attention to atrophy of the involved limb, localized the disease to the anterior part of the spinal cord, and noted the deformities of the spinal column. He also differentiated the disease from spastic paralysis in early life. Duchenne, in his treatise on electricity (1865), discussed polio, asserting his belief that the disease was due to spinal cord involvement. André Cornil (1863), and Jean Louis Prévost and Félix Alfred Vulpian (1865) demonstrated the loss of anterior horn cells in poliomyelitis, which was also confirmed by Lockhart Clarke (1868) and Charcot and Alex Joffroy (1870). The epidemic nature of polio was first noted by Oscar Medin in 1890, and the infectious nature of the polio virus was demonstrated by Otto Wickman in 1907. Karl Landsteiner and Erwin Popper (1909), and Simon Flexner and Paul Lewis (1909) transmitted the disease to monkeys. The history of poliomyelitis, including the era of vaccine development by Jonas Salk and Albert Sabin, is well reviewed by John R. Paul in *A History of Poliomyelitis* (1971).

Encephalitis

Celsus and Galen used the term *phrenitis* to describe a disorder that is now recognized as encephalitis. Throughout the Middle Ages, the term *phrenitis* was used loosely and often confused with more purulent or suppurative infections of the brain, such as meningitis. In 1790 Lucas mentioned the occurrence of lesions of the brain in measles, and in 1872 Carl Frederick Westphal suggested the name *acute disseminated encephalomyelitis* for these lesions. Adolf Strümpell (1853–1926), in his paper on acute encephalitis entitled

"Über die akute Encephalitis der Kinder" (1885), described a disease accompanied by fever, vomiting, and seizures that lasted for prolonged periods. Strümpell differentiated this condition from acute poliomyelitis. His observations were supported by Paul Möbius, who described two children, aged one and one-half and three years, with fever, loss of appetite, and somnolence. Pierre Marie felt that this process could attack the white as well as the gray matter. Strümpell also suggested that some of these cases could account for cerebral palsy in children. After the great 1917 epidemic of von Economo's encephalitis, it became evident that the neurologic symptoms and sequellae of such infections in children could be quite varied. However, it was not until the 1930s that specific viral agents were identified. Over the next half century, the role of acute and chronic viral disease in child neurology assumed major clinical importance and is reviewed in this book in the chapter introductions for those periods.

Bacterial Infections

Meningitis Although meningitis is predominantly a disease of children, it occurs at all ages. This was not appreciated by physicians of the Middle Ages because the disease was not recognized during life and autopsies were not yet done for the purposes of diagnosing such problems. There are, however, earlier references by Celsus, Galen, Avicenna, and in the Edwin Smith papyrus (2500 B.C) to illnesses resembling meningitis. The term *meningitis* was first used to signify an "inflammation caused by Traumatism of the head" by François Herpin in 1803 (Müllener, 1965, 12). In 1806 Gaspard Vieusseux described the first epidemic of bacterial meningitis that occurred in Geneva in 1805:

At the end of January, in a family composed of a woman and three children, two of the children were attacked and died in less than forty-eight hours. Fifteen days later, the disease appeared in another family in the neighborhood, composed of a father, mother and five infants, four of whom were attacked at almost the same time, and all died. . . . There appears a violent pain in the head, especially over the forehead; then there comes pains of the heart, or vomiting of greenish material, of stiffness of the spine, and in infants, convulsions. . . . Examination of the body showed most frequently a sanguinous engorgement in the brain without any particular alteration of the other viscera. (Major, 1945, 188)

Elisha North published *A Treatise on a Malignant Epidemic, Commonly Called Spotted Fever* (1811) based on the epidemic that he observed in Goshen, Connecticut, in 1807 (Major, 1945, 189). The first major advance occurred in 1887, when Anton Weichselbaum described Neisseria meningitis. Heinrich Quincke described the procedure of lumbar puncture (1891), which soon led to rapid advances in recognition of the different bacteria causing this disorder. Slawyk, for example, recognized the disease due to Hemophilus influenza (1899). Quincke's work also led to the contributions of Georges Widal, who investigated the cytology, Plant the serology, and Mastrezet the chemical composition of cerebrospinal fluid (Merritt and Fremont-Smith, 1938). The first specific effort at therapy was the introduction by Simon Flexner of anti-meningococcal serum (1907). However, successful therapy began with the discovery of sulfonamides in 1932, and their reported efficacy in the treatment of meningitis in 1937. The present antibiotic era was ushered in by Alexander Fleming's discovery of the value of penicillin and its early successful use for the treatment of meningococcal meningitis in 1943. In the 1950's meningococcal disease was treated with sulfonamides, pneumococcal disease with penicillin, and Hemophilus influenzae with chloramphenicol but, in any given patient, before the organism was identified by culture, all three antibacterial agents were administered. As ampicillin became available in the 1960's and was shown to be effective against all three pathogens, it was often used alone, until the development of resistant strains of Hemophilus influenzae appeared. More recently, immunologic identification of bacterial pathogens has led to early diagnosis of the specific agent, and newly developed antibiotics have been employed. An interesting historical review on meningitis has been written by E-R. Müllener (1965).

Brain Abscess By the early nineteenth century, brain abscesses had been described by those interested in pathology and were beautifully illustrated in many of the anatomical atlases (McHenry, 1969, 402). The first successful drainage of an abscess was performed in an adult by the French surgeon Sauveur Morand in 1768. He used trephination, dural incision, and tube drainage. William Detmold in 1850 first opened the lateral ventricles for the treatment of abscesses and the first descriptions of subdural empyemas were by John Abercrombie (1836) and Victor von Bruns (1854). The modern era of treatment of brain abscesses in both children and adults begins with the work of William Macewen and his publication of *Pyogenic Infective Diseases of the Brain and Spinal Cord* (1893). Perhaps the first extensive report solely on this problem in children was that of L. Emmett Holt (1898), in which he reviewed thirty-two cases, noting the difficulties in diagnosing brain abscesses in children and differentiating this condition from meningitis. The later work of Cyrille Courville and Johannes M. Nielsen (1934) confirmed and amplified the observations of Holt and others on the close relation in children between otitis media, and sinus or mastoid infections, and the development of brain abscesses. The history of the treatment of brain abscesses has been reviewed by J. Garfield (1978).

Tuberculous Meningitis The first documented record of tuberculosis dates back to 5000 B.C in the remains of a skeleton showing spinal involvement. Many physicians of antiquity described other illnesses that, when examined retrospectively, were likely to have been tubercular in origin. Allison reported on a Peruvian child from 800 A.D. who had Pott's disease with paraplegia (1973). The first accurate description of tuberculous meningitis was that of Robert Whytt in 1768 in *Observations on the Dropsy in the Brain*. Whytt classified this disease into three stages and, although his description is still unparalleled, he mistook the sequellae, that is hydrocephalus, for the disease itself. In 1779 C. W. Quinn used the term *acute hydrocephalus* to separate the infectious or inflammatory type of hydrocephalus from that due to congenital or chronic disorders. Martinet and Alexandre Parent-Duchâtelet separated the basal arachnitis form from the arachnitis of the convexities of the brain and observed that the basal form was more common in children (1821). The studies of Nicholas Senn, who was the first to suggest the tuberculous origin of meningitis (1825); Capuron and Chauvel, who employed the term *fièvre cérébrale* (brain fever); Fabre and Constant, who introduced the term *tuberculous meningitis* in 1835; and Guersent, who divided meningitis into tuberculous and non-tuberculous forms (1839), soon followed. Around this time, William Gerhard in the United States (1833–34) and Charles Morehead in India (1847–48) described and correlated the clinical and pathological findings in children with tuberculous meningitis. Later, contributions towards the understanding of this disorder grew dramatically, yet it was always appreciated that this disorder in children clinically presented differently than in adults (Gowers, 1893). The studies of Rich and McCordock in 1933 suggested that meningitis was due to release of bacilli from a caseous focus in either the brain or meninges because intravenous injection of the bacilli did not result in disease. However, more recent studies suggest that there probably is early hematogenous dissemination that seeds a slowly developing meningeal lesion. With the advent of streptomycin (1946), isoniazid (1956), and Rifampin (1965), treatment is now successful in most children and has been carefully studied by John Lorber (1956), Edith Lincoln (1960), and P. M. Udani (1973), among many others (see Tandon, 1978, for all uncited references).

Syphilis Syphilis and its nervous system manifestations have been well described over the past two hundred years (McHenry, 1969, 401). Theodor Rumpf in 1887 reviewed this problem in children and noted a high incidence of convulsions, death, and hydrocephalus, a finding also noted by Alfred Fournier (1876). Gowers had also observed seizures in children with syphilis (1881a). John Abercrombie, who was an assistant physician at Great Ormond Street and who wrote on hemiplegia in children, noted congenital syphilis as a cause of hemiplegia in four of fifty children examined. Bernard Marfan reported a case of hemiplegia in a five-month-old girl (1887) as did Hughlings Jackson in a ten-year-old girl with hemiplegia who previously had chorea (1868). Fournier related a case of paraplegia in a seven-year-old boy (1876). Syphilitic spinal cord disease was described by Ernst Julius Remak in 1885. Albrecht Von Graefe reported a two-year-old with a third nerve palsy. Juvenile dementia after infancy rather than congenital cerebral deficiency was discussed by Judson Bury (1883). The monograph *Juvenile Paresis* (1936) by William Menninger thoroughly reviews the childhood neurologic aspects of neurosyphilis.

NEUROCUTANEOUS SYNDROMES

A recent review in the volume entitled *Phakomatoses* from the *Handbook of Clinical Neurology* listed thirty-seven separate neurocutaneous disorders (François, 1972; Liebaldt and Leiber, 1972). Although an overview is not feasible, several historical points can be mentioned. It is interesting to realize that even though Désiré Bourneville described tuberous sclerosis in 1880 and Frederick von Recklinghausen described neurofibromatosis in 1882, it was not until 1919 that these disorders were first grouped together, when Max Bielschowsky described them as dysplasias with a tendency to blastoma formation. In 1923 J. Van der Hoeve coined the term *phakomatoses* (birth mark) for these disorders, adding Von Hippel-Lindau syndrome to this group in 1932 and Sturge-Weber syndrome in 1936. Because of both ectodermal and mesodermal involvement, Cornil in 1933 suggested the term *neuroectomesodermoses* and Oehler the term *ectomesodermal blastomatoses* (1936). Ludo Van Bogaert, however, in 1935 referred to these conditions as *congenital neuroectodermal dysplasias*, based on the idea that the most significant involvement was that of the skin and nervous system, which were both derived from the primitive ectoderm (François, 1972, 3). These disorders were also recognized as involving tumors that from one perspective contained elements representing both developmental malformations and benign tumors. Thus Putschar (1935) and Wohlwill (1946) proposed the term *hamartoses* (to deviate or miss the goal) and Paul Yakovlev and Guthrie (1931), among others, used the term *dysplasias with blastomatous tendencies* to stress the frequently observed tissue proliferation that occurs. Kissel and Beurey stressed the genetic nature of these conditions referring to them as the *genoneurodermatoses* (1953). Although these disorders are presently grouped as neurocutaneous syndromes, the specific genetic determinants of the different disorders are now just beginning to be realized: for example, neurofibromatosis has been localized to chromosome 17 (Type 1) and 22 (Type 2).

Early contributions to understanding childhood learning disorders originated from several different directions (Thompson, 1966; Critchley, 1970; Strother, 1973; Kessler, 1980). Aphasic disorders, although reported as early as 400 B.C., underwent modern scrutiny with the work of Paul Broca, Freud, Hughlings Jackson, and Henry Head (McHenry, 1969; Strother, 1973). In fact, Freud is credited with the first definite statement in the medical literature that language dysfunction may be based on innate or developmental factors (Thompson, 1966). The disorders of oral language development stem from the studies of word-deafness in adults. In James Kerr's early studies (1897), he described children "who hear well but are dumb" (Strother, 1973). Later J. H. Claiborne discussed word and tone-deafness, suggesting that they were due to congenital lesions or delayed cerebral maturation (1906). This was amplified by the studies of C. H. Town, who wrote *Congenital Aphasia* (1911), a term he attributed to Alfred Binet (Strother, 1973), and criticized by the later studies of Alexander Ewing in his monograph *Aphasia in Children* (1931).

From a separate direction, a Scottish ophthalmologist, James Hinshelwood, reported several cases in 1895 of word-blindness in adults; which was soon followed by the report of Pringle Morgan, an English general practitioner (*A Case of Congenital Word-Blindness*, 1896); and James Kerr (1897), a school physician of intelligent children with reading disabilities. Hinshelwood subsequently published a book (1900) and then his definitive monograph on the subject in 1917, *Congenital Word-Blindness*.

Samuel Orton, in his extensive studies on language and reading disorders of children, discussed many different areas, including developmental aphasia and developmental agraphia. Because of his early training in neuropathology, he had suggested several theories to account for these disabilities and also proposed approaches to treatment that are still in use today. Orton also appreciated the importance of ambidexterity, reversals when attempting to read or write, and occasional mirror reading or writing.

Another approach to understanding learning disabilities in children evolved from the studies of brain injury. The epidemic encephalitis that occurred during World War I affected a large number of children. Studies at that time concentrated primarily on behavioral disorders. The early studies of Edgar Doll, Winthrop Phelps, and Ruth Melcher (1932), and Elizabeth Lord (1937) on the psychological and learning problems of children with cerebral palsy, due presumably to birth trauma, added another dimension to studying the relation between brain injury and learning. Further formulation for the concept of brain damage that caused both retardation and learning disability were elucidated in the series of papers by A. A. Strauss and H. Werner (1938–47) culminating in the book by Strauss and L. E. Lehtinen in 1947 *Psychopathology and Education of the Brain-Injured Child*. Strauss's work also contained many formulations and suggestions for educational training and in part popularized the problem of the child who could not learn. This stimulated the growth of many local, state, and nationwide organizations and led eventually to the formation of the Association for Children with Learning Disabilities and to more active government support for special education.

While Strauss's work was garnering much attention, the concept of minimal brain damage was also receiving support. This apparently was not a new idea because in 1908, Alfred Tredgold, in his book *Mental Deficiency*, observed that in milder cases (of birth injury), the initial symptoms may rapidly subside and it is only when the child begins his schooling that deficiency is noted. (Tredgold, 1908, 194–269). Similar statements were made by Hugo Ehrenfest and Edgar Doll (Strother, 1973). Later, when Ingalls and Gordon introduced the idea of *biological gradient of disease*, this concept was eventually applied to children; and Lilienfeld, Pasamanick, and Knobloch, among others, used the term *continum of reproductive casualty* and provided extensive evidence linking abnormal maternal and fetal events with various disorders of language and behavior.

In a historical overview of minimal brain dysfunction, C. R. Strother mentions several conferences of importance that have focused attention on the problem of reading disabilities. The first, held at Johns Hopkins in 1961, concluded that the diagnosis ". . . . will continue not to depend on a single telltale sign or group of signs, but on the clinical appraisal of the whole configuration of symptoms and test findings" (Strother, 1973). Macdonald Critchley, at the second conference held in Philadelphia in 1966, called for the recognition of a specific syndrome resulting from a genetically determined constitutional disorder, realizing that there was still little agreement on a definition of developmental dyslexia (Strother, 1973). Another major advance came in 1962 at the Oxford International Study Group on Child Neurology organized by Ronald MacKeith and Martin Bax. The two major recommendations from this meeting were that the term *minimal brain damage* should be replaced by *minimal brain dysfunction*, and that greater efforts needed to be directed towards classifying the various heterogeneous groups of disorders that fell under this rubric. Agreement on the term *minimal brain dysfunction* in the United States came after the completion of a task force report sponsored by the United States Public Health Service (Clements, 1966). Two years later, the National Advisory Committee on Handicapped Children published their first annual report, which included a definition of the term *learning disability*. This foreshadowed the changes in terminology published in 1980 (and revised in 1989) in the American Psychiatric Association's *Diagnosis and Statistical Manual of Mental Disorders*, which distinguished developmental disorders of language, reading, writing and calculation from attention deficit disorders. The use of this latter terminology dated back to the studies of E. Kahn and L. H. Cohen (1934), who observed "organic drivenness" in the behavior of the brain-damaged children that they had evaluated, as well as the studies of Strauss and his colleagues (see Spreen et al, 1984, for references).

CONCLUDING REMARKS

This introduction has briefly focused on the subject matter of child neurology as it evolved from the earliest of medical times until the mid to latter part of this century. There are many topics that have only briefly been covered and others, which are of current importance, such as neonatal neurology, that have not been included. Likewise, tumors and topics particularly related to pediatric neurosurgery have been omitted as there are several recent excellent histories that have been published on these subjects (Walker, 1951; Sachs, 1952). These, to some extent, are incorporated into several of the biographical sketches of the founders who have contributed to these particular disciplines. Little has also been mentioned concerning the broader context of pediatrics and neurology during this period of growth and maturation of child neurology. Prior to each of the five chronologically oriented biographical sections, a brief overview of the principal trends and movements of these two fields has been included.

REFERENCES

References include those for both the introductory section on the history of child neurology, as well as for the five separate chapter introductions on pediatrics and neurology. The majority of these citations can be found in several of the standard reference sources, such as Abt, 1965; Garrison, 1929; Haymaker and Schiller, 1970; and McHenry, 1969. Citations prior to 1900 not listed in these sources are easily accessible through the CATLINE or HISTLINE directories of the National Library of Medicine. Neurological references after 1900 not cited above can be found in one of the following four sources: *Clinical Neurology*, edited by A. B. Baker and L. H. Baker (1975); *The Nervous System*, edited by D. B. Tower (1975); specific volumes from the *Handbook of Clinical Neurology*, edited by P. J. Vinken, and G. W. Bruyn (1960 to present); or *Brain's Diseases of the Nervous System*, edited by Sir John Walton (1985). Pediatric references after 1900 cited above can be found in one of the following three sources: Holt's *Pediatrics*, edited by H. L. Barnett and A. H. Einhorn (1968); *History of American Pediatrics*, by T. E. Cone (1979); or *History of the American Pediatric Society*, by H. K. Faber and R. McIntosh (1966).

Abt, A.F. 1965. *Abt-Garrison History of Pediatrics*. Philadelphia: W. B. Saunders Company.

Aicardi, J. 1986. Myoclonic Epilepsies of Infancy and Childhood. In Advances in Neurology. Vol 43. *Myoclonus*. Ed. S. Fahn, C. D. Marsden, and M. H. Van Woer. New York: Raven Press.

André-Thomas. 1897. *Le Cervelet, étude anatomique, clinique et physiologique*. Paris: G. Steinheil.

Ariés, P. 1962. *Centuries of Childhood. A Social History of Family Life.* Translated from the French by Robert Baldick. New York: Alfred A. Knopf.

Baker, A. B., and L. H. Baker (eds). 1975. *Clinical Neurology*. New York: Harper and Row.

Balthazar, E. E., and H. A. Stevens. 1975. *The Emotionally Disturbed, Mentally*

Retarded: A Historical and Contemporary Perspective. Englewood Cliffs, New Jersey: Prentice-Hall, Inc.

Barnett, H. L., and A. H. Einhorn (eds). 1968. *Holt's Pediatrics*, 14th ed. New York: Appleton-Century-Crofts.

Batten, F. E. 1903. Cerebral Degeneration with Symmetrical Changes in the Maculae in Two Members of a Family. *Trans Ophthal Soc U.K.* 23:386.

______. 1914. Family Cerebral Degeneration with Macular Change (So-called Juvenile Amaurotic Idiocy). *Quart J Med* 7:444–54.

Baumes, J. P. 1797. *Des convulsions dans l'enfance, de leurs causes, et de leur traitement.* Paris: C. Belle.

Benner, D. G. (ed). 1985. *Baker Encyclopedia of Psychology*, 921–27. Grand Rapids, MI: Baker Book House.

Billard, C. M. 1828. *Traité des maladies des enfans nouveaux-nés et à la mamelle.* Paris: J. B. Baillière

Brachet, J. L. 1824. *Mémoire sur les causes des convulsions chez les enfans et sur les moyens d'y remédier.* Paris: Bechet Jeune

Brett, E. M. 1983. *Paediatric Neurology*. London: Churchill Livingstone.

Bridge, E. M. 1949. *Epilepsy and Convulsive Disorders in Children.* New York: McGraw-Hill Book Co., Inc.

Byers, R., and P. R. Dodge. 1967. Huntington's Chorea in Children. *Neur* 17:587.

Caudle, F. M. 1984. History of Psychology. In *Encyclopedia of Psychology*, Vol. 2, 123–30. Ed. R. J. Corsini. New York: John Wiley and Sons.

Cazauvielh, J. B. 1827. Recherches sur l'agenesie cérébrale. *Arch gén Méd* 14:1,347.

Clarke, J. 1815. *Commentaries on Some of the Most Important Diseases of Children.* London: Longman, Hurst, Rees, Orme & Brown.

Clements, S. D. 1966. *Minimal Brain Dysfunction in Children*. Monograph No. 3. Bethesda, Md.: U.S. National Institute of Neurological Disease and Blindness.

Collier, J. S. 1899. Cerebral Diplegia. *Brain* 22:396.

Cone, T. E., Jr. 1979. *History of American Pediatrics*. Boston: Little, Brown and Company.

______. 1983. Historical trends: Evolving pediatric concepts of variation and deviation up to 1920. In *Developmental-Behavioral Pediatrics*. Ed. M. D. Levine et al. Philadelphia: W. B. Saunders Co.

Cotard, J. L. 1868. Etude sur l'atrophie cérébrale. Thèse.

Critchley, M. 1970. *The Dyslexic Child.* 2d ed. London: William Heinemann Medical Books.

Crothers, B. 1926. *Disorders of the Nervous System in Childhood.* New York: D. Appleton and Company.

Cruveilhier, J. J. 1835–42. *Anatomie pathologique du corps humaine; descriptions avec figures lithographiées et colorées des diverses alterations morbides dont le corps humain est susceptible.* Paris: J. B. Baillière.

Dejerine, J. J., and André-Thomas. 1902. *Traité des maladies de la moëlle épinière.* Paris: J. B. Ballière.

DeJong, R. N. 1982. *A History of American Neurology*. New York: Raven Press.

DeMause, L. 1974. *The History of Childhood.* New York: The Psychohistory Press.

Deutsch, A. 1946. *The Mentally Ill in America*. New York: Columbia University Press.

Dreifus, F. R., and M. G. Netsky. 1964. Progressive Poliodystrophy. *Am J Dis Child* 107:649.

Dubowitz, V. 1980. A History of Muscle Disease. In *Historical Aspects of the Neurosciences. A Festschrift for Macdonald Critchley.* Ed. F. C. Rose and W. F. Bynum. New York: Raven Press.

______. 1989. The Duchenne Dystrophy Story: From Phenotype to Gene and Potential Treatment. *J Child Neur* 4:240–50.

Dugdale, R. 1877. *The Jukes; A Study in Crime, Pauperism, Disease and Heredity.* New York: Putnam.

Dyck, P. J. 1975. Inherited Neuronal Degeneration and Atrophy Affecting Peripheral Motor, Sensory, and Autonomic Neurons. In *Peripheral Neuropathy*, 825. Ed. P. J. Dyck, P. K. Thomas, and E. H. Lambert. Philadelphia: W. B. Saunders Co..

Dyken, P. R. 1989. Viral Diseases of the Nervous System. In *Pediatric Neurology, Principles and Practice.* Ed. K. F. Swaiman. St. Louis: The C. V. Mosby Company.

Ehrenfest, H. 1922. *Birth Injuries of the Child.* New York: D. Appleton & Co.

Eldridge, R. 1970. The Torsion Dystonias. Literature Review and Genetic and Clinical Studies. *Neur* 20:1.

English, P. C. 1989. Not Miniature Men and Women: Abraham Jacobi's Vision of a New Medical Specialty a Century Ago. In *Children and Health Care, Moral and Social Issues.* Ed. L. M. Kopelman and J. C. Moskop. Boston: Kluwer Academic Publishers.

Escardo, F. 1944. La neuropediatria en el arte. *Arch Argentinos Ped* 21:257–72.

Ewing, A. 1931. *Aphasia in Children.* New York: Hafner Publishing Co.

Faber, H. K., and R. McIntosh (eds). 1966. *History of the American Pediatric Society*. New York: McGraw-Hill.

Fisher, R. G. 1951. Surgery of the Congenital Anomalies. In *A History of Neurological Surgery*. Ed. A. E. Walker. Baltimore: The Williams and Wilkins Company.

Ford, F. R. 1966. *Diseases of the Nervous System.* 5th ed. Springfield, IL: Charles C Thomas.

Ford, F. R., B. Crothers, and M. C. Putnam. 1927. *Birth Injuries of the Central Nervous System. Part 1. Cerebral Birth Injuries. Part 2. Cord Birth Injuries*. Baltimore: The Williams & Wilkins Company.

François, J. 1972. A General Introduction. In *Handbook of Clinical Neurology*. Vol. 14: *The Phakomatoses.* Ed. P. J. Vinken and G. W. Bruyn. Amsterdam: North Holland Publishing Company.

Frank, A. G., L. H. Marshall, and H. W. Magoun. 1976. The Neurosciences. In *Advances in American Medicine: Essays at the Bicentennial*, 552. Ed. J. Z. Bowers and E. Purcell. New York: Josiah Macy, Jr., Foundation.

Freud, S. 1893. *Zur Kenntnis der cerebralen Diplegien des Kindesalters*. Leipzig: Franz Deuticke.

______. 1897. *Die Infantile Cerebrallähmung*. Wien: Alfred Holder Publishing Co.

Friedreich, N. 1863, 1876–77. Über degenerative Atrophie der spinalen Hinterstränge. *Virch Arch path Anat* 26:391,433; 68:145, 70:140.

Garfield, J. 1978. Brain Abscesses and Focal Suppurative Infections. In *Handbook of Clinical Neurology*. Vol. 33: *Infections of the Nervous System*, part 1. Ed. P. J. Vinken. and G. W. Bruyn. Amsterdam: North Holland Publishing Company.

Garrison, F. 1929. *An Introduction to the History of Medicine.* Philadelphia: W. B. Saunders .

Garrod, A. E. 1908. The Croonian Lectures on Inborn Errors of Metabolism. *Lancet* 11:1, 73, 142, 214.

______. 1909. Inborn Errors of Meatbolism. London: Oxford University Press.

Goddard, H. H. 1912. *The Kallikak Family; A Study in the Heredity of Feeblemindedness*. New York: MacMillan.

Gowers, W. R. 1880. *The Diagnosis of Diseases of the Spinal Cord.* London: J. and A. Churchill.

______. 1881a. *Epilepsy and Other Chronic Convulsive Disorders: Their Causes, Symptoms and Treatment*. London: Churchill.

______. 1881b. Clinical Lectures on Birth Palsies. Lancet: 1:709–11, 759–60.

______. 1886–88. *A Manual of the Diseases of the Nervous System.* London: J. and A. Churchill.

______. 1893. *A Manual of Diseases of the Nervous System.* 2d ed. Philadelphia: P. Blakiston Son & Co.

Green, J. R. 1965. The Origins of Neurological Institutes. In *Horizons in Neurological Education and Research*, 93. Springfield, IL: Charles C Thomas.

Greenfield, J. G. 1954. *The Spino-Cerebellar Degenerations*. Oxford: Blackwell Scientific Publications.

Halpern, S. A. 1988. *American Pediatrics. The Social Dynamics of Professionalism, 1880–1980.* Los Angeles: The University of California Press.

Hammond, W. A. 1871. On Athetosis. *Med Times Lond* 2:747.

Haymaker, W., and F. Schiller. 1953. 2d ed., 1970. *The Founders of Neurology*. Springfield, IL: Charles C Thomas.

Hers, H. G., and F. van Hoof. 1973. *Lysosomes and Storage Diseases*. New York: Academic Press.

Herz, E. 1944. Dystonia. *Arch Neur Psych* 51:305.

Hinshelwood, James. 1917. Congenital Word Blindness. London: H. K. Lewis.

Holt, L. E. 1898. A Report of 5 Cases of Abscess of the Brain in Infants,

Together with a Summary of 27 Collected Cases in Infants and Very Young Children. *Arch Ped* 15: 81–105, 161–72.

Ingram, T. T. S. 1964. *Paediatric Aspects of Cerebral Palsy*. Edinburgh: E. & S. Livingstone.

Jackson, J. H. 1931. *Selected Writings of John Hughlings Jackson*. Edited for the Guarantors of Brain by James Taylor with the advice and assistance of Gordon Holmes and F. M. R. Walshe. London: Hodder and Stoughton, Ltd.

Kahn, E., and L. H. Cohen 1934. Organic Drivenness: A Brainstem Syndrome and an Experience. *NEJM* 210:748.

Kanner, L. 1964. *A History of the Care and Study of the Mentally Retarded*. Springfield, IL: Charles C Thomas.

Keating, J. M. 1891. *Cyclopaedia of the Diseases of Children*. Philadelphia: J. B. Lippincott Company.

Kessler, J. W. 1980. History of Minimal Brain Dysfunction. *Handbook of Minimal Brain Dysfunctions: A Critical View*. Ed. H. E. and E. D. Rie. New York: Wiley.

King, L. S. 1963. *The Growth of Medical Thought*. Chicago: The University of Chicago Press.

Konigsmark, B., and L. Weiner. 1970. The Olivopontocerebellar Atrophies: A Review. *Medicine* 49:227.

Lazarow, P. B., and H. W. Moser. 1989. Disorders of peroxisomal biogenesis. In *The Metabolic Basis of Inherited Disease*. Ed. C. R. Scriver et al. New York: McGraw-Hill Information Services.

Lennox, W. G. and M. A. Lennox 1960. *Epilepsy and Related Disorders*. Boston: Little Brown & Company

Levinson, A. 1943. *Pioneers of Pediatrics*. New York: Froben Press.

______. 1949. Notes on the History of Pediatric Neurology. In *Victor Robinson Memorial Volume: Essays on the History of Medicine*. Ed. S. R. Kagan. New York: Froben Press.

Liebaldt, G.P., and B. Leiber. 1972. Cutaneous dysplasias associated with neurological disorders: Synopsis and Differential Diagnosis. In *Handbook of Clinical Neurology*. Vol. 14: *The Phakomatoses*, 101–31. Ed. P. J. Vinken and G. W. Bruyn. Amsterdam: North Holland Publishing Company.

Little, W. J. 1843–44. Course of Lectures on the Deformities of the Human Frame. *Lancet* 1:5–7, 38–44, 70–74, 209–12, 230–33, 250, 257–60, 290–93, 318–20, 346–49, 353.

______. 1861. On the Influence of Abnormal Parturition, Difficult Labor, Premature Birth and Asphyxia Neonatorum, on the Mental and Physical Condition of the Child, Especially, in Relation to Deformities. *Trans Obst Soc Lond* 3:293.

Livingston, S. 1954. *The Diagnosis and Treatment of Convulsive Disorders in Children*. Springfield, IL: Charles C Thomas.

Macewen, W. 1893. *Pyogenic Infective Diseases of the Brain and Spinal Cord; Meningitis, Abscess of Brain, Infective Sinus Thrombosis*. Glasgow: Maclehose.

Major, R. H. 1945. *Classic Descriptions of Disease.* 3d ed. Springfield, IL: Charles C Thomas.

Matalon, R., K. Michals, and D. Sebesta. 1988. Aspartoacylase Deficiency and N-Acetylaspartic Aciduria in Patients with Canavan Disease. *Am J Med Gen* 29:463.

McHenry, L. 1969. *Garrison's History of Neurology.* Springfield, IL: Charles C Thomas.

______. 1980. Neurology and Art. In *Historical Aspects of the Neurosciences*, 481. Ed. F. C. Rose and W. F. Bynum. New York: Raven Press.

Meissner, F. L. 1850. *Grundlage der Literatur de Pädiatrik.* Leipzig: Fest'sche Verlagsbuchhandlung.

Menninger, W. C. 1936. *Juvenile Paresis*. Baltimore: The Williams & Wilkins Company.

Merritt, H. H., and F. Fremont-Smith. 1937. The Cerebrospinal Fluid. Philadelphia: Saunders.

Morton, L. 1983. *A Medical Bibliography (Garrison and Morton)*. 4th ed. Hampshire, England: Gowers Press.

Müllener, E-R. 1965. Six Geneva Physicians on Meningitis. *J Hist Med* 20:1–26.

Myrianthopoulos, N. C., ed. 1981. *Handbook of Clinical Neurology*. Vol. 42: *Neurogenetic Directory* part 1. Amsterdam: North Holland Publishing Company.

Neophytides, A. N. 1981. Paralysis Agitans, Juvenile of Hunt. In *Handbook of Clinical Neurology*. Vol 42: *Neurogenetic Directory*, part 1. Ed. N. C. Myrianthopoulos. Amsterdam: North Holland Publishing Company.

North, J. 1826. *Practical Observations on the Convulsions of Infants.* London: Burgess and Hill.

O'Leary, J. L., and S. Goldring. 1976. *Science and Epilepsy. Neuroscience Gains in Epilepsy Research*. New York: Raven Press.

Orth, J. 1875. Über das Vorkommen von Bilirubinking-stalten bei neugebornen Kindern. *Virchows Arch Path Anat* 63:447

Osler, W. 1889. *The Cerebral Palsies of Children.* Philadelphia: P. Blakiston.

Paul, J. R. 1971. *A History of Poliomyelitis*. New Haven: Yale University Press.

Penfield, W., and C. Erickson. 1941. *Epilepsy and Cerebral Localization.* Springfield, IL: Charles C Thomas.

Penfield W., and H. Jasper. 1954. *Epilepsy and the Functional Anatomy of the Human Brain*. Boston: Little, Brown and Company.

Peterman, M. G. 1957. Pediatric Contributions to Neurology. *JAMA* 165:2161.

Poser, C. M., and L. van Bogaert. 1956. Natural History and Evolution of the Concept of Schilder's Diffuse Sclerosis. *Acta Psych Neur Scand* 31:285.

Post, A. 1891. Infections of the Nervous System in Hereditary Syphilis. In *Cyclopaedia of the Diseases of Children,* vol. 4, 590–98. Ed. J. M. Keating. Philadelphia: J. B. Lippincott.

Prichard, J. C. 1822. *A Treatise on Diseases of the Nervous System*. London: Underwood

Ring-Mrozik, E., and T. A. Angerpointer. 1986. Historical Aspects of Hydrocephalus. *Prog Ped Surg* 20:158–87.

Rosen, G. 1944. *The Specialization of Medicine with Particular Reference to Ophthalmology.* New York: Froben Press.

Ruhräh, J. 1925. *Pediatrics of the Past.* New York: Paul B. Hoeber.

______. 1932. *Pediatric Biographies.* Chicago: American Medical Association.

Rumpf, T. 1887. *Die syphilitischen Erkrankungen des Nervensystems.* Wiesbaden: J. F. Borrmann.

Russell, D. S. 1949. *Observations on the Pathology of Hydrocephalus.* London: His Majesty's Stationery Office.

Sachs, B. 1891. Chorea. In Cyclopaedia of the Diseases of Children, vol. 4, 840–56. Ed. J. M. Keating.

______. 1895. *A Treatise on the Nervous Diseases of Children.* New York: William Wood.

Sachs E. 1952. *The History and Development of Neurological Surgery.* New York: Paul B. Hoeber, Inc.

Sachs, B., and F. Peterson. 1890. A Study of Cerebral Palsies of Early Life, Based upon an Analysis of One Hundred and Forty Cases. *J Nerv Ment Dis* 17:295.

Schultz, D. 1981. *A History of Modern Psychology.* 3d. ed. New York: Academic Press.

Schumacher, G. A. 1975. The Demyelinating Diseases. In *Clinical Neurology.* Vol 2. Ed. A. B. and L. H. Baker. New York: Harper and Row.

Scriver, C. R. et al, (eds). 1989. *The Metabolic Basis of Inherited Disease. New York: McGraw-Hill Information Services.*

Séguin, E. 1846. *Traitement moral, hygiène et éducation des idiots et des autres enfants arrières.* Paris: J. B. Ballière.

Spillane, J. D. 1947. *Nutritional Disorders of the Nervous System.* Edinburgh: E & S Livingstone, Ltd.

Spreen, O., et al. 1984. *Human Developmental Neuropsychology.* Oxford: Oxford University Press.

Stevens, L. A. 1971. *Explorers of the Brain.* New York: Alfred A. Knopf.

Strauss, A. A., and L. E. Lehtinen. 1947. *Psychopathology and Education of the Brain-Injured Child.* New York: Grune & Stratton, Inc.

Still, G. F. 1931. *The History of Paediatrics.* London: Oxford University Press.

Strother, C. R. 1973. Minimal Cerebral Dysfunction: A Historical Overview. In *Minimal Brain Dysfunction.* Ed. F. de la Cruz, B. H. Fox, and R. H. Roberts. New York: Annals of the New York Academy of Medicine 205:6–17.

Strümpell, A. 1885. Über die akute Encephalitis der Kinder (Polioencephalitis acuta, cerebrale Kinderlähmung). *Jahrb Kinderheilk* 22:173.

Stumpf, D. A. 1981. The Founding of Pediatric Neurology in America. *Bull NY Acad Med* 57:804–16.

Sturges, O. 1881. *On Chorea and Other Allied Movement Disorders of Early Life. London: Smith, Elder & Co.*

Sundius, P. 1754. *Epilepsia infantili.* Upsaliae: Stippendiar Wredianus.

Tandon, P. N. 1978. Tuberculous Meningitis. In *Handbook of Clinical Neurology*. Vol. 33: *Infections of the Nervous System*, part 1. Ed. P. J. Vinken and G. W. Bruyn. Amsterdam: North Holland Publishing Company.

Taranta, A., and G. H. Stollerman. 1956. The Relationship of Sydenham's Chorea to Infection with Group A Streptococci. *Am J Med* 20: 170.

Temkin, O. 1934. Galen's *Advice for an Epileptic Boy. Bull Hist Med* 2:179–89.

______. 1945. *The Falling Sickness: A History of Epilepsy from the Greeks to the Beginnings of Modern Neurology*. Baltimore: Johns Hopkins.

Thomasen, E. 1948. *Myotonia, Thomsen's disease (Myotonia congenita?), Paramyotonia, and Dystrophia myotonica*. Danmark: Universitetsforlaget i Aarhus.

Thompson, L. J. 1966. *Reading Disability: Developmental Dyslexia*. Springfield, IL: Charles C Thomas.

Thomsen, J. 1876. Tonishe Krampfe in willkürlich beweglichen Muskeln in Folge von ererbter psychischer Disposition (Ataxia muscularis?). *Arch Psych* 6: 706.

Tower, D. B. (ed). 1975. *The Nervous System.* A three-volume work commemorating the 25th anniversary of the National Institute of Neurological and Communicative Disorders and Stroke. New York: Raven Press.

Tredgold, A. 1908. Mental Deficiency. London: Ballière, Tindall and Cox.

Van Huffelen, A. C. 1989. A Tribute to Martinus Rulandus. *Arch Neur* 46:445.

Veeder, B. S. 1957. *Pediatric Profiles*. St. Louis: The C. V. Mosby Co.

Vinken, P. J., and G. W. Bruyn, (eds). 1969 to Present. *Handbook of Clinical Neurology*. Amsterdam: North Holland Publishing Co.

Vogt, H. 1910. *Die Epilepsie im Kindesalter mit besonderer berücksichtigung erzieherischer, unterrichtlicher und forensischer Fragen.* Berlin: S. Karger.

Wallace, S. 1984. The Evolution of Developmental Medicine. In *Child Care Through the Centuries*, 80–107. Ed. J. Culkand T. Turner. Cardiff, Wales: STS Publishing.

Walker, A. E. (ed). 1951. *A History of Neurological Surgery*. Baltimore: The Williams and Wilkins Company.

Walton, J. 1981. *Disorders of Voluntary Muscle.* 5th ed. Edinburgh: Churchill Livingstone.

______. 1985. *Brain's Diseases of the Nervous System.* Oxford: Oxford University Press.

Watson, J. D., and J. Tooze. 1981. *The DNA Story: A Documentary History of Gene Cloning*. San Francisco: Freeman.

West, C. 1871. On Some Disorders of the Nervous System in Childhood. London: Longmans, Green, & Co.

West, W. J. 1841. On a Peculiar Form of Infantile Convulsions. *Lancet* 1:724–25.

Whytt, R. 1768. *Observations on the Dropsy in the Brain*. Edinburgh: J. Balfour.

Williams, G. 1987. *The Age of Miracles: Medicine and Surgery in the Nineteenth Century*. Chicago: Academy Chicago Publishers

Wolf, J. M. 1969. Historical Aspects of Cerebral Palsy. In *The Results of Treatment in Cerebral Palsy*. Ed. J. M. Wolf. Springfield, IL: Charles C Thomas.

Zeman, W. 1970. Historical Development of the Nosological Concept of Amaurotic Familial Idiocy. In *Handbook of Clinical Neurology*. Vol. 10: *Leukodystrophies and Poliodystrophies*. Ed. P. J. Vinken and G. W. Bruyn. Amsterdam: North Holland Publishing Co.

Zeman, W., et al. 1970. The Neuronal Ceroid Lipofuscinoses (Batten-Vogt syndrome). In *Handbook of Clinical Neurology*, vol. 10. Ed. P. J. Vinken and G. W. Bruyn. Amsterdam: North Holland Publishing Co.

Zülch, K. J. 1969. The Place of Neurology in Medicine and its Future. In *Handbook of Clinical Neurology*, vol. 1. Ed. P. J. Vinken and G. W. Bruyn. Amsterdam: North Holland Publishing Co..

______. 1987. *Historical Development of German Neurology*. Berlin: Springer-Verlag.

Before the Development of Medical Specialists

FOUNDERS PRIOR TO 1800

OVERVIEW

MODERN MEDICINE identifies and classifies many distinct diseases, defining them in terms of symptoms, cause, and location. This concept of distinct disease entities, however, is of relatively recent origin. Classical and medieval medicine had not generally distinguished specific diseases but rather had been concerned with various states in sick persons (Rosen, 1944, 16). The Hippocratic and Galenic teachings stated that good health or disease depended on the balance between the four humors of blood, phlegm, and yellow and black bile; these teachings were still accepted and practiced until the seventeenth and eighteenth centuries. Diseases could be treated by restoring the humors to their proper proportion by such methods as bloodletting, sweating, venesection, scarification, cupping, or applying leeches (Cone, 1979, 24). As observed by George Rosen:

> *As long as such conceptions of disease prevailed, physicians could not, in the nature of the case, concentrate their attention on any specific seats of disease. But as soon as disease was found to be associated with local lesions in organs or in the tissues of these organs, and the existence of organ pathology could be shown to correlate with certain clinical descriptions observed at the bedside, there emerged the concept of distinct diseases, such as pneumonia, bronchitis, and the like.* (Rosen, 1944, 16)

The sixteenth and seventeenth centuries witnessed the rise of modern physical science, the growth of the modern scientific method, and the development of a mechanical philosophy and a mechanistic attitude (King, 1963, 139). Terrestrial and celestial science analyzed the motion of bodies, large and small. The microscope extended the concepts of these fields to biology and the stage was set for a new system of explanations of how particles and bodies obeyed the laws of motion and how circulation through the body could explain phases of health and disease. Isaac Newton, Marcello Malphigi, and Antonj van Leeuwenhoek were representative of the beginning of the age of enlightenment. There was a new reliance on experience and observation; learning from nature, not from books, was essential (King, 1963, 151). Francis Bacon and the new empiricism issued a novel doctrine — respect for facts tempered and elaborated by judicious reasoning. The tenets of this experimental scientific method were soon applied to the practice of medicine in recording observations and analyses of symptoms.

The first true break from Galenic medicine was the work of Theophrastus von Hohenheim, more commonly known as Paracelsus (1493–1541). He emphasized that diseases were essentially the result of external causes affecting a particular organ and producing anatomical changes. By the end of the seventeenth century, great strides had been made. William Harvey's discovery of circulation had revolutionized medicine, which still held to the Galenic humoral theory as the cause of disease. The work of Thomas Sydenham was another major turning point. His emphasis was on the gathering of knowledge about specific diseases and of classifying them by their symptoms and pathology. "By abstracting the pathological symptoms that he saw repeatedly in individual sick people, and coordinating them into separate groups, he arrived at a conception of a disease as an entity, an objective thing in itself" (Rosen, 1944, 19). These concepts were advanced by several notable physicians in the eighteenth century, such as François de Sauvages, but it was not until the first half of the nineteenth century that such thinking became instrumental in changing medicine completely. From this, pediatrics and neurology eventually emerged as distinct disciplines.

PRIOR TO THE eighteenth century, the concept of childhood as perceived today did not exist and children were not deemed worthy of much scientific or medical investigation. Philippe Ariès in *Centuries of Childhood* (1962) observed the following about children and the appearance of the modern family during this time period:

In medieval society the idea of childhood did not exist; this is not to suggest that children were neglected, forsaken, or despised. The idea of childhood is not to be confused with affection; it corresponds to an awareness of the particular nature of childhood, that particular nature which distinguishes the child from the adult, even the young adult. In medieval society this awareness was lacking. That is why, as soon as the child could live without the constant solicitude of his mother, his nanny, or his cradle-rocker, he belonged to adult society. . . . Language did not give the word "child" the restricted meaning we give it today: people said "child" much as we say "lad" in everyday speech. The absence of definition extended to every sort of social activity: games, crafts, arms. (Ariès, 1962, 128)

Although the pediatric treatises of the sixteenth and seventeenth centuries were beginning to distinguish between pediatric and adult diseases, very little was said concerning inherent psychological and emotional differences. Likewise, general cultural attitudes, as depicted by artwork during the Renaissance, perceived children to be little adults in body shape, posture, development, and social interaction (Escardo, 1944). In part, this attitude reflected a certain degree of parental expediency, due to the high infant mortality rate and the low standard of living of the general populace. There were numerous other factors that contributed to both child-rearing practices and the attitudes of physicians towards children, as expressed by Thomas E. Cone, Jr.:

Brevity of life of both parents and children, dramatic as it appears in contrast to the longevity that characterized the twentieth century, only partially explains why children and childhood were of so little importance almost until modern times. Of profound significance too was the conception of society in which the family, not the individual, was the essential unit of social organization. Promotion of family ambition and advancement of family interest, not the realization of private ambition or the achievement of personal success, were seen as the common, all-important task. Hence unlike modern society, in which personal happiness and fulfillment are regarded as the sine qua non *of a successful marriage and family life, the personal affections of husband and wife, parents and children, were of minor concern in seventeenth century England and America. In a society in which the romantic concept of marriage played so small a role, it is hardly to be expected that the parent-child relationship would be sentimentalized.* (Cone, 1983, 5)

Children of this era were subject to the complete authority of their fathers, were treated like "little adults," were sent early into the workplace, and soon became aware of the hazards and risks that faced them. It is not difficult to imagine how these societal perceptions affected the attitudes of physicians in approaching the diseases of children.

Concepts of child health did not exist and children were treated similarly to adults with purges, emetics, bleeding, and medications such as calomel, tartar emetics, quinine, and opium (Cone, 1979, 30). Sanitation remained primitive and epidemics of smallpox, diphtheria, dysentery, and scarlet fever were frequent and decimated the inhabitants of cities. The common ailments of children were mainly attributed to teething, worms, and convulsions. Until the eighteenth century, childbirth and attendance of the child afterward was relegated to midwives, but by the middle of the nineteenth century, obstetrics had become a specialty and obstetricians slowly assumed this role. It was not until the turn of this century that pediatricians began to wrest away from obstetricians the care of the newborn.

Most children were cared for by women, as physicians shunned the care of children, in part because of the high mortality rate. Children were not frequently seen by a physician until after they had been weaned and only when they were quite ill, never for well-baby care. Only the children of nobility and the upper classes received attention from the medical profession. In the seventeenth and eighteenth centuries, breast feeding by mothers or wet nurses was the only method of infant feeding. Although methods of artificial feeding began to appear, they were not fully accepted until the mid nineteenth century.

During the Middle Ages and the Renaissance, pediatrics inherited a mixed legacy from the ancient Greek, Roman, Egyptian,

Hebraic, and Islamic civilizations. The practices of infanticide, abandonment, and selling of children were slowly discouraged. The first foundling asylum was opened in 787 in Milan, Italy, and in 1523, the Hôtel Dieu in Lyon, the oldest hospital in France, first admitted children for care. Infant mortality during the sixteenth and seventeenth centuries was high. Social welfare was almost nonexistent, owing to the numerous wars and epidemics that had plagued Europe. Problems due to poor infant hygiene and nutrition were just being publicly discussed. Focus on the medical diseases of children, as opposed to discussion of infant care, began with *De morbis acutis infantum* by Walter Harris (1689), followed by the works of Nils Rosen von Rosenstein (1764), Michael Underwood (1784), William Cadogan (1750), and George Armstrong (1767). Ludwig Meissner's *Grundlage der Literatur der Pädiatrik* (1850), an exceptional compendium, catalogued the pediatric literature from 1472 to 1849 under 90 subheadings. Meissner's compilation of seventeenth-century pediatric monographs listed 18 works on infant nutrition, 69 on monsters, 2 on infantile jaundice, 6 on aphthae (mouth ulcers), 25 on infantile atrophy, 5 on dentition, 29 on intestinal worms, 8 on hydrocephalus, 3 on clubfoot, and 114 on smallpox.

Many diseases of children were first described in the seventeenth and eighteenth centuries. Among these were scarlet fever (1626), rickets (1650), cretinism (1657), dysentery (1672), diphtheritic croup (1748), varicella (1767), tuberculous meningitis (1768), pyloric stenosis (1788), poliomyelitis (1789), and achondroplasia (1791). The first journal containing articles on pediatrics was the *Archiv für die Geburtshülfe Frauenzimmer - und neugebohrner Kinderkrankheiten*, started in Jena in 1787.

Institutions devoted to the welfare and care of children had, to some extent, been in existence prior to the nineteenth century. St. Vincent de Paul was responsible for one of the major foundling homes for children, the Hospice des Enfants Trouvés (1640). The first pediatric clinic or dispensary was established by George Armstrong in 1769 in London. The first and foremost children's hospital in Europe, the Hôpital des Enfants Malades, was founded in 1802.

THE ORIGINS OF neurology can be traced to the ancient Egyptian papyri, but it was not until the time of Hippocrates (460–370 B.C.), and later Galen (131–201 A.D.), that accurate descriptions of diseases involving the nervous system were recorded. Clinical descriptions of post-traumatic contralateral hemiplegia, focal seizures, subdural hematomas, spinal tuberculosis, and epidemics of paralysis are all mentioned in the Hippocratic writings. Galen accurately described many specific brain structures and studied the neurophysiology of spinal cord transection in animals. He was cognizant of the testing of the different sensory modalities of touch, temperature, and pain. His writings contain observations on the effects of trauma, alcohol, and drugs on the nervous system. He also commented on sciatica and proposed treatments for epilepsy and aphasia.

In the Middle Ages, mental functions were thought to originate in the cerebral ventricles of the brain and vapors were believed to enter the brain through the blood vessels. William of Saliceto, a thirteenth-century surgeon and professor at the University of Bologna, proposed that the brain governed voluntary and the cerebellum involuntary motion. Mercurials were used to treat syphilis, and epilepsy was believed to be a contagious disease. The period of the Renaissance was marked by advances in neuroanatomical description typified by Gregor Reisch (1512) and particularly, Andreas Vesalius (1543). Jean François Fernel, who authored the first work on physiology, proposed the concept of reflex activity, believing that all motor acts could not be under complete willful control (1542). Clinical neurology advanced little during the Middle Ages and the Renaissance, although neurological disorders were depicted in artistic works of the times (Escardo, 1944; McHenry, 1980).

The seventeenth century was marked by impressive contributions to neurology. Thomas Willis first used the term neurology, derived from Greek and meaning the anatomy of the nervous system, in *De cerebri anatome* (1664). Willis was the first to distinguish between cranial and spinal nerves, as well as autonomic and peripheral nerves. He added to the description of the arteries at the base of the brain; believed that the brain was the organ of thought; recognized that lesions of the internal capsule caused contralateral hemiplegia; and described several neurological disorders, including myasthenia gravis and general paresis. Other anatomical descriptions were those of the lateral cerebral fissure (1637) and aqueduct (1663) of Franciscus Sylvius and the arachnoid granulations of Antonio Pacchioni (1721). The first microscopic examination of the nervous system was done by Leeuwenhoek (1677), followed later by that of Malpighi (1686). Among the principal contributions to the developing field of neurophysiology was the theory of reflex action of René Descartes (1662), the concepts of tissue irritability of Francis Glisson (1677), cerebral localization by Willis (1664), and the studies of muscle contraction by Giovanni Borelli (1681), William Croone (1644), and Jan Swammerdam (1758). Aside from several well-remembered and original descriptions, such as chorea minor by Thomas Sydenham (1686), and trigeminal neuralgia by John Locke (1677), the major clinical advances related to the studies of cerebral apoplexy were by Johann Wepfer (1658) and Gregor Nymman (1670).

Neurological efforts in the eighteenth century were primarily descriptive and categorical. The most important works were written by Hermann Boerhaave (1761) from Holland and William Cullen (1778) from Scotland. Carl Linnaeus, the renowned botanist, is believed to have written the first detailed account of aphasia (1745). The Swiss physician, Gaspard Vieusseux, who described the first epidemic of bacterial meningitis (1805), also described the clinical features of the lateral medullary syndrome due to occlusion of the posterior inferior cerebellar artery in himself. John Fothergill published original descriptions of facial neuralgia (1776) and migraine (1777–84). Simon André Tissot wrote on epilepsy, migraine, and other neurological disorders (1770–80). Alcoholic and nutritional polyneuropathies were described by John Lettsom (1787); peripheral facial paralysis by Nikolaus Anton Friedreich (1797), who was grandfather of the more famous Nikolaus Friedreich; and spinal cord compression from vertebral tuberculosis by Percival Pott (1779). Neurology at this juncture was quite subordinate to the field of general medicine. There was no published "great work" that identified neurology as a separate discipline, nor were the medical journals of the day replete with neurologically oriented papers.

The neurological problems of children prior to 1800 were overshadowed, to a large extent, by the social and hygienic problems that resulted in the high infant and child mortality rates. From the beginnings of recorded medical history, it is also probable that handicapped children were perceived similar to the mentally ill and retarded. Demonical possession, witchcraft, spiritualism, and beliefs in all types of superstitions, permeated the attitudes toward the severely afflicted child. Children born with congenital defects were perceived as monsters, those with seizures were possessed, and those with other forms of mental or physical illness had been taken by the devil or were suffering at the hands of the gods. Much of what is believed about the treatment of such children, however, is conjectural, as very little recorded history is available. For example, Leo Kanner, in his study of the history of mental retardation (1964), observed that Heinrich Laehr's *Die Literatur der Psychiatrie, Neurologie und Psychologie von 1459 bis 1799* contained no references to children with mental deficiency.

There has, however, been recognition and concern for children suffering with neurologic disease dating from Galen's *Advice for an Epileptic Boy* (Temkin, 1934). The outlines of this history have been traced in the Introduction on the history of child neurology. With the social, intellectual, and industrial changes that began in the sixteenth century, medicine changed dramatically. With this, an interest developed in childhood neurologic disorders. Representative of these beginnings were: Thomas Sydenham and his description of chorea; Nicolaas Tulp and his brief but accurate illustration of meningomyelocele; Michael Underwood's first clinical description of poliomyelitis; and Robert Whytt's description of tuberculous meningitis and hydrocephalus. (Please see the list at the end of the Introduction for references.)

THOMAS SYDENHAM

THOMAS SYDENHAM (1624–1689) (figure 1) was born in the town of Winford Eagle, Dorset. The Sydenham family, who were able to trace their roots back to the time of King John, had been politically active for many years. During the Civil War, they sided with the Parliamentarians and both of Sydenham's brothers were officers in the Roundhead army. William, the elder brother, who rose to be a colonel and later governor of Weymouth and the Isle of Wight, was also a member of Parliament, while two other brothers and Sydenham's mother were killed during those troubled years (Dewhurst, 1966).

Not much is known about Thomas Sydenham's childhood. He started his university studies in 1642 at the age of eighteen as a commoner of Magdalen Hall, Oxford, but left two months later to become a soldier in the Parliamentary army. He returned to his studies in Oxford after the town fell to the Parliamentary army. Although he graduated with a degree of M.B. (Bachelor of Medicine) in 1648, he did not establish a practice of medicine until 1661, thirteen years later. He might have continued his medical studies intermittently during those years, possibly spending some of that time at Montpellier under the Protestant physician, Charles Barbeyrac. Unfortunately, information on this presumed sojourn is based solely on the statement of M. Desault, an eighteenth-century French surgeon, who claimed that one of his friends met Sydenham in Montpellier (Dewhurst, 1966). His fragmentary formal studies of medicine were probably the outcome of his involvement with the Puritan cause and his brother's career. Following the Restoration, his brother lost political power. He subsequently died, and from then on, Sydenham devoted all his time to medicine, treating patients, teaching, and writing. In 1661 he established himself as a physician in London, later moving to Pall Mall, a prestigious area that had become populated after the Restoration. In 1663 he became a Licentiate of the College of Physicians. His practice was interrupted in 1665 when the Great Plague struck the city and Sydenham, along with other physicians, moved to the country. In 1677 he took the degree of

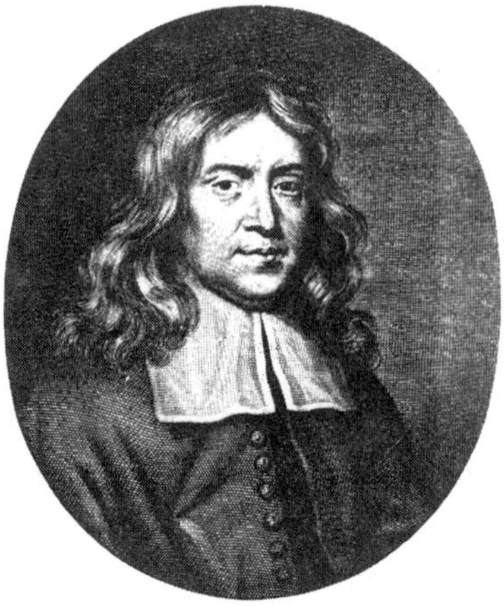

Figure 1. An engraving of Mary Beale's portrait of Thomas Sydenham (1624-1689), reproduced from the first edition of his *Observationes medicae* (1676). Taken from K. Dewhurst *Dr. Thomas Sydenham (1624-1689). His Life and Original Writing*. Berkeley and Los Angeles: University of California Press, 1966.

Doctor of Medicine in Cambridge. He continued his clinical work and writing although he was considerably limited by gout, renal calculus, and hematuria, from which he had suffered since 1654. Sydenham died at his home in Pall Mall on the 29th of December, 1689, and was buried in the Church of St. James, Westminster. He had three sons, one of whom, William, had qualified in medicine in Scotland and previously had joined his father in practice.

In 1666, when forced out of London by the plague, Sydenham completed the first edition of *Methodus curandi febers, propriis observationibus superstructa* (*Method of Treating Fevers, Based on His Own Observations*), which he dedicated to Robert Boyle, his friend and mentor in Oxford, who introduced him to epidemic diseases. The book, based on his observations of the London epidemics, consisted of four sections: continued fevers, the symptoms of continued fevers, intermittent fevers, and smallpox. It was probably written in English and later translated into Latin. A second edition was published in 1668 with the addition of a chapter on the plague. His second major book, *Observationes medicae circa morborum acutorum historiam et curationem*, appeared in 1676 and was an expanded revision of his work on fevers (Payne, 1900, 115–37). A Continental edition was published within the same year in Strassburg. The book became a major textbook of medicine, both in England and Europe. His third book, *Dissertatio Epistolaris* (1682) dealt with the treatment of confluent smallpox and hysteria. A further edition of this book was published in Geneva one year later. Sydenham's final book, *Tractatus de podagra et hydrope* dealt with gout. It was published in 1683. Other works included

Schedula monitoria (1685) and *Processus integri* (1692) (Payne, 1900, 138–57).

Two schools of medicine existed at the time of Sydenham: the School of Hippocrates and the School of the Chemists. The latter was based on tradition and authority; the former on observation. Though Sydenham accepted parts of the Hippocratic doctrine of the humors, according to which diseases were thought to result from disturbance of the four imaginary humors, his main guide and methods of diagnosis were his medical observations.

This simple recognition of the priority of direct observation and its paramount supremacy to everything else, was the proclamation of what is now an old truth, of what was then a new one and of what is always a great one (Latham, 1848).

He attempted to study diseases by recording observations without any preconceived hypotheses (Dewhurst, 1966). In a letter to his friend and pupil, John Mapletoft, Sydenham says:

The more I observed the facts of this science with an attentive eye, and the more I studied them with due and proper diligence, the more I became confirmed in the opinion which I have held to up to the present hour, that the art of medicine was to be properly learned only from its practice and its exercise. (Sydenham, *"Epistle Dedicatory to the Third Edition of His Book Medical Observations,"* in Latham, 1848, 4)

Sydenham followed these methods in his practice and teaching of medicine. He probably did not read widely on medicine, nor did he quote from or refer to previous writings. When one of his pupils, Richard Blackmore, asked what authors he should read, he was directed to Don Quixote: ". . . A very good book. I read it still."

Sydenham should be counted among the first medical epidemiologists using the Hippocratic method of observing the maladies of each season and year as a model for the London epidemics between 1661–1675. His theory of epidemic constitutions maintains that contagious diseases are influenced by cosmic or atmospheric influences that may change their types, as well as by environmental and seasonal influences. A specific influence — telluric or climatic — becomes dominant and impresses peculiar features on the clinical manifestations of diseases prevalent at that time (Rolleston, 1920; Crookshank, 1920; Greenwood, 1919). On the other hand, he objected to basic research because he thought that pathological data would confuse the physician whose only concern should be with curing diseases (Wolfe, 1961). Sydenham's unorthodox ways of practicing and teaching medicine and his critical and uncompromising attitude towards his colleagues provoked considerable antagonism in the medical establishment of his time. A faction of the Royal College favored withdrawing his license on the ground of irregular practice. In spite of many complaints in his writings of persecution, he retained the support of intellectuals and had loyal pupils who later held high positions in British medicine. He had a long and rich relationship with two of these students, John Locke and John Mapletoft, and they spread his ideas throughout England and the Continent.

Sydenham is probably one of the greatest representatives of practical medicine in England in a period that was rich with achievements in other scientific fields such as geology, botany, microscopy, zoology, anatomy, and chemistry, because of the works of Robert Hooke, John Ray, Thomas Willis, and Robert Boyle (Latham, 1848).

In addition to laying the foundation of modern clinical medicine by training physicians to carefully listen to the history of the disease and the patient's symptoms, Sydenham also stopped the use of many dangerous medicines and the practice of many dangerous therapies. He often did not dispense drugs at all and frequently prescribed fresh air, exercise, a moderate diet, and purges (Garrison, 1929). He introduced a "cooling treatment" for smallpox and Peruvian bark for agues. His "cooling treatment" for smallpox was different from the current common practice. He kept the patient out of bed as much as possible and allowed only a few bedclothes and liberal fluids — a treatment that probably saved the lives of many. He was, however, mistaken as to the etiology of this disease, regarding it as a natural process that everyone had to experience at least once during his lifetime and "as the most slight and safe of all other diseases."

Sydenham made several important contributions to pediatrics. He offered one of the earliest and most detailed descriptions of measles and is generally credited with being the first to describe and name scarlet fever, although some have suggested that he did great harm in his description by not recognizing that a sore throat was a major symptom and that this disorder was contagious. His description of the disease is as follows:

SCARLET-FEVER *(Scarlatina) may appear at any season. Nevertheless, it oftenest breaks out towards the end of summer, when it attacks whole families at once and more especially the infant part of them. The patients feel rigors and shiverings, just as they do in other fevers. The symptoms, however, are moderate. Afterwards, however, the whole skin becomes covered with small red maculae, thicker than those of measles, as well as broader, redder, and less uniform. These last for two or three days, and then disappear. The cuticle peels off; and branny scales remain, lying upon the surface like meal. They appear and disappear two or three times.* (Ruhräh, 1925, 328)

Interestingly, Sydenham was probably first to recognize several neurological complications of scarlet fever, symptoms suggesting either the development of streptococcal meningitis or perhaps a toxic or hypertensive encephalopathy:

This, however, must be borne in mind. If there occur at the beginning of the eruption either epileptic fits, or coma — as they often do occur in children or young patients — a large blister must be placed at the back of the neck, and a paregoric draught of syrup of poppies must be administered at once. This last must be repeated every night until they recover. The ordinary drink must be warm milk with three parts water, and animal food must be abstained from. (Ruhräh, 1925, 329)

Neurology occupied only a small part of Sydenham's writings. When asked why he wrote nothing concerning the diseases of the head, he answered that he "did not undertake to write upon diseases that he was uanble to cure." Nevertheless, he wrote on a few neurological and psychiatric conditions and is known for describing what came to be known as "Sydenham chorea," which is his main contribution to child neurology. His description of this entity that he called "St. Vitus' Dance" is vivid and accurate.

Sydenham twice described chorea. The fuller account, taken from *Schedula monitoria* (1686) and translated by Pechey, appears in G. F. Still's *The History of Paediatrics* :

Chorea Sancti Viti is a sort of Convulsion which chiefly invades Boys and Girls from ten years of Age to Puberty. First it shews itself by a certain

Lameness or rather Instability of one of the Legs, which the Patient drags after him like a Fool; afterward it appears in the hand of the same side; which he that is affected with this Disease can by no means keep in the same Posture for one moment, if it be brought to the Breast or any other Part, but it will be distorted to another Position or Place by a certain Convulsion, let the Patient do what he can.

If a cup of Drink be put into his Hand he represents a thousand Gestures like Juglers, before he brings it to his mouth; for whereas he cannot carry it to his mouth in a Right line, his hand being drawn hither and thither by the Convulsion, he turns it about for some time till at length happily reaching his Lips, he flings it suddenly into his mouth and drinks it greedily as if the poor Wretch designed only to make Sport. For as much as this Disease seems to me to proceed from some Humours rushing in upon the nerves which provoke such preternatural Motions, I think the curative Indications are first to be directed to the lessening of those Humours by Bleeding and Purging, and then to the strengthening of the Genus Nervosum, in order to which I use this Method (Still, 1931, 276).

The second, shorter, and probably more frequently quoted description appeared in Sydenham's *Processus integri* that was published posthumously in 1693:

ON ST. VITUS'S DANCE

This is a kind of convulsion, which attacks boys and girls from the tenth year to the time of puberty. It first shows itself by limping or unsteadiness in one of the legs, which the patient drags. The hand cannot be steady for a moment. It passes from one position to another by a convulsive movement, however much the patient may strive to the contrary. Before he can raise a cup to his lips, he makes as many gesticulations as a mountebank; since he does not move it in a straight line, but has his hand drawn aside by spasms, until by some good fortune he brings it at last to his mouth. He then gulps it off at once, so suddenly and so greedily as to look as if he were trying to amuse the lookers-on. (Latham, 1848, 2:257–59)

Sydenham's treatment of chorea, by bleeding and purging, reflects the therapeutic practices of his day. His method of containing as many as twelve ingredients in one prescription was also characteristic of his time (Levinson, 1943).

In his writings we also find a small chapter on "The Epilepsy of Children":

This may begin so early as the first month, from over frequent alvine evacuations. . . . Or it may come on during teething, between the seventh and nineteenth months, accompanied by cough, or by (what is much worse) green vomit (like that of hysteria) and diarrhea. . . . At times, the fit comes on without warning. The face becomes livid, the eyes and mouth distorted, the limbs convulsed. At times, it is indicated beforehand by a contraction of the finger, or by a fixed and strange immobility of the eyeballs. In cases where they allow a truce, the infants are drowsy until a fresh attack resuscitates them. (*Processus integri,* 1686, in Latham, Vol. 2, 1848, 284–85)

Sydenham also contributed to the field of psychiatry. In his comprehensive review on hysteria, found in his *Dissertatio epistolaris ad Guilelmum Cole, M.D.*, written in 1682, he recognized that it is a frequent condition that appears in both men and women and that it is a disorder of the nervous system that simulates an organic illness (Veith, 1956; Schneck, 1957).

Thomas Sydenham was one of the most outstanding physicians of the seventeenth century, called by some the founder of clinical medicine. Although his contribution to child neurology is only a small part of his enormous contribution to clinical medicine, it is an example of his superior diagnostic ability and the clarity and accuracy of his writings.

Yitzchak Frank
MANHASSET, NEW YORK

REFERENCES

Crookshank, F. G. 1920. First Principles and Epidemiology. *Proc Roy Coll Med* 13:159–84.

Dewhurst, K. 1966. *Dr. Thomas Sydenham (1624–1689). His Life and Original Writing*. Berkeley and Los Angeles: University of California Press.

Garrison, F. H. 1929. *An Introduction to the History of Medicine*, 269–72. Philadelphia and London: W. B. Saunders & Company.

Greenwood, M. 1919. Sydenham as an Epidemiologist. *Proc Roy Coll Med* 12:55–76.

Latham, R. G. 1848. *The Works of Thomas Sydenham, M.D. Translated from the Latin Edition of Dr. Greenhill, with a Life of the Author*. London: Printed for the Sydenham Society. Special edition, 1979, The Classics of Medicine Library, Division of Gryphon Editions, LTD, Birmingham, Alabama.

Levinson, A. 1943. *Pioneers of Pediatrics*, 39–41. New York: Froben Press.

Payne, J. F. 1900. *Thomas Sydenham*. London: T. Fisher Unwin.

Rolleston, H. 1920. The Change of Type of Disease. *JAMA* 74:1495–97.

Ruhräh, J. 1925. Thomas Sydenham. In *Pediatrics of the Past*, 321. New York: Hoeber.

Schneck, J. M. 1957. Thomas Sydenham and Psychological Medicine. *Am J Psych* 113:1034–36.

Still, G. F. 1931. Thomas Sydenham. In *The History of Paediatrics*, 276. London: Oxford University Press.

Sydenham, Thomas. 1676. *Observationes medicae circa morborum acutorum historiam et curationem*. London: G. Kettilby.

______. 1682. *Dissertatio epistolaris ad Guilelmum Cole, M.D., de observationibus nuperis circa curationem variolem confluentium necnon de affectione hysterica*. London.

______. 1686. *Schedula monitoria de novae febris ingressu*. London: G. Kettilby.

______. 1844. *Opera omnia*. Ed. Gulielmus Alexander Greenhill. London: Sydenham Society.

Veith, I. 1956. On Hysterical and Hypochondrial Afflictions. *Bull Hist Med* 30:233–40.

Wolfe, D. E. 1961. Sydenham and Locke on the Limits of Anatomy. *Bull Hist Med* 35:193–220.

NICOLAAS TULP

NICOLAAS TULP'S (1593–1674) (figure 1) first name is variously spelled in English, as "Nicolaas," "Nicolas" or "Nicholas," but his real name was Claes Pieteszoon or Nicolaus Petrus in Latin. He was born on October 11, 1593, in Amsterdam. His father was a prosperous merchant in the city and Nicolaas was the youngest of four children. He later adopted the name "Tulp," which means tulip in Dutch, because it is said that his house was decorated with tulip flowers (Goldwyn, 1961).

Tulp began his studies of medicine in 1611 at the University of

Leyden, at that time the foremost school of medicine in Northern Europe. He was enrolled as a student of medicine by the rector Snellins and his inaugural dissertation was on the relationship of body and soul. After graduation he practiced medicine and married Aafge van Voegh in 1617, who died an untimely death in 1628. In 1625 he was appointed Prelector in Anatomy at the Surgeon's Guild and in 1628 he was elected judge in Amsterdam.

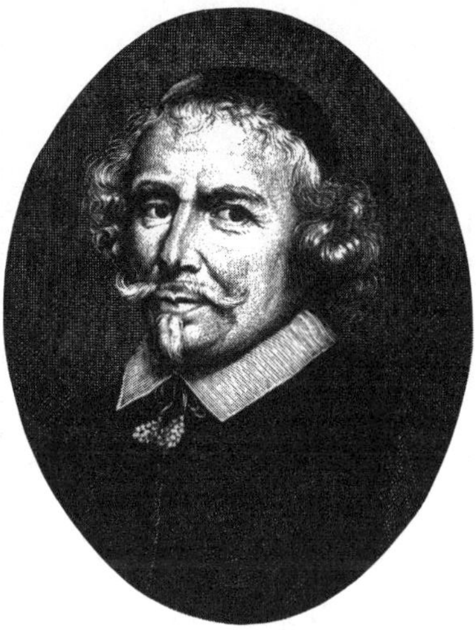

Figure 1. Portrait of Nicolaas Tulp (1593-1674). From the 1687 edition of *Observationes medicae*.

On January 31, 1631, Tulp demonstrated an anatomy dissection for the first time and, in the next year, Rembrandt painted Tulp dissecting the muscles of the arm. This is the famous painting known as *The Anatomy Lesson of Dr. Tulp* (Hecksher, 1958).

His *Observationes medicae* (*Medical Observations*), written in 1637, were first published in 1641 and reissued in many editions. The book was originally written as a practical guide for his son who had just become a doctor, and contained 228 observations. This book was based on more than twenty-five years of practice and thirteen years of professorship in anatomy and medicine and was praised by Albrecht von Haller as a "golden work." The entire work was written in Latin because Tulp was opposed to writing medical works in the vernacular that could be read by the general public who might attempt to treat themselves with disastrous results. It has, however, been partially translated into English (Scolten, 1928).

In the very first observation of the book, entitled *Calvaria fracta*, he gives the following description: "A heavy window fell down on the son of Peter de Wit, smashing his skull on the left side. The paralysis took place on the right side. But why, prithe, is the

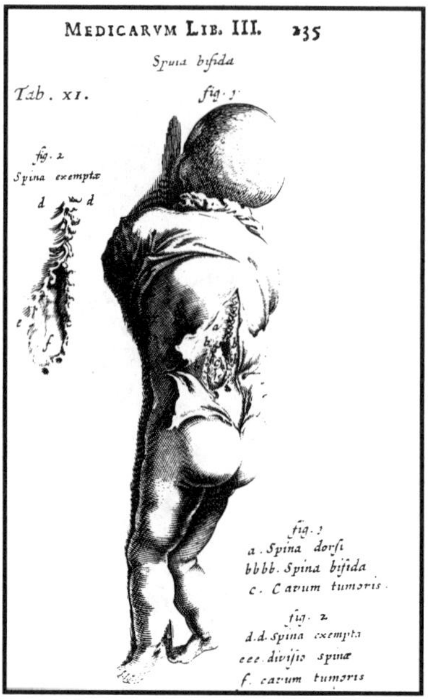

Figure 2. The first anatomical description and sketch of spina bifida from the 1687 edition of Tulp's *Observationes medicae.*

opposite side affected." Tulp was unaware of decussation of the pyramidal tract, which had been demonstrated by Galen centuries before.

Tulp's inclusion as a founder of child neurology is based on the first clear description of spina bifida, which is found in this same book. The term was coined by Tulp and has been in general use since then (Furukawa, 1987). Although this malformation had been recognized since the time of Hippocrates and later described by Vesalius (Scolten, 1928), Tulp described six cases, one a child with an extensive lumbar meningomyelocele arising from a narrow pedicle (Rickman, 1963). He recognized that the method of treatment of these tumors, which consisted of puncture of the sac and aspiration of the fluid, was commonly followed by death. His treatment differed in that he dissected the sac and ligated the pedicle. Unfortunately, the patient died some days later from infection. The dissected body of the infant is depicted in an excellent illustration (figure 2) showing the nerves and spinal defect. A combination of spina bifida and hydrocephalus was described by Morgagni (Morgagni, 1769). Other important descriptions in Tulp's book include beri-beri, epilepsia ex pollice (probably Jacksonian epilepsy), hereditary hyperhidrosis, hemorrhagia cerebri confirmed by autopsy, hydrocephalus, catalepsy, and ileocecal valve (later known as the valve of Tulp). He considered cancer contagious. He also gave a very detailed and vivid description of the orangutan, which interested him because of its resemblance to man.

Tulp retired from his professorship of the guild in 1652 and was honored with a silver-gilded tulip made especially for him (Thyssen, 1929). In 1654 he was chosen mayor and was re-elected in 1655, 1666, and 1671. He died on September 15, 1674, at the age of almost eighty-one years, having enjoyed both an illustrious medical and political career.

Tetsuo Furukawa
TOKYO, JAPAN

REFERENCES

Furukawa, T. 1987. First Description of Spina Bifida by Nicolaas Tulp. *Neur* 37:1816.

Goldwyn, R. M. 1961. Nicolaas Tulp (1593–1674). *Med Hist* 5:270–76.

Heckscher, W. S. 1958. *Rembrandt's Anatomy of Dr. Nicolaas Tulp*. New York: New York University Press.

Morgagni, G. B. 1769. *The Seats and Causes of Diseases Investigated by Anatomy* (Translated from Latin by B. Alexander.) Vol. 1: *Of Hydrocephalus and Watery Tumours of the Spine*, 244. London: A. Miller.

Rickham, P. P. 1963. Nicolaas Tulp and Spina Bifida. *Clin Peds* 2:40–42.

Scolten, A. 1928. Work of Nicolaas Tulp (1593–1674). *Med Life* 35:380–91.

Thyssen, E. H. M. 1929. Nicolaas Tulp. A Contribution to the History of the Medical Science of the Seventeenth Century (Translated from the Dutch by A. Scolten.) *Med Life* 36:394–442.

Tulp, N. 1641. *Observationes medicae.* Amsterdam: Ludovis Elzevirius.

MICHAEL UNDERWOOD

ALTHOUGH THERE IS evidence of poliomyelitis in Egyptian mummies of 3,700 B.C and in skeletons of Vikings buried in Greenland in 1000 A.D., the first accurate description of this disorder in children did not appear until 1789 and is credited to Michael Underwood. This description appeared in the second edition of his classic *A Treatise on the Diseases of Children.*

Michael Underwood (1737–1820) (figure 1) received his early education in West Moulsey, Surrey. At age sixteen, he was apprenticed to one of London's most eminent surgeons, Caesar Hawkins, who at that time served as Sergent Surgeon (personal physician) to King George II. He then studied as a house pupil at St. George's Hospital and became house surgeon in 1761 for one year before venturing to Paris, where he attended anatomy lectures. Upon his return in 1764, he received the Grand Diploma of the Company of Surgeons and began practice in both surgery and obstetrics. Underwood's reputation in obstetrics grew, and two years later he was appointed surgeon to the British Lying-in Hospital. It should be recalled that midwives attended deliveries; the presence of men was not yet common and not always welcome (Maloney, 1950). In 1783 he published *A Treatise upon Ulcers of the Legs* and several minor obstetrical works, followed in 1788 by *Surgical Tracts on Ulcers of the Legs* (Ruhräh, 1932). In 1784 he was one of very few obstetricians admitted to the Royal College of Physicians. This appointment forced his disenfranchisement from the Company of Surgeons, but had little effect on his career, which was now principally devoted to the "diseases of women and children." Although his practice gained impetus after he became physician to the Princess of Wales and attended the birth of Princess Charlotte in 1796, Underwood apparently suffered a series of major depressive episodes that impaired both his professional and social life until his death in 1820 at the age of eighty-four.

Underwood's most important work was his A *Treatise on the Diseases of Children* (1784). The book went through twenty-five editions over sixty years, was published in several languages, and is regarded as one of the important works associated with the development of modern pediatrics. The first edition was a small duodecimo volume of 288 pages and, as was the custom of the day, was addressed to both the layperson as well as members of the medical profession. However, by the fourth edition (1799) Underwood focused more on the science of medicine (Still, 1931). Underwood's awareness of his contemporaries is evident as he frequently discussed the works of Walter Harris, George Armstrong, and William Cadogan. The famous second edition appeared in 1789; a third in 1795 was issued in two volumes, followed by a fourth edition in three volumes (1799). The last edition prepared by Underwood was issued in 1819; Samuel Merriman edited the eighth in 1826, and Marshall Hall compiled one of the later revisions (1835). In the United States four separate editions were issued between 1793 and 1842. A French translation was published in 1786 and one in German in 1848. Underwood's book was the accepted standard in pediatrics for over sixty years. In contrast, Walter Harris's *De morbis acutis infantum* was available for nearly one hundred years and the work of Nils Rosen von Rosenstein (*Underratelser om barn-sjukdomar och deras bote medel*), which was originally published in Sweden, appeared in seventeen editions in eight languages between 1753 and 1851 (Ruhräh, 1932).

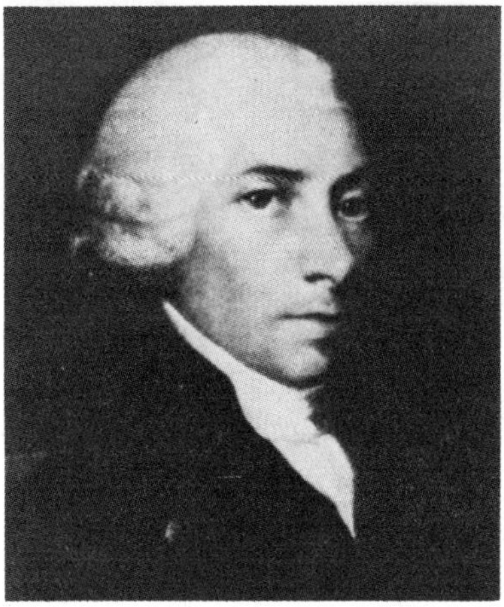

Figure 1. Michael Underwood (1737–1820).

Underwood's description of poliomyelitis is found in the second edition under the heading "Debility of the Lower Extremities" and reads as follows:

This disorder either is not noticed by any medical writer within the compass of my reading, or is not so described so as to ascertain the disease here intended. It is not a common disorder anywhere, I believe, and seems to occur seldomer in London than in other parts of the kingdom. Nor am I enough acquainted with it to be fully satisfied, either in regard to the true cause, or seat of the disease, either from my own observation, or that of others, with whom I have corresponded, except in the instance of teething or of foul bowels; and I have not myself had an opportunity of examining the body of any child who has died of this complaint. I shall therefore only describe its symptoms, and mention the several means attempted for its cure in order to induce other practitioners to pay attention to it.

If it arises from teething, or foul bowels, the usual remedies should be employed; and have always affected a cure. But the complaint as often seems to rise from debility, and usually attacks children previously reduced by fever, seldom those under one or more than four or five years old. It is then a chronical complaint, and not attended with any affection of the urinary bladder, nor with pain, fever, or any manifest disease; so that the first thing observed is a debility of the lower extremities, which gradually become more infirm, and after a few weeks are unable to support the body.

When only one of the lower extremities has been affected the above means in two instances out of five or six entirely removed the complaint; but when both have been paralytic, nothing has seemed to do any good but irons to the legs, for the support of the limbs, and enabling the patient to walk. At the end of four or five years, some have by this means got better proportion as they have acquired general strength; but even some of these have been disposed to fall afterward into pulmonary consumption, where the debility has not been entirely removed. (Underwood, 1789, 53–57.)

The clinical syndrome described by Underwood is characteristic of this disorder presumably as it existed in England. As J. R. Paul observed in *A History of Poliomyelitis*, Underwood mentioned nothing about epidemics but did emphasize the occurrence of this disorder in young children. Underwood's description in the fourth English edition (1799) is somewhat clearer and more complete, suggesting a greater clinical exposure to this disorder since his original description ten years previously.

After Underwood's clinical description, the next major advance in our knowledge of poliomyelitis was that of Jakob Heine, an orthopedic surgeon, who in 1840 helped differentiate this disorder from similar conditions of cerebral origin. Charcot, in 1870, while studying the pathology of this disorder, felt it was due to primary degeneration of the anterior horn cells. Charcot's theory had actually been preceded four years earlier by a case report of Jules

Prevost and Alfred Vulpian describing atrophy of the anterior horn in an infant with this disorder, but it was a definitive paper by John Rissler in 1888 that comprehensively reviewed the neuropathology. Charcot's concepts of the disease were also being disputed by both Adolf Strümpell and Pierre Marie, who believed that poliomyelitis represented one portion of a clinical spectrum of disorders rather than a discrete entity. With Oscar Medin's report in 1890 of the Swedish epidemics, it became clear that Charcot's hypothesis was correct. Subsequently, the studies of Ivan Wickman (1907), demonstrated human to human transmission. The studies of Kurt Landsteiner and Edwin Popper (1909), and Simon Flexner and Paul Lewis (1909), who first successfully infected monkeys with this virus, ultimately led to the later studies that identified the polio virus and the subsequent development of the vaccine. These events are thoroughly depicted by J. R. Paul in *A History of Poliomyelitis* (1971).

Underwood has long been recognized for his contribution to pediatrics, and his original clinical description of poliomyelitis has often been cited. In a way, his inclusion as a founder of child neurology is somewhat of a redundancy, and perhaps irrelevant, when one considers that the majority of the current generation of child neurologists have probably seen few, if any, children with this disorder. Yet, it is also his ability to synthesize case material and to present it as a discrete condition, that is also worth recognizing. This ability to analyze and classify clinical symptoms and signs has imbued child neurology with its distinct character.

Stephen Ashwal
LOMA LINDA, CALIFORNIA

REFERENCES

Maloney, W. J. 1950. Michael Underwood: A Surgeon Practising Midwifery from 1764 to 1784. *J Hist Med* 5:289–314.

Paul, J. R. 1971. *A History of Poliomyelitis*, 20–30. New Haven: Yale University Press.

Ruhräh, J. 1932. Michael Underwood. In *Pediatric Biographies*, 176–79. Chicago: American Medical Association.

Still, G. F. 1931. Michael Underwood. In *The History of Paediatrics*, 476–86. London: Oxford University Press

Underwood, M. 1783. *A Treatise upon Ulcers of the Legs*. London: J. Mathews.

______. 1784. *A Treatise on the Diseases of Children, with Directions for the Management of Infants from the Birth*. London: J. Mathews.

______. 1789. *A Treatise on the Diseases of Children*, 53–57. London: J. Mathews.

ROBERT WHYTT

ROBERT WHYTT (1714–1766) (figure 1) was born in Edinburgh, Scotland, on September 10. He was the second son in a family that traced their roots back to Matthew Whytt, who had been granted a land charter in 1492. Whytt's father, a lawyer after whom he was named, died six months before his birth. Upon the death of his father, his mother moved to Kirkcaldy where Whytt received his early education. He began his more formal education at St. Andrews University in 1727 and three years later proceeded to study medicine in Edinburgh, where the faculty included such luminaries as Alexander Monro, Daniel Rutherford, John Sinclair, Andrew Plummer, Charles Alston, and Robert Innes. Whytt continued his training in London under William Cheselden for two more years, then went to Paris, where he studied at la Charité and l'Hôtel Dieu. After studying in Paris, he went to Leyden to study under Bernhard Albinus and Herman Boerhaave (Still, 1931). He received his M.D. at Rheims in 1736 and this was reconfirmed the following year by St. Andrews University upon his return to Scotland. In 1738 he became a member of the Royal College of Physicians of Edinburgh.

Whytt gained recognition for being one of the first to successfully treat urinary calculi ("stone of the bladder"), which at that time, along with gout, was considered a major malady and drew much public interest. He was one of the first to isolate the "active ingredient" of a popular treatment originated by a Mrs. Joanna

Stephens; he found the ingredient to be limewater (French, 1969, 7). His observations, first reported in 1743, were subsequently published in 1752: *An Essay on the Virtues of Lime-Water in the Cure of the Stone.* In the same year he was elected a fellow of the Royal Society of London, having already been appointed to the medical faculty at Edinburgh where he took the chair of the Theory of Medicine in 1747. In 1761 he was made first physician to the King of Scotland and two years later was elected president of the Royal College of Physicians, a position he held until his death.

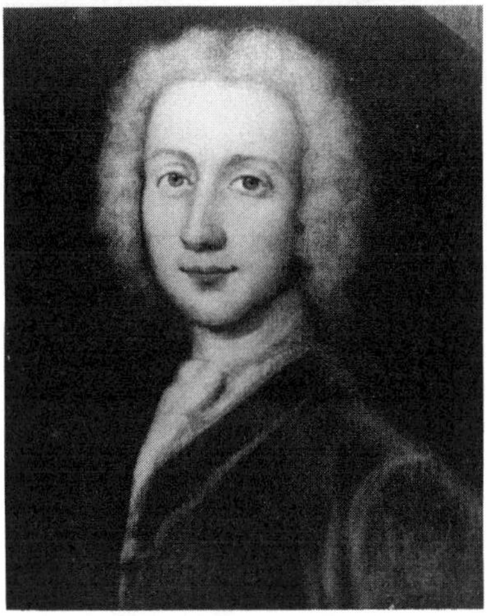

Figure 1. Robert Whytt (1714-1766).

Whytt's interests lay in the area of physiology and it is here that he made his greatest contribution to medicine by developing the concepts of neural regulation of vasomotor control. His idea of the importance of the "sentient principle" in vital and involuntary activities was presented in the first of his physiological essays "An Enquiry into the Causes which Promote the Circulation of Fluids in the Small Vessels of Animals" (French, 1969, 7). Several years later he published his "Essay on the Vital and Other Involuntary Motions of Animals" (1751), which is considered his most important contribution and which laid the basis for the concept of reflex activity. Whytt classified motion into three types: voluntary, involuntary, and mixed, and he believed in a central mechanism for their regulation. He believed that all involuntary activity could be explained either directly through the action of the stimulus upon the end organ, or indirectly through neurally mediated mechanisms at the level of the spinal cord or medulla (French, 1969, 77–92).

Whytt also believed that voluntary motions could be initiated by the immediate action of the mind. He believed in the concept of the soul as being responsible for almost all manifestations of life. To him, the soul was single, immaterial, and immortal (French, 1969). It had other unique properties because it remained in the body for a time after death and it was not completely a free agent, but acted in accordance with certain laws. Whytt's ideas about the nature of the soul, its relation to previous Aristotelian and Platonic concepts of the soul, as well as the ventricular theories as to the seat of the soul, are beautifully described in the recent work of R. K. French, *Robert Whytt, the Soul, and Medicine* (1969).

Whytt's contribution to child neurology is that of the first definitive description of tuberculous meningitis in children in *Observations on the Dropsy in the Brain*, which was actually published in 1768, two years after his death. Until Whytt described it, the disease was essentially unrecognized. Earlier observations had used the term phrenitis to describe many conditions that appeared to affect the brain by causing various types of impairment of mental function. Included in these early descriptions are case reports of probable tuberculous meningitis. In contrast, hydrocephalus had been recognized by Hippocrates, who apparently described clinical symptoms of water on the brain and suggested treatment by opening up the top part of the cranium to let out the fluid (Ruhräh, 1925). Aëtius and Paul of Aegina both mention collections of water between the skull and membranes of the brain, that is, subdural fluid collections, but not truly hydrocephalus. Celsus briefly reported on external hydrocephalus, but this term was used primarily to describe scalp edema or other subgaleal fluid collections. Both Galen and Vesalius also described several children with hydrocephalus, but the relationship to infection was uncertain. Thomas Willis observed in 1682 that fatal and incurable headaches could "follow abscesses and swellings of the envelopes of the brain, as well as plaques and tubercles of these membranes" (Ruhräh, 1925). In 1704 Duverney described in "Observations on a Dropsy of the Brain" a four-year-old-girl who died after a fifteen-day illness, and whose autopsy showed hydrocephalus and inflammation of the mesenteric glands. This work was followed by the observations of Petit in 1718, in which convulsions, lip biting, progressive stupor and pallor, spreading of the sutures, prominence of the forehead, protruding of the eyes, and swelling of the head were seen in patients whose post-mortem examination showed hydrocephalus. Sinclair (1732) from Edinburgh and Paisley (1733) from Glasgow reported several cases of hydrocephalus with intermittent fevers and Monro also described several forms of hydrocephalus. Giovanni Morgagni in 1761 described cases of hydrocephalus associated with serositis. De Sauvages de la Croix (1763) probably should be credited with the first account of tuberculous meningitis because he gave a very lucid description in a paper entitled "Eclampsia ab hydrocephalo," which was published in his *Nosologia methodica*. However, this report was not recognized until Isidore Bricheteau extracted this paper in 1829, almost sixty years after Whytt's publication. Portions of De Sauvages's work were translated by John Ruhräh in *Pediatrics of the Past*:

Eclampsia depending upon hydrocephalus, commonly called water in the brain, is a very frequent disease which carries off a considerable number of our children even in the families of the most distinguished rank. It would be very important if one could foretell it, for once existing one can hardly remedy it. It attacks children of three, four or five years, principally those who are affected with scrofula, with enlargements of the mesenteric glands, and whose parents have had syphilis. It begins by lack of appetite; the children lose their taste for everything, even their toys; they are pale, sad, capricious and of a bad humour; their pulse is small, languishing. At intervals the face becomes red as in exacerbations of acute diseases. To this there is added feebleness, a sort of languor; the head becomes very heavy and totters upon the shoulders; the mouth undergoes sudden distortion; the eyes become fixed and appear covered with a sort of cloud; the hands and some parts of the face are agitated with convulsive movements; the intellectual faculties become obscured, the patients are drowsy, and as if stupid or dull; the pulse becomes feeble, frequent, unequal, and death takes place in the space of several days. On opening the body one finds a considerable effusion of serous fluid in the ventricles of the brain. (Ruhräh, 1925, 408)

Whytt's account of tuberculous meningitis and hydrocephalus was based on his observations of twenty patients and is recorded in a forty-eight page monograph. He divided the disease into three stages depending on the condition of the pulse: quick, slow, and then rapid. Early in his monograph he clarified the definition of hydrocephalus as follows:

The hydrocephalus, or dropsy of the head, is either external or internal. The former has its seat in the cellular substance, between the skin and the pericranium, or between this membrane and the skull. In the internal hydrocephalus, the water is sometimes collected between the cranium and dura matter, or between this last and the pia matter; but most commonly is found in the ventricles of the brain, immediately below the corpus callosum: And this is not only the most frequent and fatal species of the hydrocephalus, but also that with which medical writers seem to have been least acquainted.

This was followed by Whytt's reviewing the previous observations of others and clearly differentiating chronic hydrocephalus, presumably due primarily to developmental malformations, from the acute hydrocephalus occurring with tuberculous infection:

It, may seem strange, that a dropsy of the ventricles of the brain, which in our days so frequently occurs, should have been altogether unknown to the ancients, and so little attended to by most of the moderns. The reason may be, that those patients who were carried off by this disease have been generally supposed to die of a fever ending in a coma; and in such cases the head is seldom opened.

Altho' a dropsy of the ventricles of the brain does very rarely occasion any opening of the sutures, or swelling of the head (Vesalius gives an account of the child of two years old, whose head was greatly enlarged, and in the ventricles of whose brain he found nine pounds of water; But this is an extraordinary case; and it is probable the water began to be collected soon after the child's birth, and before the sutures of the skull could offer any considerable resistance to its pressure. I shall only add here, that I have not only never observed any increase of the size of the head in the species of hydrocephalus of which I now treat, but that it is an error, though a common one, to imagine, that those children who have big heads are most liable to this disease; for all of those whom I have attended, few or none were remarkable for the largeness of their head, but several had been very sprightly, and of a delicate make.); yet in most cases it may be easily distinguished from every other disorder, by the following symptoms, which with the greatest care I have collected, in attending about twenty patients in this disease.

The next section of Whytt's monograph presents the clinical symptoms of this disorder as he separated it into three stages. I have extracted several quotes of interest to pediatricians or child neurologists.

THE FIRST STAGE (QUICKENED PULSE):

Children who have water in the ventricles of the brain begin to have many of the following symptoms, four, five, or six weeks, and in some cases much longer, before their death.

At first they lose their appetite and spirits; they look pale, and fall away in flesh; they have always a quick pulse, and some degree of fever. In some cases I have seen a hydrocephalus attended with a considerable degree of fever, which had frequent remissions, but without any order or regularity: In other cases the paroxysms came on pretty regularly in the evening, and then the disease was taken for a slow irregular nervous fever, or for one occasioned by worms. At this time, in children of five years and upwards, I have found the pulse at a hundred and ten, in others at a hundred and twenty, and in a few cases at a hundred and thirty, or even at a hundred and forty strokes in a minute; but rarely ever so full as to indicate bleeding.

THE SECOND STAGE (SLOW IRREGULAR PULSE):

During the second stage, most of the symptoms mentioned in the first continue. The sick are then unable to sit up, tho' generally they sleep little, till towards the end of this period, when they begin to grow drowsy. They moan heavily, yet cannot tell what ails them. Their eyes are often turned towards their nose, or they squint outwards, and sometimes they complain of seeing objects double. Some, towards the end of this stage, grow delirious, and cry out in a wild manner, as if they were much frightened.

THE THIRD STAGE (RAPID PULSE):

In the third stage, the patient, who before was little disposed to sleep, becomes then drowsy and comatose. When roused, he utters only a few incoherent words, and appears to be insensible. The beginning of the coma is uncertain; it is often about the end of the second stage before the pulse grows quicker for the second time; but in a few cases I have known this quickness of the pulse come on before the patients become comatose.

Frequently one eye-lid loses its motion, and afterwards the other becomes also paralytic. About this time, or rather sooner, the pupil of one or both eyes ceases to contract, and remains dilated in the greatest light. But the time of this symptom varies much: In some it happens five, six, or seven days, in others only two or three days, before they die. . . .

Before they are seized with the coma, they sometimes complain of seeing strange and frightful objects. A day or two before death, the tunica conjunctiva of one or both eyes frequently becomes inflamed; but they generally continue to hear for some days after they are blind.

In this stage, the patients are sometimes observed to be constantly raising one of their hands to their head; and are generally troubled with convulsions of the muscles of the arms, legs, or face. . . .

A day or two before death, the patient either swallows with difficulty, or not at all. Lastly, the respiration grows more frequent and laborious; and in some there is a considerable pause after every expiration. This kind of breathing I have also observed in those who have died of an apoplexy, arising from a suppression of urine.

Whytt then presents a brief summary of the autopsy findings regarding ten of his patients and he later estimates a ventricular volume of from two to five ounces:

Upon opening the heads of ten of those patients from whom I have collected the symptoms above mentioned, I found in all of them a clear thin fluid in the anterior ventricles of the brain, immediately below the corpus callosum. There was frequently the same kind of liquor in the third and fourth ventricles; but whether this is always the case, I cannot say, as I had not attended sufficiently to this circumstance. I never met with water between the dura matter and the brain, between the hemispheres of the brain, or immediately above the corpus callosum. Altho' there seems to be a communication between the two anterior ventricles; yet, in two cases, I found one of them much distended, while the other contained but little water.

The most fascinating portion of this monograph is the section in which Whytt attempts to provide a pathophysiological explanation for some of his clinical observations. It is here that one recognizes Whytt's capacity and eminence as one of the leading physiologists of his day. He provided explanations for six observations, including the loss of appetite and vomiting; aversion to light; the slow irregular pulse in the second stage; the quick pulse in the third stage; the dilation of the pupil; and the slow respirations towards the end of the disease. Extracts from two of these observations demonstrate his astuteness for observation and analysis that still forms the basis of much bedside teaching today:

THE SLOW IRREGULAR PULSE IN THE SECOND STAGE. *The motion of the heart is owing to the irritation of the returning venous blood poured into its ventricles. This irritation, however, could have no effect upon the heart, were it not for its sensibility, which depends entirely on its nerves. Wherefore, in a hydrocephalus, when the water is collected within the brain in such quantity as to press, with a considerable force, on the medullary substance, the nerves proceeding from it will in some degree lose their powers, and consequently the heart will be less sensible. And hence the pulse becomes often as slow, and sometimes slower than in a natural state, altho' there be a real fever in the body; which fever, were it not for this pressure on the origin of the nerves, would occasion a quick pulse.*

THE DILATATION OF THE PUPIL. *The contraction of the pupil is owing to the uneasy sensation excited in the retina by too much light; and hence it is, that in a dark place, or when the retina becomes insensible of the stimulus of light, the pupil is always observed to be wide. In the hydrocephalus, when the water in the ventricles presses so much on the thalami nervorum opticorum as to render the optic nerves in a great measure insensible, the retina will no longer feel the impression of light and therefore the pupil will remain dilated.*

Whytt unfortunately died two years before the publication of this monumental study and thus did not enjoy the acclaim and sense of personal accomplishment that would have been his. He suffered many personal tragedies in his life. His father died before he was born, his mother and brother died early in life, his two sons by his first marriage to Helen Robertson died in early infancy, as did eight of fourteen children from his second marriage to Louisa Balfour (French, 1969). His health began to fail about a year before his death, with symptoms suggestive of diabetes. He died at the age of fifty-two on April 15, 1766. It was his eldest son, Robert, with the assistance of Sir John Pringle, who edited and published Whytt's writings in 1768 as *The Works of Robert Whytt*, the same year his *Observations on the Most Frequent Species of Hydrocephalus Internus* was published (French, 1969).

It is now slightly more than two hundred years since Whytt first cared for children who were developing a progressive and invariably fatal disease of the nervous system that now can be successfully treated. Aside from his numerous contributions enhancing many fields of medicine and physiology, it is clear that his recognition of tuberculous meningitis in children was one of the important works that contributed to the development of pediatrics as a specialty distinct from other fields of medicine. Whytt's work on tuberculous meningitis thus also created an interest in one of the future areas of subspecialization, that is, the study of disorders of the nervous system in children.

Stephen Ashwal
LOMA LINDA, CALIFORNIA

REFERENCES

De Sauvages de la Croix, F. B. 1763. *Nosologia methodica sistens morborum classes, genera et species juxta Sydenham's mentem et botanicorum ordinem.* Amstelodami: Fratr. de Tournes.

French, R. W. 1969. *Robert Whytt, the Soul, and Medicine.* London: The Wellcome Institute of the History of Medicine.

Morgagni, G. B. 1761. *De sedibus et causis morborum per anatomen indagatis, libri quinque.* Venetiis: Remordiniana.

Ruhräh, J. 1925. Robert Whytt. In *Pediatrics of the Past*, 401–22. New York: Hoeber.

Still, G. F. 1931. Robert Whytt. In *The History of Paediatrics*, 443–49. London: Oxford University Press.

Whytt, R. 1751. *An Essay on the Vital and Other Involuntary Motions of Animals.* Edinburgh: Hamilton, Balfour and Neill.

______. 1752. *An Essay on the Virtues of Lime-Water in the Cure of the Stone.* Edinburgh: Hamilton, Balfour and Neill.

______. 1768. *Observations on the Dropsy in the Brain.* Edinburgh: Balfour, Auld and Smellie.

Willis, T. 1682. *Opera omnia.* Amstelodami: H. Wetstenium.

The Beginnings of Pediatrics and Neurology

THE EARLY NINETEENTH CENTURY

1800 – 1850

OVERVIEW

MEDICAL PROGRESS in the first half of the nineteenth century mirrored that in many other scientific fields. The invention of the stethoscope by René Laennec (1816), the ophthalmoscope by Hermann von Helmholtz (1851), and later the thermometer by Carl Wunderlich (1868), brought substance and accuracy to the bedside examination. Medicine was preoccupied with the identification and classification of diseases by symptoms, clinical signs, and pathology.

The correlation of clinical nosography with morbid anatomy and physiology was the great contribution of the Paris school of clinical pathologists during the first five decades of the nineteenth century — 1800 to 1850. Here there emerged from the confusion of the eighteenth century a relatively clear and critical picture of disease entities based upon the idea that there was a definite connection between the clinical findings at the bedside and the lesions observed in various organs at autopsy. In effect the work of the Paris school represented the fusion of two trends in medicine that hitherto had proceeded along more or less independent lines. (Rosen, 1944, 19)

The study of pathology was a great advance because it focused on specific changes in organs rather than humoral effects. Until the middle of the nineteenth century there was almost no understanding or use of statistics to correlate symptoms with specific diseases and the effects of specific treatments. Clinical laboratories for investigating disease first appeared. As a consequence of these advances, a completely new medicine was created. The continuous efforts of describing new diseases, of categorizing and determining the progression of symptoms, and of correlating clinical findings with pathology completely revolutionized clinical medicine. The significance of this change was that it ultimately provided the scientific basis for the development of specialization. The early nineteenth century still reflected physicians' ignorance of pharmacology. Treatment continued to be dependent upon bleeding, homeopathy, hydrotherapy, use of electricity, and plant remedies.

From a social perspective, the tremendous urban population shifts precipitated by the industrial revolution, created hazardous conditions of poverty, poor hygiene, and unsanitary living conditions. The mortality rate in children was exceptionally high. It was during this era that the broad movements of child care, and social, and educational reform were initiated with the development of almshouses, orphanages, asylums, and institutions. However, the care provided in such facilities was abysmal. Diets were inadequate and the spread of disease was always life threatening. At home, the industrial revolution changed the style of family living. Shifting from an economy where most people worked within the home to one in which parents and children labored in factories loosened the tight-knit structure of parental authority and exposed children to many different situations and life styles that gave them much more independence and autonomy.

PEDIATRICS

Pediatrics was influenced by changes occurring in medicine and obstetrics in France. The teachings of Marie Bichat, Jean Cruveilhier, René Laennec, Pierre Louis, and Auguste François Chomel emphasized the importance of pathology in understanding the disease progression and the use of numerical analysis to group and classify symptoms. The concept of clinical instruction by use of the case-history method and bedside teaching was implemented by Gabriel Andral and François Vallieux. Knowledge of pediatric diseases could now be disseminated in a more rigorous and thoughtful fashion. Finally, pediatric texts, such as that of Charles Michel Billard (1828), for the first time used this new approach to classify and describe children's diseases. In 1831, Adolphe Quetelet, a Belgian astronomer and statistician, began the first systematic anthropometric studies of the growth of children that are still used today. In 1838 the first chemical and physiological investigations comparing human and animal milk were begun by Johann Friedrich Simon. Additional original descriptions of pediatric diseases appeared, including hemophilia (1803), bronchitis (1808), tetany (1815), meningitis (1805), goiter (1840), pernicious anemia, and adrenal insufficiency (1849). Ludwig Meissner's Grundlage listed some 150 monographs on pediatrics published between 1800 and 1850.

Progress in lowering infant and childhood mortality rates was beginning to be made. Cholera and typhoid epidemics had resulted in such a devastating loss of life that sanitary reforms and other public health measures were introduced. The problems attendant with public education were also examined; for example, the effects of crowded classrooms, improper diet, insufficient sleep, poor hygiene, and the risk of infection, especially tuberculosis. This scrutiny was associated with the rapid growth of the first pediatric clinics and hospitals including, among many others, those at Petrograd (1834, now Leningrad), the Charité in Berlin (1834), Dresden (1834), Vienna (1837), Budapest (1839), Stockholm (1845), and Copenhagen (1846). The first periodical devoted exclusively to pediatrics, the Analekten über Kinderkrankheiten, was briefly published in Stuttgart, Germany, from 1837 to 1841. Aside from the treatise on pediatric diseases by Billard, several other notable books were published by Frederic Rilliet and Antoine Barthez (1838–43), Ernest Bouchet (1845), and Charles West (1848), covering such topics as pneumonia, intestinal hemorrhage, tuberculosis, infant nursing and nutrition, typhoid fever, paralysis, and pleurisy.

NEUROLOGY

Clinical neurology in the early nineteenth century was a very limited discipline. Practiced primarily by those in general medicine, it began to develop as a distinct entity as knowledge accumulated in the basic neurosciences. This clearly stimulated further study of nervous system diseases affecting man.

Neuroanatomy focused on elucidating the gross structure of the brain with the help of many important contributions, including those of Sir Charles Bell, who published *The Anatomy of the Brain* (1801); Johann Reil, who named the insula and characterized the lobes of the cerebellum (1807); and Luigi Rolando, who described the cerebral convolutions and sulci (1809). Franz Gall and Johann Spurzheim determined that the cerebral white matter consisted of nerve tracts and that the gray matter was the origin of mental activity (1810–19). Benedikt Stilling invented the microtome, essential for the preparation of brain tissue for examination (1824). Theodore Schwann described the myelin sheath of peripheral nerves (1838), Johannes Purkinje the cerebellar ganglion cells that bear his name (1838), and Jules Baillarger the cortical laminations (1840). Neuropathology atlases and monographs were published by John Abercrombie (1828), Robert Hooper (1828), Jean Cruveilhier (1835–42), and Richard Bright (1831).

Many advances occured in neurophysiology in the first half of the nineteenth century. Determination of the function of the anterior and posterior roots were respectively shown by Charles Bell (1811) and François Magendie (1822). Julien Legallois (1812) and Jean Pierre Flourens (1837) localized the respiratory center in the lower medullary centers of the brainstem. Flourens also showed that vision depended on an intact cortex and equilibrium on the function of the semicircular canals. The concept of the spinal cord reflex arc was further elaborated by Marshall Hall (1850). Hall also defined and conceived the term spinal shock. Charles Edouard Brown-Séquard's studies of the spinal cord demonstrated the decussation of the sensory fibers (1846). Johannes Müller developed the concept that individual sense organs gave rise to their own specific type of sensation (1826). The electrophysiological studies of Emil du Bois-Reymond provided the first clear description of the resting current present in muscles and nerves (1848). Phrenology, as proposed by Franz Gall and Johann Spurzheim, was popularized during this period, but its popularity faded as more rigorous scientific work convincingly disproved these theories. Although the studies of Alexander Monro (1783) and George Kellie (1824) had suggested that the brain's blood volume was constant, George Burrows disproved this doctrine. His studies represent the beginning of research in cerebrovascular physiology (1843–44). Frans Donner examined cerebral pial vessels under a sealed glass chamber and, with different experimental conditions such as asphyxia, observed vasodilation (1850). Forty years later, Charles Roy and Charles Sherrington proposed the idea of the metabolic and neural control of the cerebrovascular circulation (1890).

Clinical neurology also advanced. John Cooke published the first separate work on clinical neurology, *A Treatise on Nervous Disease* (1820–23). The beginning of the "modern" era of neurology is credited to Moritz Romberg's *Lehrbuch der Nervenkrankheiten des Menschen* (1840).

Cerebral apoplexy received considerable attention. Morgagni had shown intracerebral hemorrhage to be the cause of apoplexy and proposed a vascular etiology (1761). John Cheyne suggested that apoplexy could be due instead to cerebral anemia rather than congestion (1812). John Abercrombie classified apoplexy into three types and correlated the different cerebrovascular insults with clinical symptoms (1828).

The physiological concepts of epilepsy in this period were based on the prevailing misconception that irritability and sensibility were located in different areas of the nervous system. Irritability was a property of the spinal cord and brainstem, which were responsible for muscular contraction. The cerebral hemispheres were the centers of sensation and volition but not movement. Thus, Marshall Hall believed the medulla served as the origin of epilepsy (1851). It was during this period that Etienne Esquirol described *le petit mal* (1838), Louis Calmeil used the term *absence* (1824), Richard Bright described focal seizures (1836), and Robert Todd defined post-ictal paralysis (1855). Other neurological diseases were also described during this time. James Parkinson published his *Essay on the Shaking Palsy* (1817), and Jean Cruveilhier described disseminated sclerosis (1835). Moritz Romberg gave the classical description of tabes dorsalis (1846) and Amand Duchenne described progressive muscular atrophy (1849).

For the first time, extensive works solely devoted to infantile and childhood seizures appeared, written by physicians with varied medical and surgical backgrounds. Monographs by Jean Baptiste Timothée Baumes, Jean-Louis Brachet, John North, and John Clarke followed the traditional medical literary form then used, reporting series of detailed individual case histories with appended comments. Differences between seizures and convulsions were considered at great length, yet made little sense and were quite arbitrary. As seizures were the terminal event in many childhood diseases, their causes were frequently ascribed to a wide variety of conditions. On the other hand, convulsions, teething, and fever were also believed to be responsible for most ailments seen in children. This circular assignment of causation persisted for most of the nineteenth century. However, over the next hundred years, the general principles of observation, localization, and classification of diseases led to a reasonably broad understanding of the primary and secondary causes of epilepsy. The introductory section on the history of child neurology covers many of these landmark discoveries.

Hydrocephalus also consumed much of the interest of the early writers, as it was obviously a very dramatic and frightful condition that had been known since the time of classical medicine. From their work, one can appreciate that physicians such as John Cheyne, William Gerhard, Ludwig Mauthner, and Charles West had much clinical experience with this disease in young children. Their application of pathology to the clinical findings helped distinguish the acute from chronic forms as well as the inflammatory and infectious causes from those due to congenital malformations. Although their descriptions predate the modern microbial era, their writings indicate the presence of external inflammatory factors affecting the brain, aside from tuberculosis, which was already well recognized.

The great awakening of social reform that followed the French and American revolutions found in medicine many causes to champion. The mentally defective, insane, deaf-mutes, blind, and handicapped began to draw sympathy from the general public and later private and public institutions. Jean Itard is among many who brought attention to this problem, particularly in children. Although considered a founder of child psychiatry, he is included here because his experience with the Wild Boy of Aveyron is representative of the relation between neurological development and environmental experience. The works of Albert Deutsch (1946), Leo Kanner (1964), and Lloyd deMause (1974) provide several interesting historical analyses of this subject. (Please see the list at the end of the Introduction for references.)

JEAN BAPTISTE TIMOTHÉE BAUMES

JEAN BAPTISTE TIMOTHÉE Baumes (1756–1828) (figure 1) was born in Lunel, France. His father was a successful merchant. Young Baumes was educated at Sorèze, Nîmes, and, eventually, Montpellier. His early education was somewhat hampered by poor health, but he was a good student, learning several languages and becoming knowledgeable in the humanities. A biography describes him when in medical school: "Tormented by the desire to learn, his competitive spirit was so great that in a short time he could not be equaled by his rivals. His rapid rise to success astonished not only his colleagues but also his teachers" (Golfin, 1828). He received his medical degree on May 2, 1777. His drive to compete, and his apparently easy professional successes, were to become characteristic of his career.

Almost immediately after Baumes graduated from medical school his father's business in Lunel failed, and Baumes was forced to abandon plans to continue his studies in Montpellier. He moved to Saint-Gilles in July, 1777, and began the practice of medicine. Within a short time he established a reputation as a highly skilled clinician and began to publish his clinical observations in the *Journal de médecine de Paris*; the first of these papers appeared in 1780. This success prompted his family and friends to urge him to return to Lunel, and he soon left Saint-Gilles to con-

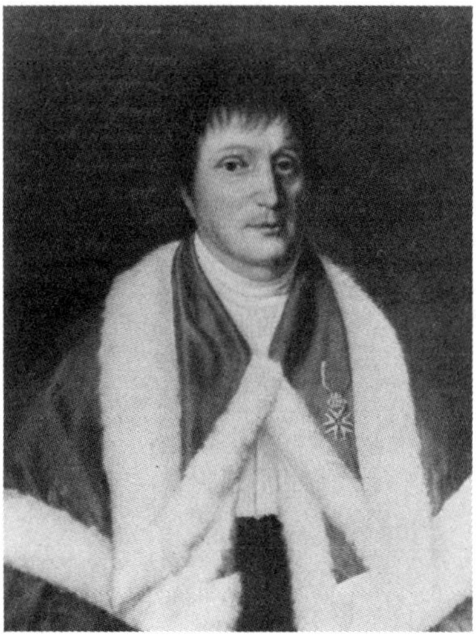

Figure 1. Portrait of Jean Baptiste Timothée Baumes (1756–1828).

tinue his practice in his hometown. His stay there was brief, for he was soon lured away to the city of Nîmes.

The people of Nîmes were eager to have him. His pride and ambition were enhanced by the insistent entreaties of the town notables, and Baumes decided to accede to their wishes. He quickly earned their approval, trust, respect, and admiration, but in this new theater, Baumes began to experience the drawbacks inseparable from success: the hate and harassment of jealous men. Nevertheless, he was sure of his genius and confident in his popularity; the attacks of his enemies served only to intensify his love of study, to increase his determination, and to encourage his research and writing (Golfin, 1828).

Between 1782 and 1790, Baumes wrote a number of articles and monographs that he entered in competition for prizes offered by the Royal Society of Medicine in Paris. He received awards for "Sur les accidens de la dentition" (1782), "Sur la phthisie pulmonaire" (1783), "Sur les maladies populaires" (1783), "Sur l'usage du quinquina, administré dans les fièvres rémittentes" (1785), "Sur les maladies épidémiques" (1786), "Sur les scrophules ou écrouelles" (1788), "Sur les émanations des eaux stagnantes et le desséchement des marais" (1789), "Sur les topographies médicales" (1790), and "Sur le rachitis" (1790). The Paris School of Medicine awarded him an honorable mention for "Sur les vers" (1780), and prizes for "Sur les convulsions" (1785), "Sur l'ictère des nouveau-nés" (1786), "Sur le carreau" (1787), and "Sur les maladies convulsives de l'Amérique" (1787). This succession of well-received papers prompted the Royal Society of Medicine to consider asking him to remove himself from competition. In 1791 he won another major competition and was named by Louis XVI to a faculty chair at the School of Medicine of Montpellier.

The teaching of medicine was initiated at Montpellier in the tenth century; it received its legal charter as a school of medicine in 1220. Nearly six centuries later, on August 12, 1792, the revolutionary government of the new republic revoked its charter, and for three years the school had no legal existence. The faculty, however, kept the school going, and it was during this period that, for the first time in France, true bedside teaching was initiated. In 1794 Baumes established the first medical clinic in France. As clinic head, his responsibilities were to observe and record the symptoms and signs of patients, to select those particularly suited for teaching purposes, to perform autopsies, to direct the laboratories and to aid other professors in their research, and to administer the general affairs of the clinic (Euzière, 1927). In 1805 Baumes helped form the Society of Practical Medicine.

Baumes was highly regarded as both a teacher and a clinician, and he attracted a large number of disciples and patients. He documented his observations of specific and various diseases in scientific publications, and toward the end of his life he devoted much of his time to writing a six-volume book, *Nosologie clinique, ou traité complet de médicine pratique interne et externe* (*Clinical Nosology, or Internal and External Practical Medicine*). Because of his deteriorating health and compulsion to revise the text to keep it up-to-date, this project was never completed. Unfortunately, the original draft of this major opus was lost and never published. Baumes suffered from a slow progressive disease of unknown nature, and died at the age of seventy-two on July 19, 1828.

Baumes's first work relevant to pediatric neurology, *Des convulsions dans l'enfance, de leurs causes et de leur traitement* (*On Convulsions in Infants, Their Causes and Their Treatment*), was published in Nîmes in 1789. The book was translated and published in German in 1791, and in Italian in 1797. A second edition was published in Paris in 1805. Baumes conceived his book as a compendium of all the various ideas that had been advanced concerning childhood convulsions; his objective was to identify all the different kinds of convulsions, their various causes, and their prevention and treatment. In the book he defines convulsions as involuntary contractions of muscle fibers and points out that these contractions may be either tonic or clonic in type. This broad definition results in the inclusion of nonepileptic behavior such as trismus, colic, hiccups, and even vomiting and strabismus. He was clearly aware of epileptic convulsions, but in the text it is difficult to determine when he is referring to phenomena he believed to be epileptic. This problem is evident in his discussion of foods as a cause or precipitant of convulsions. For instance, he discussed the fact that pieces of meat, chestnuts, or truffles, if fed to a child at the time the teeth first appear, will cause problems because the child cannot chew such food properly. Such food, he says, will therefore pass almost whole into the stomach and cause hiccups and vomiting. In the same context, he described a child with "epileptic" convulsions caused, he thought, by excesses of fruit and milk and cured by purging. A few paragraphs later he insisted that the treatment for epileptic convulsions should be quite different from that for other types of convulsive attacks. The latter should be treated with evacuants such as chicory syrup, peach flower syrup, apples, or rhubarb, whereas epileptic convulsions should be treated with an infusion of rhubarb and powdered tin salts or bismuth, or even an infusion of wild valerian.

Baumes believed that all convulsions reflected a hereditary tendency. This genetically determined diathesis rendered the child extremely sensitive to all sorts of provocations that could trigger a convulsion, for example, bad digestion, loud noise, and bright light. Children are particularly susceptible to convulsions, he thought, because of an inherent delicateness of their nervous and muscular systems and "softness" of their solid parts. He believed that the tendency to convulsions diminished as the solidity of the soft parts of the body increased. He maintained that convulsions were more prevalent in warm regions, such as America, where body fibers are more soft and limp! It is easy to understand, therefore, his beliefs that too soft a schooling disposed a child to convulsions, that the best treatments were cold baths for children and daily tepid baths for newborns, that exercise was important, and that newborns should move their legs and should not be swaddled. He felt that meat and other solid foods were important in the child's diet and that too liquid a diet led to weakness. Beef and chicken bouillon were all right in moderation, as was wine, if diluted with water and sugared. He believed that susceptibility to convulsions could be increased by excessive activity, especially around the time of the second dentition. Lack of exercise and other deficiencies during pregnancy and problems during the birth process were prone to cause a susceptibility to seizures, as were poor health habits.

Environmental factors he considered to be quite important; variations in barometric pressure and climate, particularly low pressure and hot summers, were thought to increase the incidence of seizures. Heat, Baumes said, stimulates the nerves, and high humidity, combined with heat, sends many "exhalations" into the air that may adversely affect the body. Thus, people who live in warm climates have a general disposition to convulsions, especially of the "stomach and intestines."

Clothing was also considered to be a factor. He felt that the swaddling of infants does not permit sufficient body movement, making the infant too hot, and inhibiting perspiration, all of which predispose the child to, or possibly cause, convulsions. The use of hoods for infants, particularly if the drawstring is tight, produces pressure on the brain and impedes circulation of the blood. Garments that cover the entire body should be avoided because "they will impede breathing."

Baumes also believed that convulsions could be caused by bad breast milk. Adverse factors in the milk, such as increased acidity, could result from fasting, hard work, or excessive passion. He considered sexual activity to be good, in moderation. He also believed that weaning too early (deprivation of milk) could cause epileptic seizures.

In a section on physical and mechanical irritants, he pointed out that various poisons such as arsenic and lead may cause convulsions and recommended that purgatives, emetics, narcotics, and mercury be avoided. He recognized that fever could cause or precipitate convulsions and that the attacks may occur only when a child is febrile. He recommended that evacuants and quinine rubdowns and arsenic acid dissolved in distilled water be used for treatment.

Perhaps one of the most interesting discussions in Baumes's book concerned strabismus, which he apparently classified as a tonic convulsion. He recommended that one eye of the infant be covered "to force the weak one to work." His discussion of epilepsy comes near the end of his book. He wrote that the convulsions may be either partial or generalized, either tonic or clonic, and that there is usually a loss of consciousness. He stated, however, that epilepsy is of infinite variety and nuance, and that internal organs may be involved by producing involuntary urination or defecation and contraction of the diaphragm. Baumes knew that encephalitis and hydrocephalus may be associated with epileptic convulsions. He also noted that epilepsy often had its onset near the time of puberty and that such seizures may cease spontaneously within a short time.

Eighteenth-century medicine in France was not distinguished by great physicians and scientists. It was, however, a period of gradual emancipation from theological dogma and metaphysical theories. It was not until the nineteenth century, the age of Marie François-Xavier Bichat, René Laennec, Claude Bernard, and Louis Pasteur, that, for the first time, careful observation and the establishment of facts took precedence over theory and metaphysical conjecture. It is within this frame of reference that Baumes's book on childhood convulsions should be viewed. It was the first book to be devoted entirely to childhood convulsions, and it appeared more than thirty years before the first publication of such a book in English, that of John North in 1826.

Peter Kellaway

Eli M. Mizrahi
HOUSTON, TEXAS

REFERENCES

Baumes, J. B. T. 1789. *Des convulsions dans l'enfance, de leurs causes et de leur traitement.* 1st ed. Nîmes.

______. 1805. *Traité des convulsions dans l'enfance, de leurs causes et de leur traitement.* 2d ed. Paris: Méguignon l'aîné.

Euzière, J. 1927. Le centenaire de la création des chefs de clinique. *Aesculape* 17:110–12.

Golfin, P. H. 1828. *Notice biographique sur M. Baumes, professeur à la Faculté de Médecine de Montpellier.* Montpellier: V. Picot.

JEAN-LOUIS BRACHET

JEAN-LOUIS BRACHET (1789–1858) was born in Gavos in the Rhone valley near a village that bears his family name. The Brachets were an old and respected family in this region and could afford to provide Jean-Louis with a good education. Choosing medicine for a career, he enrolled at the age of seventeen in the Hôtel Dieu at Lyon. Seven years later, in competition with his peers, he won the appointment of surgeon intern. While at Lyon, Brachet was an aide and disciple of several of the distinguished physicians of the day, including Guillaime Dupuytren and Jean-Nicolas Corvisart. Both were true clinicians and keen observers who bothered little with theory. Corvisart is regarded as the first to initiate the teaching of semiology. Brachet completed his internship in five years and almost immediately was named adjunct surgeon at the Hôtel Dieu. At that time, France was defending itself against the invading armies of Russia and Austria. Soon after Paris surrendered to the Russians, Lyon was taken by the Austrian army (April 11, 1814). Napoleon abdicated and was banished to the isle of Elba. At the age of twenty-five, Brachet was appointed surgeon to Napoleon in exile.

During the previous year, Brachet devoted himself to the study of epidemic diseases, particularly typhus, which was raging in France as a consequence of the war. He himself was stricken by typhus in 1814 and was unable to continue in his duties to the exiled emperor. After what appears to have been a stormy course, he survived and returned to live with his family while he recuperated. Brachet lived for another forty-four years, devoting himself to medical practice in the hospitals of Lyon and to his favorite activity, the study of experimental physiology and pathology. His interests were a product of the remarkable age in which he lived. It was a time in France when Marie François-Xavier Bichat was developing biology into a true science based on the conjoint study of morphology and physiology, and the science of experimental medicine was in the process of development by the great innovators, François Magendie and Claude Bernard. At the same time, Corvisart and, most importantly, René Laennec were laying the foundations of modern clinical medicine. The modern concept in medicine that only facts confirmed by experimentation should be believed as true was first enunciated, when Brachet was fifty-three, by Magendie in his *Phénomènes physiques de la vie (Phenomena Particular to Living Bodies)* (1842).

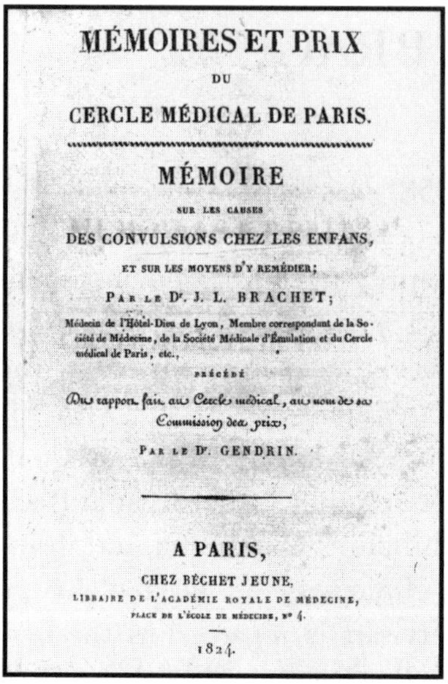
MÉMOIRES ET PRIX
DU
CERCLE MÉDICAL DE PARIS.

MÉMOIRE
SUR LES CAUSES
DES CONVULSIONS CHEZ LES ENFANS,
ET SUR LES MOYENS D'Y REMÉDIER;
PAR LE Dr. J. L. BRACHET;
Médecin de l'Hôtel-Dieu de Lyon, Membre correspondant de la Société de Médecine, de la Société Médicale d'Émulation et du Cercle médical de Paris, etc.,
PRÉCÉDÉ
Du rapport fait au Cercle médical, au nom de sa Commission des prix,
PAR LE Dr. GENDRIN.

A PARIS,
CHEZ BÉCHET JEUNE,
LIBRAIRE DE L'ACADÉMIE ROYALE DE MÉDECINE,
PLACE DE L'ÉCOLE DE MÉDECINE, No 4.
1824.

Figure 1. Title page of Brachet's prize-winning book, one of the first on convulsive disorders in children.

Brachet wrote on many subjects, ranging from his first paper in 1813 on the movement and dilation of the heart to hepatic glycogenesis. He wrote a book on hydrocephalus (1818) and a treatise on the physiology of the ganglionic nervous system (1830). His major contribution to child neurology was one of the first books to be published on convulsive disorders of children. For this book, *Mémoire sur les causes des convulsions chez les enfans, et sur les moyens d'y remédier* (Brachet, 1824) (figure 1), he was awarded the annual prize of the Cercle Médical of Paris. A revised and enlarged edition was published in 1837 in Paris, Lyon, and Montpellier. In 1840 he was named a Chevalier of the Légion d'Honneur by Louis-Philippe. He died in Lyon on April 10, 1858.

Brachet's book on childhood convulsions was at the time considered a benchmark work and "a light which served to illuminate several obscure and unknown aspects of the psychology of the nervous system" (Potton, 1859). For the first time, convulsions were considered to be phenomena resulting from an irritation or modification of the central nervous system. Brachet defined convulsions as all violent movement that is involuntary and transient, involving a more or less large number of the voluntary muscles and occurring with or without loss of consciousness. He distinguished, as did Baumes before him, between idiopathic and symptomatic convulsions. Unlike his predecessor, however, he was more restrictive in what he considered to be convulsions. Baumes, he wrote ". . . will never convince me that colic, strabismus, icterus, etc., are convulsions" (1824).

Brachet noted that a convulsive movement could affect only one part of the body and that there might be a progressive spread to other parts of the body "one after another." However, he distinguished what he called epilepsy from convulsions: epilepsy had its origin in the brain and its membranes, whereas convulsions originated in the spinal cord and its membranes. Loss of consciousness always occurred in epileptic seizures and lasted throughout the attack but occurred in convulsions only during the most violent period of the paroxysms and ended before the convulsion was over. He believed epilepsy to be almost invariably incurable, that it had no known cause, and that attacks increased in number and severity with age. Convulsions, on the other hand, he believed were curable and indeed disappeared after a certain age; they had a physical, physiological, or psychological cause that could be determined. Chorea (St. Vitus' dance), for instance, he classified as a convulsive disorder.

Brachet closed his manuscript with a review and critique of various treatments. Among his more useful recommendations was that narcotics such as henbane and hemlock should be considered as not only uncertain in their effects but dangerous! He regarded human cranium, chalk, crayfish eyes, hippopotamus teeth, ivory, and precious stones as inert substances with negative if any action. It is not surprising that Brachet considered epilepsy to be incurable, because his treatments must have been totally ineffective. Zinc oxide, he thought, was good for momentary relief but not effective if the symptoms persisted. Opium and morphine were good "in certain situations." Camphor, musk, amber, and castoreum were useful for their calming effects, as was a solution of ammonia. Purgatives such as Corinthian grapes, chicory syrup, and almond oil were useful in certain cases but were "not for general use." Ethers and anodynes administered in a sugar cube were good for stopping spasms and convulsions. As William Lennox commented in his monograph on epilepsy, "Disheartening is the thought (as one thinks of patients with seizures throughout the ages) that for more than two millennia the medicines and the treatments prescribed by outstanding physicians were without value" (Lennox and Lennox, 1960). Brachet had been dead for more than fifty years before the first truly effective anticonvulsant drug, phenobarbital, was introduced by Alfred Hauptmann in 1912 (Hauptmann, 1912). Bromide, which was the first agent to have a verified antiepileptic action, was introduced by Sir Charles Locock the year before Brachet's death, but because of its limited antiepileptic properties and its devastating effect upon mental function and the skin, bromides were little used after the introduction of phenobarbital.

Peter Kellaway

Eli M. Mizrahi
HOUSTON, TEXAS

REFERENCES

Brachet, J. L. 1818. *Essai sur l'hydrocéphalite ou hydropisie aiguë des ventricules du cerveau*. Paris: Gabon.

______. 1824. *Mémoire sur les causes des convulsions chez les enfans, et sur les moyens d'y remédier*. Paris: Bechet jeune.

______. 1830. *Recherches expérimentales sur les fonctions du système nerveux ganglionnaire, et sur leur application à la pathologie*. Paris: Gabon.

______. 1837. *Traité pratique des convulsions dans l'enfance*. 2d ed. Paris: Germer-Baillière.

Hauptmann, A. 1912. Luminal bei epilepsie. *Münch med Wschr* 59:1907–9.

Lennox, W. G., and M. A. Lennox. 1960. *Epilepsy and Related Disorders*. Vol. 1. Boston: Little, Brown, and Co.

Potton, F. F. A. 1859. Notice historique sur la vie et les travaux de Jean-Louis Brachet. *Ann soc méd Lyon* 2:5–56.

JOHN CHEYNE

A SCION OF distinguished physicians dating back to the 1500s on both sides of his family, John Cheyne (1777–1836) (figure 1) belonged to that influential group of nineteenth-century physicians who were known as the "Irish School." It included Robert Adams, Abraham Colles, Dominic Corrigan, Robert Graves and William Stokes (O'Brien, Crookshank, and Wolstenholme, 1984). Cheyne is best remembered today for that sinister cyclic breathing pattern that he described (Cheyne, 1818) and to which attention was recalled a generation later by William Stokes (Stokes, 1846). An interest in children's diseases, along with compiling case records with post-mortem studies of acute encephalopathies and hydrocephalus, led to his publication of *An Essay on Hydrocephalus Acutus, or Dropsy in the Brain*. This work establishes his place in the history of child neurology (Cheyne, 1808).

Cheyne's autobiography appeared in his *Essays on Partial Derangement of the Mind in Supposed Connexion with Religion*, which was published posthumously by his son (Cheyne, 1843). In this work, Cheyne detailed that he was born in Leith, a seaport suburb of Edinburgh on the 3rd of February, 1777. He attempted to gain a classical education but, because his teaching was at the hands of failed tutors, these attempts were abortive. At the age of thirteen, he was assigned medical tasks by his physician father that consisted of caring for his more destitute patients. Apparently thriving in these responsibilities, the youth supplied them with medicines, bled them and dressed wounds, and reported to his father on their conditions. At fifteen he unofficially attended medical lectures at the University of Edinburgh. He dined and clubbed with the medical students and quickly discovered that his prior amateurish medical observations and training by his father caused him to be equally as well acquainted with medical subjects. He presented himself to the professors for examination, passed easily, and obtained his medical degree in June 1795. Cheyne then joined the Royal Regiment of Artillery as assistant-surgeon. He was present when the Irish rebelled against British rule at the

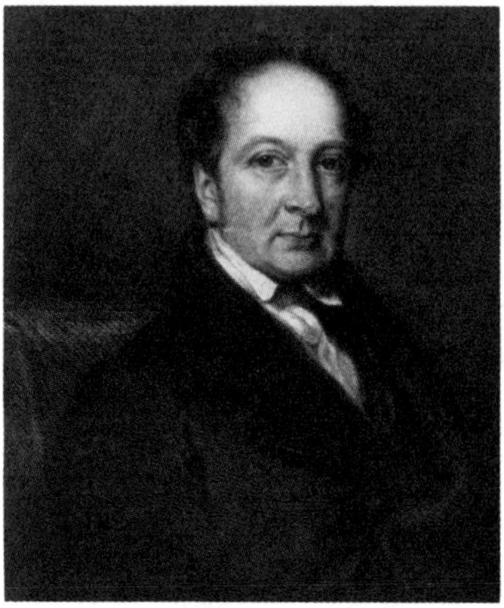

Figure 1. Dr. John Cheyne (1777–1836) painted by Rev. William Deane. A copy of this painting hangs in the Royal College of Physicians of Ireland, 6 Kildare Street, Dublin 2, Ireland.

Battle of Vinegar Hill in 1798; this experience lent him some later expertise in military medicine.

In 1799 he returned to Leith to take charge of the Ordinance Hospital and also assisted in his father's practice. He developed a note-keeping system and recorded cases that were of greatest clinical interest. When he "foresaw that a disease would end unfavorably," he took measures to ensure the family's permission to open the body. At this period he befriended Charles Bell, who was beginning his own pathological studies, which would lead to Bell's future eminence. After Cheyne obtained autopsy permission, he observed Bell's dissection, learning much from him and became convinced that Bell was "a man of genius."

Cheyne directed his attention principally to children's diseases. When epidemics arose, he studied the best monograph he could find on the subject. He consulted with his most experienced medical colleagues and compiled case books with extensive notes. His appreciation of pathology distinguished his literary labors. He published on children's diseases, such as croup (Cheyne, 1801), bowel complaints, jaundice in newborns, and weaning (Cheyne, 1802).

In the preface of his important treatise on acute hydrocephalus, Cheyne admitted that the physician's duty was to be cautious in making hypotheses because knowledge of disease is very imperfect. And, appropriately, reviewing this work leads the modern reader to conclude that many of the patients who survived, which Cheyne diagnosed as hydrocephalus acutus, probably had acute encephalitis and/or cerebral edema. The children did not have enlarged heads. Those symptoms that suggested hydrocephalus acutus to Cheyne included gradually worsening headache with emesis, abdominal pains and characteristic stools, ". . . . at first clayey; as the disease advances they become of a gelatinous consistence, dark green, of a sickly smell, sometimes as dark as tar" (Cheyne, 1808). Cheyne recognized that Robert Whytt diagnosed hydrocephalus earlier (Whytt, 1768); mistakenly Cheyne stated that "hydrocephalus was not known as a distinct disease before 1768" (Cheyne, 1808). Vesalius was one among other early investigators who described hydrocephalus. In the second edition of his momentous *De humani corporis fabrica*, published in 1555, Vesalius noted a young girl to have a head larger than any man's. The fluid was described as not being collected between the skull and the exterior membrane, but within the cavity of the brain itself. Nine pounds of water was removed from the ventricles at autopsy (Vesalius, 1555).

Many of Cheyne's autopsy cases of hydrocephalus seemed to be tuberculous, because they had mustard-seed-sized tubercles, caseous depositions in the viscera, and the ventricles contained excess fluid — "from two to six ounces of lipid serum" (Cheyne, 1808). Modern studies reveal that the average volume of each lateral ventricle varies between two to thirty-nine cubic centimeters, or one ounce or less (Newton and Potts, 1978). Cheyne observed that, although it would seem that tapping enlarged cerebral ventricles to reduce the fluid pressure would seem appropriate, "this operation, which has often been performed by ignorant men, is generally almost immediately productive of fatal consequences." Blood letting seemed to work best for Cheyne.

Cases of Apoplexy and Lethargy with Observations upon the Comatose Diseases was published in 1812. In this work, he made observations on stroke patients. He noted that elderly people's internal carotid arteries lose their contractile and distensile power owing to a boney or earthy matter depositing within their coats. He believed that apoplexy resulted from stress, alcohol, and tobacco, usually in people aged forty to sixty years. He knew that children were much more likely than adults to survive hypoxia without paralysis.

Following nine years of practicing medicine, studying pathology, and collecting cases for his above publications, Cheyne decided to leave Scotland and search for a position elsewhere in Great Britain. This move was apparently due to an excess of political disputes within Edinburgh's medical community at that time and he was "anxious for an opportunity of distinguishing myself more than of securing a large income" (Cheyne, 1843). While his wife Sarah, whom he married in 1804, and with whom he fathered sixteen children, temporarily moved in with her mother and physician father until he found a position, Cheyne visited Dublin (Cheyne, 1931). There he found the "profession respected. . . and the labourers liberally rewarded," and he set up practice in March 1809. In 1811 he was appointed as physician to the Meath Hospital. This led to a professorship of the practice of physic at the College of Surgeons in Dublin. This school supplied medical officers to the army and navy during the long Napoleonic Wars. His military medical experience apparently so enriched his lectures that great crowds of surgeons and assistant-surgeons of the local garrison attended. These courses and his daily attendance at the Meath Hospital, along with his private practice, filled his days.

Personally, Cheyne was ambitious and astute in acquiring popularity, public favor, and the respect of his colleagues. He said in his autobiography that he studied the characters and the ethics of those most prominent in his profession. He prided himself on the fact that he was able to forbear professional disputes and criticisms directed at himself, thus living "to see my opponents becoming steady and useful friends." His professional political savvy surfaced because, after he had located in Dublin, he was the first physician to meet regularly with apothecaries in medical consultation (Ormsby, 1888). He was extremely attentive to his relationships with his peers and his patients and their families. He emphasized that he never was critical of other attending physicians, no matter how deserving of criticism. When requested by a patient to recommend a surgeon, physician, or apothecary, he was always careful to provide names of three or four men of established character. He made it a rule never to acquaint anyone, not even members of his own family, with the names of his patients and he was cognizant not to inflame the ill will of patients by paying unnecessary visits.

In October 1815 Cheyne was appointed one of the physicians to the House of Industry, a hospital two miles from his home. Here he visited upwards of seventy patients daily, most laboring under fever, of whom eight or ten demanded careful physical examination. Competent nurses accompanied these rounds and advised him as to which patients did or did not require more than a glance. He was thus able to complete rounds in an hour. Cheyne recorded that these rounds, in addition to the one hour walk each way to and from his home in Merrion Square, physically exhausted him. Because he felt that these other duties infringed on his own private practice ("In 1812 my fees amounted to 472 pounds . . . in 1816 [fees] yielded me 1,710 pounds."), he resigned both his professorship at the College of Surgeons and his charge at the Meath Hospital.

In 1817 Cheyne and Edward Percival formed the Clinical School and the Museum of Morbid Anatomy at the House of Industry Hospital, but by 1820 Cheyne resigned from the House of Industry and was appointed Physician-General at the General Military Hospital, "the highest medical rank in Ireland. . . . I felt that I had fully attained the object of my ambition." Obviously proud of his economic growth and success, Cheyne continually updated the readers of his autobiography on the expansion of his private practice; he remarked that the average annual yield from his practice over the next ten years was five thousand pounds. Cheyne alludes to an underlying chronic illness of an unspecified type when he stated in his autobiography that if it weren't for his naturally weak constitution, "always injured by fatigue of body or anxiety of mind," he could have added fifteen hundred pounds more to each year's income (Cheyne, 1843).

By age forty-eight, Cheyne's prosperous practice was finally stultified by failing health, a "nervous fever." Following a long and arduous day of patient visits, he would have to rest at night before taking supper. Observing so much sickness around him, he began to comprehend the nature of his own illness, and described it as "a climacteric disease . . . slowly executing its appointed mission" (Cheyne, 1843). Resting as much as possible by leaving town frequently, and by getting friends to share his practice, the progress of his disease was retarded, which allowed him to continue some medical work in Dublin until 1831 when the practice "became an intolerable burden; my sleep was broken and unrefreshing; in the morning I was languid and dispirited, and in the evening I had a high degree of nervous fever."

Upon Cheyne's retirement to England, forty-five of the most

eminent physicians then practicing in Dublin jointly signed a letter expressing their deepest felt sentiments of esteem for his virtues, exemplary professional character, extensive knowledge, and sound practical judgement. A letter of similar vein was sent to him on April 9, 1831, signed by "The Apothecaries of Dublin."

His retreat was an estate named Sherington Manor, in Newport Pagnell, fifty miles north of London on today's M1 motorway in Buckinghamshire. There he consulted the sick local villagers, and undertook to write some articles on croup, epilepsy, epidemic gastric fever, and laryngitis (Forbes, Tweedie, and Connolly, 1832); he also included an article on wakefulness, a subject of which he felt highly qualified, since he was unable to obtain restful sleep (Forbes, Tweedie, and Connolly, 1832).

Because he lost vision in his right eye due to cataract formation and his chronic illness, Cheyne gave up the practice of medicine in 1833. A very intimate friend and colleague, Dr. Adair Crawford, visiting Cheyne in 1833, described Cheyne's pulse as habitually over one hundred, that he suffered much from thirst, and at night from wakefulness (*Med Times Gaz*, 1857). The progress of the disease continued uninterrupted. Mrs. Cheyne noted, "I could hardly conceive life to remain under such emaciation . . . but he was sustained as he could take nourishment. His mind loses its power of continued thought, from weakness and drowsiness, but it is unimpaired, and as firm on the matter of religion as when in full vigor" (*Med Times Gaz*, 1857). Following bed confinement for six weeks because of "mortification of the lower extremities," Cheyne died on January 31, 1836 (Cheyne, 1843).

Biographical and obituary notices highlight Cheyne's very deep religious feelings toward which his weakened energies were directed in his last years. His *Essays on Partial Derangement of the Mind in Supposed Connexion with Religion* discussed what we now conceptualize as psychosomatic phenomena. Cheyne argued the necessity of relieving mental illness before physical symptoms could be cured (Cheyne, 1843). He directed this work to clergymen in order to help them understand how to best place divine truth before their flock and have their congregation accept it: "A melancholic or hypochondriacal patient (has little hope of accepting divine truth) until the bodily disease, with which the mental delusion is connected, is cured or relieved." In this fascinating work, Cheyne discussed psychological mechanisms; parietal lobe dysfunction, such as anosognosias he observed in stroke patients; receptive aphasias with retained reading abilities; Dr. John Hunter's half-hour experience in 1789 of symptoms that were highly suggestive of transient global amnesia; and many other accurate clinical insights.

The eight-to-eleven-year history of progressing fatigue and exhaustion, thirst, cataracts, weight loss, and terminal "mortification of the lower limbs" suggests the adult onset type of diabetes mellitus and its attendant complications as the cause of Dr. John Cheyne's slow demise.

Lance Fogan
PANORAMA CITY, CALIFORNIA

REFERENCES

Cheyne, A. Y. 1931. *The Cheyne Family in Scotland.* Eastbourne: V. V. Sumfield.

Cheyne, J. 1801. *Essays on the Diseases of Children with Cases and Dissections. Essay I, of Cyanche trachealis, or Croup.* Edinburgh: Mundell, Doig and Stevenson.

______. 1802. *Essays on the Diseases of Children with Cases and Dissections. Essay II. On the Bowel Complaints, More Immediately Connected with the Biliary Secretion, and Particularly of Atrophia ablactatorum, or Weaning Brash.* Edinburgh: Mundell and Son.

______. 1808. *An Essay on Hydrocephalus acutus, or Dropsy in the Brain.* Edinburgh: Mundell, Doig and Stevenson.

______. 1812. *Cases of Apoplexy and Lethargy with Observations upon the Comatose Diseases.* London: Underwood.

______. 1818. A Case of Apoplexy in Which the Fleshy Part of the Heart was Converted into Fat. *Dublin Hos Rep* 2:216.

______. 1843. *Essays on Partial Derangement of the Mind in Supposed Connexion with Religion.* Dublin: Wm. Curry, Jun. and Co.

Forbes, Tweedie, and Connolly. 1832. *The Cyclopedia of Practical Medicine.* Vol. 1, 5. London: Sherwood, Gilbert, and Piper, and Baldwin and Cradock.

______. 1857. Men of the British School — No. 4 — John Cheyne. *Med Times Gaz*: 17–20, 41–43, 69–79.

Newton, T. H., and D. G. Potts. 1978. *Radiology of the Skull and Brain.* Vol. 4: *Ventricles and Cisterns.* St. Louis: Mosby Co.

O'Brien, E., A. Crookshank, and G. Wolstenholme. 1984. *A Portrait of Irish Medicine.* Dublin: Ward River Press Ltd.

Ormsby, L. H. 1888. *Medical History of the Heath Hospital and County Dublin Infirmary*. Dublin: Fannin and Co.

Stokes, W. 1846. Symptoms Referable to the Respiratory Function. *Dublin Quart Jour Med Sci* 2:73–85.

Vesalius, A. 1555. *De humani corporis fabrica*. Libri septum. Basel: Joannis Oporini.

Whytt, R. 1768. *Observations on the Dropsy in the Brain*. Edinburgh: Balfour, Auld and Smellie.

JOHN CLARKE

JOHN CLARKE (1761–1815) (figure 1), son of a surgeon of the same name, became an exceptional lecturer in midwifery, whose fame as a "medical discoverer" rests on his contributions to the care of children (Stephen and Lee, 1908, 434) and his original description of laryngismus stridulus and its association with tetany. Born in the latter part of the eighteenth century, he was ushered into an "age of theorists and systematists" where new medical disciplines were begat by great innovative minds, including pathological surgery by John Hunter, preventive inoculation by Edward Jenner, public hygiene by Leslie Carl Frank, embryology by Etienne Wolff and medical bibliography by Albrecht von Haller (Garrison, 1923, 75). During Clarke's brief fifty-four years, a marked change occurred in the health and well-being of children as "the interest in infantile mortality as a phase of national depopulation was the starting point of the new social science of infant welfare" (Garrison, 1923, 84). Clarke and his contemporaries saw the dreadful death rate for children under five in London decrease by half, from 63 deaths per 100 children to 31.8 per 100, largely due to changing attitudes on hygiene and nutrition during infancy, as well as the emergence of a science of child care in the nineteenth century, which evolved to include care for the newly born, the prematurely born, and even the unborn, in the latter twentieth century.

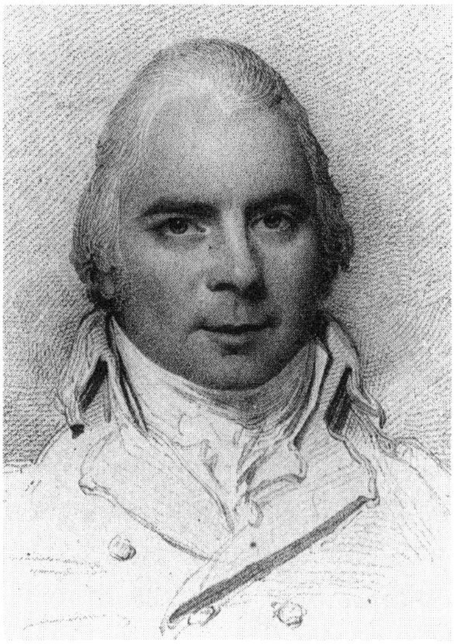

Figure 1. John Clarke (1761-1815).

Clarke was born in Wellingborough, Northamptonshire in 1761. He was initially educated at St. Paul's School, followed by his formal medical education at St. George's Hospital. After becoming a member of the Corporation of Surgeons, he began practice in Chancery-Lane, and also lectured on midwifery at the private medical school founded by William Hunter. Clarke quickly enjoyed the reputation of an extraordinary teacher and practitioner, described as "a good classical scholar, a man of indomitable industry and perseverance" with "a promptitude in action and a fertility of resources which obtained for him the confidence of patients and the admiration of the profession" (Munk, 1878). He received a license in midwifery from the College of Physicians in 1787 and four years later obtained the degree of Doctor of Medicine. After being chief midwifery practitioner of London for several years, Clarke moved to the west end to consult on the diseases of women and children, after giving his practice to his brother, Sir Charles Mansfield Clarke. He spent several more years as physician to the lying-in hospital on Store Street and the Asylum for Female Orphans and as lecturer on midwifery at St. Bartholomew's Hospital, before semi-retiring from practice due to organic disease of the stomach and ascites, from which he died in August, 1815.

Clarke's contributions to the literature of child neurology include two papers read before the Royal Society and three books. The earlier works deal with Clarke's developing interest in obstetrics based on his extensive clinical experience (Clarke, 1788; Clarke, 1793).

John Clarke's 198-page tome, *Commentaries on Some of the Most Important Diseases of Children*, was never completed because of his death in 1815. The pages that exist, however, deal mostly with neurological problems, including convulsions, phrenitis, idiocy, paralysis, and epilepsy. One-third of Clarke's unfinished opus was related to convulsions and their management. Clarke differed from other writers of the day, such as Michael Underwood, insisting that convulsions "are never an idiopathic disease, but may generally be traced to some pre-existing cause" (Clarke, 1815, 84). Naive to electrical and neurochemical aspects of brain function, Clarke was convinced that "in every case of convulsion (be the remote cause whatsoever it may) the brain is at the time organically affected, either directly or indirectly" (Clarke, 1815, 90). Clarke believed the classical theories of convulsion arising from the ventricles, and explained the association between convulsions and non-neurologic entities, such as teething, by their effects on the brain due to changes in pressure caused by alterations of blood flow to the vessels of the head.

Clarke's therapeutic measures for convulsions were in keeping with his theories that convulsions were related to an organic brain process often due to pressure from alterations of blood flow. He agreed with classical authors that convulsions with teething should be treated by scarifying the gums, but decried the use of "popular and empirical nostrums, under the specious names of Fit Drops, and C" and questioned the use of antispasmodic medicines, stating "it may be well worth enquiry to ascertain whether the merits of the antispasmodic class of medicines have not been overrated, and whether they have not continued to be employed rather through a deference to authority rather than from any decisive proof of their efficacy" (Clarke, 1815, 111). Clarke was a strong advocate of purgatives, however, recommending evacuations using glyster, calomel, senna with manna, and tincture of jalap. He also believed that "in the greater number of cases, where convulsions occur, the head is overloaded with blood, it will be right to take away blood by leeches, by cupping, or by opening the external jugular vein" (Clarke, 1815, 106). This practice was later challenged by John North and others and gradually lost favor. Other measures of the day included the use of inhaled alkali, such as ammonia, and the application of cold water to the face and head.

Of particular note in Clarke's *Commentaries* is the description of "a peculiar species of convulsions in infant children," similar to descriptions of tetanus in infancy, reintroduced by Joseph Clarke (no relation) twenty-six years earlier (Still, 1931, 490), but different enough to realize an entirely new syndrome, which was to be embellished with the name "tetany" by Lucien Corvisart (Singer and Underwood, 1962, 535) thirty-seven years after Clarke's death.

There is one case of convulsive affection, which is more apt to be overlooked than any other, because the symptoms are not at first very violent, so as to attract the attention of parents or nurses. It is often mistaken and treated as some other disease, even by medical men; and the true character of it has been little known, even to practitioners generally conversant with infantile disorders; it is therefore less likely to be detected by those who have bestowed little or no attention upon them.

This convulsive affliction occurs by paroxysms, with longer or shorter intervals between them, and of longer or shorter duration in different cases, and in the same case at different times.

It consists in a peculiar mode of inspiration, which it is difficult accurately to describe.

The child having had no apparent warning, is suddenly seized with a spasmodic inspiration, consisting of distinct attempts to fill the chest, between each of which a squeaking noise is often made; the eyes stare, and the child is evidently in great distress; the face and the extremities, if the paroxysm continues long, becomes purple, the head is thrown backward, and the spine is often bent, as in opisthotonus; at length a strong expiration takes place, a fit of crying generally succeeds, and the child, evidently much exhausted, often falls asleep.

In one of these attacks a child sometimes, but not frequently, dies. . . .

. . . As the breathing is affected by these paroxysms, the complaint is generally referred to the organs of respiration, and it has been sometimes called chronic croup; but it is very different from croup, and is altogether of a convulsive character. . . .

. . . Accompanying these symptoms, a bending of the toes downwards, clenching of the fists, and the insertion of the thumbs into the palm of the hands, and bending the fingers upon them, is sometimes found, not only during the paroxysm, but at other times.

Clenching the fist with the thumb inserted into the palm of the hand, often exists for a long time in children, without being much observed, yet it is always to be considered as an unfavorable symptom, and frequently is a forerunner of convulsive disorders, being itself a spasmodic affection. . . .

. . . Convulsions of this description seldom, if ever, occur after the expiration of the third year of the child's life, and not often in children which have lived by sucking. . . . (Clarke, 1815, 86–89)

Although Clarke's explanations for convulsions are burdened with the misconceptions of the eighteenth century, his description of tetany is indeed apart from other convulsions, croup and "nine-day fits" and describes in particular detail the laryngospasm accompanying tetany, its prevalence in artificially fed infants, and its paradoxically low mortality. Other physicians added observations and introduced methods for detecting minor degrees of affliction. These physicians included John North (1826), who observed the association between the peculiar convulsions of tetany and the presence of rickets; Armand Trousseau (1868), who produced carpopedal spasm by compressing the brachial artery; and Frantisek Chvostek (1876), who described the characteristic grimace by tapping the facial nerve. In time, laboratory investigations of parathyroid disease in animals and the effects of calcium metabolism merged with clinical observations of tetany. Nevertheless, it was a full century after Clarke's enlightening description that work by Ferdinand Kehrer identified tetany in the newborn period to be responsive to calcium (1913) and investigations by John Howland and William McKim Marriott (1917) elucidated the role of hypocalcemia in this condition.

John Clarke's volume, although unfinished, served as a useful text of the day, a dramatic expression of the importance of neurologic disorders in childhood disease, a treatise on maladies of the brain that invited comment, both favorable and unfavorable, from contemporaries and their students, and an initial clinical description of an important clinical entity with multisystem implications. His abbreviated career reflected a burgeoning growth in the influence of the science of infant welfare, to which today's practitioners owe a great admiration.

Larry E. White
NORFOLK, VIRGINIA

REFERENCES

Chovstek, F. 1876. Beiträge zur Tetanie. *Wien med Presse* 17:1201–3, 1225–27, 1253–58, 1314–16.

Clarke, J. 1788. *An Essay on the Epidemic Disease of Lying-In Women in 1787–88.* 4 vols. London: J. Johnson.

______. 1793. *Practical Essays on Pregnancy and Labour and the Diseases of Lying-In Women.* 8 vols. London: J. Johnson.

______. 1815. *Commentaries on Some of the Most Important Diseases of Children.* London: Longman, Hurst, Rees, Orme & Brown.

Garrison, F. 1923. A System of Pediatrics. In *History of Pediatrics.* Philadelphia: W. B. Saunders Co.

Howland, J., and W. Marriott. 1917. Observations upon the Calcium Content of the Blood in Infantile Tetany and upon the Effect of Treatment by Calcium. *Quart J Med* 11:287.

Kehrer, F. 1913. Die geburtshilflichgynakologische Bedentung der Tetanie. *Arch Gynaek* 99:372.

Munk, W. 1878. *The Roll of the Royal College of Physicians of London*, Volume 2. London: The Royal College of Physicians of London.

North, J. 1826. *Practical Observations on the Convulsions of Infants.* London: Burgess and Hill.

Singer, C., and E. Underwood. 1962. *A Short History of Medicine.* New York: Oxford University Press.

Stephen, C., and S. Lee. 1908. *Dictionary of National Biography.* Volume 4. London: Smith, Elder, & Company.

Still, G. 1931. *The History of Paediatrics: The Progress of the Study of Diseases of Children up to the End of the 18th Century.* London: Oxford University Press.

Trousseau, A. 1868–1872. *Lectures on Clinical Medicine Delivered at the Hôtel-Dieu, Paris.* P. Victor Bazire, ed. London: New Sydenham Society.

WILLIAM GERHARD

IN THE UNITED STATES, pediatrics began to develop as a separate specialty in the middle of the 1800s. The first book on infant feeding, entitled *Maternal Physician*, was written in 1810. George Logan's *Practical Observations on Diseases of Children* (1825) and William Potts Dewees's *Physical and Medical Treatment of*

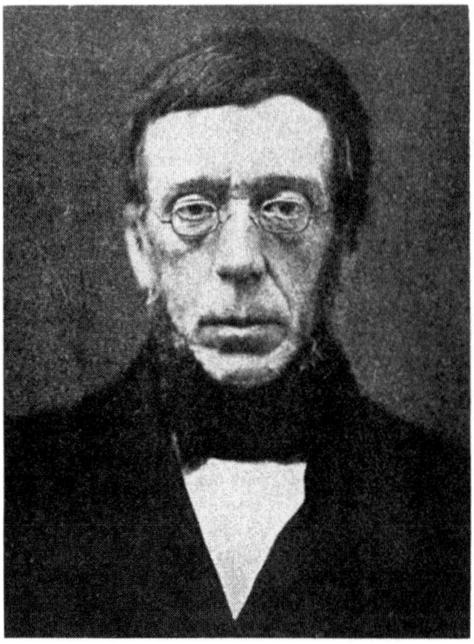

Figure 1. William Wood Gerhard (1809-1872).

Children (1825) were among the first treatises in this specialty and were soon followed by one of the early classic texts by David Francis Condie, *The Diseases of Children* (1844). Training in pediatrics centered in Philadelphia and New York, where the first institution devoted to children, the New York Nursery and Child's Hospital, opened in 1854. Some of the first academic and clinical faculty appointments were those of Abraham Jacobi, appointed as Professor of Diseases of Children at New York Medical College in 1850, and Job Lewis Smith as Professor of Diseases of Children at Bellevue Hospital in 1861.

Neurology also had its beginning in the United States around the time of the Civil War, primarily due to the influence of Silas Weir Mitchell and William Alexander Hammond. There had been isolated writings in the early 1800's by physicians such as James Jackson, John Ware, John Kearlsy Mitchell, Robley Dunglison, and Theodore Beck (DeJong, 1982, 4). However, it was the contributions of Benjamin Rush, considered the Father of American Psychiatry, Amariah Brigham, psychiatrist and author of the first American book dealing with neurology, entitled *An Inquiry Concerning the Diseases and Functions of the Brain, Spinal Cord, and Nerves* (1840); and Charles Edouard Brown-Séquard, the neurophysiologist, who laid the foundations for the development of neurology. The subsequent need to evaluate and treat war related neurological injuries spurred a period of rapid growth, the appearance of several clinical centers in neurology, and stimulated many individuals to become interested in the diseases of the nervous system. At the same time, interest in child neurology was also beginning. Bernard Sachs, Abraham Jacobi, William Norton Bullard, Sarah McNutt, and Edouard Séguin are known, in part, for their interest and contributions to this field at the turn of the century. It is of interest then, to recognize the early contribution of William Gerhard who, in 1834, published "On the Cerebral Affections of Children," a comprehensive study of tuberculous meningitis in children.

William Wood Gerhard (1809–1872) (figure 1) was born in Philadelphia of German and Moravian descent. His great-grandfather, Frederick Gerhard, emigrated from Darmstadt in 1737 and settled in Berks County, Pennsylvania. His grandfather, Conrad, moved to Philadelphia and his father, also William Gerhard, was born there in 1774. His mother, Sarah Wood of Salem County, New Jersey, was descended from the Gill family of Northern Ireland. As a child, Gerhard was described as having a remarkable love of books (Stewardson, 1874). He was once missing at dinner time despite an intensive search of the family's house and grounds. He was found upstairs in an unoccupied room in a closet filled with old books, stretched out on the top shelf and so absorbed in reading that he had not heard the dinner bell or the repeated calls for him.

Gerhard graduated from Dickinson College in 1826 and completed his medical studies under the direction of Dr. Joseph Parrish at the University of Pennsylvania in 1830. The subject of his dissertation was the topical application of medicines for surface wounds and blisters, and was based on the case material that he had gathered at the Philadelphia Almshouse. His thesis was quite unusual because it consisted of a considerable collection of observations about treatments that he cautiously and rigorously analyzed, in contrast to the more typical dissertation of the day that had little data and many loose assertions. This thesis foreshadowed the style and character of many of his future investigations.

Gerhard went to Paris in 1831 where he studied under Auguste François Chomel, Gabriel Andral, and Pierre Louis. Because of the earlier influences of Marie François Bichat and François Broussais, many of the physicians of the Paris school were devoted to careful observation of diseases at the bedside and dissecting rooms, content to determine such points as could be rigidly deduced from slowly accumulating facts, without attempting to launch into general hypotheses. Fortunately for Gerhard, he had the opportunity to study with several of the most thoughtful and rigorous of such investigators, especially Pierre Charles Alexandre Louis (1781–1872). Louis opposed the arbitrary doctrines of Broussais and was one of the first to use medical statistics in evaluating the importance of symptoms and disease manifestations (Abt, 1959). Louis greatly impressed the American medical students studying in Europe and, between 1830 and 1840, a number of these students came under his guidance. Among these were Henry Bowditch, Oliver Wendell Holmes, and George Shattuck from Boston; Alonzo Clark and Valentine Mott from New York; and George Norris, Alfred Stille, and William Pepper from Philadelphia.

As was expected, Gerhard spent a number of hours each day in the hospital examining patients and carefully collecting data that he believed useful for both himself and medicine. His first paper, coauthored with Casper W. Pennock, was entitled *Observations on the Cholera in Paris* and was published in 1832 (Pennock and Gerhard, 1832). He then confined himself almost exclusively to the Hôpital des Enfans Malades, which contained upwards of five hundred beds for children, ranging in age from two to sixteen years. Here he accumulated material for a series of interesting papers that he began while still in Paris and completed upon returning to Philadelphia. The first of these was an essay containing a description of a number of fatal cases of smallpox in children. Another was based on his careful observations of pneumonia in children that contributed largely towards establishing the different characteristics of the clinical course and pathology of pneumonia in children compared to adults.

On returning to Philadelphia in 1833, Gerhard became resident physician at the Pennsylvania Hospital. There he demonstrated that the continued fevers seen in numerous children in the United States were identical to the typhoid fever that he studied in Paris. When an epidemic of typhus broke out in Philadelphia in 1836, he showed that this was different from typhoid fever and similar to that seen in Edinburgh and Paris. The honor of discovering typhus had been divided among Perry of Glasgow, Lombard of Geneva, Gerhard and Pennock of Philadelphia, and Shattuck of Boston, but according to William Osler, Gerhard's papers in the *American Journal of the Medical Sciences* (1834) were the first in any language to give a full and satisfactory account of the clinical and anatomical distinctions that were later recognized and accepted (Waterson, 1971).

In 1838 Gerhard was appointed assistant to the well-known

James Jackson and soon had a reputation as an excellent and commanding lecturer, especially on diseases of the chest and thorax. In fact, in 1840, the medical students at the University of Pennsylvania presented him with a series of resolutions expressing their "high estimate of the value of clinical instruction, his eminent qualifications for imparting such instruction, and particularly upon his truly scientific and practical manner of elucidating disease, and his unequalled skill in illustrating the diseases of the thoracic organs" (Stewardson, 1874, 478). Gerhard was elected president of the Pathological Society of Philadelphia in 1838, and in 1842 published his best-known work *Diagnosis, Pathology, and Treatment of Diseases of the Chest*, which went through four editions.

Gerhard suffered two severe attacks of typhoid fever, the first in 1837 and the second, more serious, in 1843. This second attack left him partially disabled and necessitated an extended trip to Europe the following summer. Upon his return, he continued teaching and practicing at the Pennsylvania Hospital and helped begin the university clinics. He continued lecturing, seeing patients, and publishing, primarily in the *Medical Examiner*, of which he was one of the editors. His later works dealt with such topics as spotted fever, typhoid fever, typhus, and several other clinical topics. Retiring in 1868, he traveled to Europe, again visiting his mentor, Pierre Louis, who was then eighty-seven years old. Gerhard married late in life and had three children. He died on April 28, 1872 from an "attack of apoplexy." Stewardson (1874) described him as having "uniform steadiness with which he devoted himself to clinical teaching . . . placid in temper, kind and generous in his feelings, genial and gentle in his manners."

In 1834 Gerhard published the first extensive paper in the United States dealing with child neurology. His article, "On the Cerebral Affections of Children," appeared in two parts in the *American Journal of the Medical Sciences* and was based on his clinical experience at the Hôpital des Enfans Malades in Paris. In the first part, Gerhard published the details of ten children he examined. This part was preceded, however, by his concerns about the acquisition of objective and unbiased clinical data.

The cerebral affections of children are too rare for collecting a large mass of personal observations in a year's study. . . . This little personal experience will be perhaps partially compensated by the absence of all preconceived notions as to the nature, relative importance of symptoms or frequency of lesions in these cases; many of the observations are incomplete, none of them are perfect, but they have all been collected without the desire of confirming any previous opinion, or of reaching other results than such as will be warranted by rigorous deductions. I have avoided examining the works upon these affections, and I have even abstained from comparing my own observations with each other, believing that during a series of observations I should pursue the safer course to avoid all risk of forming a premature opinion upon a subject still intricate and obscure. . . . Such a method of study seems to me the only means of arriving at truths which subsequent experience will confirm, instead of the vague notions thrown out by one author and rejected by his successor as false and untenable. (Gerhard, 1834, 313)

Each case history averaged four to five pages of text, providing an almost daily account of the child's symptoms and physical findings and was followed by a description of both the general pathology and neuropathology found at autopsy. Gerhard concluded each case with a clinicopathological observation. An example from Case IV, Stephanie Erlemont, age five and one-half years is typical:

The rigidity of the right arm was one of the first symptoms noticed, and at the very commencement was sufficiently marked to attract the attention of the parents. . . . The left side of the body was frequently the seat of strong convulsive movements, and in the last two days offered a degree of rigidity as great as the right side. No delirium was noted; the intellectual faculties were very obtuse, but still retained on the fifth day. . . . Passing to the anatomical lesions we find very few traces of an affection of the cerebral mass; the granulation in the fossa of Sylvius (more abundant on the right side) were [sic] *abnormal, but whether they are to be regarded as the product of the acute affection, or as gray tuberculous granulations, is not perfectly certain.* (Gerhard, 1834, 338)

In part 2 of his paper, Gerhard tabulated the findings of his own ten patients plus an additional twenty that he collected primarily from colleagues but also from several other published case reports. In addition to the name, age, sex, and systemic findings, the tables included the neuropathology of the meninges, ventricles, and the "cerebral substance."

The last portion of his paper is an analysis of other clinical symptoms of these patients. Vomiting, cephalalgia, constipation, convulsions, muscle rigidity, paralyses, diminished sensibility, pupillary dilation, dulling of intelligence with the eventual lapsing into coma, and slowing of the pulse were present in varying degrees in all patients. Gerhard concluded that all these infants suffered from tuberculous meningitis. In reviewing his tables, it is clear that many of them did not suffer from hydrocephalus. He thus independently contradicted the well-known earlier studies by Robert Whytt. It will be recalled that Whytt's paper dealt primarily with hydrocephalus due to tuberculous meningitis. Without wishing to comment on Whytt's work, of which presumably he would have been aware, Gerhard also clearly demonstrated that the cerebral symptomatology could occur solely on the basis of the tuberculous involvement of the nervous system without the development of hydrocephalus.

It is interesting to note that, prior to concluding his paper, Gerhard discussed his differential diagnosis of five other disorders he had seen that could mimic tuberculous meningitis. These included typhoid fever, a mass at the base of the brain, a parenchymal tuberculoma, and two other disorders which, by their description, resemble bacterial meningitis and brain abscesses.

Considering that these papers on cerebral affections in children were written in 1834, sixty years before child neurology was "born" in the United States with the publication of Bernard Sachs's famous text, one can appreciate Gerhard's contribution to child neurology. Perhaps had he been of a slightly later generation, when both pediatrics and neurology became credible specialties in the United States, he would have been able to enlighten us with other objective observations.

Stephen Ashwal
LOMA LINDA, CALIFORNIA

REFERENCES

Abt, I. 1959. History of Pediatrics. In *Brennemann's Practice of Pediatrics*. I. McQuarrie and V. C. Kelley, eds., 1:21–22. Hagerstown, Maryland: Harper & Row.

Brigham, A. 1840. *An Inquiry Concerning the Diseases and Functions of the Brain, Spinal Cord, and Nerves*. New York: G. Adkard.

Condie, D. F. 1844. *The Diseases of Children*. Philadelphia: Lea & Blanchard.

Dejong, R. N. 1982. *A History of American Neurology*. New York: Raven Press.

Dewees, W. P. 1825. *Physical and Medical Treatment of Children*. Philadelphia: H. C. Carey & Lea.

Gerhard, W. W. 1834. On the Cerebral Affections of Children. *Am J Med Sci* 13:313–59, 14:99–111.

______. 1837. *On the Typhus Fever Which Occurred in Philadelphia in 1836, Showing the Difference Between This and Typhoid*. Philadelphia.

______. 1842. *Diagnosis, Pathology, and Treatment of Diseases of the Chest*. Philadelphia: Haswell & Barrington.

Logan, G. 1825. *Practical Observations on Diseases of Children, Comprehending a Description of Complaints and Disorders, Incident to the Early Stages of Life, and Method of Treatment*. Charleston: A. E. Miller.

Pennock, C. W., and W. W. Gerhard,. 1832. *Observations on the Cholera in Paris*. Philadelphia: J. R. A. Skerrett.

Stewardson, T. 1874. Biographical Memoir of William W. Gerhard. *Trans Coll Phys Phil* 4:473–81.

Waterson, D. 1971. William Wood Gerhard. In *Dictionary of American Medical Biography*, H. Kelly and W. Burrage, eds., 460. Boston: Milford House. Reprinted from first edition of 1928.

Whytt, R. 1768. *Observations on the Dropsy in the Brain*. Edinburgh: Balfour, Auld and Smellie.

JAKOB HEINE

JAKOB HEINE (1800–1879) (figure 1) was born in the town of Lauterbach in the Black Forest of Germany. Little information survives concerning his childhood, which occurred in an age of post-Enlightenment intellectual fervor, as well as social and political turbulence. His family was apparently well educated and hard working. Jakob's father, Martin Heine, was a blacksmith and farmer who developed and taught improved agricultural methods. He also was the inventor of an exercise bed. Similar systematic and innovative approaches were taken by other members of the family toward solving problems in mechanical engineering, physical rehabilitation, and medicine. Jakob's uncle, Johann Heine, was a pioneer in the field of orthopedic rehabilitation and Bernard Heine, Jakob's cousin, was the first surgeon to do an osteotomy to straighten bones. Thus it is little wonder that quite early in his life, Jakob Heine demonstrated a keen interest in science. Perhaps more importantly, he demonstrated an aptitude and a willingness to work.

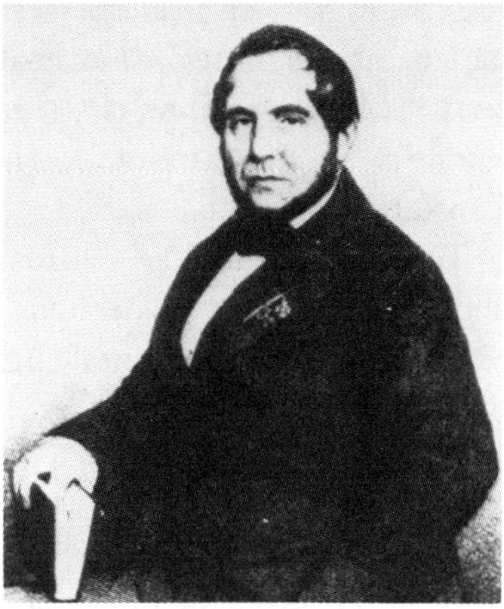

Figure 1. Jakob von Heine (1800–1879). From Ebstein, E., "Jacob [sic] V. Heine. Ein Gedenkblatt zu seinem 50. Todestag," in *Der Chirurg*, 1118. Berlin: Springer Verlag, 1929.

Jakob Heine's decision to study medicine was heavily influenced by his uncle, who was a distinguished orthopedist and maker of orthotic appliances. He moved to his uncle's home in Würzburg after graduating from the Alpirsbach Latin School at age twenty-three. Theological studies quickly gave way to the study of medicine. Heine obtained practical experience on the wards of the Carolinenanstalt, an important orthopedic hospital of which his uncle was founder and administrator. He finished his doctoral thesis in 1827 and then worked as an assistant in pathology to both Johann Schonlein and Cajetan Textor (Heine, 1968). Heine applied himself to the investigation of the anatomic pathology of crippling diseases of childhood.

After just eighteen months of assistantship, the government of Baden Württemberg commissioned Heine to found a hospital for the treatment of orthopedic illnesses. This facility was built at Bad Canstatt, in order to take advantage of local springs that were well known for their healing powers. Heine built pools to contain these waters, as well as facilities for exercise, physical therapy, manufacture of prosthetic appliances, and orthopedic surgery. He designed, modified, and built a variety of mechanical devices for support or exercise of crippled limbs and twisted backs. As many of his patients were young, he provided therapists for them during the period that they were at Bad Canstatt for rehabilitation. For more than thirty-five years, Heine enlarged and improved his hospital, attracting patients from a wide area. He systematically gathered records of the clinical history and physical examination of each patient. Keen observation enabled him to recognize and characterize sporadic poliomyelitis as a specific disease afflicting a small minority of the lame and crippled children who arrived at Bad Canstatt.

This achievement is the more remarkable if both the incidence and contemporary understanding of this illness are considered. Large epidemics of poliomyelitis had not yet appeared until several decades after Heine described his cases. Sporadic poliomyelitis was an uncommon illness, poorly distinguished from cerebral palsy, encephalitis, and even rickets. The earliest unmistakable accounts are those found in Michael Underwood's *Treatise on the Diseases of Children* (1789) and Giovanni Monteggia's *Instituzione Chirurgiale* (1813). Both note the association of fever and the sudden onset of clinically variable paresis in teething infants and young children. Underwood was republished in several English as well as German editions, but Heine cited neither of these predecessors. John Abercrombie further characterized the illness as one of motor paralysis with sparing of sensation (Abercrombie, 1828). Contemporary investigations by Charles Bell and François Magendie demonstrated that isolated loss of motor function could be produced in animals if the anterior gray horn of the spinal cord was disrupted. Abercrombie suggested that teething paralysis might follow such a lesion in humans.

Cases of teething paralysis were sufficiently rare that the occurrence of four cases in the country practice of John Badham during the summer of 1834 prompted him to publish an account and a request for information concerning the cause and treatment. The German reprint of this account, published in 1836, prompted Heine to publish his personal experience of twenty-nine cases as a book-length monograph in 1840 entitled *Beobachtungen über Lähmungszustände der untern Extremitäten und deren Behandlung* (Report Concerning a Laming-Illness of the Lower Extremities and Its Management). Although Heine had evaluated his patients for rehabilitation four to fourteen years after the onset of their paralysis, he discerned characteristic historical and clinical features that distinguished what he called "infantile paralysis" from other recognized causes of "childhood laming." These observations were en-

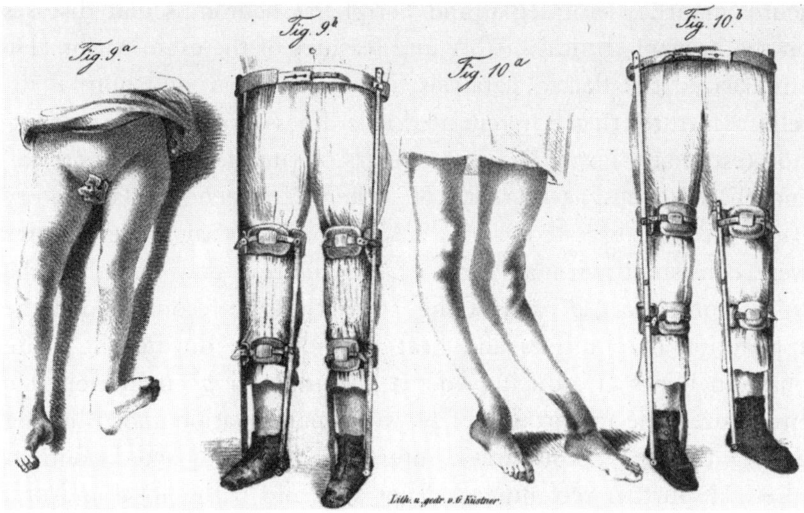

Figure 2. An example of one of several illustrations from *Beobachtungen über Lähmungszustande* (1890) showing Heine's use of long-leg braces for the treatment of poliomyelitis.

larged in his subsequent monograph *Spinale Kinderlähmung* (Spinal Child-Laming), published in 1860.

Heine observed that the disease usually afflicted strong, healthy children between the ages of five and thirty-six months. The onset was usually, but not always, marked by systemic illness. Approximately 75 percent experienced fever, 60–70 percent vomiting, 50–60 percent convulsions, 25–40 percent irritability, 25–35 percent difficulty teething, and 5 percent scarlet fever prior to the rapid onset of flaccid paralysis, usually of the lower extremities. Transient impairment of bowel and bladder function was noted in less than 10 percent of cases. Mental status was impaired transiently, if at all, in association with high fever or convulsions, and there were no sensory deficits after the first few days. Neither respiratory compromise nor death are described in association with the acute phase of illness. The paralysis reached its nadir within the first few days, followed by improvement. Limbs that remained paralyzed for more than a few months did not recover and became wasted, cold, and blue. Nearly half of the children developed monoparesis, one-third paraparesis, and one-fifth hemiparesis, with variable involvement of the trunk and neck. Scoliosis developed in one-third of Heine's patients. He did not describe muscle-stretch reflexes.

Heine clearly distinguished poliomyelitis from cerebral palsy, acute infantile hemiplegia, and peripheral neuromuscular diseases on the basis of clinical history and features of the examination. He emphasized the flaccid paralysis, intact sensation, and normal intellect, features that differentiated this illness from spinal compression (especially Pott's Disease), abscess or tumor, as well as stroke, encephalitis, and a variety of other "transient inflammatory pareses." He suggested, as had Abercrombie, that these features were consistent with a lesion of the anterior gray horns of the spinal cord. On the basis of this conviction, he recommended the application of poultices and heat to the spine during the acute phase in hopes of reducing edema and improving circulation. He emphasized the importance of physical manipulation and splinting during the early post-paretic interval in order to avoid contractures. He further recommended hot and cold baths, local and oral stimulants (camphor and strychnine), and specially tailored exercises (gymnastics and massage), which could be continued for as long as improvement was experienced. Irremediable contractures were treated with tenotomies, employing the subcutaneous methods pioneered by Louis Strohmeyer in 1833. Ultimately, patients were fitted with short or long leg braces for ambulation (figure 2). His monograph included lithographic illustrations of exercise equipment and braces. A century of experience with epidemic poliomyelitis was to add little to this rational program of therapy.

Heine's first volume was widely read and controversial. Moritz Romberg praised Heine's achievement in 1840. The Irish physician, Henry Kennedy, as early as 1841, attempted to discount Heine's view that childhood paralyses could be caused by spinal cord lesions. Heine was not cited in West's 1843 monograph on "morning paralysis" but was criticized in West's pediatric textbook, as well as in an article in the London Medical Gazette. The French physicians, Richard de Nancy and François Rilliet, were unable to find abnormalities of the spinal cord in several cases that came to autopsy and criticized Heine's failure to provide any pathologic evidence for his spinal localization of the neurologic findings. Yet less than six cases of poliomyelitis came to autopsy prior to 1870. Indeed, the characteristic pathologic changes were overlooked in several of these cases prior to the definitive work of Charcot and his colleagues (Paul, 1971, 40–60).

Heine's therapeutic views were apparently widely circulated and he certainly attracted many referrals. His 1860 monograph reports a personal experience with more than one hundred and twenty cases, a remarkable number considering the fact that the first sizeable European epidemic did not occur until 1887 (Medin, 1890). The data reported in this monograph resemble in general outline the observations made in 1840. Heine reviewed the controversy concerning localization, reaffirming his belief that the lesion was in the anterior gray horn of the spinal cord. He marshalled the evidence available from autopsies and animal experimentation, fully aware that such information was scant and inconclusive. He relied particularly on Schiff's demonstration that damage to the anterior gray substance of the cord could produce paralysis without sensory loss below the level of the lesion. His views were vindicated by the pathological investigations of Charcot, Vulpian, Parrott, and Joffroy in 1870. (Charcot and Joffroy, 1870; Parrott and Joffroy, 1870; Vulpian, 1870).

The title page of the 1860 monograph reports the many honors accorded Heine — Jakob von Heine as he was now known, as a mark of personal distinction. He was named a Privy Counsellor and Knight of the Order of the Crown of Baden-Württemberg and a Knight of the Imperial Russian Order of St. Wladimir. He was a member of the medical societies of Baden-Württemberg, Pest, Warsaw, and Othen. His therapeutic techniques were widely practiced and served a particularly important role in the management of epidemic poliomyelitis, which made its appearance in the late nineteenth century (Rurâh and Mayet, 1917). Fittingly, poliomyelitis became Heine-Medin Disease, linking Heine's name with that of Oscar Medin, the earliest great figure who studied the epidemic form of the disease. Heine was accorded the singular honor of producing a distinguished successor in the person of his own son, Karl, who became Professor of Orthopedics at the University of Prague.

Jakob von Heine retired from his Orthopedic Institute in 1865 and died on November 12, 1879.

Waltraud Schrank

Robert S. Rust
ST. LOUIS, MISSOURI

REFERENCES

Abercrombie, J. 1828. *Pathological and Practical Researches on Diseases of the Brain and the Spinal Cord.* Edinburgh: Waugh and Innes.

Badham, J. 1834–35. Paralysis in Childhood. *Med Gaz* 17:215.

Charcot, J. M. and A. Joffroy. 1870. Cas de paralysie infantile spinale avec lésions des cornes antérieures de la substance grise de la moelle épinière. *Arch physiol norm path* 3:134.

Heine, J. 1968. *Neue Deutsche Biographie.* Historical Commission of the Bavarian Academy of Sciences. Berlin: Duncker and Humblot, 8:282–83.

______. 1840. *Beobachtungen über Lähmungszustände der untern Extremitäten und deren Behandlung.* Stuttgart: Koehler.

______. 1860. *Spinale Kinderlähmung.* Stuttgart: Koehler.

Medin, O. 1890. En epidemi af infantil paralysi. *Hygiea* 52:657.

Monteggia, G. B. 1813. *Instituzione Chirurgiale.* 2d ed. Vol. 1. Milano: Giuseppe Maspiro.

Parrott, J. and A. Joffroy 1870. Note sur un cas de paralysie infantile. *Arch physiol norm path* 3:309.

Paul, J. R. 1971. *A History of Poliomyelitis.* New Haven: Yale University Press.

Ruhräh, J. and E. E. Mayer. 1917. *Poliomyelitis in All Its Aspects.* Philadelphia: Lea and Febiger.

Strohmeyer, L. 1833. Die Durchschneidung der Achillessehne, als Heilmittel des Klumpfusses, Kagazin geselschaft. *Mag Fur des Heilklinik* 39:195.

Underwood, M. A. 1789. *A Treatise on the Diseases of Children.* 2d ed. London: Printed for J. Mathews.

Vulpian, A. 1870. Cas d'atrophie musculaire graisseuse datant de l'enfance; lésions des cornes antérieures de la substance grise de la moelle épinière. *Arch physiol norm path* 3:316.

West, C. 1843. On Some Forms of Paralysis Incidental to Infancy and Childhood. *Lond Med Gaz* 32: 829.

JEAN ITARD

AN ENIGMATIC AND lonely-ten-year-old boy, the child known as the Wild Boy of Aveyron was captured in a forest located in the south of France, on the boundaries of the districts of Tarn and

Aveyron, at the beginning of the year 1800. Because it was thought he had always been completely wild, he was taken to Paris where scientists would attempt to clarify which part of his psychological life pertained to education and, on the other hand, which pertained to nature. At least, physicians asked the question in those explicit terms, and some of them still do.

No one knows how long the Wild Boy of Aveyron lived alone in some sort of hut he had built with branches and twigs where he withdrew at night. It was discovered because of large amounts of feces near the site. Entirely nude, he ran away when people approached, thus rendering his capture difficult. People had to stalk him for several days and caught him as he was picking acorns, his favorite food. However, he escaped. Fifteen months later, around mid July 1799, three hunters met him again, caught him and took him to their home. He stayed a few weeks in Lacaune, but tiring of the bad treatment inflicted by the woman who was looking after him, he again escaped. Dressed in the rags of an old shirt that had been given him in July, the child begged his food from isolated farms. He also was seen digging in the ground and picking potatoes, turnips, and acorns that he would eat raw. He was never seen near habitations until January 8, 1800, when at dawn he was discovered at St. Sernin-sur-Rance at the home of citizen Vidal, a wool dyer. The local government representative immediately named the boy "St. Sernin" and transferred him to the civil hospice of St. Afrique, a more secure place. Upon arrival he looked hunted, haggard, exhausted, and he bit anyone who tried to hamper his will. He resented wearing clothes or shoes; he strolled about endlessly and, after having walked for some time, put his hands on the ground and ran. He refused to lie in bed, always had a side-long glance, looked at no one and, at the first sign of severity, looked as if his soul was veiled with uncertainty that he feared to show. Shameless, he relieved himself anywhere. He also responded with devotion when hugged or when he received signs of physical affection.

At the end of January 1880, he was transferred to Rodez and lived with Father Bonnaterre, professor of natural history at the Ecole Centrale. At the time of the boy's arrival at Rodez, the minister of the interior, Lucien Bonaparte, Napoleon's brother, announced that he would claim the unfortunate boy if his parents

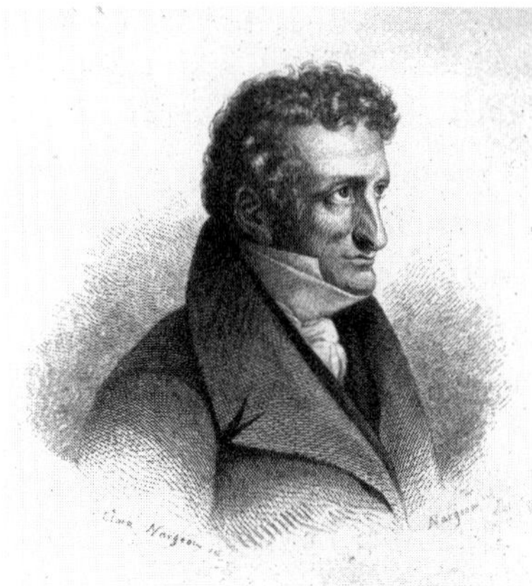

Figure 1. Jean Itard (1774–1838).

could not be found. Also, the Société des Observateurs de l'Homme, a society that included almost all scientists who had survived the revolution, announced that it would be very important for the progress of human sciences to ascertain if, indeed, the condition of a man left to himself was totally adverse to the development of intelligence and an affective life.

The Société had designated a commission to report on the condition of the boy, consisting of Joseph Marie Degerando, Georges Cuvier, and Philippe Pinel. On November 29, 1800, Pinel delivered his report. The auditorium was full, as Pinel was greatly respected. In his recent book on mental alienation, he had developed and explained the basis and methods as well as the therapeutic successes of the moral treatment of madness, a treatment he would now call psychotherapy. During this famous meeting, a young medical student, Jean Marc Gaspard Itard (1774–1838) (figure 1) listened to the clinical report of the great Pinel. His presentation was simple; many traits and instinctive behaviors of the boy could be compared not only with those of pets, but also with those of wild animals. Since, by many other features, he could also be compared to the young idiots of the Salpêtrière and Bicêtre, Pinel was not afraid to draw some obvious conclusions that he intended to develop during a further meeting. As Itard was the health officer of the Institute for Deaf-Mutes, he decided immediately to apply psychotherapy to the boy.

During his first six months in Paris, the boy's state of mind and health deteriorated; he spent his time alone, refused all contacts, walked sometimes in the alleys, upright, rocking, but most often he remained in a squatting position in the corners of walls or fences. He gained a tremendous amount of weight, eating everything that was available.

The young health officer hoped to return the boy to society by the following means: the child would be given a particular treatment and regimen that Itard would prescribe and the execution of which would be supervised by a woman who would remain with him permanently. This treatment was a form of training based upon the development of the senses that Maria Montessori developed a century later. The authorities at that time suggested, however, that the Wild Boy be placed at Charenton, one of the three asylums in Paris that could provide for his needs. Itard opposed this and quickly wrote his initial report "De l'Éducation d'un homme sauvage, ou des premiers développements physiques et moraux du jeune sauvage de l'Aveyron" (1801). This long analysis gave Itard the opportunity to give a name to the boy; he chose "Victor" because the boy appeared to express love and tenderness each time someone pronounced a word with the vowel *o*. In fact, the origin of the name is more poetic — it was found in a very popular novel by Ducray-Duminil that was published in 1796 and considered to be the archetype of melodrama and romanticism. The title of this novel and play was on everyone's lips: *Victor, ou l'enfant de la forêt*. It should also be mentioned here that a popular story and legend of the times involved Louis XVII, who was supposed to have escaped death and lived in the woods awaiting better times and his eventual return to the throne; a story which may explain the subject and popularity of the play, and furthermore of Victor himself.

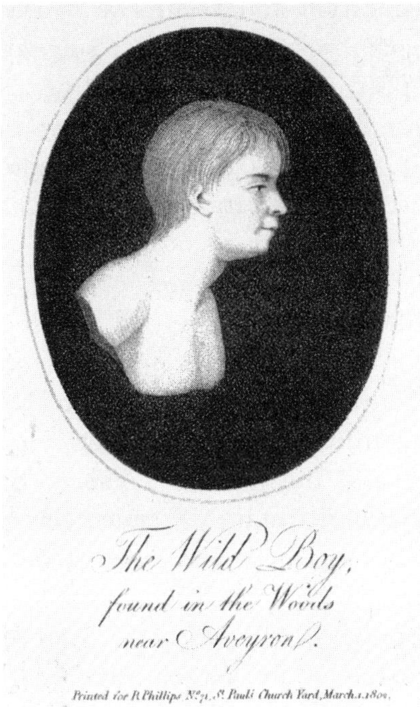

Figure 2. Victor, the Wild Boy of Aveyron.

The response to Itard's report was overwhelming and he translated it into English immediately (1802). It also succeeded in postponing the transfer of Victor to Charenton. Itard spent the summer of 1806 writing his second memoir on the boy. It was a status report but also the evidence of the end and the failure of the education and treatment of the adolescent who seemed to have gone back to his former stage of brutishness (Itard, 1807). Victor spent his days alone, strolling about mechanically in the garden of the institute or curled up and tormented by his nascent sexuality. It was indeed the noisy demonstrations of his sexuality that made the administration decide to get rid of the young man, who was now twenty years old.

At the beginning of July, 1811, Victor and his caretaker, Madame Guerin, settled almost across the street from the institute for the Deaf-Mutes in the crumbling building of the Feuillantines Convent, deserted since the Reign of Terror. There in a modest cabin, the public life of St. Sernin, who was also called Joseph or Victor, but was best known by the name of the Wild Boy of Aveyron (figure 2), ended. He died at the Impasse des Feuillantines seventeen years later at the beginning of 1828, totally forgotten and without having ever spoken. No one knows where he was buried.

Jean Marc Gaspard Itard (1774–1838) was born in Oraison, north of Marseille, the third child but the only one who survived. His father, a baker in Oraison, entrusted little Jean Marc Gaspard to his own brother, Jean-François, priest at the Riez cathedral, some fifteen kilometers from his native village. Itard was taught at the seminary of this town and finished his studies at the Oratorians of Marseille. He had just begun to work in a bank in Marseille when he was caught up in the popular uprising of 1793. He barely escaped participating in the uprising, thanks to his uncle Jean-François's intervention, who cleverly made him enlist as a third-class surgeon at the Toulon Military Hospital. There Itard heard of the dreadful circumstances of his uncle's death while fleeing the sack of the Riez cathedral. He had escaped through the mountains but, wounded and exhausted, fell into a precipice and was crushed on the ice of the river. Itard was nineteen years old when this happened.

At the military hospital of Toulon, Itard followed a course given by the renowned surgeon, Dominique Larrey. It was then that his interest in medicine began. He accompanied the famous surgeon on his return to Paris. Second-class surgeon at the Val-de-Grâce until 1805, he resigned from this position when he was offered the position of a major assistant-surgeon for the eleventh regiment stationed in Utrecht.

It was not difficult for him to resign. He was indeed already famous because of his attempt at educating and treating Victor. He had published his first report on this "very interesting creature" in 1801 and suddenly found himself propelled into a leading position in the scientific world. He was a tireless and persistant worker and published on numerous topics. From 1801 to 1807 he wrote several reports on the Wild Boy of Aveyron. In 1802 he translated Doctor Willich's *Domestic Hygiene.* From 1810 to 1820, he published numerous articles, including twenty or so titles for a medical sciences dictionary (Gineste, 1981). In 1821 he wrote a handbook on ear diseases and hearing impairment and in 1827, with his friend Jean Etienne Esquirol, an annotation of Hoffbauer's translation of legal medicine regarding the insane and deaf-mutes.

As Itard was publishing these works, he also climbed the social ladder, signalled by his election to the Légion d'Honneur in 1814 and to the Academy of Medicine in 1822. At the same time, he suffered from increasing pain, probably Pott's disease, which early on bent his body and from which he had suffered since he was at least thirty. He appeased his condition by spending his last days in a country house of the Beausejour Park in Passy, one of the most chic suburbs of Paris, where he had Chateaubriand and Rossini for neighbors. It was there that he died at three o'clock in the morning on July 5, 1838.

Itard's acute clinical observations allowed him to discover psychological differential diagnosis of the deaf-mutism that he had described as early as 1801 in his first printed report on Victor. He achieved a clearer understanding of the causes of these problems in his brilliant 1828 memoire from the Royal Academy of Medicine, "Mutism Produced by Lesions of Intellectual Functions," in which were shrewdly described what we would call today "speechless psychoses."

Itard was a young medical student in 1800 at the time of the Wild Boy's arrival in Paris. In addition, he was one of Philippe Pinel's favorite students along with Esquirol; they attended the master's courses at the Salpêtrière in the insane women's ward. Esquirol will remain for future generations the founder of Western psychiatry. At the time of the Wild Boy's arrival in Paris, Esquirol and Pinel started the moral treatment of madness, which we call psychotherapy today. In this environment, and according to Itard's own acknowledgement, the assuming of the responsibility for the Wild Boy was nothing but an extremely long psychotherapy session.

This first instance of psychotherapy cannot be evoked without speaking of the theoretical and practical conditions that made it possible. Pinel's famous gesture of unchaining the insane at Bicêtre in 1793 is from this point of view very progressive. This symbolic gesture in the middle of the French Revolution conveyed the perception that the insane are men and women like everybody else, an idea that was a result of the Revolution. Unfortunately, according even to Pinel, it is not he who removed the chains; this myth, as celebrated as the taking of the Bastille or the battle of Valmy, was the work of his son and great grandnephew, a long time afterward. Nevertheless, this indicates to us that something was happening in the minds of these "psychiatrists" during the French Revolution.

Itard's contributions can be viewed from several perspectives. From the psychiatric point of view, he conceived of the perception of madness as a potentially integral part of normal psychological life. "The limits which separate reason from madness, good from evil of our moral existence, are placed very much by chance and in an arbitrary manner, here by the doctor and there by the moralist and are liable to vary" (Gineste, 1988). Therapeutically, Itard's framework of a continuum between normalcy and psychiatric illness provided an approach to different forms of treatment.

Lesser known is Itard's description of the first case of Gilles de la Tourette syndrome (1825). The patient, the Marquise de Dampierre, had motor tics involving her hands and arms that began at age seven. She was thought to be suffering from overexcitement and mischief and as the movements became more frequent she was subject to reprimand and punishment (Goetz and Klawans, 1982, 2). Her tics became generalized, severe, and lasted her entire life. Almost sixty years later, in 1884, she was seen by Charcot, having already been examined by many neurologists. Although Itard did not attempt to link this case with other patients having tics, his emphasis was on differentiating this disorder from other cases of chorea.

Itard was also recognized by the French Academy of Sciences for his contributions to the educational sciences in his attempts to train Victor. He had proved that even a severe mental defective could be improved to some extent by appropriate training (Kanner, 1964, 16). His experiments and work marked the beginning of a long drive toward developing the limited potentials of the developmentally disabled. Shortly before his death in 1838, Itard handed down the results of his researches and experiments to Edouard Séguin, who subsequently became a leader in the educational reform movement for the handicapped in both Europe and the United States (Deutsch, 1946, 337).

Thierry Gineste
PARIS, FRANCE

Stephen Ashwal
LOMA LINDA, CALIFORNIA

REFERENCES

Deutsch, A. 1946. *The Mentally Ill in America.* New York: Columbia University Press.

Gineste, T. 1981. *Victor de l'Aveyron, dernier enfant sauvage, premier enfant fou.* Paris: Le Sycomore.

______ 1988. Pour célébrer le cent-cinquantenaire de la mort d'Itard. *Frénésie, Revue de la Société internationale d'Histoire de la psychiatrie et de la psychanalyse.* Vol. 6.

Goetz, C. G., and H. L. Klawans. 1982. Gilles de la Tourette Syndrome. In *Gilles de la Tourette Syndrome,* 1–16. Ed. A. J. Friedhoff and T. N. Chase. New York: Raven Press.

Itard, E. M. [J. M. G.] 1801. *De l'Education d'un homme sauvage, ou des premiers développements physiques et moraux du jeune sauvage de l'Aveyron.* Paris: Goujon.

______. 1802. An Historical Account of the Discovery and Education of a Savage Man; or the First Developments, Physical and Moral, of the Young Savage Caught in the Woods near Aveyron, in 1798. London: Richard Phillips.

Itard, J. M. G. 1807. *Rapport fait à S. E., le Ministre de l'Intérieur sur les nouveaux développements et l'état actuel du sauvage de l'Aveyron.* Paris: Imprimerie impériale.

______. 1821. *Traité des maladies de l'oreille et de l'audition.* Paris: Méquignon-Marvis.

______. 1825. Mémoire sur quelques fonctions involontaires des appareils de la locomotion, de la préhension et de la voix. *Arch gén méd* (Paris) 8:385–407.

______ 1827. *Annotation HOFFBAUER J. C. Médecine légale relative aux aliénés et aux sourds-muets, ou les lois appliquées aux désordres de l'intelligence.* Paris: Baillière.

______. 1828. Mémoire sur le mutisme produit par la lésion des fonctions intellectuelles. *Acad Roy Méd* 1:3–18.

______. 1842. *Traité des maladies de l'oreille et de l'audition.* 2ème éd. (posthume). Paris: Méquignon-Marvis Fils.

Kanner, L. 1964. *A History of the Care and Study of the Mentally Retarded.* Springfield, IL.: Charles C Thomas.

Willich, A. F. M. 1802. *Hygiène domestique, ou l'art de conserver la santé et de prolonger la vie.* Translated by J. M. G. Itard. Paris: Ducauroy.

LUDWIG WILHELM MAUTHNER

ADVANCES IN medical knowledge in the early 1800's involved the development of separate branches of medicine and surgery. Medical specialization that had begun in medieval times had fallen into oblivion but was revived again and a number of specialties became independent. Thus, internal medicine and surgery became separate specialties and pediatrics became independent from internal medicine and obstetrics. As part of this phenomenon, the first children's hospital was established in Paris in 1802. Louis XVI had appointed the Hôtel Dieu commission (1775) consisting of Jacobus René Tenon (1724–1816), Antoine Lavoisier (1743–1794) and Pierre Laplace (1749–1847) to investigate the public health problems of France. One of their recommendations was the establishment of separate hospitals for children and subsequently the Maison de l'Enfant Jésus was transformed into the Hôpital des Enfans Malades, which contained three hundred beds. Since then children have been treated in either separate facilities or separate wards within the hospital setting. The second children's hospital was established some thirty years later in St. Petersburg (Leningrad). In the following years several other children's hospitals were organized.The third institution of this kind was founded by Ludwig Wilhelm Mauthner in Vienna in 1837 (Szabo, 1976).

Mauthner's importance to child neurology is based on his writing the first comprehensive book in this field in 1844.

Ludwig Wilhelm Mauthner (figure 1) was born on October 14, 1806, in the small provincial town of Gyor, Hungary. Mauthner began his studies in 1823 and was admitted to the military medical college of Vienna, the Joseph Academy, founded in 1785. He graduated in 1831 and then spent several years in military service as a physician and assistant in the Academy clinic (Kirchenberger, 1913). During several epidemics of cholera and typhus, Mauthner became known for his hard work and administrative abilities. He was subsequently promoted to regiment director at the Academy. He published his first paper in 1834 on the epidemic of typhoid fever that had occurred during the winter of 1831–32.

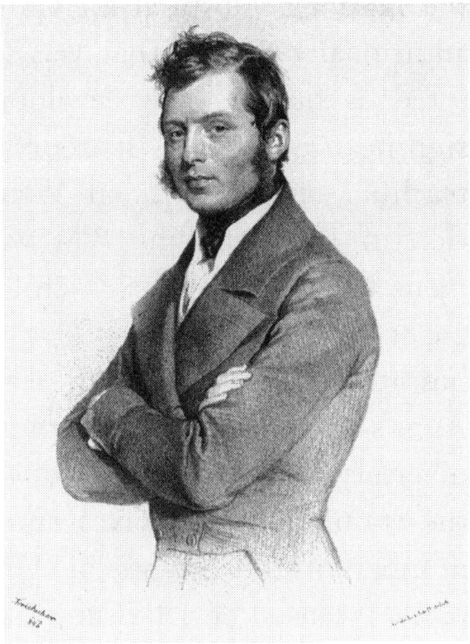

Figure 1. Ludwig Wilhelm Mauthner (1806–1858). Lithograph by Joseph Kriehuber, Vienna, 1846.

After leaving military service, Mauthner worked as a clinical assistant. In 1837 he established in Schottenfeld, a suburb of Vienna, the world's third children's hospital, the Institute for Poor and Sick Children, consisting of a twelve-bed facility. Mauthner was a gifted and kindly man. At his own expense he started the hospital in rented rooms that also served as the outpatient clinic. Mauthner made morning and afternoon rounds with an assistant and careful observations were recorded at the bedside. His assistant recorded the patients' histories, maintained the pharmacy, and covered for Mauthner when he was unavailable. The dispensary clinic was conducted daily and apparently physicians from all over Europe attended. Autopsies were performed with great care and interesting specimens were produced in colors by the artists of the Joseph Academy where they were preserved. Mauthner's endeavors in this area were soon acknowledged and sponsored by the Empress Maria-Anna and in 1842 the hospital became known as the National Hospital for Children. The hospital also acquired an additional building that was staffed by the Sisters of Charity who acted as nurses. The development of this hospital was of great significance because it represented the beginning of organized teaching of pediatrics in Vienna. Mauthner started such instruction in 1839 and in 1844 was given permission by the government to demonstrate sick children in clinical lectures based on his paper "Die pflege Gesunder und kranker Kinder." In 1848 the hospital was moved into a new building and was named the Saint Anna's Hospital. This hospital recently celebrated its 150th anniversary (Krepler and Gadner, 1988). Here Mauthner organized the training of midwives and pediatric nurses. At that time the number of inhabitants of Vienna was over half a million. The patient census of 1848 at the hospital included over six hundred inpatients and two hundred outpatients. In appreciation of Mauthner's work the Imperial Court granted state support for the hospital in 1849 and in 1850 it became affiliated with the University of Vienna as the University Department of Pediatrics (Krepler and Gadner, 1988). By that time Saint Anna's Hospital had fifty beds, twenty of which were used for the teaching of pediatrics. The following year Mauthner was appointed Extraordinary Professor of Diseases of Children.

Mauthner had lectured in the field of pediatrics since 1839 and continued to publish a wide variety of scientific papers. Early in his career he showed a great interest in hydrotherapy, publishing such papers as *Die Heilkrafte des Kalten Wasserstrahls mit einem Rückblicke auf die Geschichte und mit besonderer Rucksicht auf das Staubregenbad und Kalte Bader* ("The Healing Power of Cold Watersprays with a Retrospective Review of Cold Baths and Dustspray Baths") (1837). Mauthner also had a great interest in pediatric nutrition. He not only formed and headed an organization concerned with this problem but also published several lay and scientific papers in this area, including *Kinder-Dietetik, Eine Anleitung zur naturgemässen Pflege und Erziehung des Kindes* (Children's Diets, a Guide to Natural Care and Education of the Child) in 1853. This book appeared in three editions and was also translated into French. His publications appeared in the *Osterreichische Zeitschrift für Kinderheilkunde* (The Austrian Journal of

Pediatrics) of which he was one of the editors. Mauthner died at the age of fifty-two on April 8, 1858.

The Saint Anna's Hospital that Mauthner founded has had a long and illustrious history in pediatrics. Franz Mayr (1814–1816), who succeeded Mauthner as director of the St. Anna's Hospital, was considered the founder of clinical pediatrics in Vienna. He began to categorize the symptoms and courses of different pediatric illnesses, wrote several monographs dealing with scarlet fever, measles, congenital syphilis, and conducted the training of nurses that Mauthner had initiated. Hermann Wiederhofer (1832–1901), who followed Mayr, developed a clinical school of pediatrics in Vienna that was highly regarded. Wiederhofer was instrumental in developing isolation wards for the care of children with diphtheria and scarlet fever, developed large quantities of the Liebig's milk-malt soup that was distributed in the outpatient clinics, and wrote several classical papers, including one on intussusception. Over the ensuing generations many famous Austrian pediatricians trained or directed the hospital founded by Mauthner. Among these were Alois Monti (1839–1909), who wrote on spinal cord hemorrhage; Theodor Escherich (1857–1911), who had distinguished himself with his work on gastrointestinal infections; Ernst Moro (1874–1951), who wrote on colic of the nervous infant and after whom the "Moro" reflex describing the infantile grasp response was named; and Clemens Pirquet (1874–1929), one of the outstanding figures of the early twentieth century in pediatrics and infectious disease.

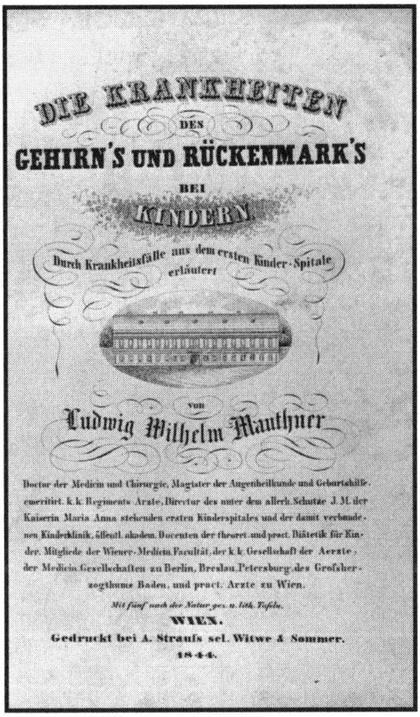

Figure 2. Title page of the first published textbook in the field of child neurology (1844).

Mauthner's contribution to child neurology is of great interest because it has not been recognized in most of the standard works on either the history of pediatrics or neurology. He is the author of the first text in this field, entitled *Die Krankheiten des Gehirn's und Rückenmark's bei Kindern* (*Diseases of the Brain and Spinal Cord in Children*), published in 1844 in Vienna (figure 2). This 446-page book is similar in both style and organization to many of today's standard texts. His interest in this area was based on extensive clinical experience as noted in his Foreword:

From the rich treasure of 15,836 cases which were observed before 1847, with clinical details, I chose the illnesses of the brain and spinal cord of children for a special treatise, partly because of the special significance of these organs, and partly because of the great difficulty, even experienced physicians find in the practical diagnosis and therapy of these pathological conditions.

Mauthner's attention to detail, his appreciation of the difficulties in collecting such clinical material and having it accepted in the scientific community at large is clearly present and still a concern of the child neurologist of today:

Even though I have not spared any effort or sacrifice in the course of this difficult job, I was still hesitant for a long time to publish it, fearing that through some hasty conclusion I will bring shame to science and that I could not stand up to the contemporary demands of such copious material. Our times make it unusually difficult for the practicing physician to rise to the present standard of science with the vast revolution of knowledge to learn and appreciate.

Mauthner's book is organized into two major sections with fourteen chapters as follows:

I. Diseases of the brain in children
    1. Brain Congestion
    2. Brain Apoplexy
    3. Brain Inflammation
    4. Acute Hydrocephalus
    5. Brain Edema
    6. Brain Atrophy
    7. Dropsy and Brain Hydatids
    8. Tuberculosis of the Brain
    9. Softening of the Brain
    10. Convulsions

II. Diseases of the Spinal Cord
   1. Spinal Congestion
   2. Spinal Cord Apoplexy
   3. Spinal Cord Inflammation
   4. Spinal Spasms

In these chapters, descriptions of many disorders that confront us today were carefully described with many detailed clinical histories, responses to treatments, and the results of pathological examinations. Intracranial hemorrhage, meningitis, encephalitis, Sydenham chorea, and hydranencephaly are among many of the disorders that are included. In the section on spinal cord apoplexy Mauthner provided the first description of spinal cord hemorrhage in the newborn due to traumatic delivery and tearing of the spinal cord (Mauthner, 1844, 403). In addition, Mauthner included several illustrations on the pathology of the nervous system from some of the autopsies that he performed. This primarily included examples of bacterial meningitis associated with scarlet fever and tuberculous meningitis.

Mauthner makes some interesting observations. In his discussion of cerebral apoplexy, or what we now consider either severe cerebral ischemia or hemorrhage, he notes the following:

> . . . *The risk and the incidence of apoplexy in newborns and infants would even be much higher if the communication between the scalp's and the brain's blood vessels were not remarkably increased compared to the adult.* (Mauthner, 1844, 44)

Such observations suggest that Mauthner was aware of the fact that infants appear to tolerate asphyxial insults to a greater degree than adults and he alludes to one contributing factor, that of the role of the leptomeningeal circulation.

Mauthner later discusses some of his observations on meningitis and one can appreciate his attempts at correlating pathology with the clinical state of his young patients:

> . . . *If the meninges are inflamed, the feeling of pain is in most cases non-localized. Except in otitis media, which is commonly caused by propagation of inflammation of the inner ear to the dura mater, and which causes shooting and pulsating pains, you will not be able to differentiate between the localization of pain and the infected area of the brain. . . . The pain caused by meningitis has characteristic effects on children, such as agitation and crying.*

This behavior even worsens their pain, so that they may become angry and irritable. Their entire temper changes. Accompanying their headache, you find an extremely increased tenderness of the entire body; thus, they react against the lightest movement, they startle at the faintest noise. Their state of suffering is usually marked in their features showing distortion and debility.
(Mauthner, 1844, 74)

A final example from Mauthner's book is that of an interesting table that he included. This table summarized his opinion on how one can differentiate cerebral from systemic disease in the lethargic or obtunded child:

	LETHARGY DUE TO BRAIN DISEASE	LETHARGY DUE TO SYSTEMIC OR ABDOMINAL DISEASE
1.	Progressive increase in drowsiness.	Periods of sleeplessness before drowsiness.
2.	Easily awakened and remains so. The temperature of the head is evenly elevated.	Easily awakened but falls back to sleep immediately. Posterior part of head is warmer.
3.	Awakens spontaneously or to light noise.	Sleeps the entire day without waking.
4.	Head remains unmoved, children spontaneously touch their head.	Hide their heads under pillow, turn head automatically and cross hands over belly. Eyes half closed.
5.	Eyes closed, sometimes open and stare.	Eyes half closed.
6.	Deep sighing and groaning, abdomen collapses, respiratory irregularities.	Lies quietly, occasionally murmur, abdominal girth increases.
7.	Pulse is slow, hard and small.	Weakened pulse.

(Mauthner, 1844, 117)

Mauthner's legacy to succeeding generations of physicians caring for children with neurological disorders is another good example of the way physicians have strived to classify diseases into orderly and understandable patterns. Although overshadowed by those who followed him in Vienna, Mauthner's contributions to both pediatrics and child neurology are substantial, and he deserves recognition as one of the founders of child neurology.

Stephen Ashwal
LOMA LINDA, CALIFORNIA

ACKNOWLEDGMENTS

I wish to thank Christine Fischer (a visiting medical student from Hamburg, Germany), Dr. Laszlo Mate, my mother (Elizabeth Ashwal), and uncle (Mr. Eric Glucksman), for their assistance with translation. In addition, Dr. H. Gadner from the Saint Anna Kinderspital in Vienna was kind enough to send me the Commemorative book celebrating the 150th anniversary of St. Anna's Hospital, as well as the photograph of Dr. Mauthner.

REFERENCES

Biographisches Lexikon. 1932. *Ludwig Wilhelm Ritter Mauthner von Mauthstein*, 127. Berlin: Urban and Schwarzenberg.

Kirchenberger, S. 1913. Ludwig Wilhelm Ritter Mauthner von Mauthstein. In *Lebensbilder hervorragender osterreichisch-ungarischer Militär-und Marineärzte*. Vienna: Joseph Safar.

Krepler, P. and H. Gadner. 1988. *Das Kind und ein Arzt, 150 Jahre St. Anna-Kinderspital*. Wien: Facultas Universitätsverlag.

Mauthner, W. L. 1834. Bemerkungen über das typhöse Fieber mit Nasenbrand (Vulgo Blaunase), welches im Winter 1831–32 unter dem Militär in Galizien epidemisch geherrscht hat. *Hufeland's Journal*. Berlin.

______. 1837. *Die Heilkrafte des kalten Wasserstrahls mit einem Rückblicke auf die Geschichte und mit besonder Rucksicht auf das Staubregenbad und kalte Bader*. Wien: Strauss.

______. 1844. *Die Krankheiten des Gehirn's und Rückenmark's bei Kindern. Durch Krankheitsfälle aus dem ersten Kinder-Spitale erläutert*. Wien: A. Straufs sel. Witwe and Sommer.

———. 1853. *Kinder-Dietetik, eine Anleitung zur naturgemässen Pflege und Erziehung des Kindes.* Wien: Gerold.

Szabo, G. Y. 1976. Professor W. L. Mauthner, M.D. (1806–1858), Pediatrician, the Great Son of Györ. International Congress of The History of Medicine, 24th Budapest. *Acta Budapest:* 441–42.

JOHN NORTH

JOHN NORTH (1790–1873), one of the original three hundred Fellows of the Royal College of Surgeons, specialized in midwifery and the diseases of women and children. Although he was a well-known London practitioner in his time, few details are known about his life, apart from what may be gleaned from obituary notices. Nevertheless, he deserves to be remembered by pediatric neurologists, for he wrote the first monograph in the English language on the "convulsions of infants." Since antiquity, writers had usually mentioned fits or convulsions in texts on child care, but the earliest monographs were by two French physicians: Jean Baptiste Timothée Baumes's *Traité des convulsions dans l'enfance* (1789), and Jean-Louis Brachet's *Mémoire sur les causes des convulsions chez les enfans* (1824). In England, John Clarke dedicated more than half of his *Commentaries on the Most Important Diseases of Children* (1815) to reflections on various types of convulsions and epilepsy. Then in 1826, John North's *Practical Observations on the Convulsions of Infants* was published.

John North was born in 1790 to Benjamin North of Woodstock and Mary Churchill North, the daughter of Bartholomew Churchill of Todmorden (Plarr, 1930). As was true of many surgeons at that time, he began his professional career in the army as assistant surgeon in the Oxfordshire militia. At the close of the Peninsular War, he was stationed in Bristol where he was responsible for the health of recruits and of French prisoners. In 1814 he left the army to practice in London, devoting his attention to midwifery and the diseases of women and children and achieving a large and successful practice by the 1830s. He married twice, first to a Miss Lyster of Dublin, then to a Miss Karie of London, who survived him. He died on March 6, 1873, at the age of eighty-three.

In addition to his book on infant convulsions, North wrote several professional papers and was editor of the *London Medical and Physical Journal* from 1829 to 1830. During the 1830s, he was appointed lecturer on the diseases of women and children at the Westminster Hospital School and then to the Middlesex Hospital in 1838. He was popular with his students, who found his lectures lively, clear, and concise. In the 1830s, North was one of the foremost practitioners of medicine in London. In December 1843, he was elected as a Fellow of the Royal College of Surgeons. However, at about this time, he came into a considerable fortune and retired from medical practice and teaching. How he spent the remaining thirty years of his life is unrecorded, except that he continued to dwell in his professional residence in Gloucester Place, where he died.

According to one obituary notice (Obituary, 1873), North had great physical and mental energy and was thoroughly independent in thought and speech — ". . . indeed, he was occasionally too brusque to be pleasant." This trait of candor, even bluntness, infuses the text of *Practical Observations on the Convulsions of Infants*. Whereas most eighteenth- and early nineteenth-century medical authors were opaque, verbose, and interminable theorists, North wrote simply and clearly, avoided speculation, admitted ignorance, and actually dealt with practical matters, such as distinguishing between types of convulsions and the extent of treatment required. Also, perhaps in keeping with his character, he did not hesitate to criticize other authors with whom he disagreed. Literary polemics were then almost standard practice, yet his repeated censure of John Clarke seems ill-placed, because the latter could not defend himself, having died in 1815.

Nonetheless, North's main bone of contention with Clarke was over a critical issue. In his *Commentaries*, Clarke stated that "in every case of convulsion (be the remote cause whatsoever it may), the brain is at the time organically affected, either directly or indirectly . . ." (Clarke, 1815, 90). North took exception to the concept of inevitable organic damage because, in most autopsies of children who had died of convulsions, no brain lesions were found, and because the acceptance of such a principle entailed the use of drastic therapy in all instances (North, 1826, 44). Clarke had recommended full depletive treatment, including clysters, various purgatives such as calomel and senna and, to relieve excessive blood flow to the brain, leeches to the head and lancing of the external jugular vein. North intimated that Clarke had "a striking influence upon the opinion of the present day" and, as a consequence, physicians administered depletive therapy with even more enthusiasm than Clarke would have sanctioned.

In North's opinion, "in most cases of convulsions there is some functional disturbance of the brain." Organic disease could be the cause, or the consequence, of fits, but this was far from admitting its constant presence. More likely, according to North, a state of temporary cerebral irritation was due to the effect of distant lesions. His main example was teething, classically associated with convulsions. Here, and in other instances of local irritation, drastic general depletive measures were unnecessary because usually local treatment, such as lancing the gums, would stop the fits.

His book provides other insights into the ideas and therapies of the time. As was then commonplace, he believed that some children were constitutionally predisposed to convulsions. More unusual, perhaps original, was his observation that convulsions were frequently associated with rickets (Shanks, 1948). The following is a quote illustrating this belief:

In rickety children the size of the head is disproportionately large; and, from the general symptoms of rachitis, it is evident that the head and spinal marrow are considerably affected; the brain increases rapidly in size, the senses are usually very acute, and convulsions are very frequent attendants of this distressing malady. (North, 1826, 12)

Early on he also stated that very young infants were subject to "a peculiar species of convulsive affection termed trismus nascentium" (North, 1826, 56) consisting of spasmodic rigidity of muscles, particularly those of the lower jaw. Dr. Abraham Colles of Dublin believed this condition to be due to suppuration of the umbilical cord (Colles, 1818), but North doubted this interpretation because sepsis of the cord was a common occurrence, yet he and many of his contemporaries had never seen a case of trismus. He accepted contemporary opinion that convulsions associated with eruptive fevers, such as measles, smallpox, and scarlet fever, were due to "sympathy" between the brain and affections of the skin. No mention was made of raised body temperature as a cause of convulsions; this concept would have to await the reintroduction of clinical thermometry in the 1860s. North did record James Currie's assertion, made in the late eighteenth century, that a cold bath was most efficacious in arresting fits, whatever their cause (Currie, 1797, 115). Currie's advocacy of clinical thermometry and cold bathing was ignored by his contemporaries who, like North, thought it dangerous to plunge a sick baby in cold water. Warm bathing was, however, acceptable treatment for convulsions.

North carefully distinguished epilepsy from simple convulsions. He disagreed with contemporary authorities who suggested that the two conditions were reciprocally convertible into each other. He admitted that simple fits, if frequently repeated, might degenerate into epilepsy with lamentable consequences. Yet he doubted that the reverse was true, for he had never seen a "case of epilepsy lose its distinctive characters and pass into simple convulsions" (North, 1826, 221).

The final two chapters addressed "a spasmodic affection of the chest and larynx in young children, accompanied by general or partial convulsions." John Clarke had already provided a description of this syndrome — carpopedal spasm and laryngismus stridulus foreshadowing convulsions (Clarke, 1815). North made reference to his predecessor's findings in an earlier paper (1825), again to disagree with Clarke's diagnosis of organic brain damage and to propose milder therapy. The symptoms were frightening, but North had never seen a case end fatally. By the following year, when his book was published without any mention of Clarke on this point, North had witnessed one death but continued to stress that full recovery was the usual outcome. Oddly enough, although North had found convulsions frequently to be associated with rickets, he made no further mention of this association in these final chapters on carpopedal spasm and laryngismus stridulus. Indeed, he believed painful teething to be the most common cause of this particular type of convulsion.

In many instances it may be difficult, and perhaps impossible, to assign the probable cause of this frequent variety of convulsive affection. I have no doubt that it is in many cases immediately connected with painful dentition. . . . In several instances I have known all the above symptoms gradually disappear upon the appearance of teeth; and instant relief will be frequently afforded if the teeth are sufficiently advanced to admit of the gums being freely divided. (North, 1826, 260)

Teething would continue to be held responsible for most of the ills of later infancy right through the nineteenth century. Only very gradually would it be realized that teething usually coincided with weaning, and that the food provided to replace breast milk was the more probable culprit.

North's book received mixed reviews. Lengthy notices with fulsome praise were published in 1826 by the *London Medical and Physical Journal* and by the *Medical-Chirurgical Review*. But the *Lancet* was brief and dismissive, finding North's criticism of Clarke pedantic and unnecessary (*Lancet*, 1826). The polemic created much interest at the time for, although dead for more than ten years, Clarke was still held in high esteem, while North also had vocal disciples. His greatest gift to his contemporaries may have been his reiterated contention that most babies with convulsions need not be assaulted with calomel, leeches, and the lancet.

Elizabeth Lomax
LOS ANGELES, CALIFORNIA

REFERENCES

Baumes, J.B.T. 1789 *Traité des convulsions dans l'enfance, de leurs causes et de leur traitement.* 1st ed. Nîmes

Brachet, J. L. 1824 *Mémoire sur les causes des convulsions chez les enfans, et sur les moyens d'y remédier*. Paris: Bechet jeune.

Clarke, J. 1815. *Commentaries on Some of the Most Important Diseases of Children.* London: Longman, Hurst, Rees, Orme & Brown.

Colles, A. 1818. On the Cause of the Disease Termed Trismus nascentium. *Dublin Hosp Rep* 1:285–91.

Currie, J. 1797. *Medical Reports, on the Effects of Water, Cold and Warm, as a Remedy in Fever and Febrile Diseases*. Liverpool: Cadell and Davies.

Lancet. 1826. Practical Observations on the Convulsions of Infants. (London) 10:265–68.

London Medical and Physical Journal. 1826. Practical Observations on the Convulsions of Infants. 55:486–502.

Medico-Chirurgical Review. 1826. Practical Observations on the Convulsions of Children. (London) Ser. 2, 5:149–68.

North, J. 1825. Observations on a Peculiar Species of Convulsions in Children. *Lond Med Phys J* 53:39–42, 284–87.

______. 1826. *Practical Observations on the Convulsions of Infants.* London: Burgess and Hill.

Obituary. 1873. John North, F.R.C.S. *Med Times Gaz* (London) 1:318.

Plarr, V. G. 1930. *Plarr's Lives of the Fellows of the Royal College of Surgeons of England.* Revised by Sir D'Arcy Power. Bristol: John Wright.

Shanks, R. A. 1948. The Historical Background of Convulsions in Childhood. *Arch Dis Child* (London) 23:281–89.

FRIEDRICH TIEDEMANN

FRIEDRICH TIEDEMANN (1781–1861) (figure 1), one of the pioneering German anatomists and physiologists, is perhaps best known to both pediatricians and child neurologists for his studies of the developing fetal central nervous system. It would not be an oversimplification to state that much of our current understanding of fetal brain development is directly traceable to his early investigations.

Born on August 23 in Cassel, Germany, Tiedemann's introduction to academics came at a very early age. His father, Dietrich Tiedemann, a philosophy and psychology professor of considerable repute, was a recognized authority of his time on the development of intelligence. It is perhaps due to his father, more than anyone else, that Friedrich Tiedemann's early interest in academics developed. The intellectually rich environment of the university served to further stimulate and mold his curiosity, ultimately establishing his desire for pursuing a career in medicine. This same environment also instilled within him a mature understanding of science. This understanding was later reflected in the careful,

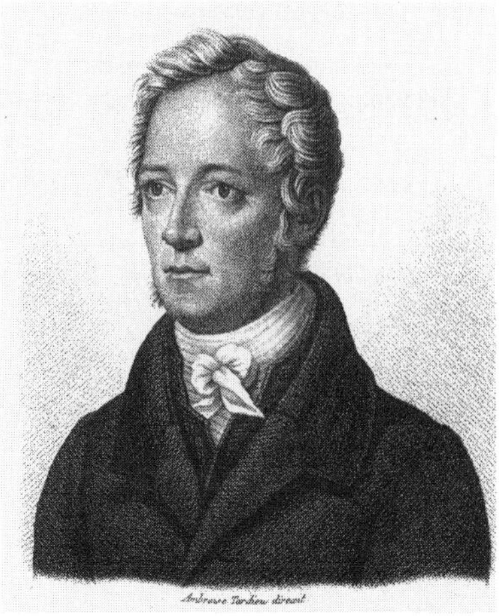

Figure 1. Friedrich Tiedemann (1781–1861).

methodical approach to research that became the hallmark of his later work.

His formal education in medicine began in the latter part of the 1700s when he entered the Marburg Gymnasium, where he concentrated on medical theory. By 1804 he completed his studies, but, due to the loss of his father from a contagious illness, was determined never to practice clinical medicine. Instead, he left Germany and moved to France where he pursued postgraduate studies in physiology with Franz Gall, concentrating on comparative osteology and craniology. The phrenological theory of Gall (and to a lesser extent Johann Spurzheim) proposed a direct relation between intellectual functioning and the shape of the cranium which, in turn, was thought to be determined by the pattern of cortical convolutions. The outward displacement of the cranium was proposed to directly reflect the extent of cortex devoted to intellectual or moral functions. Although phrenological theory was incorrect, it nonetheless was based on solid anatomical observation, and, more importantly, served as an important impetus for later studies of the relation between structure and function. Importantly for Tiedemann, this exposure to phrenology focused his interest on the development of the central nervous system, with special emphasis on the ontogeny of neocortical maturation.

Perhaps equally instrumental during this time were Tiedemann's studies with Baron de la Cuvier, the founder of comparative anatomy, and the French naturalist Jean Baptiste Lamarck, the premier theorist on structural development at that time. Each of these individuals were to have a profound effect on the later theoretical orientation and empirical direction of Tiedemann's research. During this time period he was recognized for his earlier study detailing the central nervous system of the pigeon, later published as a collected series (Tiedemann, 1826).

This work prompted his appointment in 1806 to the Landshut Medical Faculty as Professor and Chair of Anatomy and Zoology.

During his tenure at Landshut he continued studies on brain development, which were correlated with his father's previous studies on the development of intelligence, and published several major works on the classification of mammalian and avian species. Additionally, he advanced the current understanding of comparative physiology and anatomy by publishing several compendiums on the cardiovascular system of teleosts and large reptiles, and the lymphatic vessels and respiratory systems of birds (*Anatomie des Fischerzens*, 1809). For his work on sea echinoderms he was awarded a prize by the prestigious Academy of Sciences of Munich and Berlin, and elected a member to the same body in 1816 (Tiedemann, 1826).

Not only did Tiedemann excel in comparative physiology and anatomy but he also distinguished himself in his studies of the human fetus. For example, he was the first to correctly demonstrate the separation of fetal and maternal blood. His pioneering work on human fetal cerebral anatomy resulted in his book *Anatomie und Bildungsgeschichte des Gehirns im Fötus des Menschen, nebst einer vergleichenden Darstellung des Hirnbaues in den Thieren* (*The Anatomy of the Foetal Brain, with a Comparative Exposition of its Structure and Function*). This work was originally published in 1816 and was dedicated to the German physiologist Johann Friedrich Blumenbach. One of the important contributions of this work was its careful analysis of fetal cortical development. It is here that Tiedemann took exception to the proposal of Gall and Spurzheim, that the brain (prosencephalon, mesencephalon, and rhombencephalon) developed from the spinal cord. Tiedemann cogently argued that rather than developing from "spinal marrow" (spinal cord), the brain develops as an elaboration of the walls of the cerebral vesicles. Beyond this he also recorded other aspects of brain growth. These included: description of the crossing of the pyramidal tract in the embryo, growth of the peripheral nerves, and the upward shift of the developing spinal cord. Perhaps the most important contributions of this major work were his observations on the development of the sulci and gyri of the neocortex. For example, he was the first to correctly describe the order of development of the main, secondary, and tertiary fissures during the first trimester of gestation.

In 1816 Tiedemann changed academic positions and accepted a position as professor of Anatomy and Physiology at the University of Heidelberg. This resulted in his close collaborations with the renowned chemist Leopold Gmelin. This blending of two different backgrounds, the chemistry of Gmelin with the anatomy and physiology of Tiedemann, resulted in advances in several areas of medicine. Most notable among these were Tiedemann's and Gmelin's studies on the passage of materials between the stomach and small intestines, as well as examinations of the digestive process itself. Prominent among their works at this time were their thorough investigations of the biliary system (Tiedemann and Gmelin, 1826–27). International recognition of these and other works prompted Tiedemann's appointment as corresponding member of the French Academy of Sciences, and his later induction as a Fellow of the Royal Society in 1832.

His studies on the digestive system continued until 1835 when failing vision forced Tiedemann to seek help with his academic work from his son-in-law. Even though impaired with this handicap, he nonetheless continued to publish his research. For example, in 1837 he published his book *On the Brain of the Negro Compared with that of the European and the Orangoutang* (Tiedemann, 1837). In this work he countered many of the then current notions of human racial differences. Employing standard empirical techniques to measure cranial vault size and cortical areas, he concluded that there was no intellectual difference between the various human races. More importantly, he argued that the subservient state of some races could not be justified based on presumed assumptions of intellectual inferiority.

Following the political uprisings in Germany between 1848 and 1849, little information is available about the further activities of Tiedemann. We do know that a medal was struck to commemorate the fiftieth anniversary of his doctorate, while his last academic publication was a work on the history of tobacco. His death was recorded in Munich on January 22, 1861.

Friedrich Tiedemann was clearly a man of many talents who published in a variety of fields and held positions at many of the prestigious universities of his time. The field of pediatric neurology is clearly indebted to his early studies on fetal brain development. It is these pioneering studies that served as the important impetus and foundation for much of the later work in developmental neurobiology that was conducted in the twentieth century.

The focus on structure-function relationships, established by Gall and others under the philosophy of phrenology, were advanced and elevated to academic levels by Tiedemann and his contemporaries (Gall and Spurzheim, 1810–19). For the first time this empirical approach to the study of the brain provided a proper and powerful perspective to understanding the functioning of the central nervous system. Although this was clearly a major achievement in its own right, the second major achievement of Tiedemann's work was the intensive use of comparative studies. The insight into mechanisms of neural development and organization derived from other species became one of the major trademarks of Tiedemann's work, the implicit assumption being that the mechanisms of neural development observed in one species would not vary significantly across species, and would at the very least be suggestive of human development. This combination of comparative observation and use of empirical techniques became much of the mainstay of later research in the nineteenth and twentieth centuries. For example, this can be traced in the later works of Wilhelm His (1904), S. Ramon y Cajal (1928), and Charles S. Sherrington (1906) in their examinations of neocortical development, cellular morphology, and neural functioning. It is impressive to realize that the concepts in neurology that are today regarded as "classical" were not fully developed until the later part of the 1800's, after the death of Tiedemann. Many of the ideas implicit in Tiedemann's writings were to be formally advanced later by His, Cajal, Sherrington, and their contemporaries as a theoretical framework for neuron function. Thus, based in part upon Tiedemann's research, the neuron doctrine proposed that the neuron is composed of three functional parts: the cell body, the dendrites, and the axon. Moreover, transmission of information was viewed as one way (the "dynamic polarization" of Cajal) through the soma and dendrites via synapses, and sending impulses out through the axon. Each neuron was conceptualized to integrate information, with the motor neuron activating specific muscle groups (the "final common pathway" of Sherrington). The earlier works of Tiedemann describing the structural organization of the human brain and it stages of development became the foundation upon which these concepts were developed.

Even the more contemporary findings on neocortical organization by such individuals as Le Gros Clark, Lorente de No, and Korbinian Brodmann, or the more recent advances in cortical functioning made by Vernon Mountcastle, and David Hubel and Thorsten Wiesel, can trace their achievements back to the early observations and techniques of Tiedemann (Bonin, 1960). His application of comparative anatomy and physiology to the study of the human brain offered new insights into its development and function. It is because of his painstaking methodology and influential theoretical concepts of medicine that we enjoy the advancements made in this field today.

Suzanne L. Miller
MONTICELLO, MINNESOTA

Michael Kirby
LOMA LINDA, CALIFORNIA

REFERENCES

Bonin, G. von. 1960. *Some Papers on the Cerebral Cortex.* Springfield: Charles C Thomas.

Cajal, S. Ramón y. 1928. *Degeneration and Regeneration of the Nervous System.* Translated by R. M. May. London: Oxford University Press.

Gall, F. J. and J. C. Spurzheim. 1810–19. *Anatomie et physiologie du système nerveux en général et du cerveau en particulier*. Paris: Schoell.

His, W. 1904. *Die Entwickelung des menschlichen Gehirns während der ersten Monate.* Leipzig: S. Hirzel.

Sherrington, C. S. 1906. *The Integrative Action of the Nervous System.* New Haven: Yale University Press.

Tiedemann, F. 1809. *Anatomie des Fischerzens*. Landshut: J. Thomann.

______. 1816. *Anatomie und Bildungsgeschichte des Gehirns im Fötus des Menschen, nebst einer Einervergleichenden Darstellung des Hirnbaues in den Thieren*. Nürnberg: Stein.

______. 1823. *The Anatomy of the Foetal Brain, with a Comparative Exposition of its Structure and Function*. Translated by W. Bennett. Edinburgh: CarFrae.

______. 1826. *Specielle Physiologie.* Heidelberg: K. Gross.

______. 1837. *Das Hirn des Negers mit dem des Europäers und Ourang-Outangs verglichen.* Heidelberg: K. Winter.

Tiedemann, F. and L. Gmelin. 1826–27. *Die Verdauung nach Versuchen.* Heidelberg: K. Gross.

CHARLES WEST

IN THE MID NINETEENTH CENTURY pediatrics in England was just emerging as a separate branch of medicine. Its devebp - ment was greatly affected by several major trends that profoundly influenced the medical thinking of the day. The epidemics of cholera, dysentery, typhoid fever, and smallpox were associated with an incredibly high infant mortality. Of the 19,560 deaths recorded in London in 1815, more than one-third were reported in children under age five. Sanitary reforms, including a variety of programs directed at public health improvements, attention to infant hygiene and nutrition, and the development of health care facilities for children were implemented to combat the devastating epidemics that periodically swept through England, Ireland, and the Continent. Another major trend was the development of clinical bedside teaching. Originated by the French, brought to Ireland in the 1820's and shortly therafter to England, its later effect on the teaching of pediatrics was profound. New diseases were described and new systems of medical thinking and teaching evolved. In the center of these changes, from the pediatric perspective, and considered one of the pioneers of English pediatrics of this period was Charles West, author of *On Some Disorders of the Nervous System in Chidhood*, published in 1871.

Charles West (1816–1898) (figure 1) was born in London and received his early education in his father's school in Amersham. His father, a Baptist lay preacher, moved his family to Buckinghamshire from London when Charles was five years old and later to Amersham (Obituary, 1898). Young West was apprenticed to a general practitioner when he was fifteen where he became adept at compounding medicines and developed a lifelong interest in literature, especially Shakespeare. In 1833 he entered St. Bartholomew's Hospital as a medical student and received several prizes for his outstanding work (Clavering). Two years later he transferred to the University of Bonn in Germany and then went to Paris for several months of training (Abt, 1923). He completed medical school in September 1837 in Berlin, where he received his degree.

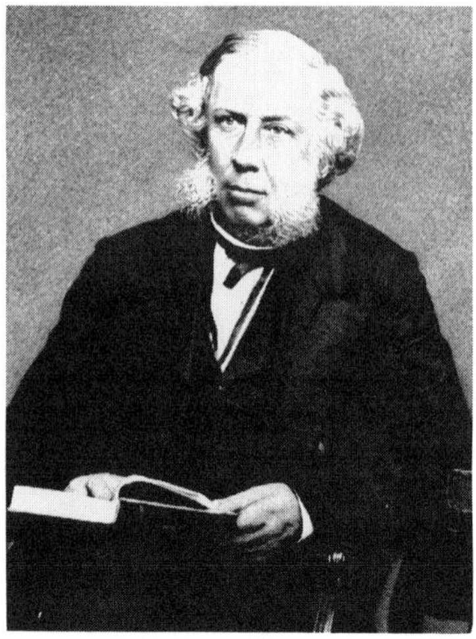

Figure 1. Charles West (1816–1898).

West returned to London for more training and experience in the practice of medicine. In 1842 he was appointed to the Royal Infirmary for Children on Waterloo Bridge Road and in 1845 lectured in midwifery at the Middlesex Hospital. He presented a series of lectures on diseases of children at Middlesex Hospital that became the basis of his writings on children. This series was published in 1848 as the *Lectures on the Diseases of Infancy and Childhood*. It was based on West's notes of 600 patients and 180 autopsy examinations that he had done. It passed through seven editions and was translated into almost every European language and into Arabic. By the fifth edition, West had based his findings on the analysis of 1200 hundred recorded cases and 400 autopsies that had been collected from 30–40,000 infants and children that he had examined during his previous 26 years of practice. This work, along with the published lectures on midwifery delivered at St. Bartholomew's Hospital, was the foundation of his fame (Abt, 1923).

His focus on the nervous system of children is evident in this work, in which the second through twelfth lectures were on diseases of the brain and nervous system: congestion of the brain; cerebral hemorrhage and cephalhematomas; inflammatory affections of the brain; acute hydrocephalus; simple inflammation of the brain; chronic hydrocephalus; hypertrophy and atrophy of the brain; hydrocephaloid disease; diseases of the spinal cord; and finally, night terrors, epilepsy, chorea, paralysis, and facial hemiplegia (West, 1848).

The following excerpt is from West's second lecture and indicates his unusual interest in the nervous system diseases of infants and children.

Gentleman — It can scarcely be necessary to assign many reasons for beginning this course of lectures with the study of diseases of the nervous system. The subject, although beset with many difficulties, has always engaged much attention; partly, no doubt, from the natural tendency of the human mind to inquire most curiously into those truths that seem most hidden; but still more from the alarming nature of many of the symptoms that betoken disturbance of the nervous system, and from the frequently fatal issue of its diseases. But besides the general interest and importance of these affections, at whatever age they may occur, their extreme frequency in early life gives them an additional claim on our notice. (West, 1848, 27)

Charles West did not originally describe salaam convulsions as is sometimes erroneously reported. Salaam convulsions were first reported by W. J. West in the *Lancet* in 1841 and the case reported concerned his own child.

West attempted to convert the Royal Infirmary for Sick Children from a scattered group of dispensaries into a cohesive hospital unit for sick children (Abt, 1923). Apparently, the professional jealousy of his colleagues prevented this transition from taking place. The true reason for these difficulties with his medical colleagues is not evident. However, the recorded facts suggest that he had unusual intellectual ability and energy, was a superb clinician, well organized in all of his efforts, and a very good writer.

West transferred his interest to other areas of London and with the assistance of Sir Henry Bence-Jones established the Hospital for Sick Children in Great Ormond Street in 1852. West visited hospitals in London, corresponded with continental children's hospitals and, through the social prestige of a benefactor, secured financing for the project in Great Ormond Street. The hospital, consisting initially of ten beds, was located in a house that had once been occupied by Richard Meade. The Wests supplied all the furnishings and Charles organized the accounting system, the diet table, a special fund, a system of boarding-out cottages, a museum of anatomy, wrote the catalogue, started an infant nursery and was physician-in-chief in addition to his many other duties (Abt, 1923). He also established a school of pediatric nurse training. His interest in this subject, along with an outline of nursing duties and obligations, is recorded in *How To Nurse Sick Children*, which he published anonymously in 1852. Training in this hospital nursing school is now considered the premier experience in this field in England. Charles Dickens lived near the Great Ormond Street Hospital and was very active in fund raising for the institution, although he apparently was not a close personal friend of West. Several of his speeches were published and his speech at the anniversary festival of the Hospital for Sick Children in February, 1858, is considered another specimen of Dickens's genius (Abt, 1923). By 1860, 691 inpatients and over 12,000 outpatients were treated. The growth since then has remained remarkable.

The Lumleian Lectures were presented by West in 1871 and published as *Some Disorders of the Nervous System in Childhood.* Lecture One discussed neuralgia and epilepsy. Lecture Two was concerned with chorea and paralysis. Lecture Three dealt with the disorder and loss of the power of speech plus some discussion of mental and moral peculiarities and their disorders (West, 1871).

An example of West's clinical acumen can be seen in the following description, taken from the first lecture, about petit mal epilepsy, a disorder which, at that time, was considered rare:

In the adult we are familiar with attacks of slight epilepsy — the petit mal, as it is termed — which yet we know tend none the less surely to develop into the characteristic epileptic paroxysm, and which, indeed, we regard with perhaps even more solicitude than the regular epileptic convulsion, as far as their influence on the intellectual powers is concerned. In childhood such attacks are at least as common preludes to epilepsy as in the adult, and are the more deserving of attention from their very liability to be overlooked. That a grown person should stand for a few seconds, his eye fixed on vacancy, that he should suddenly stop in the midst of an unfinished sentence, or pause with no obvious reason in the act of writing, or of eating, or of drinking, at once attracts notice, its repetition excites alarm. In the child, however, such things are apt to be overlooked, or to be called bad habits, or to be passed by with some commonplace unmeaning observation which consoles the friends, and with which the doctor too often feels himself relieved from the duty of careful inquiry and close observation. I believe, however, not only that such an onset of epilepsy is at least as common in the child as in the adult, but that an imperfect suspension of consciousness — the child knowing in what passes, though unable to speak — is not very uncommon; and further that it is far from unusual to have the early stage of epilepsy in childhood announced by sudden incoherent talking for a few seconds, or a wild look — a cry of surprise, or a short fit of almost hysterical sobbing announcing the close of the paroxysm. (West, 1871, 37)

Although bromides had been reported for use in the treatment of seizures by Sir Charles Locock in 1857 and by Sir Edward H. Sieveking in 1858 (McHenry, 1969), West also applied its use to children:

It were worse than idle before such an audience as I have the honor to address to go over the commonplaces of medical practice, but I may be expected to say something as to my experience of specifics for epilepsy. I have tried all, or almost all, in favor of which any reasonable evidence could be adduced, and all have failed. The only one which has appeared to me to exert any specific power over epilepsy is the bromide of potass, and in a few instances its results have been most remarkable. It hardly ever fails to arrest the frequency of attacks; now and then it has seemed entirely to prevent them; and the crucial test of arresting fits by bromide of potass — of suspending the remedy and seeing the fits return, and of once more putting a stop to them by the resumption of the medicine, has on some occasions reestablished its value beyond question. In the great majority of cases, however, the amendment has not entirely maintained itself; the system has after a time become habituated to the remedy, and after several augmentations of the dose, each of which has seemed to renew that old influence, I have been compelled to discontinue it in consequence of the depression of the pulse, the general loss of power, and the appearance of the peculiar pustular eruption which occasionally follows its long-continued use. In other cases, too, the agent which at first worked wonders, ceased to have any influence. The constitution tolerated the increased dose, but so did the disease; the patient continued to take the medicine, but the fits, though once controlled, returned after a time just as before. (West, 1871, 45)

In the second lecture, West presented his analysis of sixty-six children with chorea and described their clinical presentation, progression, and the association of rheumatic symptoms in sixteen of these patients. He rightly stated that there was no relation between the severity of rheumatic symptoms and the intensity or duration of chorea. He noted that the facial grimacing seen in chorea usually began at the same time as did disorders of swallowing and speech. This was helpful, according to West, in differentiating the "grimacing of nervous children" from a choreiform disorder. West was also very interested in the language disturbances that occurred in childhood chorea, which he believed were not simply due to loss of muscular power or abnormal tongue movements but to some central effect on intellectual processing. The remaining sections of the second lecture review some of the well-recognized "paralytic disorders," including sections on diptheria, rickets, and other chronic diseases; disorders associated with painful extremities, particularly hip-joint disease; paralysis seen in the developmentally delayed ("paralysis of the idiot"); chorea; cerebral tubercles; tumors; and finally "essential paralysis," that is, poliomyelitits.

The third lecture in this series focused principally on disorders of speech and is of interest because it represents one of the earliest child neurological discussions of this topic. West recognized that "the date at which children begin to talk varies very greatly" and that "it by no means constantly follows that tardy acquirement of the power of speech implies a deficiency of intelligence." His first concern in such cases was deafness and he admonished his audience that "it is not easy in early childhood to ascertain the existence of congenital deafness." Another group of children with delayed speech were those with some degree of intellectual retardation, referred to in West's time in England as "backward children," and in France as "les enfants arrières." West recognized the parallel in such children in the delay of language and motor and social development. West also described the phenomena of loss of acquired language in conjunction with chorea, typhoid fever, and one or two children who presumably had encephalitis. West also is perhaps the first to describe the acute onset of aphasia associated with right hemiplegia in a child. This was observed in a five-year-old girl after an attack of "sunstroke, followed by coma of a fortnight's duration." The child's intelligence was described as normal, her receptive language appeared intact but she was only capable of uttering "dah." She was periodically seen by West and two years later had minimally recovered, being able to speak a few single words and repeat some phrases. The section on language disorders concludes with the description of the temporary loss of speech that West observed in several children, which he was at a loss to explain.

In 1875 West resigned as senior physician to the Hospital for Sick Children on Great Ormond Street but refurnished the new hospital in its entirety and donated his library and pathological drawings (Abt, 1923). The material is intact and is now located in the archives section of the hospital library and is listed in a catalogue published by that institution (Payne).

Because of bad health, West moved to Nice in 1880 and practiced there for five years. Returning to London, he began a private practice on Harley Street and had no problem procuring patients, but he was not accepted on the staff of the local hospitals. Following some years of ill health interspersed with travel, he died in Paris on March 19, 1898. The *British Medical Journal* gave three pages to his obituary and the length of this article indicates their respect for his contributions to medicine (Obituary, 1898, 921). West himself, in a very reflective passage from his work, aptly summarized his thoughts about his life and his contributions:

A moment's satisfaction may be pardoned me in thankfully acknowledging these evidences that my toil has not been fruitless. But it is with no feeling of flattered vanity that I now lay down my pen. The revision in mature age of the labors of one's youth must, with most persons, minister to self-reproach rather than to self-satisfaction. The same unsolved problems meet one's eye now as met it years ago; one's deficiencies are felt more deeply; they seem graver and less excusable as the time for remedying them passes by; one longs for the leisure gone, for the energies of former years, which one fancies, coupled with the soberness of advancing life, might help to add something more and better to the common store of knowledge. (West, 1865, preface)

Lucius Waites
DALLAS, TEXAS

Stephen Ashwal
LOMA LINDA, CALIFORNIA

ACKNOWLEDGMENTS

Special thanks to Mr. R. J. Lunnon, Honorary Deputy Archivist, and the staff of the Department of Medical Illustration, The Hospital for Sick Children, Great Ormond Street, London, for their kind cooperation in making some of this material available.

REFERENCES

Abt, I. A., ed. 1923. *Pediatrics,* Vol. 1, 89–90, 120. Philadelphia: W. B. Saunders and Co.

Clavering, R. A. n.d. Dr. Charles West and the Founding of the Children's Hospital in Great Ormond Street. Unpublished manuscript. London: Archives of the Hospital for Sick Children, Great Ormond Street.

McHenry, L. C. 1969. *Garrison's History of Neurology*, 396. Springfield, Illinois: Charles C Thomas.

Obituary. 1898. Charles West, M.D., F.R.C.P.. *Brit Med J* 1:921–23.

Payne, W. W., comp. n.d. *The West Library Catalogue, The Hospital for Sick Children, Great Ormond Street.* London: Joseph Collard and Sons.

______. 1870. Speeches, Letters, and Sayings of Charles Dickens, 49–51. New York: Harper and Brothers.

West, C. 1848. *Lectures on the Diseases of Infancy and Childhood.* London: Longman, Brown, Green and Longmans.

______. 1852. *How to Nurse a Sick Child.* London: Longman, Brown, Green, and Longmans.

______. 1854. *An Enquiry into the Pathological Importance of Ulceration of the Os uteri.* Croonian Lectures. London: Longman, Brown, Green, and Longmans.

______. 1865. *Lectures on the Diseases of Infancy and Childhood.* 5th ed. London: Longmans, Green, Longman, Roberts, and Green.

______. 1867. *Lectures on the Diseases of Women.* 3d American ed. from 3d English ed. (1864). Philadelphia: H. C. Lea.

______. 1871. *On Some Disorders of the Nervous System in Childhood, being the Lumleian Lectures Delivered at the Royal College of Physicians of London in March 1871.* London: Longmans, Green and Co.

West, W. J. 1841. On a Peculiar Form of Infantile Convulsions. *Lancet* 1:724–25.

The Growth of Pediatrics and Neurology and the Beginnings of Child Neurology

THE LATE NINETEENTH CENTURY

1850 – 1900

OVERVIEW

THE MODERN SCIENTIFIC MOVEMENT in medicine, which began in the early nineteenth century, attained its full stride in the latter half of the century. Whereas the early clinical investigations of the French School were based on the bedside systematic study of disease, emphasis shifted towards the laboratory as microbiology, physiology, and chemistry provided completely new and exciting knowledge of health and disease. Rudolf Virchow's *Cellularpathologie* (1858) set in motion a novel way of looking at the body as "a cell-state in which every cell is a citizen," diseases being "merely a conflict of citizens in this state, brought about by the action of external forces" (Garrison, 1929, 570). While Louis Pasteur investigated fermentation (1857) and putrefaction (1862), demonstrating the existence of bacteria, Robert Koch showed for the first time, in his studies of the anthrax bacillus, that a definite infectious agent was caused by a specific microbial agent. Koch later studied the etiology of traumatic infectious disease (1878) and reported on his discovery of the tubercle bacillus and the bacterial spread of disease (1882). At the same time, Joseph Lister showed that carbolic acid was an effective antiseptic agent in surgery (1867) and Ignaz Semmelweis published his famous treatise on the causes and treatment of puerperal sepsis (1861), followed nineteen years later by Pasteur's discovery that this was due to streptococcal septicemia. Coupled with the earlier introductions of ether (1842, 1846) and chloroform (1847) anesthesia and later that of blood transfusions (1867, 1901), these discoveries led to the modern era of surgery and obstetrics. They ultimately provided a foundation for the development of pediatrics as a separate field, including the diagnosis and treatment of childhood infectious disease and the surgical correction of many congenital anomalies. Based on the work of Claude Bernard in France and Johannes Müller and Carl Ludwig in Germany, physiology became an important specialty. Laboratories for physiology, chemistry, and pharmacology were established as each of these fields became separate disciplines. The latter half of the nineteenth century saw the implementation of blood-chemistry testing and the clinical use of the Roentgen ray, developments which allowed physicians to use the laboratory for diagnosing and treating living patients rather than having to wait for the results of postmortem pathology.

Two of the most important trends in medicine that began during the latter half of the nineteenth century were the institutionalization of patient care and the change in the perception and treatment of patients with mental disorders. The emergence of hospitals from unsafe and dirty habitats of the poor and dying to the modern, fully equipped, technologically based facility has had an extraordinary impact on all phases of medicine. It provided the arena for the development of all medical specialties, gave impetus to the formation of nursing as an important profession, and helped centralize and standardize medical education. An example of this is the practice of midwifery which, over a period of time, yielded to that of hospital-based obstetrics. With the growth of the nineteenth-century social welfare movements, a new and more positive attitude towards the insane and mentally disabled developed. Perhaps the two most important trends in this regard were the slow and difficult process of humanizing the living conditions of such patients and the attempts at understanding and classifying the different forms of mental disease of these afflicted inmates. The work of Philippe Pinel early in the century and later that of Jean Martin Charcot stand out in this regard. Charcot's individual and systematic examination of the five thousand inhabitants of the Salpêtrière permitted him to continue Pinel's work of distinguishing the insane from mentally subnormal and gave him the opportunity to contribute a great deal to the current overall conceptualization of clinical neurology. These events had an important influence on the future development of child neurology.

PEDIATRICS

Infant nutrition, growth and development, and infectious disease were the primary concerns of those physicians interested in the "diseases of children," "pediatry," "pediology," and by the turn of the century, "pediatrics." This was the era of Robert Koch, Louis Pasteur, the introduction on a wider scale of the smallpox vaccine, and the discovery by Pierre Roux in 1887 of diphtheria antitoxin. The importance of these advances and those following the introduction of antibiotics almost a half century later are appreciated when one realizes that the infant mortality rate in the first year of life varied between 25 and 50 percent. In foundling homes the rate was as high as 75 to 90 percent. By age twelve the overall mortality rate for children was close to 50 percent. However, as pointed out by Guy Williams, there was some optimism about the future of children:

Once safely born, a baby at the end of the nineteenth century would have ahead a much better chance of surviving infancy than a child of a similar age in the early 1800s. The custom of swaddling infants in tight restrictive clothes had virtually disappeared during the century, under the influence of a number of pioneers who encouraged lighter, freer coverings. The use of powerful drugs such as laudanum to quieten {sic} babies had gradually been discontinued, too, though inquests in 1837–8 had still shown that fifty-two infants out of a total of a hundred and eighty-six had perished, primarily, through the administration of opium. The rubber nipple, patented in 1841, had solved many of the problems of feeding away from the breast; and substances much more suitable than "pap" (bread or flour soaked in milk or in water) were being used as food, largely due to the lead given by the great German chemist Justus von Liebig (Williams, 1987, 87).

The latter half of the nineteenth century was marked by the

ascent of Germany and England as leading centers for the care and study of children. The German school of pediatrics was primarily responsible for the development of laboratory methods for investigation of pediatric diseases. Max Rubner and Johann Heubner published the first work on the average daily food requirements of the normal and malnourished infant (1898–99). Infant formulas, milk stations, and special milk dairies were created in many countries by pediatricians concerned with improving infant nutrition. Theodore Escherich recognized the importance of intestinal bacterial pathogens as the cause of infantile diseases (1884). Many diseases were described in this period, including syphilitic pseudoparalysis (1872), infantile purpura (1872), infantile scurvy (1875), megacolon (1887), celiac disease (1888), and juvenile rheumatoid arthritis (1896).

Charles Darwin's *On the Origin of Species* (1859) and *The Descent of Man* (1871) quickly had a profound impact on the study of childhood development and helped to kindle the eugenics movement as did the work of Gall and Spurzheim. By the early twentieth century, the emerging science of child development depicted childhood as a sequence of discrete stages, each with its own behavioral expectations. Writers of both religious and secular texts agreed that the early years were highly consequential for the individual's character and eventual standing in society. The association of childhood with original sin, pervasive in eighteenth-century Calvinist thought, gave way to a new attitude in the nineteenth century. Children were perceived as precious, malleable, and in need of adult guidance and protection (Halpern, 1988, 37).

The social reform and child welfare movements gained momentum and in large part were responsible for the emergence of pediatrics as a distinct field of medicine. The first extensive studies of myopia and other visual problems of children were published by Hermann Cohn from Breslau (1867), based on his examinations of 10,600 school-age children, although Albrecht von Graefe had proposed surgical treatment of strabismus in 1857. School hygiene remained an important issue. School lunches were mandated by law in France in 1882. Throughout Europe, England, and the United States, many clinics, homes, and institutions were opened for orphans, the handicapped, and the chronically ill. Charles West organized the opening of the Hospital for Sick Children at Great Ormond Street in 1852. Two years later, the Child's Hospital and Nursery, the first American facility solely for children, opened in New York City, followed by the Children's Hospital of Philadelphia (1855). Throughout Europe more than fifty children's hospitals were inaugurated during the period between 1850 and 1900 (Abt, 1965). Children's hospitals and asylums contributed to the emergence of pediatrics in a number of different ways. They provided a concentration of case material for the investigation of children's disorders and served as training centers where practitioners gained experience in the treatment of children's diseases. Medical facilities for the young created a specific need for physicians capable and willing to care for such patients. The bulk of papers written by pediatricians of this era were based on clinical case material gathered from observations in the hospital setting.

Professional pediatric organizations were formed during this era. The first pediatric societies arose in Germany (1883) and Russia (1885). In 1887 the American Medical Association created a pediatric section and the following year, the American Pediatric Society was formed; its first two presidents were Abraham Jacobi and Job Lewis Smith. This was soon followed by the founding of similar organizations in France (1899), and England (1900). Journals devoted solely to pediatrics appeared in Austria, France, Germany, Italy, Russia, and the United States (Abt, 1965).

NEUROLOGY

The period between 1850 and 1900 is considered by many to be the golden age of neurology. Neurological traditions still stemmed from internal medicine, yet several great schools of clinical neurology developed: in France, that of Jean Martin Charcot and Amand Duchenne; in England, John Hughlings Jackson and William Gowers; in Germany, Wilhelm Erb and Hermann Oppenheim; and in the United States, Silas Weir Mitchell and Charles Mills. One of the major forces that caused neurology to become a separate entity was the evolution of neuropathology as a separate discipline, which is credited to Charcot in France, but neuropathology also flourished in Germany during this era. Among the numerous neuropathological observations made during this period were the description of general paresis and senile dementia by

Alois Alzheimer (1897, 1904) and the pathology of spinal cord trauma by Heinrich Obersteiner (1888).

The latter half of the nineteenth century also saw impressive gains in neurohistology based on the work of Rudolf Virchow (1854); Joseph von Gerlach, Sr. (1858); Camillo Golgi (1873); Vittorio Marchi (1885); Franz Nissl (1885); and Carl Weigert (1895). Wilhelm His, who originated such terms as dendrite, neuropil, neuroblast, and spongioblast, concentrated on the embryogenesis of the nervous system (1889). Louis Ranvier, in one of the first histology texts of the nervous system, described the famous node of interrupted myelin sheath that bears his name (1878). Heinrich Waldeyer formulated and named the concept of the unit structure of the nervous system to be the "neuron," consisting of the nerve cell and its processes (1891). This concept was based in part on the earlier investigations of isolated nerve degeneration of Augustus Waller (1850). Waldeyer helped to end an almost century-old controversy between those who believed the brain to be a vast reticular network in which nerve impulses traversed almost all cells and those who argued that neural activity was transmitted from one cell to another. The exquisite and extensive studies of Ramon y Cajal supported this latter concept (1899–1904). Around this time, Vladimir Betz described the large pyramidal cell of layer five of the cerebral cortex that bears his name (1894).

Claude Bernard also made major contributions, which were his description of the origins and functions of the cervical sympathetic nervous system and the examination of the vasomotor innervation of blood vessels (1858). The concept of synaptic transmission, suggested initially by Luigi Galvani (1792), was further studied by Emil du Bois Reymond (1848–84) and Charles Sherrington (1897). Sherrington also performed extensive studies of the distribution of spinal nerve root motor function (1892) and outlined the sensory dermatomal distribution (1894). Sherrington's work, summarized in *The Integrative Action of the Nervous System* (1906), accorded him recognition as the founder of modern neurophysiology. Herman Helmholtz made the first measurements of nerve conduction velocity in 1850. Robert Remak is credited with developing the modern concept of the autonomic nervous system (1838). Walter Gaskell demonstrated its different divisions and postulated two antagonistic systems, one excitatory and one inhibitory (1886, 1916). The work of John Langley incorporated this concept into sympathetic and parasympathetic divisions (1894, 1921). Cortical localization of motor function was proven by the electrode stimulation experiments of Eduard Hitzig and Theodor Fritsch (1870) and around the same time Hermann Munk suggested the presence of a post-rolandic sensory cortex (1868). These studies culminated in the meticulous cortical electrophysiological mapping by David Ferrier (1876). Over the next seventy-five years, these investigations were extended and correlated with the brain's cytoarchitecture by Victor Horsley, Charles Sherrington, John Fulton, Wilder Penfield, Paul Bucy, Derek Denny-Brown, and many others.

The modern era of neurochemistry began with the studies of Johann Thudichum, who characterized many of the sphingolipids of the nervous system. He summarized these investigations in one of the most fundamental texts of neurology *A Treatise on the Chemical Constituents of the Brain* (1884). His work laid the foundation for later studies involving the detection of specific lysosomal storage diseases. In a different area, the first studies of brain oxidative metabolism in which the arteriovenous difference in oxygen content was measured and reported by Leonard Hill and D. N. Nabarro in 1895.

Clinical neurology was able to shed centuries of confusion and mature into an active, systematic, and comprehensive discipline. Perhaps the best examples of this process relate to the new knowledge and theories about apoplexy and epilepsy. Investigation of apoplexy was based on the microvascular anatomical studies of the brainstem by Henri Duret (1873) and Otto Heubner, who demonstrated the presence of the leptomeningeal anastamotic circulation (1874). Charcot (1866) and Abel Bouchard (1872) advanced the idea that miliary aneurysms could rupture and cause intracranial hemorrhage. From a different perspective, Hans Chiari advanced the idea that occlusive disease of the extracranial vessels could cause cerebral symptoms (1905). The investigations of John Hughlings Jackson and William Gowers ushered in the modern era of the theoretical understanding and clinical classification of epilepsy. Jackson believed epilepsy to be an expression of a discharging neuronal lesion (1863); Gowers proposed the most complete and useful clinical classification of seizure types (1881). Sir

Charles Locock reported on the use of bromides for the treatment of epilepsy (1857).

This was also an era of extremely dominant personalities in neurology, best typified by Jean Martin Charcot (1825–1893). His contributions were multiple. His legendary didactic clinical Tuesday Lessons, held for many years at the Salpêtrière, attracted a worldwide audience of outstanding physicians interested in neurology. His clinicopathological correlations were important in developing concepts of cerebral localization. Among his numerous clinical contributions were the first definitive descriptions of multiple sclerosis (1868), amyotrophic lateral sclerosis (1869), and with Pierre Marie, one of the major forms of genetically determined demyelinating neuropathies (1886).

There were many other important clinical discoveries made during this time. Jean Landry described ascending paralysis in 1859. Amand Duchenne, aside from his exhaustive studies of the physiology and pathology of muscle disease, differentiated tabes dorsalis from other paralytic diseases and suggested its syphilitic etiology (1859). Prosper Menière described labyrinthine vertigo (1861) and Paul Broca, expressive aphasia (1861). George Huntington published his classical description of hereditary chorea (1872). Carl Wernicke in 1881 described hemorrhagic polioencephalitis. Heinrich Quincke introduced the lumbar puncture (1891), Anton Weichselbaum first discovered the meningococcus (1887), and Johann Heubner isolated it from cerebrospinal fluid (1896).

Neurologists also promoted their own organizations and finally obtained academic appointments. The first association of neurologists was the New York Neurological Society (1872), followed three years later by the establishment of the American Neurological Society, the first national organization of neurologists. The Société de Neurologie de Paris was founded in 1899. The first department of neurology was established in 1871 at the University of Pennsylvania. In Paris, Charcot obtained the first independent chair of neurology in 1882. In England, the Hospital for the Paralyzed and Epileptic, founded in 1860 at Queen's Square and soon known as the National Hospital, became the center of British neurology and home to such luminaries as John Hughlings Jackson, William Gowers, David Ferrier, and later S. Kinnier Wilson, and Gordon Holmes. In Germany the influence of psychiatry affected the independence of neurology, yet physicians such as Wilhelm Erb, Hermann Oppenheim, and Nikolaus Friedreich made significant contributions. Several major neurology journals were also established during the last quarter of this century, including the *Archiv für Psychiatrie und Nervenkrankheiten* (1868), the *Journal of Nervous and Mental Disease* (1876), *Brain* (1878), *Revue neurologique* (1878), and *Deutsche Zeitschrift für Nervenheilkunde* (1891).

CHILD NEUROLOGY

Modern child neurology had its clinical origins in the latter half of the nineteenth century. As this was the "golden age" of adult neurology, one of the major benefits was the attention directed towards related disorders in children, primarily in France, Germany, and England. Thus Charcot and many of those he trained made fundamental contributions reflecting his wide variety of interests. Charcot's observations on muscular atrophy led to the combined studies with Pierre Marie and the description of a form of hereditary neuropathy (1886); his involvement with hysteria and movement disorders led to his collaboration and some say bequeathing of a disease to Georges Gilles de la Tourette (1885). Others, such as Désiré Bourneville (1880), Augusta Klumpke (1885), and Jules Dejerine (1893), made important contributions to child neurology based on the firm foundation of neuropathology gleaned while students of Charcot. Bourneville, who founded the first day school for special instruction of defective children in Paris, and Edouard Séguin were both very active participants in the care of institutionalized children with neurological disorders. Bourneville is also well remembered for his description of tuberous sclerosis. Charcot's contemporary, Amand Duchenne, clearly laid the foundation for almost all subsequent studies of neuromuscular disease, both in adults and children, through his methodical clinical examinations, electrical stimulation studies, and correlative histopathology.

In Germany and Austria, the ascent of neuropathology, which helped separate neurology from psychiatry, was of particular importance to child neurology. The studies of Sigmund Freud on infantile cerebral paralysis (1891, 1893, 1897); Wilhelm Erb on brachial plexus injury (1874), muscular dystrophy (1884) and myotonic dystrophy (1886); the original observations of the weak hypotonic infant by Guido Werdnig (1891, 1894), Johann Hoffmann (1893, 1897, 1900), and Hermann Oppenheim (1900); the studies of spinal dysraphism by Friedrich von Recklinghausen (1886) and Hans Chiari (1895); and the studies of spinocerebellar degeneration by Nikolaus Friedreich (1876), are all good examples of neuropathology as it applied to the evaluation of children with these disorders.

In England a more functional and clinically oriented approach was in progress, as evidenced by two of the most eminent neurologists of this period, John Hughlings Jackson and William Gowers, and their contribution to many areas of child neurology, most importantly epilepsy, cerebral palsy, and chorea. The contributions of several other important figures of this period who were not neurologists included those of William Little (cerebral palsy, 1861), John Langdon Down (trisomy 21, 1866), Octavius Sturges (childhood chorea, 1881) William Day (headaches, 1887), and William Macewen (cerebral infections, 1893). In the United States there was a long hiatus between William Wood Gerhard's *On the Cerebral Affections of Children* (1834) and the clinical contributions of William Osler (1889, 1894) and Bernard Sachs (1895).

Overall, it appears that child neurology was just beginning to develop as a particular subspecialty and that its origins at this juncture were patterned primarily by the events and discoveries happening in adult neurology. It was not until the early twentieth century that the social, hygienic, and educational reform movements, coupled with the emergence of pediatrics and the advances in scientific knowledge, had an unalterable and positive effect on the direction and growth of child neurology. (Please see the list at the end of the Introduction for references.)

DÉSIRÉ MAGLOIRE BOURNEVILLE

DÉSIRÉ MAGLOIRE BOURNEVILLE (figure 1) was born on October 21, 1840, in Garencières, Normandy. His ancestors were Normandy farmers and his father was a small land owner. The young Bourneville studied medicine in Paris and became an intern of the hospitals of Paris: Bicêtre, Salpêtrière, St. Louis, and Pitie. He volunteered his medical services in Amiens during the severe cholera epidemic of 1866 and, in recognition of his unselfish effort, this city bestowed on him a gold watch (Benda, 1969). He returned and completed his medical studies in 1870.

Bourneville also volunteered as ambulance surgeon to the 160th battalion of the National Guard during the Franco-Prussian War (Benda, 1969). He became a medical officer of the field hospital Jardin des Plants. At the end of the war, he courageously protected hospitalized wounded soldiers from their violent revolutionary political enemies and thus helped avoid a confrontation. This was an early indication of Bourneville's quixotic character later to appear in his battles for the laicization of hospitals.

Bourneville was Charcot's pupil at the Salpêtrière. In his early university years, he was also influenced by Noel Pascal, Claude Bernard, and particularly by the psychiatrist, Louis Delasiauve, who later became his mentor at the Bicêtre. In 1870 he wrote his graduate thesis on thermometry in cerebral hemorrhage and other brain maladies (Bourneville, 1870). In 1879 Bourneville became physician to the pediatric service at the Bicêtre, a position he kept until his compulsory retirement in 1905. He organized his service according to Charcot's methods. Early in his career he developed an interest in patients with mental subnormality and was a pioneer in the development of their education.

Bourneville's early interest and dedication to medical writing led him in the year 1872 to publish Charcot's lectures under the title *Leçons sur les maladies du système nerveux faites à la Salpêtrière.* He was a contributor to the extraordinary journal *Iconographie photographique de la Salpêtrière.* After the Franco-Prussian War, he

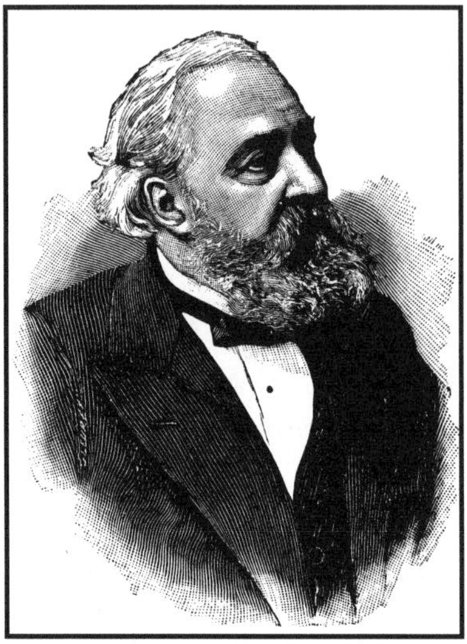

Figure 1. Désiré Magloire Bourneville (1840–1909).

founded and edited, until two years before his death, the weekly medical journal *Le progrès médical*. He used this periodical to defend vigorously his medical and political beliefs. In 1880, under Charcot's tutelage, he started the new journal *Archives de neurologie* and one year later he founded another journal *Année médicale.* He also published annual reports under the title *Recherches cliniques et thérapeutiques sur l'épilepsie, l'hystérie et l'idiotie* (Bourneville and d'Olier, 1881), a treasure of neuropathological observations with which he established his reputation as the leading European authority on all that concerned mentally retarded children (Obituary, 1909).

The greatest contributions of Bourneville were medico-pedagogic. Bourneville reorganized the education and training of mentally retarded patients at Bicêtre (Bourneville, 1892a) and created in Vitry, near Paris, a private institution for defective children of upper social classes (Bourneville, 1890; 1892a; 1892b). As a reformer, he met with much hostility when he attempted to remedy the deteriorated conditions of old hospitals. He became involved in politics as a result of his continuing efforts to benefit mentally defective patients. For seven years he served on a municipal council and in 1883 was elected representative of a Parisian sector to the Chamber of Deputies. He was then able to introduce legislation to improve the education of nurses employed by hospitals and asylums. He helped to reorganize the obstetrical services and created a body of obstetrical physicians, or *médecins-accoucheurs* (Bourneville and Blondeau, 1881). His quest for all these improvements often brought him to confrontation with some of his colleagues who opposed his views on hospital specialization. He was then exposed to misrepresentation and abuse from reactionary colleagues and politicians who opposed his progressive views and regarded him as an iconoclast, the "anticlerical type," as Léon

Daudet called him. However, he remained loyal to his principles and was always firm in defending them (Bourneville, 1881).

Although Bourneville dedicated his life to helping mentally defective patients, he is better known to medicine, and particularly to child neurology, for one major contribution to neuropathology. In 1880 he gave a detailed report of the neurologic symptoms and gross cerebral pathology of a previously unknown disease (Bourneville, 1880). His seminal paper published in the *Archives de neurologie* is entitled "Sclérose tubéreuse des circonvolutions cérébrales: Idiotie et épilepsie hémiplégique." Unknown to Bourneville was Friedrich von Recklinghausen's brief paper presented to the Obstetrical Society of Berlin in 1862 describing the pathologic findings in the heart and brain of an infant who had died shortly after birth: several myomata of the heart and a great number of scleroses of the brain were found when an autopsy was performed.

The patient described in Bourneville's first paper on tuberous sclerosis was a fifteen-year-old girl who had been having seizures since early infancy that only involved her eyes. At age two years, the seizures became more generalized. She had never been able to walk or talk. At the age of three years, she was admitted to la Salpêtrière with intractable seizures and mental retardation. When last examined at age fifteen, she had a right spastic hemiplegia and facial skin lesions described as a "confluent vesiculopapular eruption of the nose, cheeks, and forehead" and recognized as "acné rosacée et pustuleuse." She also had many skin tags ("petit molluscum") on the neck. Bourneville describes a seizure that occurred at the end of the examination as follows:

Her eyes rolled up and to the left; her arms were rigidly held against the chest, the right more than the left. Immediately after, there were clonic movements of the right limbs and at the same time rapid convulsions of both upper eyelids. Finally, there was stertorous breathing and bloody froth appeared at her mouth. (Bourneville, 1880)

For several months this girl continued to have many seizures and on May 7, 1879, she was found dead in her bed.

Postmortem examination disclosed raised, opaque, whitish areas in many of the cerebral convolutions. Bourneville summarized his findings with this conclusion: "In one word, we are dealing with a hypertrophic sclerosis of portions of the circumvolutions" (Bourneville,

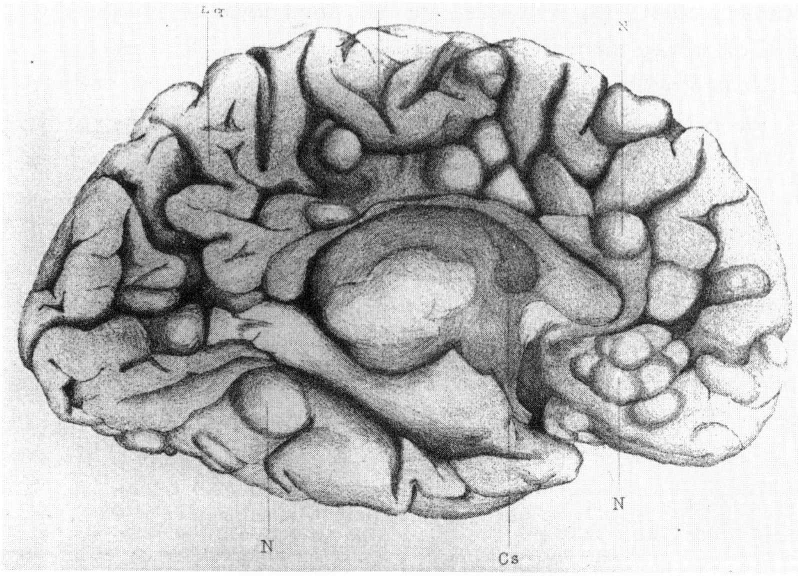

Figure 2. Drawing of brain specimen showing cerebral lesions seen in tuberous sclerosis, originally plate 7 from Bourneville and Brissaud, 1881.

1880). There were also lesions of the corpus striatum consisting of white sclerotic islands that contrasted with the gray background of the basal ganglia. The kidneys had many whitish hard round masses protruding 3 to 5 centimeters over the surface that when sectioned had the appearance of "cancerous tissue."

One year after his first paper, Bourneville published a second pathological observation in association with Brissaud (Bourneville and Brissaud, 1881). The patient was a boy admitted to the Bicêtre at age four; he had been experiencing right-sided seizures since the age of four months. He had walked at the age of two and at four could speak but only one syllable that he repeated incessantly. His seizures increased in frequency and severity. He had a loud cardiac murmur, cyanosis, and pulmonary rales. He stopped eating and drinking and died shortly thereafter on January 6, 1880. Postmortem examination disclosed sclerotic hypertrophic cerebral convolutions as reported in the fifteen-year-old patient. Brain sections demonstrated ventricles of normal size but their lateral walls were covered with many small sclerotic tumors, 2 to 5 millimeters in diameter, bunched together like grapes (figure 2). The heart was large, its ventricular wall hypertrophic, and the pulmonary infundibulum was practically obliterated. Microscopic examination of the cerebral cortex disclosed a paucity of neurons and an excess of glia in the sclerotic gyri but not in the depths of the sulci. Bourneville and Brissaud suggested that the cerebral lesions were due to a chronic inflammatory process of very slow evolution.

The significance of Bourneville's contribution is appreciated today, more than ever, because tuberous sclerosis of the brain and involvement of other organs with hamartomas are frequently recognized in living patients because of the technological advances in organ imaging. At the time of Bourneville's death in 1909, he had only begun to recognize the relation between one type of skin lesion, the facial angiofibroma, then called "adenoma sebaceum," and the cerebral disease. Today it is estimated that the prevalence of tuberous sclerosis is near one in ten thousand, that is, ten to fifteen times greater than estimated ten years ago. The challenge remains: one hundred and ten years after Bourneville's discovery, the pathogenesis of his disease is still a mystery.

Manuel R. Gomez
ROCHESTER, MINNESOTA

REFERENCES

Benda, C. E. 1969. Désiré Magloire Bourneville (1840–1909). In *The Founders of Neurology*. 2d ed. Ed. W. Haymaker and and F. Schiller, 410–413. Springfield, IL: Charles C Thomas.

Bourneville, D. M. 1870. Études de thermométrie clinique dans l'hémorragie cérébrale et dans quelques autres maladies de l'encéphale. Graduate thesis. Paris.

______. 1880. Sclérose tubéreuse des circonvolutions cérébrales: Idiotie et épilepsie hémiplégique. *Arch neur* (Paris) 1:81–91.

______. 1881. *Laicisation de l'assistance publique.* Paris.

______. 1890. *Rapports . . . sur le compte et les budgets de l'Asile de Villejuif et sur la fondation Vallée*. Paris: Imprimeries réunies.

______. 1892a. *Histoire de la section des enfants de Bicêtre (1879–92)*. 2d ed. Paris: *Le progrès médical*.

______. 1892b. *Histoire de la fondation Vallée*. 2d ed. Paris: Bicêtre.

Bourneville, D. M., and A. R. Blondeau. 1881. *Des services d'accouchements dans les hôpitaux de Paris*. Paris: A. Delahaye and E. Lecrosnier.

Bourneville, D. M., and E. Brissaud. 1881. Encéphalite ou sclérose tubéreuse des circonvolutions cérébrales. *Arch neur* (Paris) 1:390–412.

Bourneville, D. M., and H. d'Olier. 1881. *Recherches cliniques et thérapeutiques sur l'épilepsie, l'hystérie et l'idiotie. Compte rendu du service des épileptiques et des enfants idiots et arrières de Bicêtre pendant l'année 1880*. Paris: A. Delahaye.

Charcot, J. M. 1872–93. *Leçons sur les maladies du système nerveux faites à la Salpêtrière*. Ed. D. M. Bourneville Paris: A. Delahaye.

Obituary. 1909. *Brit Med J* 1(1909): 1519.

Von Recklinghausen, F. 1862. Ein Herz von einem Neugeborenen welches mehrere theils nach aussen, theils nach den Hohlen prominirende Tumoren (Myomen) trug. *Verh Ges Geburtsch* 25 Marz. 20:1–2.

JEAN MARTIN CHARCOT

FEW PEOPLE were as influential and important in the development of neurology as Jean Martin Charcot (1825–1893) (figure 1). This French medical genius took the nascent field of neurology and, by the close of his brilliant career, had defined many of its boundaries. He both asked and answered many of neurology's most important questions.

Charcot was born in Paris and early in his life wavered between the choice of a career in medicine or art. Finally deciding on a medical career, he continued to use his abilities as a talented caricaturist and combined an artistic view of his work with advancing science. Charcot began and ended his medical career at the Hôpital de la Salpêtrière where he worked primarily in the field of neurology. In 1848 when he began at the Salpêtrière, he was exposed to approximately 6,000 welfare inmates with innumerable unclassified conditions. Through careful study, observation, and description, he was able to define numerous new conditions and bring order out of chaos. His talent at nosology was perhaps his greatest contribution to the field of both adult and child neurology. He transformed the Salpêtrière into a world-class institution for neurological study and, by the time he died, had established clinical neurology as an autonomous discipline (Guillian, 1959; McHenry, 1969).

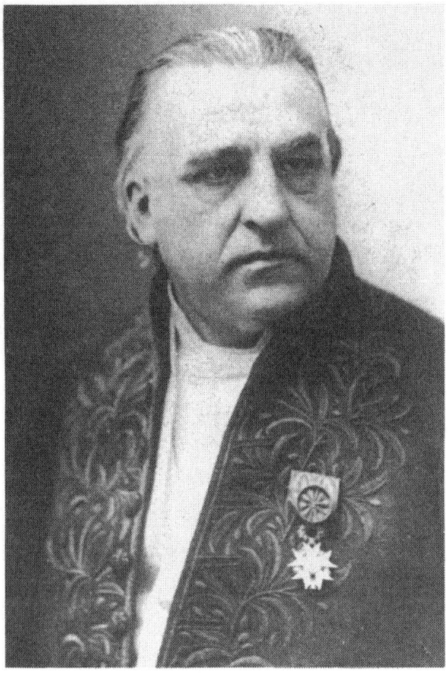

Figure 1. Jean Martin Charcot (1825–1893).

He became an intern at age twenty-three, but for nine years worked under Pierre Rayer in the areas of pathology and medicine. He wrote on diseases of the liver, lungs, and kidneys. At age thirty-six he won his aggregation and was appointed medical superintendent at the Hôpital de la Salpêtrière. He was a masterful blend of observing clinician, rigorous scientist, and artist. He worked with Alfred Vulpian, became a distinguished neuropathologist, and took the Chair of Pathological Anatomy in 1872. In 1881 he published his book *Leçons sur les maladies du système nerveux faites à la Salpêtrière* (*Lectures on the Diseases of the Nervous System Delivered at the Salpêtrière*). Indeed, according to McHenry, this date marks the founding of neuropathology as a separate branch of pathology (McHenry, 1969). Charcot distinguished multiple sclerosis from Parkinsonism and firmly established multiple sclerosis as an entity (Charcot, 1868a). In 1882 he was appointed first professor to occupy the chair of diseases of the nervous system. His concept of neuroanatomy included that of cerebral localization. He described the arthropathies found in tabes dorsalis, still known today as Charcot joints. He named and first described amyotrophic lateral sclerosis (Charcot, 1868b, 1869, 1874).

One of Charcot's major contributions to child neurology is the paper he and Pierre Marie published in 1886 on peroneal muscular atophy. In this paper they described five children and one additional case report of Schultze. Their first patient, Maxime W., was typical of the clinical syndrome (figures 2a, b). He was seen at age nine years with a four-year history of inturning his feet. The child had foot drop, moderately severe atrophy and weakness of the legs, milder arm involvement, and depressed deep tendon re-

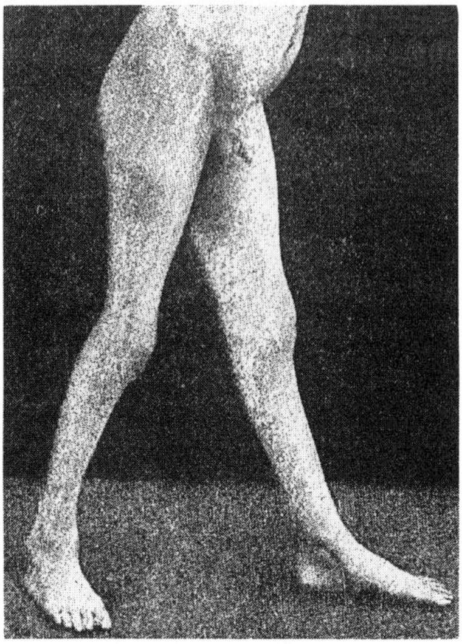

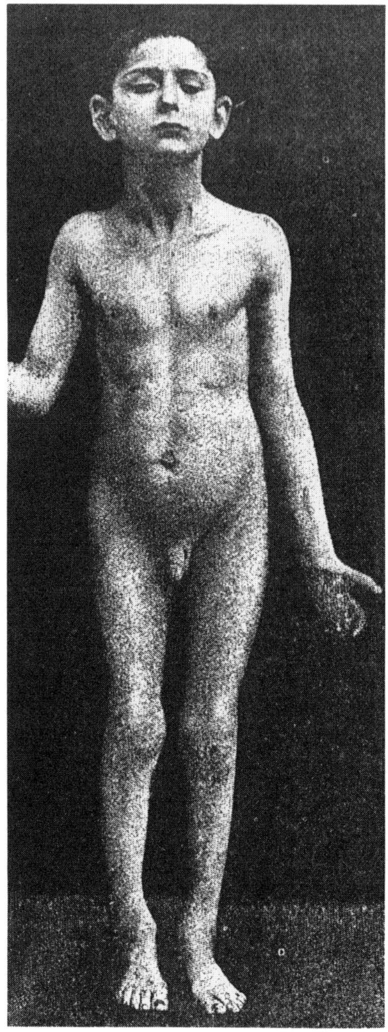

Figures 2a, 2b. Maxime W., a nine-year-old boy who suffered from progressive atrophy and weakness. His brother, age three years, had a similar disorder. This was Charcot and Marie's first patient with Charcot-Marie-Tooth disease (Charcot and Marie, 1886). Figure 2a on left was originally figure 1 in this paper; figure 2b was originally figure 2.

flexes. His brother, aged a little over three years, had similar atrophy. There were no pathological studies accompanying this report but Charcot and Marie summarized the symptoms of these patients; we recognize these symptoms today as "Charcot-Marie-Tooth disease." They also observed that sensation was usually, but not always, intact, and that signs of vasomotor instability were present. H. H. Tooth's much more extensive description in his Cambridge thesis *The Peroneal Type of Progressive Muscular Atrophy* was published the same year and earned his eponymic inclusion in this disorder that now has the less glamorous but scientifically more accepted name of hereditary motor sensory neuropathy, Type I.

Charcot, with Alex Joffroy, also formulated the concept that poliomyelitis was due to progressive degeneration of the anterior horn cells and expressed the idea that an "irritation" suddenly seized anterior horn cells in the spinal cord, causing these cells to cease functioning (Charcot and Joffroy, 1870). He and Joffroy also demonstrated that progressive muscular atrophy was due to loss of anterior horn cells (Charcot and Joffroy, 1869). Charcot was one of the first to describe ankle clonus in 1862. Toward the end of his career, Charcot became known for his work on hysteria, laying the groundwork for Janet and Freud (McHenry, 1969).

This extraordinary man made other contributions to the field of child neurology. Included among these contributions was his work on delineating the clinical presentations of childhood neuromuscular diseases, primarily forms of muscular dystrophy and atrophy. These investigations appeared serially in a collection of papers and lectures from 1874 to 1895 (Charcot, 1874; 1881a–d; 1895). Charcot substantially influenced Duchenne, introducing him to the techniques of microscopy and the value of histologic study of muscle tissue. Charcot also emphasized heredity as a cause of many neurologic disorders, particularly the childhood muscular atrophies (Charcot, 1881d). This shift in focus was the basis for much later work in the field of child neurology.

Charcot had many indirect influences in the area of child neurology. His emphasis on keen observation and reclassification and his work on nosology did much to advance the study of neurology. However, probably the most important contribution Charcot made to the field of child neurology was his influence on his pupils. He was a masterful and scholarly teacher and his Tuesday lectures were landmarks of clinical observation, into which he carefully integrated the latest scientific theories (Goetz, 1987). Among those who studied with Charcot were Edouard Brissaud, Joseph Babinski, Désiré Bourneville, Henri Duret, Ludwig Edinger, Sigmund Freud, Georges Gilles de la Tourette, Aleksei Kozhevnikov, Pierre Marie, Georges Marinesco, William Osler, Edward Constant Séguin, and Bernard Sachs.

An example of Charcot's clinical and didactic skills as it applies to child neurology can be seen in one of his Tuesday lessons (Charcot, 1872) as extracted from the recent translations by C. G. Goetz (1987, 73–77). Charcot had reviewed some of the basic concepts of chorea and was now in the process of taking a history and examining a twelve-year-old girl with Sydenham chorea:

So, we have a case of chorea. This young girl, so calm in appearance, continually moves her fingers and keeps her two feet as close to one another as possible to control involuntary leg movements. I am also told she originally was a bit aphasic. Her tongue has choreic movements, and from time to time, she involuntarily utters a tiny sound. How long has she been ill?

MOTHER *One month.*

CHARCOT: *Is this the first time?*

MOTHER: *Yes.*

CHARCOT: *Where did it begin?*

MOTHER: *The hands.*

CHARCOT: *Both simultaneously?*

MOTHER: *Yes, but over the last two days the movements are more severe.*

CHARCOT: *What does she do, is she in school?*

MOTHER: *She works with me.*

CHARCOT: *Has she had joint pains or rheumatism?*

MOTHER: *She has never complained of pain.*

CHARCOT: *Does her father have joint problems?*

MOTHER: *Yes, Doctor.*

CHARCOT: *Did he, to your knowledge, ever stay in bed for five to six weeks for such joint pains?*

MOTHER: *Four months, Doctor.*

CHARCOT: *Rheumatism is part of the past history of this case. . . . Alright, for this young girl, clearly we have identified an arthritic influence, in relationship to her chorea. And now to see if there is more. What does her father do?*

MOTHER: *He works in a glass factory heating glass.*

CHARCOT: *He is exposed to high heats and suffers from rheumatism. We must not simply conclude that the chill related to these abnormal temperature exposures is the underlying cause of his rheumatism. No, we want to identify the hereditary influences that must be there if we search. Does your husband have brothers?*

MOTHER: *Two.*

CHARCOT: *Where do they live?*

MOTHER: *One in Boulogne, the other in Paris.*

CHARCOT: *Do you know them?*

MOTHER: *Yes.*

CHARCOT: *Are they ill?*

MOTHER: *No.*

CHARCOT: *They have no neurologic problems?*

MOTHER: *No, Doctor.*

CHARCOT: *I do not bother asking her whether other family members have chorea, since neurologic entities hardly ever are passed on from generation to generation in the same form. Hence, never look for locomotor ataxia or even general paresis to be transmitted from a patient to a child. No, instead each generation may modify the expression of the familial illness. . . .*

(Now Charcot addresses the patient.)

Now, my child, would you like to say something? (The child says nothing.) Now watch her hand movements increase. She fears she will be unable to keep such movements in check. These movements are so bizarre that some say they must be made on purpose, like a clown at the circus, specifically to make people laugh, "more circulatorum" to use Sydenham's expression. She slaps her feet with no fixed rhythm, showing quite clearly the completely different character of this arrhythmic chorea from that of a rhythmic chorea of which I spoke earlier. What is your name?

PATIENT: *Leonie.*

CHARCOT: *Here is a pen; please write your name and where you live. (As she does, her foot taps throughout the task.) She has not written a single complete word. One of her fingers lifts up involuntarily. She looks at me with pleading eyes to ask me to relieve her of this suffering for her chorea is truly troublesome. Her tongue and lips move about irregularly and impede her speech. (The young girl shyly responds.)*

PATIENT: *I live in Cité de la Chappelle.*

CHARCOT: *See how her speech is a bit explosive. Have you been biting your tongue?*

PATIENT: *Yes.*

CHARCOT: *I do hope this problem abates. So here is a case of chorea presenting with this very particular lip and tongue movement. (Turning to the mother) Does she sleep?*

MOTHER: *Very little. When she awakens her movements disrupt the sheets and blankets. She grabs the pillow and flings it into the air.*

CHARCOT: *So her personality is a bit affected, a mild delirium. This case is rather interesting. Chorea almost always provokes personality changes with temporary mental decline. I have seen multilingual patients who during the chorea could only use one language, a sort of selective aphasia demonstrating their weakened intellectual state. . . . (Turning again to the mother) Is she subject to nervous attacks?*

MOTHER: *Yes, many.*

CHARCOT: *Does she cry or laugh inappropriately?*

MOTHER: *Her personality is altogether changed since the illness began.*

CHARCOT: *(Addressing an intern) Check her pain sensation.*

INTERN: *It is normal.*

CHARCOT: *Listen to her heart.*

INTERN: *It is regular.*

CHARCOT: *The patient's chorea is of significant intensity, not so much in the limbs, but in her face. And accompanying this is a change in personality, giving this case a rather special character. Now, we must turn to the care of the patient. What can we tell her and what is her prognosis? Chorea is almost always benign and resolves spontaneously in two to three months. There are some significant exceptions. We all know that adult-onset chorea is more serious than childhood chorea, most importantly, chorea during pregnancy. Also, regardless of patient age, chorea is dangerous to the patient's health if the movements become so prominent and wild that he cannot sleep. Fortunately, such severe chorea is rare. However, when one is faced with such cases, the physician's position becomes particularly uncomfortable, first because he has little to offer therapeutically and second because it is especially disheartening to see a condition that usually has no long-term consequences turn malignant and deadly.*

This complex man brought to his clinical studies his many artistic talents. Writing in collaboration with Paul Richer, Charcot's artistic skills were best seen in his two volumes *Les Difformes et les malades dans l'art* (Charcot, 1889) and *Les Démoniaques dans l'art* (Charcot, 1897). While changing the landscape of neurology, he established the first great institution of neurology at the Salpêtrière. While on vacation in 1893, Charcot died suddenly at the age of sixty-eight. His legacy, however, remains.

Mark S. George
CHARLESTON, SOUTH CAROLINA

Stephen Ashwal
LOMA LINDA, CALIFORNIA

REFERENCES

Charcot, Jean Marie. 1868a. Histologie de la sclérose en plaques. *Gaz hôp* (Paris) 41:554, 557, 566.

______. 1868b. Sur quelques arthropathies qui paraissent dépendre d'une lésion cerveau ou de la moëlle épinière. *Arch physiol norm path*, 1:161.

______. 1869. Ataxie locomotrice progressive; arthropatrie de l'épaule gauche, résultats nécroséopiques. *Arch phys norm path* 2:121.

______. 1872. *Leçons sur les maladies du système nerveux faites à la Salpêtrière*. Paris: A. Delahaye.

______. 1874. Des amyotrophies spinales chroniques. *Progrès méd* 2:573.

______. 1881a. *Lectures on the Diseases of the Nervous System*. London: The New Sydenham Society. Reprinted 1962, New York, Haffner Publishing Company under the auspices of the Library of the New York Academy of Medicine.

______. 1881b. *Lectures* . . . Vol. 3. Lecture 14: Nosographical Revision of the Amyotrophies, 165. Ed. MM Marie and Guinon.

______. 1881c. *Lectures* . . . Vol. 2. Lecture 11: Chronic Spinal Amyotrophies. Protopathic Spinal Progressive Muscular Atrophy (Duchenne-Aran Type), 163.

______. 1881d. *Lectures. . .* Vol 3. Lecture 14: Nosographical Revision of the Amyotrophies, 164.

______. 1889. *Les Difformes et les malades dans l'art.* Paris: Lecrosnier and Babe.

______. 1895. *Contribution à l'étude de l'atrophie musculaire progressive type Duchenne-Aran.* Paris: Félix Alcan.

______. 1897. *Démoniaques dans l'art.* Paris: Delahaye and Lecrosnier.

Charcot, J. M., and A. Joffroy. 1869. Deux cas d'atrophie musculaire progressive avec lésions de la substance grise et des faisceaux antéro-latéraux de la moelle épinière. *Arch phys norm path* 2:744.

______. 1870. Une observation de paralysie infantile s'accompagnant d'une altération des cornes antérieures de la substance grise de la moelle. *Compte rend Soc Biol* (Paris) 1:312.

Charcot J. M. and P. Marie. 1886. Sur une forme particulière d'atrophie musculaire progressive souvent familiale débutant par les pieds et les jambes et atteignant plus tard les mains. *Rev méd* 6:97–138.

Goetz, C. G. 1987. *Charcot, the Clinician: The Tuesday Lessons.* New York: Raven Press.

Guillian, G. 1959. *J. M. Charcot, (1825–1893): His Life — His Work.* Translated by Pearce Bailey. New York: Paul B. Hoeber.

McHenry, L. C. 1969. *Garrison's History of Neurology.* Springfield, Illinois: Charles C Thomas.

Tooth, H. H. 1886. *The Peroneal Type of Progressive Muscular Atrophy.* London: H. K. Lewis.

HANS CHIARI

HANS CHIARI (figure 1) was born in Vienna on November 4, 1851, the son of gynecologist Johann Baptist Chiari. Chiari studied pathology in Vienna under Carl Rokitansky (1804–1878) and received his degree in 1875 (Fischer, 1932). Vienna, at that time, was the center of medical progress. This was in no small measure due to the presence of Rokitansky, who was the foremost pathologist of his time. He is reported to have performed over 30,000 autopsies (Long, 1965). Rokitansky is known for developing a systematic necropsy method that is still in use today and for defining disease in terms of anatomic involvement rather than as lists of symptoms. To be trained by such a man was to be at the forefront of medical knowledge. Richard Heschl (1824–1881) assumed control of the department of pathologic anatomy following Rokitansky's retirement in 1875. Heschl made significant contributions on pulmonary infarction, the calcification of ganglion cells, and the staining characteristics of amyloid (Long, 1965). Chiari was his assistant until Heschl's death in 1881 and then moved to Prague, where he succeeded Edwin Klebs as professor of pathology. While in Vienna, Chiari became known for his detailed pathologic observations and his skill at teaching, but it was in Prague that the Austrian pathologist's best-known work was performed. He remained there until 1906 before moving to Strassburg, where he died on May 6, 1916.

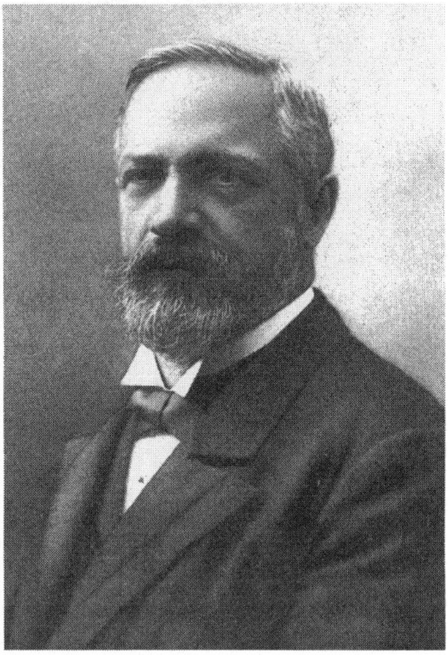

Figure 1. Photograph of Hans Chiari (1851–1916) at age 57 from the Festschrift honoring his twenty-fifth year as a Professor.

The scope of Chiari's interest was wide and his contributions extend beyond neurology. Chiari was the first to describe choriocarcinoma in 1877 (Morton, 1970) and gained eponymous fame for his work on the Budd-Chiari syndrome. The Budd-Chiari syndrome, characterized by thrombosis of the hepatic vein, was first mentioned by Lambron in 1842 and then discussed by Budd in the 1846 edition of his book on liver disease, but a clinical and pathologic explanation of the syndrome was finally provided by Chiari in 1899 (Durham, 1963). Other areas of interest included the effects of syphilis on the stomach (1891) and aorta (1906) (Morton, 1970). He also wrote a history of pathology (1903), considered to be the best modern history of pathology at that time (Garrison, 1929).

Although best known in neurology for his work on hindbrain anomalies, Chiari contributed other observations as well. In 1884 Chiari described the fist case of traumatic pneumocephaly (Walker, 1951). In an autopsy specimen, he traced a fistula from the ethmoid sinus to an air-filled cavity in the frontal lobe. Mistakenly, however, he implicated

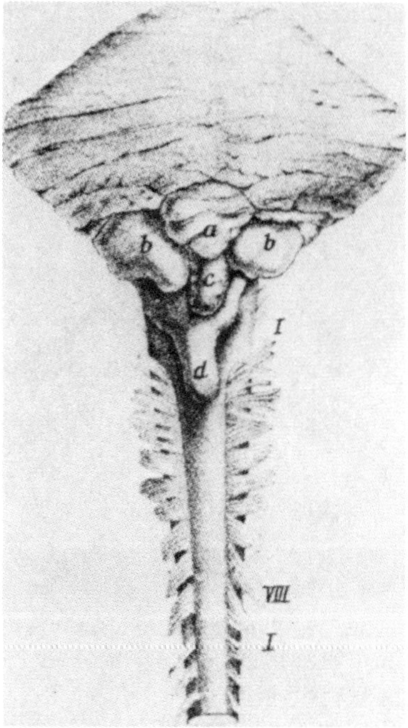

Figure 2. Chiari's illustration of the Type 2 malformation from his 1896 article "Über Veranderungen des Kleinhirns." Note that the fourth ventricle (d) and vermis (c) are displaced caudally and the upper cervical roots run upward to their foramina.

sneezing as the causative factor. More significantly, Chiari (1905) proposed that atherosclerosis of the carotid bifurcation could be responsible for intracranial embolism (McHenry, 1969). Prior to this time, diseases of the extracranial blood vessels were not thought to be a significant cause of cerebral embolism. Nine years later, Ramsey Hunt described the effect of carotid artery occlusion, confirming Chiari's hypothesis. Chiari also described platybasia, but his report followed Virchow's by approximately twenty years (McHenry, 1969).

Chiari's major achievement and principal contribution to child neurology was his pathologic study and classification of congenital brainstem abnormalities associated with hydrocephalus. The initial report in 1891 presented at the 64th meeting of the Association of German Naturalists and Physicians described his findings from autopsies performed at the Kaiser Franz Joseph Children's Hospital in Prague (Chiari, 1891; for an English translation see Wilkens, 1976). He separated the malformations into three groups and noted that a full description would subsequently be published. His major analysis followed five years later when he described the findings in sixty-three patients with hydrocephalus and confirmed his groupings (Chiari, 1896; Ogryzlo, 1942). Currently, we divide the anomalies into four types. Type 1 is associated with elongation of the cerebellar tonsils and the medial portions of the inferior cerebellar lobes so they extend into the upper part of the cervical canal. There is no medullary displacement associated with Chiari Type 1. Chiari described fourteen cases of the Type 1 malformation. The ages of his subjects ranged from three months to sixty-eight years and the majority of the subjects were adults. All of his Type 1 patients had hydrocephalus and one had a meningomyelocele. Type 2 includes caudal displacement of the pons, medulla, and vermis into the upper part of the cervical canal, elongation of the fourth ventricle and frequently a lumbar meningomyelocele (figure 2). Type 2 is also known as the Arnold-Chiari malformation. Chiari described seven cases of the Type 2 malformation with the ages of the subjects ranging from birth to six months. Hydrocephalus and spina bifida were present in all seven cases. There were five cases with a meningomyelocele, one case with a meningocele and one had spinal rachischisis. In Type 3 there is inferior displacement of the brainstem with herniation of the cerebellum and a meningoencephalocele, and Type 4 consists of cerebellar hypoplasia. Chiari described only a single case of the Type 3 malformation in a five-month-old infant. He did not describe the Type 4 malformation.

Although speculative, Chiari's interest in hindbrain anomalies may have been kindled by Rokitansky's fourteen-year study of congenital defects of the cardiac septum. Rokitansky's monograph appeared in 1875, the year Chiari received his doctoral degree, and was hailed as his greatest work (Long, 1965). Perhaps Chiari felt by studying congenital neurologic malformations he could make a contribution analogous to Rokitansky's work on the heart.

Chiari's seminal role in the development of this classification scheme is not disputed; however, he was not the first to describe the Type 2 malformation. This distinction belongs to John Cleland who, in 1883, described the anomaly eight years prior to Chiari's first paper (Carmel and Markesbery, 1972). Cleland, a British anatomist and surgeon, described his findings on the autopsies of nine infants and two chick embryos and proposed that the primary cause of this condition was dysgenesis of the brainstem. His speculations on the etiology proved prescient, but Chiari's view that hydrocephalus was the initiating event long held dominance. Cleland was all but forgotten. Julius Arnold (1835–1915), a German pathologist, reported his findings in an infant with multiple congenital anomalies in 1894 (Fischer, 1932). One of the anomalies was a Chiari Type 2 malformation. This became known as the Arnold-Chiari malformation as a result of subsequent work by Schwalbe and Gredig, who worked in Arnold's laboratory in Heidelberg (Carmel and Markesbery, 1972). Arnold's claim to the malformation is certainly less strong than Cleland's but it is unlikely that there will be a change in the eponym at this time. It is also clear that it would not be an overstatement to simply refer to these anomalies as Chiari malformations.

The malformations described by Chiari evoked little interest until 1935 when Russell and Charles Donald reported that in ten consecutive cases of patients with spina bifida and hydrocephalus they also found Chiari Type 2 malformations. They further speculated that the hindbrain anomaly was the cause of the hydrocephalus. Perhaps because of the potential for treatment by advances in neurosurgical technique, this paper generated more interest than Chiari's original work and was soon followed by publications on pathogenesis, premorbid diagnosis, and neurosurgical management (Penfield and Coburn, 1938; Adams, Schatzki, and Scoville, 1941; Ingraham and Scott, 1943). Since the 1930s the Chiari malformations have remained a topic of intense interest. By 1906 Chiari's major contributions to medical science were complete, but he remained active as a teacher and pathologist. At the time of his death in 1916, he was scheduled to be a principal speaker at the German war pathologists conference in Berlin, but he died following an attack of angina pectoris (Aschoff, 1916). He was sixty-four years old.

James R. Burke

E. Wayne Massey

DURHAM, NORTH CAROLINA

REFERENCES

Adams, R. D., R. Schatzki, and W. B. Scoville. 1941. The Arnold-Chiari Malformation. *NEJM* 225:125–131.

Arnold, J. 1894. Myelocyste, Transposition von Gewebskeimen und Sympodie. *Beitr path Anat allg Path* 16:1–28.

Aschoff, L. 1916. Obituary of Hans Chiari. *Beitr path Anat allg Path* 62:402.

Bamberger-Bozo, C. 1987. The Chiari II Malformation. In *Handbook of Clinical Neurology*. Vol. 50, 403–12. Ed. P. J. Vinken and G. W. Bruyn. Amsterdam: North Holland Publishing Company.

Carmel, P. W. and W. R. Markesbery. 1972. Early description of the Arnold-Chiari Malformation. *J Neurosurg* 37:543–47.

Chiari, H. 1891. Über Veranderungen des Kleinhirns in Folge von Hydrocephalie des Grosshirns. *Dtsch med Wschr* 17:1172–75.

______. 1896. Über Veranderungen des Kleinhirns, des Pons und Medulla oblongata in folge von kongenitaler Hydrocephalie des Grosshirns. *Dtsch Akad Wiss* Wien 63:71–116.

______. 1905. Über das Verhalten des Teilungswinkels der Carotis communis bei der Endasteritis chronic Deformans. *Verh dtsch path Ges* 9:326.

Cleland, J. 1883. Contribution to the Study of Spina Bifida, Encephalocele, and Anencephalus. *J Anat Physiol* 17:257–91.

Dittrich, P. 1908. *Festschrift Herrn Hofrat Prof. Dr. Hans Chiari.* Vienna and Leipzig: Wilhelm Braumuller.

Durham, R. H. 1963. *Encyclopedia of Medical Syndromes.* New York: Paul B. Hoeber, Inc.

Fischer, I. 1932. *Biographisches Lexicon*. Berlin: Urban and Schwarzenberg.

Garrison, F. H. 1929. *An Introduction to the History of Medicine.* 4th ed. Philadelphia: W. B. Saunders Co.

Ingraham, D. F. and H. W. Scott. 1943. Spina Bifida and Crania Bifidum. *NEJM* 229:108–14.

Long, E. R. 1965. *A History of Pathology*. New York: Dover Publications, Inc.

McHenry, L. C. 1969. *Garrison's History of Neurology*. Springfield, IL: Charles C Thomas.

Morton, L. T. 1970. *A Medical Bibliography* (Garrison and Morton). Philadelphia: J. P. Lippincott Co.

Ogryzlo, M. A. 1942. The Arnold-Chiari Malformation. *Arch Neur Psych* 48:30–46.

Penfield, W., and D. F. Coburn. 1938. Arnold-Chiari Malformation and its Operative Treatment. *Arch Neur Psych* 40:328–36.

Russell, D. S., and C. Donald. 1935. The Mechanism of Internal Hydrocephalus in Spina Bifida. *Brain* 58:203–15.

Walker, A. E. 1951. *A History of Neurologic Surgery*. Baltimore: Williams and Wilkins.

Wilkins, R. H. 1976. The Arnold-Chiari Malformation. *Arch Neur* 25:376.

EDWARD COPEMAN

EDWARD COPEMAN (1809–1880) (figure 1) was born in Great Witchingham, Norfolk, England. He began his studies of medicine with a local surgeon, Mr. Arthur Brown of Norwich, and after two years, when Brown died, transferred to Mr. John G. Crosse, an eminent surgeon of the time. During this appren-

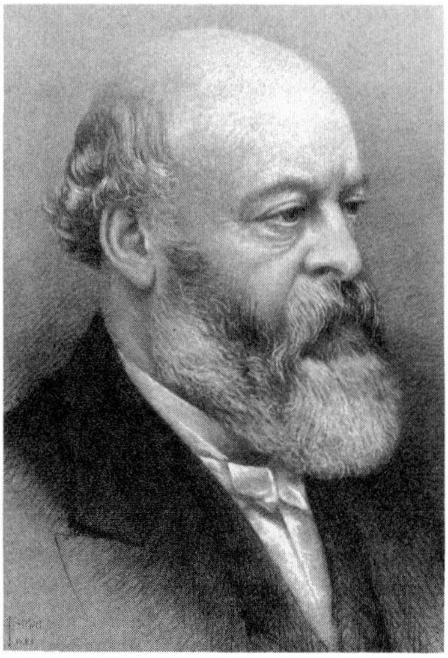

Figure 1. Edward Copeman (1809–1880).

ticeship he served as a "dresser" (medical student) at the Norfolk and Norwich Hospital. He then studied at St. George's Hospital in London and in 1831 became a licentiate of the Apothecaries' Society and, one year later, a member of the Royal College of Surgeons. Soon afterwards, he was elected House Surgeon to the Norfolk and Norwich Hospital and subsequently went into private practice in Coltishall, Norfolk. In 1845 he passed his examinations and became a fellow of the Royal College of Surgeons and in 1847 received his Doctor of Medicine from King's College, Aberdeen. Subsequently he became a member (1859) and then fellow (1871) of the Royal College of Physicians of London.

Copeman had an extensive practice but his principal services were as physician to the Norfolk and Norwich Hospital, a position he held from 1851 to 1878. He was highly regarded as an obstetrician, but was also on the staff of the Norwich Eye Infirmary and one of the founders and first physicians on the staff of the Jenny Lind Hospital for Children, named after the famous singer known as "the Swedish Nightingale," who helped raise substantial monies for this institution. Among his other achievements were his position as president of the East Anglia Branch of the British Medical Association, national president of the British Medical Association in 1874, fellow of the Obstetrical Society of London, and president of the Norwich Pathological Society.

Copeman was an enthusiastic lover of music and a violoncello player of considerable ability. He was very active in the management of the local Norfolk and Norwich music festivals for many years for which, upon resigning these responsibilities, he received a "handsome tea and coffee service" by the Lord Lieutenant and leading citizens of the county (Obituary, 1880a). Copeman was also active in community affairs, serving as a local magistrate of the city. He was described as a "warm friend," "a most upright man," and "was held in high esteem by all classes" (Obituary, 1880b). Copeman led a very active life and was busily engaged in medical practice up until the day before his death at age seventy-one on February 25, 1880.

Copeman's medical writings were quite extensive and varied. He wrote on several medical subjects including apoplexy, diphtheria, and intestinal obstruction, but he was mainly interested in obstetrics. He edited *Crosse's Cases in Midwifery*, and published several papers, including "Records of Obstetric Consultative Practice," "Illustrations of Puerperal Fever," and "On Flooding After Delivery." He received some degree of obstetrical fame locally for advocating uterine dilatation as a treatment for vomiting of pregnancy, an ineffective practice which in modern obstetrics would not be utilized because of the risks of introducing infection or precipitating premature delivery.

Copeman's inclusion in a book dedicated to the Founders of Child Neurology is based on his *Report on the Cerebral Affections of Infancy with a Few Comments and Practical Remarks*, published in 1873. It is, perhaps, the fourth independent and separate work in English that deals with the wide variety of clinical disorders that now encompass what is perceived as the field of child neurology. Charles West's *Disorders of the Nervous System in Childhood* had been published two years previously in 1871. Copeman's work also predated two lesser-known monographs, one by Walter C. Dendy entitled *On the Cerebral Diseases of Children with Regard to Their Early Manifestations and Treatment* (1848) and a second by Valentine Duke, published in Dublin in 1849 that was entitled *An Essay on the Cerebral Affections Occuring Most Commonly in Infancy and Childhood: Including Notices of Their History, Causes, Diagnosis, Prognosis and Treatment.* This ninety-page unreferenced monograph had received the Council Prize Essay at the annual meeting of the provincial Medical and Surgical Association held in Bath, England in 1848. It most likely was used by Copeman as a model for his own work. Copeman's monograph predated the more comprehensive, and what is considered the first textbook in English on child neurology, Bernard Sach's *A Treatise on the Nervous Diseases of Children*, by slightly more than twenty years (Sachs, 1895).

Copeman's monograph is primarily a historical review of the

field of child neurology by a physician with an obstetrical bent who obviously showed concern for the infants and children whom he delivered and cared for. The preface of this work demonstrates many of the previously attested qualities of this man:

The object of the following report is to offer as complete a description as possible of the phenomena and treatment of a class of diseases which cannot fail to enlist the sympathies of all who have to deal with them in practice. I have myself profited by the study required for compiling it and would fain believe that others who may be induced to read it carefully, will not retire from the task without having derived an amount of information in this very interesting department of medicine, which will repay them for the little time and trouble occupied by its perusal. Should this be so, the labour required for its production will not have been in vain. (Copeman, 1873)

Copeman's review begins with the comments on infantile seizures in *De Morbis acutis infantum* by Walter Harris (1715). He notes that Harris "recommends bleeding under certain circumstances but only in the intervals between the convulsive fits, and not during the fit." Harris also strongly advocated the use of simple pharmaceutical remedies for the treatment of seizures rather than the complicated mixtures that had little scientific basis. To this Copeman remarks:

Indeed for many years after his time the art of prescribing continued complicated and indefinite, and it was left for the present generation to separate the good from the bad, to choose the former and discard the latter; for although physicians of the present day employ a more exhaustive range of medicinal agents than Dr. Harris advised, yet they approach much nearer to the simplicity of his method, particularly with reference to patients of tender years. (Copeman, 1873, 4)

Copeman then mentions one of the first descriptions of hydrocephalus by Dr. George Armstrong in *An Account of the Diseases Most Incident to Children* (1767). Armstrong noted that hydrocephalus internus was a cause of seizures in children and he reviewed three cases, including one of his own, in which the patitents were treated with calomel that demonstrated the "curability" of this disease, though the disease probably resolved itself. These reviews were followed by a concise summary of the next important work in the field of child neurology, that of

Robert Whytt's *Observations on the Dropsy of the Brain* (1768), the first definitive description of tuberculous meningitis in which Whytt noted both the presence of hydrocephalus and the progression of the disease through three stages.

Copeman then proceeded to mention several other minor works by Fothergill, Percival, and Quinn, and discussed in depth Joseph Lieutaud's *Synopsis* (1770) and the well-known pediatric treatise of Michael Underwood (1784), both of which discussed the different causes of hydrocephalus and epilepsy. Had Copeman read the second edition of Underwood's work (1789), he might have also mentioned the first description of polio. It is worth mentioning that Copeman's observations of infants with "inward fits" is in contradistinction to that of Underwood. Copeman, noting what we would call minor motor or myoclonic seizures, believed these to be of grave consequence; Underwood chose to minimize their significance considering them to be due to "wind upon the stomach" or "chronic croup" (Copeman, 1873, 23).

Then followed an extensive discussion of Joseph Capuron's *Traité des maladies des enfans* (1813) in which detailed descriptions of convulsions and their causes are given, and mention is made of epilepsy and its hereditary nature. "Ataxic or nervous fever," which Pinel had named "cerebral fever" and which we recognize as bacterial meningitis, is considered as well as congenital hydrocephalus. Although Copeman had no comment, he extracted the following from Capuron's work concerning the treatment of hydrocephalus:

> *Lecat proposed paracentesis or puncturing the cephalic tumor, but it was rejected as a rash proceeding by Camper. The operation could not restore the brain to a healthy state, when that organ had been partially or entirely destroyed. It has also been recommended to apply a circular bandage round the head, to oppose by gentle pressure the separation of the bones of the cranium; but this method has always proved either injurious or insufficient.* (Copeman, 1873, 39)

Thus Copeman was not only a thoughtful clinician willing to try unusual methods to treat devastating diseases, but he was also well aware of their limitations. The works of Carmichael Smyth (1814), James M. Coley (1813), and John Clarke (1815) are also mentioned. In Clarke's *Commentaries on Some of the Most Important*

Diseases of Children, Copeman extracted the following clinical observations of what appears to be cerebral herniation and to which he later adds his own observations:

The state of the pupil now begins to be altered — as the retina becomes less sensible, the iris is more expanded; but, in the first instance, it often has a vibratory motion, consisting of alternate contractions and relaxations quickly repeated, especially upon sudden changes in the intensity of light falling upon the eye. Afterwards, the expanded state of the pupil becomes more permanent, till at length the iris will not contract in the smallest degree when the strongest light is brought close to the eye; and the child then becomes altogether blind. Whilst these changes are going on in the vision the muscles which direct the eye are also affected. Those which turn the eyes outwards are weakest, therefore lose their power in the greatest degree, and one or both of the eyes are turned towards the nose, and squinting is the consequence.
(Copeman, 1873, 50)

Copeman, in response to the above, makes the following observations from his own experience of autopsied cases, findings that we now consider as a very purulent form of bacterial meningitis, with extensive arachnoidal compression of the optic nerves causing the loss of pupillary responses:

The writer has seen the optic nerves entirely embedded in a sheath of coagulating lymph, extending backwards to the thalami nervorum opticorum, and to the medulla oblongata, from which it has been easy to detach considerable portions of laminated coagulating lymph. (Copeman, 1873, 53)

The remainder of Copeman's monograph deals with two other exceptional pediatric volumes and focuses primarily on hydrocephalus. These include James Risdon Bennett's *The Causes, Nature, Diagnosis, and Treatment of Acute Hydrocephalus, or Water in the Head* for which he received the Fothergillian Gold Medal in 1842, and the section on "Cerebral Diseases of Infancy" in the monumental pediatric work by Barthez and Rilliet, published in 1843. Copeman's summary is balanced and complete, but too extensive to review here. He concludes his book by providing several additional personal cases, recognizing others who have contributed to the understanding of neurological disorders of children, and finally summarizing several major observations and points of discrepancy that he extracted from his review.

Copeman is representative of many exceptional physicians who made substantive contributions in fields of medicine where little was known. These contributions were not by making a new discovery, but by helping to review and organize information, by stressing the importance of clinical observation, by correlating clinical symptoms with pathology, and by having the force of character to publish such information for the education of their colleagues and ultimately the welfare of children with such disorders. His book not only imparts a wealth of information about the field of child neurology in the nineteenth century, but his personality and character reflect a thoughtful and concerned physician.

Stephen Ashwal
LOMA LINDA, CALIFORNIA

ACKNOWLEDGMENTS

I wish to thank Dr. Anthony Batty Shaw, Emeritus Physician and Archivist of the Norfolk and Norwich Hospital, for providing much of the personal information about Dr. Copeman, as well as furnishing the portrait photograph.

REFERENCES

Armstrong, G. 1767. *An Account of the Diseases Most Incident to Children from Their Birth till the Age of Puberty; With a Successful Method of Treating Them.* London: T. Cadell.

Barthez, A. C. E., and F. Rilliet. 1843. *Traité clinique et pratique des maladies des enfants.* Paris: Alcan.

Bennett, J. R. 1843. *The Causes, Nature, Diagnosis, and Treatment of Acute Hydrocephalus, or Water in the Head.* London: S. Highley.

Capuron, J. 1813. *Traité des maladies des enfans, jusqu'à la puberté.* Paris: Croublebois.

Clarke, J. 1815. *Commentaries on Some of the Most Important Diseases of Children.* London: Longman, Hurst, Rees, Orme and Brown.

Coley, J. M. 1813. *A Practical Treatise on the Remittent Fever of Infants with Remarks on Hydrocephalus internus or Water in the Brain, and Several Other Diseases.* London: G. Nicholson.

Copeman, E. 1873. *A Report on the Cerebral Affections of Infancy with a Few Comments and Practical Remarks.* Norwich: Fletcher and Son.

Dendy, W. C. 1848. *On the Cerebral Diseases of Children, with Regard to Their Early Manifestations and Treatment*. London: John Churchill.

Duke, Valentine. 1849. *An Essay on the Cerebral Affections Occuring Most Commonly in Infancy and Childhood: Including Notices of Their History, Causes, Diagnosis, Prognosis and Treatment*. Dublin: Fannin & Co.

Harris, W. 1715. *De morbis acutis infantum.* Amstelodami: J. F. Bernard.

Lieutaud, J. 1770. *Synopsis universae praxeos medicae*. Paris: Vincent.

Obituary. 1880a. *Brit Med J* March 6, 382.

Obituary. 1880b. *Lancet* March 6, 384.

Sachs, B. 1895. *A Treatise on the Nervous Diseases of Children*. New York: William Wood.

Smyth, J. C. 1814. *A Treatise on Hydrocephalus, or Dropsy of the Brain.* London: J. Callow.

Underwood, M. 1784. *A Treatise on the Diseases of Children with Directions for the Management of Infants from the Birth.* London: J. Mathews.

West, C. 1871. *On Some Disorders of the Nervous System in Childhood.* London: Longmans, Green and Co.

Whytt, R. 1768. *Observations on the Dropsy in the Brain.* Edinburgh: J. Balfour.

WILLIAM HENRY DAY

THE YEARS 1850 to 1900 were a very active period in British neurology. In 1855, John Russell Reynolds (1828–1896) published his textbook on neurologic diseases. The National Hospital for the Paralyzed and Epileptic in Queen's Square, London, was founded in 1860. Both John Hughlings Jackson (1935–1911) and William Gowers (1845–1915) were on the faculty of the National Hospital. Gowers's *Epilepsy and Other Chronic Convulsive Diseases* appeared in 1881 and his *A Manual of Diseases of the Nervous System* appeared in 1886. Though not as well remembered as Reynolds, Jackson, and Gowers, William Henry Day (1832–1907), a prominent physician of that time, wrote extensively about disorders of childhood and is most noted for his writings on headaches in children.

William Henry Day was born on November 30, 1830, at

Wantage. He started his medical education in Bristol but transferred, completing his studies at King's College in London, where he received the diploma of Member of the Royal College of Surgeons in 1854. His first medical experience was as an assistant surgeon during the Crimean War. He was present during the siege of Sebastopol and the attack on the Redan. After the war, he returned to England and was appointed consulting physician to the Samaritan Free Hospital for Women and Children. He received his M.D. from St. Andrews in 1857 and was elected a member of the Royal College of Physicians in London in 1867.

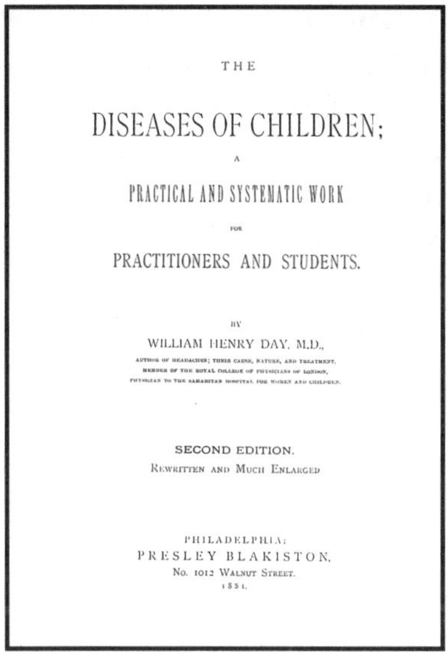
THE

DISEASES OF CHILDREN;

A

PRACTICAL AND SYSTEMATIC WORK

FOR

PRACTITIONERS AND STUDENTS.

BY

WILLIAM HENRY DAY, M.D.,

AUTHOR OF HEADACHES; THEIR CAUSE, NATURE, AND TREATMENT,
MEMBER OF THE ROYAL COLLEGE OF PHYSICIANS OF LONDON,
PHYSICIAN TO THE SAMARITAN HOSPITAL FOR WOMEN AND CHILDREN.

SECOND EDITION.

REWRITTEN AND MUCH ENLARGED

PHILADELPHIA:
PRESLEY BLAKISTON,
No. 1012 WALNUT STREET.
1881.

Figure 1: Title page from the American edition of Day's *Diseases of Children*, 1881.

While at the Samaritan Hospital, he frequently presented papers to the medical societies of London. He was a fellow of the Royal Medical and Chirurgical Society, a member of the Pathological and Clinical Societies, and a member and secretary of the Harveian Society. Between 1862 and 1888, he contributed frequently to the *British Medical Journal*, *Lancet*, and *The Practitioner*. The medical directory and obituaries in 1907 listed as particularly noteworthy his presentations on the cerebral complications of typhoid fever in children (Day, 1875a); the pulmonic and cardiac complications of abdominal tumors with remarks on bloodletting (Day, 1875b); and intestinal obstruction in the child, successfully treated with belladonna and gradual injection of warm water into the rectum (Day, 1879). His writings covered a wide range of topics, including neuralgia of the uterus (Day, 1862); gastrodynia (Day, 1865); teething and diarrhea (Day, 1873); neurosal affections of the heart in children (Day, 1878a); and posttraumatic meningitis (Day, 1883). For child neurologists, he should be remembered for his textbooks on diseases of children and for his extensive writings on headache.

Day's *Essays on Diseases of Children* was published in 1873. It consisted of a collection of seven essays with an introduction, the essays having been previously read before the Harveian Society of London. In this text, he covered disability , remittant fevers, a case of obscure cerebral disease, croup, laryngeal and tracheal irritation, and headaches. Reviewers of that time were particularly impressed with the chapters on headaches. They were described as "interesting and instructive" ("Notes," 1873) and "exceedingly practical" ("Review," 1873).

His next work *The Diseases of Children: A Practical and Systematic Work for Practitioners and Students* appeared in 1881 (figure 1). This was a much more complete monograph and served as an update of Charles West's *Diseases of Children*. In this book, one can see both his interest in public health and his conservative approach to treatment. Early in the introduction, he says:

It is a mystery that children can be raised at all in some of our great cities and towns, on account of the impurity of the air they breathe, and the insanitary conditions of the hovels they inhabit. Better accommodations must be provided for the poor if we would lessen the waste of infant life.
(Day, 1881b)

He also notes later in the introduction that "medicines are foreign to the system and should be avoided when possible, it being better to trust to food than to physic." As Day was a clinician and not a basic researcher, the sections on neurologic diseases of children reflect both his clinical experience and his reading of the literature of his day. In his section on meningitis, he divides the forms into simple leptomeningitis, tubercular meningitis, and chronic basilar meningitis. His section on predisposing and etiologic factors in meningitis starts like a modern text, listing trauma, focal head, and face infections, especially otitis media, sepsis, epidemics, pneumonia, and whooping cough, but ends by listing extremes of heat, cold, and immoderate reading. He provides long descriptions of the presenting symptoms and signs of each form of meningitis, though his sections on therapy are limited. He states that tuberculous meningitis is uniformly fatal and the treatment can only be supportive for simple leptomeningitis. He recommends decreasing vascularity with antimony and soothing of the inflamed centers with iodide of potassium, careful use of chloral hydrate, and cold compresses. In a departure from West, he states that leeches are "not very satisfactory and can scarcely be advocated in young children, the loss of blood not being well born [sic]." His chapters on seizures depend particularly on the works of Reynolds, Jackson, and Edward Sieveking. He includes sections on hydrocephalus; vascular accidents, which he lists as congestion of the brain; chorea; retardation; night terrors; and diseases of the spinal cord. In a section concerning paralysis, he talks about brachial plexus palsies; Duchenne's palsy; and infantile paralysis, which he describes as an illness that starts as a febrile disorder and ends with paralysis and wasting, with atrophy of the anterior horn cells. He also mentions facial neuralgia from petrositis.

The reviewers' reception of the text was varied. The reviewer for the *British Medical Journal* found it valuable for its extensiveness and for its discussions of treatment ("Reviews," 1881a). The reviewer from *Lancet* had a number of criticisms about the sections on therapy and concluded that this volume was best seen as a compilation of information for the practitioner but not a book to be recommended to students and it was not considered "to have advanced the study of children's diseases" ("Reviews," 1881b).

Both now and during his own time, Day is best known for his work on headaches. His first report "Headaches in Children," appeared in the *British Medical Journal* as an abstract of a paper read before the Harveian Society (Day, 1872). There followed "On the Treatment of Different Forms of Headaches" (Day, 1875c), "Clinical Lecture on Some Points in the Pathology and Treatment of Headaches" (Day, 1878b), and a two-part series entitled "Clinical Lecture on Some Varieties of Nervous Headaches," (Day, 1880, 1881a). His text "Headaches: Their Nature, Causes and Treatment" appeared first in 1877 and then underwent several revisions, the fourth edition appearing in 1888 . At the time, his text received uniformly good reviews. The second edition was listed as "useful though unpretending" ("Review," 1878), and the fourth edition was described as both practical and valuable ("Notices," 1888; "Review," 1889).

His works on headaches consisted particularly of clinical descriptions and suggestions on therapy. Day stated that "views regarding the pathology of nervous headache are vague and indefinite." In his considerations of pathophysiology, he did divide headaches into three categories: those caused by anemia versus hyperemia of the brain, those resulting from dysfunction of nervous tissue or blood vessels, and those due to "absorption into the blood of poisonous matters" and reflections of organic diseases of the stomach or kidneys. In the final edition of his text on headaches, he lists eleven types of intracerebral headaches and three forms of headaches of extracerebral origin. The headaches of childhood were divided into seven categories. The first, cerebral headaches, were posttraumatic headaches and headaches due to acute or chronic meningitis. The second category was gastric headaches. This seems to be a combination of two of his adult categories, both sympathetic and dyspepsic, or sick, headaches. The descriptions are basically that of migraine, though he only rarely uses the term "megrim." He insists on a nervous system origin of these headaches as opposed to the gastric origin postulated by other writers of his time. He states that though the disturbance can arise elsewhere, the real cause is in the nervous system and that the vomiting is a reflex from irritation of the brain. The third category he lists is epileptic or congestive headaches. In this category he describes photophobia, a throbbing headache with flushing of the face and fullness of the brain, following seizures. He also notes that the same type of headache may be associated with cardiac disease, citing an example of a child with mitral insufficiency. The fourth form is febrile headaches, also known as active hyperemia or congestion. He describes these as dull, frontal or temporal headaches, always due to an increase in cerebral blood flow. The fifth category is nervous headaches. This form of headache he feels is particularly related to either overtaxing school work or environmental stresses. He noted that nervous headaches can be due to neuralgia, for example originating from dental problems, but states that this is much less common in children than in adults. His recommendation for therapy of nervous headaches is enforced rest, fresh air, cod liver oil, and quinine, with iron if anemia is present. His sixth category is "headache depending on some intrinsic change in the cerebral membranes or tissues of the brain." In this category, he describes children usually from the poor strata of society who become progressively more debilitated, usually presenting first with frontal headache and later with lethargy, listlessness, fretfulness, and restlessness. He attributes this to anemia and often to rickets, and recommends pure air and wholesome food, combined with bromide when the child is excessively restless, and with quinine or iron during the period of recovery. His final category is organic headaches, under which he lists mass lesions, including tumors and tuberculosis.

After retirement, Dr. Day spent his last years on his estate at Holly Hill in Meopham, Kent. He died on October 22, 1907. He was described in the *British Medical Journal* as a "kindly, genial, and hospitable man," whose "loss will be regretted by a large circle of friends" (Obituary, 1907). He continues to be remembered in child neurology for his pioneering work in headaches in children. A brief description of his work appeared in the *American Journal of Psychiatry* (Harms, 1967). Recent references to his writings on headaches in children have appeared in Rothner's discussions on headaches in children, and in Hopkins text on headache (Rothner, 1978; Hopkins, 1988).

David W. Dunn
INDIANAPOLIS, INDIANA

REFERENCES

Day, W. H. 1862. Severe Neuralgia of the Uterus Following Premature Labor. *Brit Med J* 1:5–7.

______. 1865. Gastrodynia. *Lancet* 1:332.

______. 1872. Headaches in Children. *Brit Med J* 2:523.

______. 1873. Teething and Diarrhea. *Brit Med J* 2:111.

______. 1873. *Essays on Diseases of Children*. London: Churchill.

______. 1875a. Cerebral Complications of Typhoid Fever in Children. *Brit Med J* 1:222.

______. 1875b. Practical Observations on the Pulmonary and Cardiac Complications of Abdominal Tumors: With Remarks on Bloodletting after Surgical Operations. *Brit Med J* 1:588.

______. 1875c. On the Treatment of Different Forms of Headaches. *Lancet* 1:853–55.

______. 1877. *Headaches: Their Nature, Causes, and Treatment*. London: Churchill.

______. 1878a. Neurosal Affections of the Heart in Children. *Practitioner* 21:190–202.

______. 1878b. Clinical Lecture on Some Points in the Pathology and Treatment of Headache. *Brit Med J* 2:715–17.

______. 1879. Intestinal Obstruction in a Child. *Brit Med J* 1:810–11.

______. 1880. Clinical Lecture on Some of Varieties of Nervous Headache. *Brit Med J* 1:116–18.

______. 1881a. Clinical Lecture on Some Varieties of Nervous Headache. *Brit Med J* 1:224–27.

______. 1881b. *The Diseases of Children*. Philadelphia: Blakiston.

______. 1883. Spinal Meningitis in a Child Following Spinal Concussion: Recovery. *Lancet* 1:770.

______. 1888. *Headaches: Their Nature, Causes, and Treatment*. 4th ed. London: Churchill.

Harms, E. 1967. Pioneer in Studies of Juvenile Headaches: William Henry Day (1830–1907). *Am J Psych* 123:1456–67.

Hopkins, A. 1988. *Headache: Problems in Diagnosis and Management.* Philadelphia: W. B. Saunders.

______. 1873. Notes on books: *Essays on Diseases of Children. Brit Med J* 2:402.

______. 1888. Notices of Books: *Headaches: Their Nature, Causes, and Treatment.* 4th ed. *Lancet* 2:1132.

______. 1907. Obituary. William Henry Day, M.D. St. Andrews, MRCP, MRCS. *Brit Med J* 2:1192–93.

______. 1873. Review: *Essays on Diseases of Children. Practitioner* 11:436–39.

______. 1878. Review: *Headaches: Their Nature, Causes and Treatment*. 2d ed. *Practitioner* 20:277.

______. 1889. Review: *Headaches, Their Nature, Causes, and Treatment*. 4th ed. *Brit Med J* 1:658.

______. 1881a. Reviews and Notices: *The Diseases of Children. Brit Med J* 1:923–24.

______. 1881b. Reviews and Notices of Books: *The Diseases of Children. Lancet* 2:416–17.

Rothner, A. D. 1978. *Headaches in Children*: A Review. *Headache* 18:169–75.

JOSEPH JULES DEJERINE

THE NAME OF DEJERINE conjures up a legacy of classic eponymic syndromes: facioscapulohumeral dystrophy (Landouzy-Dejerine), progressive hypertrophic interstitial neuritis (Dejerine-Sottas), olivopontocerebellar atrophy (Dejerine-André-Thomas), and the thalamic syndrome (Dejerine-Roussy). Dejerine was not only a prolific writer but also a much sought-after teacher whose students later distinguished themselves by their own contributions to adult and child neurology.

Joseph Jules Dejerine (1849–1917) (figure 1) was born of French parents in Geneva, Switzerland, where his father was a carriage proprietor. He thoroughly enjoyed his childhood in the provincial Swiss atmosphere. Swimming, boxing, and fishing on Lake Leman seem to have been far more attractive pastimes in his childhood than academic studies. This relaxed and carefree atmosphere changed once he became attracted to biology and comparative anatomy. In 1871, at the age of twenty-two, Dejerine decided to pursue clinical studies. Because Geneva lacked suitable facilities for clinical study, his obvious choice was Paris. He secured an introduction to Alfred Vulpian from Jean-Louis Prevost and set out for the metropolis of Paris in a third-class compartment. France was recovering from the recent painful defeat in the 1870 war against Germany and was looking for stability. Paris at that time was a city in turmoil because of war and revolution. It was fortunate indeed for Dejerine that the next two years were politically stable under Adolphe Thiers's presidential rule. Such were the circumstances in which Dejerine set out to reach his goal under Vulpian's direction. He ultimately proved to be Vulpian's most distinguished pupil.

Vulpian, himself a pupil of Jean Pierre Flourens, was a distinguished physiologist and later an eminent pathologist. He succeeded Jean Cruveilhier to the chair of pathological anatomy in the Faculty of Medicine of Paris. He and Jean Martin Charcot had taken over the medical services at the Salpêtrière in 1862. Vulpian was studying the degeneration and regeneration of nerves and the effects of drugs on the nervous system. Dejerine was no doubt influenced by these investigations in Vulpian's laboratory. He

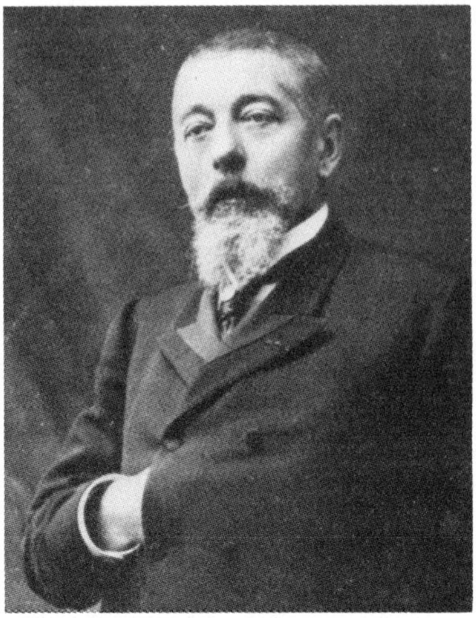
Figure 1. Joseph Jules Dejerine (1849–1917).

graduated in medicine in 1879 and advanced steadily, holding many important appointments. He was the first Chief of Clinic at the Bicêtre and also Professor of the History of Medicine and Clinical Medicine. Dejerine moved to the Salpêtrière in 1895 and in 1908 was elected to the French Academy of Medicine. In 1910 he succeeded to the Chair of Neurology at the Salpêtrière, held first by Charcot and later by Fulgence Raymond. He became the Professeur de Clinique des Maladies du Système Nerveux à la Faculté de Medicine at the Salpêtrière.

The Salpêtrière, situated on the left bank of the river Seine, in the eastern outskirts of Paris near the Gare d' Orléans Austerlitz, has an interesting history. Louis VII built it in 1603 as an arsenal for the manufacture of gunpowder, for which it was used for almost half a century. This was sufficient time for the Parisians to associate these buildings with *saltpêtre*, the principal ingredient of gunpowder, thus referring to the building as the Salpêtrière. In 1656 this complex of buildings was converted by St. Vincent de Paul into an asylum for the old, homeless and infirm women, abandoned prostitutes, and the insane. By the beginning of the nineteenth century, it was a city within a city, consisting of almost forty-five buildings with streets, squares, gardens, and a beautiful old church. There, pioneers like Phillipe Pinel, Jean Esquirol, and François Baillarger, embarked on their studies in psychiatry and boldly struck off the shackles that for centuries had held these unfortunate inmates in bondage.

Dejerine made good use of the clinical material available at the Bicêtre and later at the Salpêtrière. Many a student was attracted to Dejerine because of his keen intellect and unbounded energy as well as his unique ability to produce sense out of chaos. His students, collaborators, and colleagues at various times included Louis Landouzy, Jules Sottas, Gustave Roussy, Hippolyte Bernheim,

Théophile Alajouanine, Otfrid Foerster, Nehemie Vialet, André-Thomas, and Robert Bing.

Dejerine's contributions to child neurology are numerous. He identified facioscapulohumeral muscular dystrophy as a separate and distinct entity, describing it with Louis Landouzy in a series of papers from 1884 to 1886. In these reports, they differentiated this form of muscular dystrophy from the progressive muscular atrophy of Aran-Duchenne, stressing its onset in infancy, predilection for facial involvement, familial occurrence, and myopathic rather than neuropathic degeneration. In one family, five of the nine members were affected. An example of one member, Eugene L., is illustrated in figure 2. Seen at age twenty-one, he first developed symptoms at age three, initially with abnormal facial expression. Typically, the clinical description was very detailed and extensive, as can be seen in the following portion extracted from that accompanying the photograph:

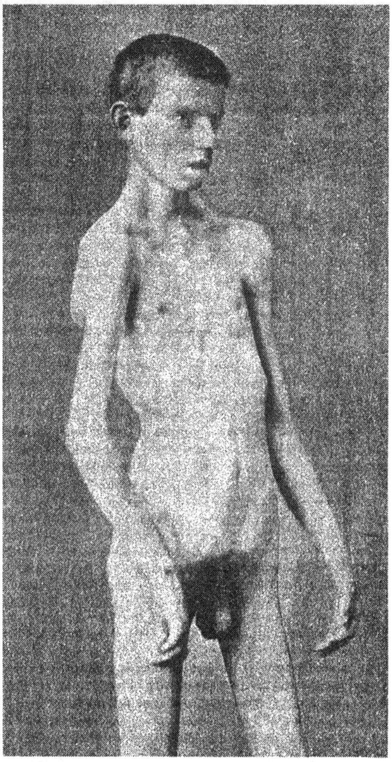

Figure 2. A patient with severe atrophy due to muscular dystrophy, as reported by Landouzy and Dejerine in 1885.

ACTUAL STATE, ON THE DAY OF ENTRY —*The face is very characteristic, having the expression of an idiot, which is unfortunate as he is quite intelligent. The skin of the face is smooth; without folds or wrinkles when he tries to show some facial expression; the mouth is formed in a particular fashion, with little movement when he tries to mimic. At rest, his cheeks are widened: the two lips are prominent, the lower one stretched and rolled in the shape of a chamber pot, the upper one is more protruding. L. . . . is not able to pucker or round out his lips. When he tries to whistle, he tries to pucker his lips but they stretch out. L. . . . when finally, with effort does whistle it is only during inspiration and not expiration. When he tries to smile, he smiles differently than the rest of the world, he smiles with spreading his upper lip with the opening accentuated and a nasolabial sound. He smiles crosswise, with widening of his cheeks and at the same time his lower lip curls under his upper lip. . . .* (Landouzy and Dejerine, 1885, 96)

Another of Dejerine's major contributions to child neurology was his report with Jules Sottas on progressive hypertrophic interstitial neuropathy in 1893 and again with André-Thomas in 1906. It should be noted that Rudolf Virchow (1855), Nikolaus Friedreich (1873), and Gombault and Mallet (1889) described isolated cases of this disorder prior to the 1893 publication of "Sur la névrite interstitielle hypertrophique et progressive de l'enfance." In this paper, Dejerine and Sottas described two siblings, a girl whose symptoms began in infancy, and her brother whose onset was at age fourteen. The children had club feet, kyphoscoliosis, generalized weakness and atrophy with greater severity distally, muscle fasciculations, decreased reaction to electrical stimulation, areflexia, sensory loss, incoordination, nystagmus, and abnormal pupillary responses. Neither of the parents was affected. At the time of death of one of the siblings at age forty-five, severe foot deformities were present and ambulation had been lost. The peripheral nerves were found to be enlarged, firm, and gelatinous. The myelin sheath was found to be thin or absent, and surrounding these abnormal fibers, they described a cuff on hypertrophic connective tissue. Dejerine and Sottas suggested, incorrectly, that the etiology of this disorder was due to the hyperplastic endoneurium that constricted and damaged nerve fibers (Dyck, 1975). However, little has been added to their original clinical or pathological description since that time.

Delineation of olivopontocerebellar atrophy, reported with André-Thomas in 1900, is also a masterful contribution to the field of neurology, reflecting both the interest in cerebellar function of André-Thomas and the expertise in pathology of Dejerine. The 1906 description of the thalamic syndrome with Roussy is reminiscent of the earlier work with Vialet. These papers highlight Dejerine's pioneering role in the study of the localization of brain function. He had first shown in 1891, and again with Vialet in 1893, that word blindness may occur as a result of lesions of the supramarginal and angular gyrus. In 1906 the authors reported the pathologic lesion producing the thalamic syndrome. Almost twenty years later Charles Foix, Paul Masson, and Pierre Hillemand demonstrated occlusion of the thalamogeniculate branches of the posterior cerebral artery as the most common cause of this syndrome. Dejerine later became interested in the functional disorders of the nervous system and developed his ideas of psychotherapy. He felt that the personality of the therapist was of extreme importance. Perhaps his greatest contributions are the *Anatomie des centres nerveux* (1895–1901), and the *Sémiologie des affections du système nerveux* (1914). In collaboration with Ernest Gauckler, he also published a book on psychiatry (Dejerine and Gauckler, 1911). The English translation of this book, *The Psychoneuroses and Their Treatment by Psychotherapy* by Smith Ely Jelliffe, was published in 1913.

Dejerine met Augusta Klumpke while she was studying in Paris and they were married in 1888. Mme. Klumpke's family was from San Francisco and the bride was given away by Professor Hardy with Professor Landouzy as her second witness. Dejerine and Mme. Klumpke were a close couple. They entertained students on Sunday nights on a regular basis. Dejerine maintained close ties to his Swiss homeland and maintained a home at Thalgut, near Bern, where he returned regularly for vacations, rest, and reflection. He and his wife took pleasure in guiding their daughter's career in medicine, like those of many other students. The Dejerines were two intellectual giants working together, each inspiring and helping the other throughout their married life. After Dejerine's death on February 26, 1917, Mme. Klumpke carried on his work with the assistance of their daughter, who was also a physician.

Bhuwan Garg
INDIANAPOLIS, INDIANA

ACKNOWLEDGMENTS

I wish to thank Ms. Nisha Garg for her help in translating some of the French manuscripts.

REFERENCES

Bing, R. 1918. Jules Dejerine (1849–1917). *Schweizer Arch Neur Psych*, 314–15.

Dejerine, J. J. 1886. *L'Héredité dans les maladies du système nerveux.* Paris: Asselin et Houzeau.

______. 1892. Contribution à l'étude anatomo-pathologique et clinique des différentes variétés de cécité verbale. *Compt rend Soc Biol* (Paris), 61–90.

______. 1914. *Sémiologie des affections du système nerveux.* Paris: Masson et Cie.

Dejerine, J. J., and A. Dejerine-Klumpke. 1895–1901. *Anatomie des centres nerveux.* Paris: Rueff et Cie.

Dejerine, J. J., and E. Gauckler. 1911. *Les manifestations fonctionnelles des psychoneuroses: leur traitement par la psychothérapie.* Paris: Masson.

______. 1913. *The Psychoneuroses and Their Treatment by Psychotherapy.* Translated by Smith Ely Jelliffe. Philadelphia: J. B. Lippincott.

Dejerine, J. J. and G. Roussy. 1906. Le Syndrome thalamique. *Rev neur*, 521–32.

Dejerine, J. J., and J. Sottas. 1893. Sur la névrite interstitielle, hypertrophique et progressive, de l'enfance. *Compt rend Soc Biol* (Paris), 63–96.

Dejerine, J. J., and André-Thomas. 1900. L'Atrophie olivo-ponto-cérébelleuse. *Nouvelle Iconographie de la Salpêtrière*, 330–70.

______. 1906. Sur la névrite interstitielle hypertrophique et progressive de l'enfance. *Nouvelle Iconographie de la Salpêtrière*, 477–509.

______. 1909. *Maladies de la moelle épinière*, 787. Paris: Libraire J. B. Baillière et Fils.

Dejerine, J. J., and N. Vialet. 1893. Contribution à l'étude de la localisation anatomique de la cécité verbale pure. *Compt rend Soc Biol* (Paris), 790–791.

Dyck, P. J. 1975. Inherited Neuronal Degeneration and Atrophy Affecting Peripheral Motor, Sensory, and Autonomic Nerves. In *Peripheral Neuropathy*, 856. Ed. P. J. Dyck, P. K. Thomas, and E. H. Lambert., Philadelphia: W. B. Saunders.

Foix, C., and P. Hillemand. 1925. Les Syndromes de la région thalamique. *Presse méd* 33:113–17.

Foix, C. and A. Masson. 1923. Le Syndrome de l'artère cérébrale postérieure. *Presse méd* 31:361–65.

Friedreich, N. 1873. Eigene Beobachtungen. In *Über progressive Muskelatrophie*, 11. Berlin: Hirschwald Verlag.

Gombault, A., and R. Mallet. 1889. Un cas de tabes ayant débuté dans l'enfance: autopsie. *Arch méd exp anat path* 1:385.

Haymaker, W. and F. Schiller. 1970. *The Founders of Neurology.* Springfield, IL: Charles C Thomas.

Landouzy, L., and J. J. Dejerine. 1884. De la myopathie atrophique progressive (myopathie héréditaire), débutant dans l'enfance, par la face, sans altération du système nerveux. *Compt rend Acad Sci* 98:53.

______. 1885. De la myopathie atrophique progressive sans neuropathie, débutant d'ordinaire dans l'enfance, par la face. *Rev méd* 4:6.

______. 1886. Contribution à l'étude de la myopathie atrophique progressive (myopathie atrophique progressive, A type scapulo-humeral). *Compt rend Soc Biol* (Paris), 478–81.

Mackay, F. H., and E. Legrand. 1936. Jean Martin Charcot. In *Neurological Biographies and Addresses*. Foundation Volume. London: Oxford University Press.

McHenry, L. C. 1969. *Garrison's History of Neurology*. Springfield, IL: Charles C Thomas.

Virchow, R. 1855. Ein Fall von progressiver Muskelatrophia. *Virchows Arch path Anat* 8:537.

MADAME AUGUSTA DEJERINE-KLUMPKE

MADAME AUGUSTA DEJERINE-KLUMPKE (figure 1) was born on October 15, 1859, in San Francisco, California, to John Gerard Klumpke and Dorothea Tolle Klumpke. She was one of four sisters, all of whom displayed great talents in either the arts or science. One became an artist; another a musician; the third a doctor of science (Bailey and Bishop, 1944). Augusta Klumpke lived in California until age eleven. Her parents later separated; Mrs. Klumpke retained custody of the children and moved to Europe, first to Germany and then Switzerland. Augusta Klumpke was a good student and demonstrated an aptitude for the sciences. She had not thought about medicine as a career until her mother read her an article about a woman who had a career in medicine. From that day forward, Mademoiselle Klumpke could think of nothing else but being a doctor (Lipinska, 1930; Satran, 1974). This was no small ambition. Women were rarities in the medical profession, medicine not being considered a profession "becoming" of a woman.

After graduating from Lausanne with a baccalaureate degree, Augusta left for Paris, because neither Lausanne nor Geneva had

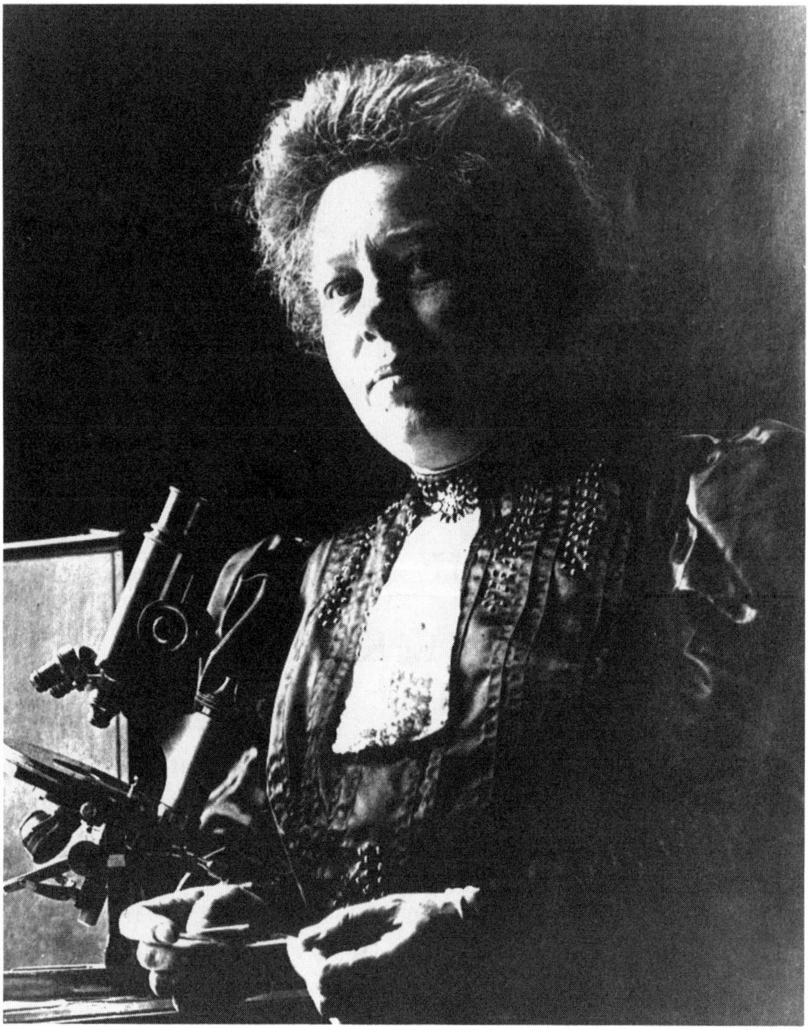

Figure 1. Madame Augusta Dejerine-Klumpke (1859–1927) in the laboratory.

facilities for the study of medicine. Having arrived, however, she was not encouraged to pursue medicine. In fact, Alfred Vulpian (her future mentor) actively discouraged her. The objections were overruled and Klumpke was allowed to enter medical school along with several other women (Lipinska, 1930; Jelliffe, 1928). Once in medical school, Klumpke's instructors recognized her intelligence, courage, and perseverance.

She was encouraged to enroll in the competition for an externship by one of her instructors, but was refused authorization by

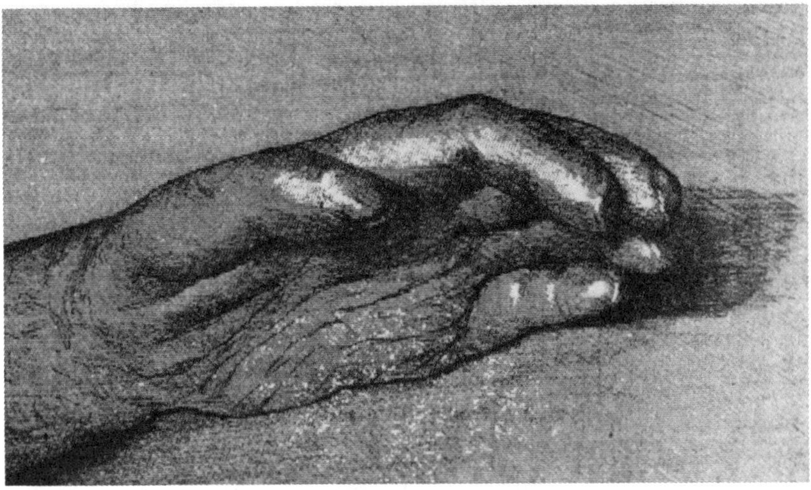

Figure 2. The wasted hand of one of the adult patients presented in "Contribution à l'étude des paralysies radiculaires du plexus brachial" (1885) showing severe paralysis and atrophy.

the Director of Public Assistance. However, in 1881, due to a campaign by Blanche Edwards (a fellow woman classmate), women were allowed to compete for an externship. Both Mlles Edwards and Klumpke succeeded in passing their written and oral examinations but were not received warmly by their peers. On the contrary, it was made clear that they were not welcome. One can imagine, then, the resistance they met when they expressed a desire to participate in the more prestigious internships. Again, Blanche Edwards led a vigorous campaign to allow women to participate in internships by writing letters to medical journals and visiting political and academic leaders. The women students eventually circulated a petition to the faculty members asking for their support. Forty members originally signed the document but virtually all backed down at special meetings held by the Societies of Physicians and Surgeons of the Hospitals of Paris. Dejerine, Klumpke's future husband, and Louis Landouzy, the future dean of the Faculty of Medicine, held firm in their support (Satran, 1974). Many reasons were given as to why women were not qualified. For example, it would take too long for a woman to dress into her petticoats when called for a medical emergency. Also, women were not physiologically suited for the demands of medicine. The

French government was ultimately forced to step in. Fortunately, Paul Bert, Minister of Public Instruction, was a leftist radical who favored the emancipation of women. In 1884 Bert issued a decree allowing women to compete for internships (Jelliffe, 1928). This created quite a stir in Paris, but Mademoiselle Klumpke performed her role as intern flawlessly.

Mlle Klumpke's recognition in child neurology comes primarily from her article, published in 1885, that describes the different types of brachial plexus paralyses (Klumpke, 1885, 591–616). In this article, she described in great detail the clinical characteristics and anatomy of the different types of paralyses that involve the brachial plexus (figure 2). She thus became the first person to separate the superior and inferior types of brachial plexus palsies and understand their anatomic and clinical differences. She recognized that these types of paralyses were subsequent to violent trauma to the upper and/or lower part of the shoulder as a result of a fall, compression of the subclavicular area by a strap, forceps delivery, or arthritis of the fifth or sixth cervical vertebral bodies. In child neurology, one primarily sees infants with this problem following a difficult delivery. In her article, she discussed primarily adults, but also recognized the infantile problem.

The article describes in clear detail the clinical differences between the classic Duchenne-Erb paralysis (superior type) and the inferior type of brachial plexus paralysis (later known as Klumpke's paralysis).

Whereas the troubles of sensation are non [null] or little marked in the superior type, they are almost never missing in the total paralysis nor in the inferior radicular paralysis. The anesthesia is complete on the hand and on the forearm. In most cases, it extends to one or two fingers in width above the elbow, limited there by a line more or less irregular. Sometimes it invades the arm, but it is the external and posterior region, until the level of the deltoid insertion which alone presents troubles of sensation. The skin of the internal region of the arm, the one of the shoulder, remains in effect always undamaged, as long as we are dealing with a lesion rigorously limited to the brachial plexus. . . . There is another symptom which is mentioned in all the observations, pathognomonic symptom so to speak, of the lower radicular paralyses, symptoms that one does not find again in the total paralyses evolving toward the Duchenne-Erb type: these are oculo-pupillary phenomena.

These phenomena, which are constant in every paralysis that is truly inferior radicular, are characterized by miosis, by the shrinking of the palpebral slit (gap), and in some cases by the shortness and by the retraction of the ocular globe. In three observations, we have, moreover, noticed the flattening of the cheek on the side corresponding to the paralysis. (Klumpke, 1885, 596–97)

Klumpke's and her colleagues' clinical observations were very important, especially the observation of the ocular-pupillary changes. Her curiosity and quest for new knowledge led her to perform a series of experiments on dogs in order to identify the corresponding anatomic lesion that results in the ocular-pupillary phenomenon. These dissections were also described in this article and summarized as follows:

In summary, the oculo-pupilar phenomena happened only during the tearing up of the inferior roots or during the section of the same roots at the level of the hole of conjugation, that is to say each time that the section or tearing up have dealt with the branch communicating with the dorsal nerve. (Klumpke, 1885, 603)

Her medical thesis was also excellently researched, concentrating on polyneuritis, particularly lead polyneuritis (Dejerine-Klumpke, 1889).

In 1888 Mlle Klumpke married Jules Dejerine, who was already highly regarded as a neurologist, and the two formed a dynamic collaborative team. Together they published innumerable pathological studies, first in the pathology lab at the Bicêtre and then at the Salpêtrière. Their insistence on continuous serial sectioning of the whole brain, along with their attention to detail, meticulous dissections, and ingenuity in presentation resulted in a comprehensive, systematic book of neuron topography entitled *Anatomie des centres nerveux* (Dejerine and Dejerine-Klumpke, 1895; Lipinska, 1930; Jelliffe, 1928). An immense number of pathological studies followed this treatise. Among the most outstanding anatomic presentations were descriptions of: 1) secondary degeneration following lesions of the cortex; 2) the connections of the red nucleus; 3) aberrant pathways of the pyramidal tract; and 4) cuneus fibers in the corpus callosum (Jelliffe, 1928). Their pathologic studies initiated a series of research projects by such notable students as André-Thomas, Gustave Roussy, Jean Lhermitte, and Jean Alexandre Barré.

With the outbreak of World War I, Mme Dejerine-Klumpke took care of the wounded at the Salpêtrière and Les Invalides. She not only performed these clinical duties but also published various articles on the treatment of traumatic cerebral injuries and the indications for the surgical treatment of spinal cord lesions (Lipinska, 1930). She and her husband also entertained frequently at their house near Bern, France, on the River Aar. Mme Dejerine-Klumpke, in particular, was known for her warmth, kindness, and hospitality. The death of her husband in 1917 was hard for her, as they were very close (Spiller, 1928). After his death, she began collaborating with her daughter, studying the osteopathies of spinal paraplegics. In 1920 she established the Dejerine Foundation, thus guaranteeing that the Paris Faculty of Medicine would have a modern pathology laboratory, museum, and library (Jelliffe, 1928).

Mme Dejerine-Klumpke died in 1927 at the age of sixty-eight. Dejerine-Klumpke's studies in neurological sciences have contributed greatly to our knowledge of the central nervous system. She was a remarkable woman, a pioneer on many different levels. A story told by Gustave Roussy exemplifies her compassion, courage, and perseverance. While Roussy was visiting Drs. Dejerine-Klumpke and Dejerine at their home in Bern, a woman fell into the nearby river Aar. Dr. Dejerine jumped into the swiftly flowing water to save the woman but was threatened with drowning himself. Mme Dejerine-Klumpke threw herself into the water, fully clothed, and rescued them both. According to Roussy, anyone who saw the seething, foaming river could not doubt the stamina, strength, and courage of this woman who helped guide the evolution of modern neurology (Jelliffe, 1928).

Mary Zupanc
MADISON, WISCONSIN

ACKNOWLEDGMENTS

Special thanks to Allaoua Toumi, of the University of Wisconsin French Department, for his assistance with the translation of Mme Dejerine-Klumpke's texts.

REFERENCES

Bailey, H., and W. J. Bishop. 1944. *Notable Names in Medicine and Surgery*. London: Lewis.

Dejerine, J., and A. Dejerine-Klumpke. 1895. *Anatomie des centres nerveux*. Paris: Rueff et Cie.

Dejerine-Klumpke, A. 1889. Des polyneurites en général et des paralysies et atrophies saturnines en particulier. Thèse. Paris: Félix Alcan.

Jelliffe, S. E. 1928. Madame Dejerine-Klumpke. *J Nerv Ment Dis* 67(6):644–47.

Klumpke, A. 1885. Contribution à l'étude des paralysies radiculaires du plexus brachial. *Rev méd* 5:591–739.

Lipinska, M. 1930. *Les Femmes et le progrès des sciences médicales*, 165–69. Paris: Masson.

Satran, R. 1974. Augusta Dejerine Klumpke. First Woman Intern in Paris Hospitals. *Ann Int Med* 80:260–64.

Schutta, H. S. 1984. Verbal communication. From the Department of Neurology, University of Wisconsin, Madison.

Spiller, W. G. 1928. Madame Dejerine-Klumpke. *Arch Neur* 20(1):193–94.

JOHN LANGDON HAYDON DOWN

JOHN LANGDON HAYDON DOWN (1828–1897) (figure 1) was born at Tor Point in Cornwall, Great Britain. His father was from Derry, Northern Ireland, while his mother (Hannah Haydon) was from North Devonshire. Hannah's father (John Haydon) married Jane Langdon and thus John Langdon Haydon Down inherited three surnames from his parents. Down had two sons, Percival and Reginald. The latter was the father-in-law to the famous Lord Brain of London. Down's sister, Jane Elizabeth, had a grandson, Sir Geoffrey Keynes, who married the granddaughter of Charles Darwin. They eventually had a son who married the daughter of Lord Edgar Adrian, co-recipient of the 1932 Nobel prize with Charles Sherrington, for their work on nerve impulses and synapses. Thus, the twentieth-century descendants of the Down family have incorporated genetic material of Darwin, Brain, and Adrian (Penrose and Smith, 1967).

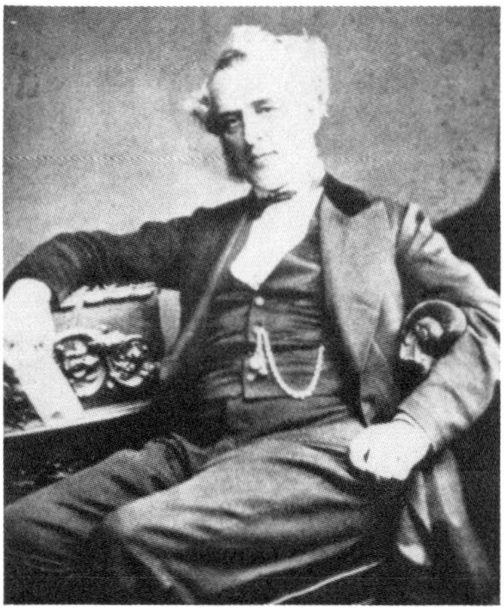

Figure 1. John Langdon Haydon Down (1828–1897).

Down was educated in the local schools of Devonshire until he was fourteen, when he became an apprentice to his father, who was the town's apothecary. It was during this apprenticeship that he learned chemistry and developed his keen interest in science. By age eighteen he had left his father and home and travelled to London to search for a better laboratory position. He first worked at the Pharmaceutical Society Laboratory where he earned his first award in organic chemistry. During this time he came in contact with many notable scientists, including Michael Faraday, whom he assisted in several of his early experiments with gasses during the 1850's. In 1853 Down left his career in chemistry and began his medical training at the London Hospital where he earned many honors and medals for his work with patients and with pharmaceuticals.

Medical education in London during the nineteenth century was mainly in the hands of individual doctors who taught anatomy and pharmacy at the hospitals. The students received all their clinical education by walking around the wards with the leaders of the great institutions. During Down's time of training, these great men included Thomas Addison (1793–1860), Thomas Hodgkins (1798–1866), Richard Bright (1789–1858), James Paget (1814–1899), William Ferguson (1808–1877), and James Simpson (1811–1870). Specialization became an accepted fact in the nineteenth century as the amount of medical knowledge expanded and the invention of newer surgical instrumentation became more difficult to learn (Lyons and Petrucelli, 1978).

In 1858, having completed his training with honors and having many opportunities to work with the most noted physicians in London, Down took a surprise appointment as superintendent of the newly formed Earlswood Asylum for Idiots in Surrey, south of London. His interest and compassion for the mentally afflicted were not apparent in his medical papers or lectures that he gave during his medical training. In some of his later writings, however, he reflects on a private pilgrimage that he made to one of the first residential homes for the mentally retarded in Abendberg, Switzerland, when he was a medical student. He describes how he found the patients in a state of grave physical and mental neglect. This image must have remained as a vivid memory during his clinical training years at the London Hospital.

England enacted legislation in the thirteenth century which was aimed to provide elementary management for "idiots." This essentially protected them and provided care for their basic needs. This legislation distinguished them from insane individuals who could be criminally prosecuted. It was not until the early nineteenth century that countries in Europe began to establish schools and homes for the feeble-minded. Edouard Séguin founded a school for idiots in Paris in 1837. The first asylum for idiots in England was founded privately at Park House in Highgate (1840). The home and program was such a huge success that a second asylum was established at Essex Hall in Colchester in 1849 (Penrose, 1954).

It became necessary in England to combine patients from two smaller residential institutions in nearby Highgate and Colchester into a larger residence that was opened in Surrey in 1858. The search for a director and superintendent of this institution was in progress when Down finished his medical training. Down took this position with enthusiasm, interest, and dedication. While at Earlswood, Down published very little and was mainly concerned with classifying the large case load of patients with mental idiocy. With his skills as a clinician and anatomist, he wrote and lectured on various clinical cases that he encountered. Some of his case reports include patients with agenesis of the corpus callosum, muscular dystrophy, and adiposo-genital dystrophy, which he called *polysarcia* (Wolstenholme and Porter, 1967).

The extent of genetic knowledge in 1858, as Down began his medical career, was heavily influenced by Darwinian theory of pangenesis (each body cell sheds gemmules into the bloodstream, which are then transported to the testis or ovary to form gametes), and Lamarkian theory (acquired characteristics induced by the environment can be inherited by the offspring in the absence of the environmental stimulus). Gregor Mendel began his isolated seven year study of the garden pea in 1857 in a small monastery in Vienna and would report his findings and theory of segregation in 1865, just one year before Down's paper on Mongolism. Unfortunately, Mendel's work would not be accepted or appreciated until after 1900. Discoveries and descriptions of fertilization and nuclear chromosomes were not introduced into the literature until after 1870 (Sinnott and Dobzhansky, 1958; Sturtevant, 1965; Connor, 1978).

Down's classical description that bears his name today was published in the *London Hospital Reports* in 1866. It was entitled "Observations on the Ethnic Classification of Idiots." Ironically, Séguin also published a case report of a syndrome that he labeled "Furfuraceous Cretinism" in 1866. Séguin attempted to distinguish it from his previously described case of an endemic thyroid deficiency syndrome seen in his patients who resided in Paris. Thus in 1866, the two superintendents at the largest residential institutions in northern Europe coincidentally described the same syndrome of idiocy that would remain as the dominant cytogenic disorder in the world today.

Down's historic paper was directed to his goal of ". . . making a classification of the feeble minded by arranging them around various ethnic standards. . . ." Down had seen a large number of mentally retarded patients, both at the Earlswood asylum and in his clinical exposure at the large London Hospital during his first eight years of work there. He commented that "a considerable portion [of the patients] can be fairly referred to one of the great divisions of the human family other than the class from which they have sprung." His three-page report dealt mainly with the very large number of "idiots" that resembled the Mongolian family. He stated "So marked is this [resemblance], that when placed side by side, it is difficult to believe that the specimens compared are not children of the same parent." His clinical description of their features is almost exactly the same as the descriptions printed in textbooks today.

The hair is not black, as in the real Mongol, but of a brownish colour, straight and scanty. The face is flat and broad, and destitute of prominence.

The cheeks are roundish, and extended laterally. The eyes are obliquely placed, and the internal canthi more than normally distant from one another. The palpebral fissure is very narrow. The forehead is wrinkled transversely from the constant assistance which the levatores palpebrarum derive from the occipitofrontalis muscle in opening of the eyes. The lips are large and thick with transverse fissures. The tongue is long, thick, and much roughened. The nose is small. The skin has a dirty yellowish tinge, and is deficient in elasticity, giving the appearance of being too large for the body. (Down, 1866, 261)

Down Syndrome has a current incidence of 1/800–1000 live births each year. Down claimed that this "Mongolian type of idiocy" occurred in more than ten percent of the cases that were presented to him at Earlswood. Down attempted to explain this form of mental retardation by a regression from the Caucasian race to another ethnic group, Mongol. Down stated "it is difficult to realize that these patients are from European parents. They have characteristic features of another race. There can be no doubt that these ethnic features are a result of degeneration" (Lane and Stratford, 1985).

Down published very little after this report. In 1887 he published a book *On Some of the Mental Affections of Childhood and Youth* in which he described several case reports of children with a variety of mental and physical ailments (Down, 1887). However, his initial goal to further classify congenital idiots ended with his subgroup of Mongols. He continued at the Earlswood Home where he was joined by his two physician sons, Reginald and Percival, who took over the responsibilities of the home following their father's death in 1897. In 1959, some ninety years after Down described his "Mongolism idiocy," Jerome LeJeune discovered an extra chromosome in patients with Down Syndrome, which marked the beginning of a new era in medical genetics (Penrose and Smith, 1967).

Down was a pioneer for the mentally defective in the mid 1800s and voiced his objection to the concept of inferiority of ethnic races during that time. He claimed that if a mentally defective member of a white race could show the racial features of a non-white race, it proved that racial differences were not specific. He used these arguments to speak out against the proponents for slavery in the United States and supported the concept of unity of mankind. Down certainly was a pioneer in the medical ethics of the mentally retarded. Personal communications indicate that Down had a grandson who had Down Syndrome, but this child was born after Down's death (Smith, 1988).

Thomas Sullivan
OAK BROOK, ILLINOIS

REFERENCES

Connor, J. M., and M. A. Ferguson-Smith. 1987. *Essential Medical Genetics*, 1–7. Oxford: Blackwell Scientific Publications.

Down, J. L. H. 1866. Observations on an Ethnic Classification of Idiots. *Lond Hosp Clin Lec Rep* 3:259–62.

______. 1887. *On Some of the Mental Affections of Childhood and Youth, Being the Lettsomian Lectures Delivered Before the Medical Society of London in 1887, Together with Other Papers.* London: J. & A. Churchill.

Lane, D., and B. Stratford, editors. 1985. *Current Approaches to Down's Syndrome*, 3–6. New York: Praeger.

Lyons, A., and R. Petrucelli. 1978. *Medicine, An Illustrated History*, 495–547. New York: Harry A. Abrams, Inc.

Penrose, L. S. 1954. *The Biology of Mental Defect*. London: Sidgwick and Jackson, Ltd.

Penrose, L. S., and G. F. Smith. 1967. *Down's Anomaly*. Boston: Little Brown and Company.

Séguin, E. 1866. *Idiocy and Its Treatment by the Psychological Method*. New York: Wood and Company.

Sinnott, E., L. Dunn, and T. Dobzhansky. 1958. *Principles of Genetics*, 1–33. New York: McGraw-Hill.

Smith, G. F. 1988. Personal communication.

Sturtevant, H. H. 1965. *A History of Genetics*, 1–25. New York: Harper and Row.

Wolstenholme, G. E. W., and R. Porter. 1967. *Mongolism*, 1–5. Boston: Little Brown and Company.

GUILLAUME BENJAMIN AMAND DUCHENNE

OUR KNOWLEDGE of the life of Duchenne derives from the accounts provided by only a handful of scholars. Except for a brief notice of his life and works (Lasègue and Straus, 1875) and various short biographical notices in French and English journals that appeared shortly after his death (Poore, 1883), few details were initially recorded. It was Joseph Collins of New York who appreciated this paradoxical circumstance of nonrecognition and who, after visiting France to contact surviving friends and family members of Duchenne and to examine letters and records, wrote a *Biography and an Appreciation* (Collins, 1908). A fuller account of Duchenne's life, much of which was contributed by Paul Guilly, appeared in Jean Lhermitte's address nominating Duchenne for posthumous election to the French Academy of Medicine (Lhermitte, 1946). The above sources appear to have provided most of the material for Henry Viet's lecture in 1948 and for Olin Chamberlain's splendid, brief vignette in *The Founders of Neurology* in 1953.

Guillaume Benjamin Amand Duchenne (1806–1875) (figure 1) was born on November 18th, in the seaport of Boulogne, France. His father was from a long line of seafarers and two years previously had been awarded the Croix de la Légion d'honneur by Napoleon for his skill in the command of a gunship in a battle with the English. Guillaume, the second of four sons, was expected to maintain the family tradition by following a career at sea, but during his college education at Douai, he developed a keen interest in science and decided to study medicine. At the age of twenty he entered the University of Paris, where among the faculty members were such prominent figures as René Laennec, Guillaume Dupuytren, François Magendie, and Jean Cruveilhier. Collins tells us that in the course of his medical studies he formed the habit of making notes of everything he thought, heard, or saw that he wished to remember. While he had a particular interest in conducting dissections with his own hands, formal writing was a chore for him, as evidenced by a very mediocre thesis on the sub-

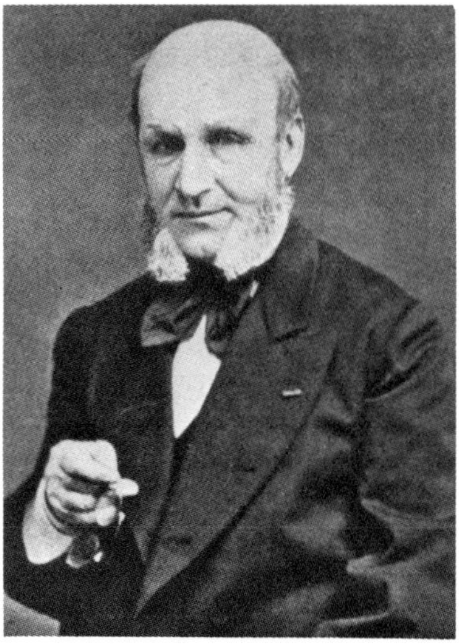

Figure 1. Guillaume Benjamin Amand Duchenne de Boulogne (1806–1875).

ject of burns. Immediately upon graduation he returned to Boulogne to establish himself in general practice. His practice grew rapidly, in part because of the high standing of the Duchenne family in the community, and also because of his thoughtful, considerate manner toward his patients. He was married in 1831 but a very happy life abruptly changed two years later when his wife died following the birth of a son. Not only did he endure profound grief, but he was also blamed for negligence in caring for his wife by his mother-in-law, who took his infant son away. The circumstances conspired to diminish Duchenne's professional stature; his wealthy clientele abandoned him and a small remaining practice left him with much time on his hands. In his professional surcease he remained alert to advances being made in medicine, in particular, the use of electric current as a therapeutic modality. Lhermitte writes that in attempting to cure a case of neuralgia by means of "electropuncture" Duchenne observed that the application of the current caused an isolated contraction limited to a cluster of muscles (Lhermitte, 1946). The observation marked a turning point in his career.

The effect of electric current on the human body had been a subject of interest to physicians throughout Europe since the introduction of the Leyden jar in 1745. However, the discovery of the induction coil in 1831 by Michael Faraday in England, and independently by Joseph Henry in the United States that same year, gave a new impetus to studies on its applications in medicine. Jean Baptiste Sarlandière's use of electropuncture had fascinated Duchenne during his student days but, aware of occasional abscesses that resulted and sensitive to the pain that it caused the patient, Duchenne employed the procedure with great reservation in his practice. On learning of the induction coil as a simple means of inducing a brief, apparently harmless, percutaneous discharge, Duchenne's interest in this procedure was rekindled. He familiarized himself with the designs of several of the instruments made throughout Europe and proceeded to construct some of his own. The new technology so fascinated him that it provided a stimulus to resume his professional life in spite of his personal devastation and social isolation. In 1839 he married his cousin, a widow, and in 1842 he moved back to Paris where he felt he would have access to a wider variety of conditions suitable for study with this new electrical technique. His home at 21 Boulevard des Italiens (now occupied by the building of the newspaper, *Le Monde*) housed an office for seeing patients, a shop for fabricating instruments, a study, and a dark room for making his own photographs.

Duchenne's introduction into the Parisian community of physicians was not easy. His Boulognese manner and characteristic dialect marked him as an outsider and seemed to catalyze a skepticism from the other physicians about opinions he expressed and the validity of his observations. His manner sometimes generated ridicule. Charles Brissaud related that the ladies of the Salpêtrière, on seeing Duchenne carrying the mahogany box containing his instruments, would say "here comes the little old man with his box of tricks." Most of the chiefs of the various hospital services had established their careers in pathologic anatomy and would use their superior knowledge in this area to diminish his credibility in clinical discussions. Duchenne was well aware of his limited expertise in the traditional disciplines but was confident that the observations being made by him in living subjects were of equal importance and complementary to those in morbid anatomy. He never sought or received a hospital appointment but preferred the freedom to follow his patients and to seek out new subjects for study in all the hospitals in Paris. In the exploratory years in which he employed the induction coil he focused particular attention on the design and manner of application of his electrodes. "Rhéophores" as he called them, if properly moistened, permitted the passage of current without causing any appreciable cutaneous sensation. Pairs could be applied to a group of muscles and, if they were fabricated to permit their placement in a body orifice, they made internal stimulation possible. Unlike the procedure employed in electropuncture, piercing of the skin was not necessary, so that he had little difficulty in inducing patients with a wide variety of illnesses to participate in his clinical trials. On the basis of accumulated anecdotes, Duchenne was persuaded of the therapeutic value of this new form of electrical stimulation for a number of conditions, especially those involving weakness or paralysis, but he also acknowledged its failure to alter outcome in other disorders, such as blindness, deafness, and constipation. He reported occasional adverse reactions, including syncope or sustained gastric pain, following esophageal stimulation. On one occasion he gave intermittent precordial shocks to a lifeless infant born after a prolonged labor (Duchenne, 1872, 137). This resulted in temporary restoration of respiration and color but repeated shocks were unsuccessful in saving the infant's life.

In 1847 Duchenne first presented an account of his methodology and summarized observations made on a wide range of conditions. This presentation was expanded and appeared in the widely circulated *Archives générales de médecine* in 1850. In the years that followed, new material was added together with elaborate illustrations and the work became a monumental volume of over eight hundred pages that was published in 1855. This volume, which marked the end of his professional obscurity, was to pass through three editions and to be translated into both English and German.

However fascinated Duchenne may have been in conducting his studies, he had a warm concern for the welfare of his patients. He was comfortable to visit the homes of the poor and to join with those who stood around a stove, chatting, joking, and feeling no concern about being paid for his services. Indeed, he often gave money away. Many likened him to Saint Vincent de Paul, the priest who had founded organized charity in France two hundred years previously. While he was comfortable in communicating with ordinary people, he was awkward in expressing himself among professional colleagues. He expounded his ideas badly, with diffuse explanations that contrasted with the precision of his clinical observations and the conclusions that could be drawn from them. Quaint mannerisms are said to have marked his delivery, an explosive "Bon!" often punctuating his account of successful experiments. Collins writes that Armand Trousseau would take over an explanation and "with incomparable verbal facility portray the ideas to which Duchenne had been trying to give expression. The latter, recognizing them as his own, would glow with satisfaction and pride to see them appear in a brilliant light. . . " (Collins, 1908). Free of any hospital appointment, administrative responsibility, or teaching assignment, Duchenne gave his entire energies to his investigations and care of his patients. Collins further relates that he was often so occupied and preoccupied that he forgot his appointments. Once invited to dinner by Baron Hausemann, the distinguished official and planner of the city of Paris, he presented himself in evening dress eight days after the event and it was with great difficulty that he was made to understand that the dinner had taken place the week before.

It became clear to Duchenne over the years that the value of faradic stimulation to restore motor function was limited but that it was a useful tool in the study of muscle function. It was in the orderly pursuit of these studies that Duchenne became a founder of neurology and indeed, child neurology, inasmuch as paresis and paralysis were major manifestations of the diseases of children of the day. Poliomyelitis and diphtheritic paralysis were rampant; few physicians took any interest in the cerebral palsies, and the many varieties of neuromuscular disease that appeared in infancy and childhood went undifferentiated. Among his observations was the role of trauma to the brachial plexus at delivery and the resulting palsies affecting the arm and hand (Duchenne, 1872). This observation preceded the writings of Wilhelm Erb by several years, the person now most often identified with this disability (Poore, 1883, 210). Duchenne's reputation grew because of the comprehensive nature of his writings and the new observations that he meticulously recorded. As time passed he became highly respected, even in the halls of the Salpêtrière. Jean Martin Charcot, nearly twenty years his junior, was to consider him his master.

The form of muscular dystrophy that is now identified with Duchenne's name is derived from his account of thirteen personally studied cases, the first of which he had reported in the second edition of his book, *Electrisation localisée* (1861). Some authors have chosen to apply the hyphenated eponym, Aran-Duchenne, to this sex-linked childhood myopathy. This is not appropriate. Aran's paper in 1849 (which includes an account of cases donated by Duchenne) is concerned with a heterogeneous group of adults with progressive muscular atrophy (Aran, 1849).

It should be mentioned that the first accurate and detailed description of Duchenne dystrophy is actually that of Edward Meryon who, in 1852, described four affected boys from the same family with this disorder. Until recently, this account was not recognized (Meryon, 1852; Dubowitz, 1980). Of further interest is the recent biographical study of Paul Broca by Francis Schiller, which mentions Broca's 1851 neuropathological observations of fatty degeneration of muscle in a patient with club foot. Schiller suggests that this report of muscular dystrophy may be earlier than that of Meryon (Schiller, 1979).

The five papers of Duchenne's that appeared in *Archives générales de médecine* in 1868 are comprehensive clinical accounts of "la paralysie musculaire pseudohypertrophique" in which the many features of the disease are compared and contrasted with other paralytic disorders. The earlier published single case had resulted in fifteen other cases being reported between 1861 and 1866 by various authors, mostly in Germany where, to Duchenne's surprise, he seemed to be more appreciated than in France. Some of these authors described the pathologic changes in the affected muscle fragments that had been obtained by biopsy. While Lhermitte credits Duchenne with the introduction of the biopsy, Duchenne himself refers to the bold initiative of Wilhelm Griesinger and Theodore Billroth (Griesinger, 1865). These well-known physicians had employed a device to obtain pieces of muscle in living subjects, but its use was immediately attacked on ethical grounds. It invariably produced a severe diffuse infection with a purulent discharge that took weeks to heal and was considered to have placed the patient's life in jeopardy. Duchenne, keenly sensitive to the ethical issue, was determined to circumvent the problem. He redesigned the German "harpon de Middeldorph" to have a smaller bore with the cutting edge meticulously sharpened. This could be drawn back after insertion into the muscle and then advanced to slice a small fragment of tissue (figure 2). A key provision in the instructions for its use was that it be maintained in alcohol. This was no prescience of Robert Koch's report of the relation between microorganisms and wound infections, which appeared more than a decade later, but simply a caveat to prevent rusting of the finely crafted instrument. Cleanliness was emphasized in order to eliminate adventitious debris from confounding the interpretation of the biopsied tissue. Unaware of the dual role of these measures,

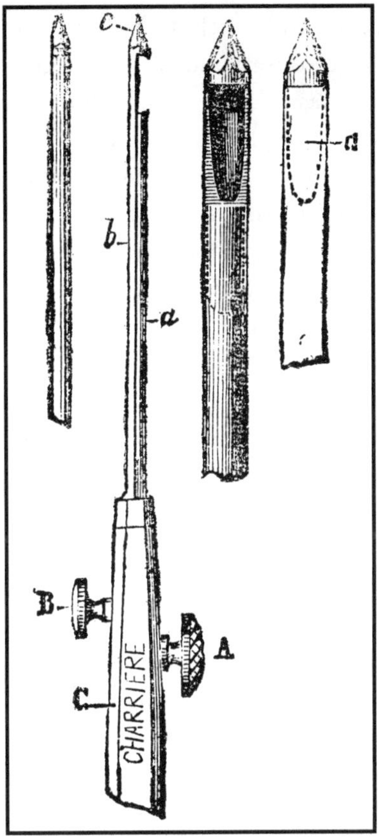

Figure 2. Drawing of the instrument used by Duchenne to perform muscle biopsies. In the closed position (extreme left) it could be inserted into the tissue as a stylet; when in place a part (a) could be retracted from the handle to open a small chamber to clip a piece of muscle when the instrument was withdrawn.

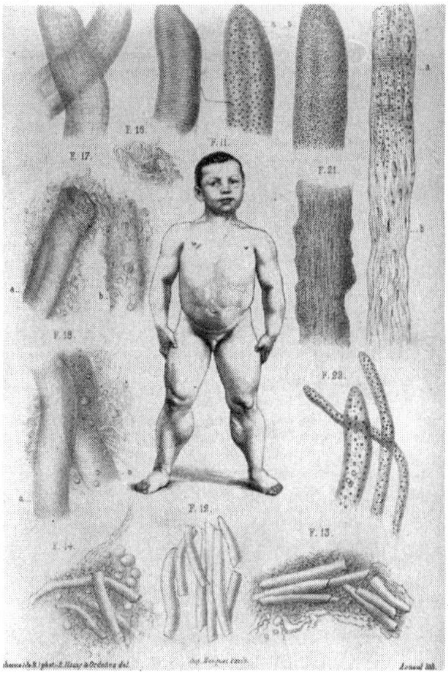

Figure 3. A lithograph from the same paper as that from which figure 2 was taken, "Recherches sur la paralysie musculaire . . .," *Arch gén méd* 11: 204. At the bottom are the separate figures illustrating early (center) and late changes (on either side) in biopsied muscle at low magnification; the remainder of the figures are at higher (200x) magnification and also show changes at various stages of the disease. These are contrasted with the findings in normal muscle (figure 19, at the top).

Duchenne claimed he never had any prolongation in wound healing and that pain caused by the introduction of the needle was minimal. The biopsy, which could be repeated in the course of the disease, was useful in staging its natural course and in demonstrating that the stage had to be taken into account when interpreting the microscopic findings (figure 3). The five papers in 1868, complete with illustrations (one of which appears in figure 4), detailed descriptions of the disease and its invariably fatal outcome in the

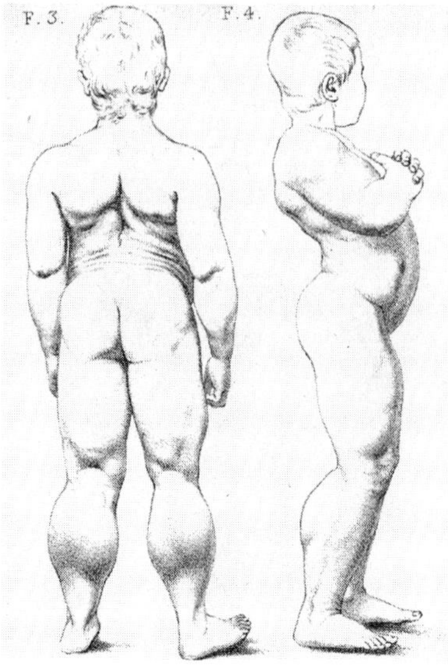

Figure 4. The Herculean appearance of a child with "la paralysie musculaire pseudo-hypertrophique" as depicted in drawings at the beginning of the second of Duchenne's series of papers published in 1868.

young, and a scholarly review of others' observations, are recognized as classic descriptions of the disease (Duchenne, 1868).

The application of faradic stimulation to paralyzed muscle groups was clearly the forerunner of electromyography. Its application in facial paralysis permitted him to differentiate between central and peripheral lesions. Duchenne used this technique to also study poliomyelitis, another disorder common in children, which he referred to as "la paralysie atrophique graisseuse de l'enfance." The failure to obtain responses in muscles affected in poliomyelitis as he had also observed in crush injuries of the spinal cord, led him to reason that the atrophy that followed polio must be the result of disease in the anterior horn cells (Duchenne, 1872, 381–437). Although this thesis had been developed by Heine in 1840 on the basis of histological findings, most writers clung to the vague, traditional concept of "essential paralysis" in which the atrophy was attributed to disuse. That the anterior horn cell destruction was the cause of the paralysis in poliomyelitis was only to be confirmed by Charcot, among several others, ten years later (Charcot and Joffroy, 1870).

In his efforts to sort out the many other forms of paralysis with the aid of the induction coil, Duchenne was less successful. He then turned to employing it in a meticulous examination of the action of individual muscles of the face. Volunteers, including children, would pose before the camera with electrodes held in place by the author and, on simultaneous triggering of current and shutter, the induced facial expression was captured. In his two-volume work entitled *Méchanisme de la physionomie humaine ou analyse électrophysiologique de l'expression des passions*, seventy-four photographs, all taken and processed by Duchenne himself, depict moods ranging from intense religious feeling to buffoonery (Duchenne, 1862). Many of the legends are minidramas of the life situations befitting the iatrogenic countenances. Some discussion is given to the muscle interplay imputed to underlie the expression of subjects of well-known works of art. In a final, more mundane, lengthy undertaking, Duchenne addresses a readership, which was to be primarily orthopedists, and describes the individual action of each muscle of the body. By combining electrical stimulation, in both human and animal subjects, with mechanical models, he provides a description of the muscles that participate in localized movements. This last major work, published in 1872, was translated into German in 1885 and into English in 1949.

Duchenne's energetic life and productive career were sharply curtailed by the events of the Franco-Prussian war and the bitter siege of Paris. He had wished to join his relatives in the military struggle but because of his age could only take consolation in caring for the sick and wounded and providing what food he could for the many who faced starvation. In one year he lost his wife, his brother, and his son, who had become a physician and moved to Paris. In the few years that followed, Duchenne became enfeebled, presumably from cerebral arteriosclerosis, and died suddenly of a cerebral hemorrhage in September, 1875, at the age of sixty-nine. A newspaper recorded that "the least known and least important member of society could not have had a more insignificant funeral procession" (Collins, 1908), and that scarcely a score of friends accompanied the body to the grave. Had Duchenne anticipated this humble marking of his passing, he probably would not have been disappointed. Years previously, when asked to accept an honorary position, he is said to have replied "No, my only ambition is that I shall not die, living always in my works. There are those who have all honors today, but later they will be forgotten, while my work will still live" (Collins, 1908). Indeed it has, in fifty-seven publications, three of which are classics.

Charles Kennedy
BETHESDA, MARYLAND

ACKNOWLEDGMENTS

I gratefully acknowledge the assistance of Isabelle Henrion and David Ko in translating sections of Duchenne's original papers, the courtesy of Dr. Joel Premont and Dr. Therese Jay in making available the portrait of Duchenne from the Académie de Médecine in Paris, and the help of Alison Tannenbaum in preparing the photographs.

REFERENCES

Aran, F. A. 1849. Recherches sur une maladie non encore décrite du système musculaire (atrophie musculaire progressive). *Arch gén méd* (Paris) 24:5–35.

Chamberlain, O. B. 1953. Guillaume Benjamin Amand Duchenne (1806–1875). In *The Founders of Neurology*. Ed W. Haymaker. Springfield, IL: Charles C Thomas.

Charcot, J. M., and A. Joffroy. 1870. Cas de paralysie infantile spinale avec lésions de cornes antérieures de la grise de la moelle épinière. *Arch phys norm path* (Paris) 3:134.

Collins, J. 1908. Duchenne of Boulogne, A Biography and an Appreciation. *Med Rec* (NY) 73:50–54.

Dubowitz, V. 1980. History of Muscle Disease. In *Historical Aspects of the Neurosciences. A Festschrift for Macdonald Critchley*. Ed F. C. Rose, and W. F. Bynum. New York: Raven Press.

Duchenne, G. B. A. 1855. *De l'électrisation localisée, et de son application à la pathologie et à la thérapeutique.* Paris: Baillière.

______. 1862. *Méchanisme de la physionomie humaine ou analyse électrophysiologique de l'expression des passions.* Paris: Renourd.

______. 1868. Recherches sur la paralysie musculaire pseudohypertrophique ou paralysie myosclérosique. *Arch gén méd* (Paris) 6 sér., 11:5–25, 179–207, 305–21, 421–43, 552–88.

______. 1872. *A Treatise on Localized Electrization, and Its Application to Pathology and Therapeutics*. Translated from the 3d ed. by Herbert Tibbits. London: L. Hardwicke.

______. 1949. *Physiology of Motion Demonstrated by Means of Electrical Stimulation and Clinical Observation and Applied to the Study of Paralysis and Deformities.* Translated and edited by E. B. Kaplan. Philadelphia: Lippincott.

Griesinger, V. W. 1865. Ueber Muskelhypertrophie. *Arch Heilk* 6:1–13.

Lasègue, C., and I. Straus. 1875. Duchenne (de Boulogne), Sa vie scientifique et ses oeuvres. *Arch gén méd* (Paris) 26:687–715.

Lhermitte, J. 1946. Duchenne de Boulogne en son temps. *Bull Acad Méd* (Paris) 130:745–55.

Meryon, E. 1852. On Granular and Fatty Degeneration of the Voluntary Muscles. *Med-Chir Trans* 35:73–84.

Poore, G. V. 1883. *Selections from the Clinical Works of Dr. Duchenne (De Boulogne)*, 9–20. London: The New Sydenham Society.

Schiller, F. 1979. *Paul Broca, Founder of French Anthropology, Explorer of the Brain*, 94–95. Los Angeles: University of California Press.

Viets, H. R. 1948. The History of Neurology in the Last One Hundred Years. *Bull NY Acad Med* 24:772–83.

WILHELM HEINRICH ERB

WILHELM HEINRICH ERB (1840–1921) (figure 1) was in many respects the German counterpart of Jean Martin Charcot in France or Sir William Gowers in England. He was the most influential neurologist in Germany in his day. Although we hear more about Charcot and the French school of neurology at the close of the last century, Erb's contributions to neurology, particularly child neurology, may have been as important. He was the first to describe the myotatic reflex and to use the reflex hammer, now frequently viewed as the symbol of the specialty, in his physical examination. Erb was a pioneer in the systematic use of reflexes as part of the neurologic examination. It was through his efforts that, for the first time, neurology was established as part of the undergraduate medical school curriculum. He was one of the founders of the *Deutsche Zeitschrift für Nervenheilkunde* in 1891. His publications include 273 papers on a variety of subjects, nearly one quarter of them devoted to non neurological topics in internal medicine (Viets, 1953; McHenry, 1969). His neurological contributions included papers on progressive muscular dystrophy (Erb and Schultze, 1879; Erb, 1884); upper brachial plexus palsy, or Duchenne-Erb paralysis (Erb, 1877); progressive spastic spinal paralysis, or Erb-Charcot disease (Erb, 1894); myasthenia gravis (Erb, 1879); as well as diseases of the peripheral nerves, spinal cord, and medulla oblongata. He published important monographs on a number of topics including

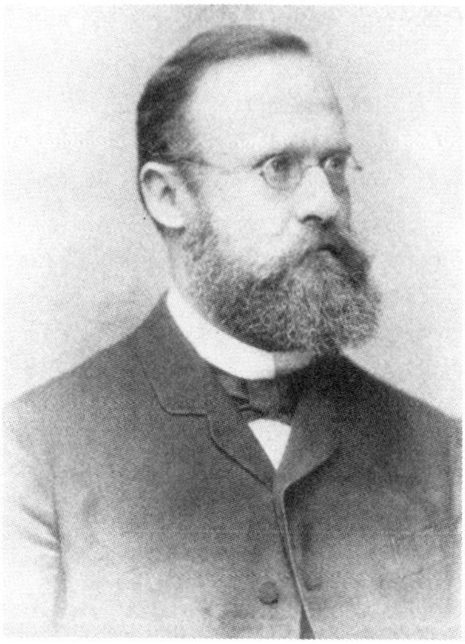

Figure 1. Wilhelm Erb (1840–1921), taken after he had assumed the directorship of the Medical Clinic at Heidelberg in 1883.

the use of reflexes in the evaluation of nervous system disease, tabes dorsalis, myotonia congenita (Thomsen's disease), and muscular dystrophy (Kuh, 1922). Erb was also the author of three major texts, all considered among the best available in their day.

Born on November 30, 1840, in Winnweiler (Bavaria) as the son of a forester, Erb was said to have developed a rugged constitution and a remarkable capacity for work as a result of his early childhood. His propensity to lose his temper as well as the rather colorful language he displayed when he did is also attributed to his youthful exposure to the outdoors and outdoorsmen. Perhaps his custom of giving his best effort for each patient regardless of their origin or the nature of their complaint also stemmed from his childhood appreciation for the common man.

Erb studied medicine at Heidelberg, Erlangen, and finally at Munich, where he received his doctorate in 1864. After receiving his degree, he became an assistant in pathology to Ludwig von Buhl in Munich. Shortly, an offer of an assistantship under Nikolaus Friedreich brought him back to the University of Heidelberg. In Heidelberg he worked under Friedreich as an instructor in the medical clinic until 1880. Erb left Heidelberg to become professor ordinarius and director of the Medical Polyclinic at Leipzig in 1880. He lived in Leipzig only three years, returning to Heidelberg in 1883 after the death of Friedreich to assume the directorship of the medical clinic of Heidelberg and remained there for the duration of his career. Friedreich exerted a profound effect on Erb's development and the direction of his scientific work, stirring in him an interest in peripheral nerve diseases and disorders involving the spinal cord and medulla oblongata.

Erb's reputation as a teacher was equal to his reputation as a scientist. He was said to have had a gift for arousing the interest and enthusiasm of his pupils, which certainly induced a number of his trainees to choose neurology as their area of special interest. Numbered among his pupils are several of the outstanding neurologists in Germany in the early twentieth century. Although he never expected more of his pupils than he was willing to give himself, his capacity for work was legendary, earning him a reputation as a stern and demanding mentor. Erb was always impeccably groomed, extremely punctual, and not one to ignore the hierarchy of academic medicine of the day. Still, he was known to be kind and thoughtful on a personal level, often going out of his way to help a student, colleague, or friend. He was felt to be fair, even handed, and always willing to help his pupils. Among his more famous students were Robert Remak, Friedrich Schultze, and Max Nonne (Viets, 1953).

Although Erb enjoyed an international professional reputation as a clinician, which brought patients from many countries to his clinic, his private life was not as rewarding. His first wife and two of his four sons died before him. He was said to become despondent when a third son was killed on the first day of World War I. He also was greatly upset by the war and by the desperate condition that his country found itself in during the later stages of it. These factors combined to make his later years somewhat unhappy. His death was said to have been the result of an attack of syncope that overcame him while listening to Beethoven's Eroica, one of his favorite pieces of music.

Among his many scientific contributions Erb (simultaneously with Carl Westphal) described the myotatic reflex and noted the abnormality of the reflexes in tabes dorsalis in 1875 (Erb, 1875; Westphal, 1875). He later confirmed the syphilitic origin of tabes dorsalis by the application of statistical methods (Erb, 1903). Considered a major expert on diseases of the spinal cord, he was one of the first to point out the possibility of causes for progressive spasticity other than syphilis (Erb, 1894).

Early descriptions of traumatic injury to the upper brachial plexus (Erb's or Duchenne-Erb palsy) were made by both Duchenne and Erb. Duchenne was the first to recognize that the traction injury to the brachial plexus could occur during the birth process (Duchenne, 1872). Both Duchenne and Erb described the use of electrical stimulation in the study and characterization of the injury (Erb, 1877). Duchenne's work with electrodiagnosis and electrotherapy stimulated what would become a major area of interest for Erb. He used electrodiagnostic techniques to study many diseases of the peripheral nerves and described the test of brachial plexus degeneration, which used stimulation of the nerve trunks at the location known now as Erb's point (Erb, 1868). He also described what was later to be called "Erb's phenomenon," that is, increased irritability of the motor nerves in tetany (Erb, 1872). Erb felt that electrodiagnosis should have a major place in neurology. He also felt strongly that it was the duty of neurologists to strive for effective treatments for the various diseases of the nervous system. He held out the hope that electrotherapy might prove to be useful in various neurological and mental diseases. The failure to develop practical uses for electrotherapy was one of his major professional disappointments.

Erb also wrote about muscular dystrophy. He coined the term "progressive muscular dystrophy" and distinguished this type of muscular dystrophy from other myopathies and dystrophies. He published a 200-page monograph on the muscular dystrophies that initially appeared in the *Deutsche Zeitschrift für Nervenheilkunde* in 1891 and later as a separate monograph (1891a, b). In it he reviewed a voluminous amount of clinical material on the muscular dystrophies, particularly a slowly progressive form affecting the shoulder and humeral muscles. For many years this was known as Erb's type, or the "juvenile form" of muscular dystrophy. Erb also provided the first clear distinction between the spinal muscular atrophies and progressive muscular dystrophy (Erb and Schultze, 1879; Erb, 1884). The first clear description of progressive spastic spinal paralysis and the categorization of this as one of the types of motor neuron disease is also credited to Erb (Erb, 1894).

One of Erb's major contributions to child neurology was his study of myotonia congenita (Erb, 1886). Erb was the first to systematically study its pathogenesis, reporting twenty-eight patients and classifying them into three groups: those with typical myotonia, those appearing similar but with atypical features, and those with myotonia and other nervous system involvement. He also described increased irritability of the muscles of patients with myotonia congenita and reported the first characteristic pathologic changes on muscle biopsy. This was an important observation, as previous investigators had only reported normal findings.

Perhaps Erb's greatest contribution was his work to establish neurology as a legitimate specialty and an area deserving of inclusion in the medical school curriculum. He believed that it was impossible for even the interested internist to keep abreast of the rapidly expanding knowledge of the nervous system and said in an address delivered in 1880:

One need hardly have to argue in detail that the only possible scientific, and the most fruitful work on the pathology of the nervous system needs to be specialized nowadays. Total devotion of a man and the consecration of all his powers is required in order to attain even approximate mastery of this huge field. (Viets, 1953)

He was among the first proponents of the systematic examination of signs and symptoms in physical diagnosis and to include the utilization of tendon reflexes in this process. As such he was one of the first physicians anywhere to carry a reflex hammer with which to examine his patients. Although he met stiff resistance, he was able, through persistent efforts, to get a course in neurology included in the undergraduate medical curriculum at the University of Heidelberg. Furthermore, he was able to achieve some recognition for neurology as an acceptable medical specialty through persistent coercion of his colleagues at medical meetings throughout Germany and Europe (Viets, 1953).

Although Erb was primarily interested in general neurology, his contributions to pediatric neurology are many, as have been described. The brachial plexus injury (Erb's palsy) due to obstetrical trauma to the newborn was not what Erb described. He actually described adult patients with a stretch injury of the upper brachial plexus as an example of the use of reflex activity in the localization of lesions of the nervous system. Nevertheless, he was aware of Duchenne's demonstration of birth injury as one of the potential causes of this "obstetrical paralysis." His work with muscular dystrophies, myotonia congenita, and other diseases affecting children, as well as his efforts on behalf of the discipline of neurology in general, certainly earn him the right to be included among the founders of child neurology.

John Bodensteiner
MORGANTOWN, WEST VIRGINIA

Duchenne, G. B. A. 1872. *De l'électrisation localisée, et de son application à la pathologie et à la thérapeutique*, 353–67. 3d ed. Paris: J. B. Baillière & Fils.

Erb, W. 1868. Zur Pathologie und pathologischen Autonomie peripherischer Paralysen. *Dtsch Arch klin Med* 4:535–78.

______. 1872. Zur Lehre von der Tetanie: Über die Prufung der electrischen Erregbarkeit motorischer Nerven. *Arch Psych Nervenkrankh* (Berlin) 4:271–316.

______. 1875. Über Sehnenreflexe bei Gesunden und Ruckenmarkskranken. *Arch Psych Nervenkrankh* 5:792–802.

______. 1877. Über eine eigentumliche Localization von Lahmungen im Plexus brachialis. *Verh naturh-med Ver Heidelberg* 1:130–37.

______. 1879. Über einen neunen, wahrsheinlich bulbaren Symptomencomplex. *Arch Psych Nervenkrankh* (Berlin) 9:336–50.

______. 1884. Über die "juvenile form" der progressiven Muskelatrophie und ihre Beziehungen zur sogenannten Pseudohypertrophie des Muskeln. *Dtsch Arch klin Med* 34:467–519.

______. 1886. Die Thomsen'sche Krankheit. Leipzig: F. C. W. Vogel.

______. 1894. Über hereditare Spinalparalyse. *Dtsch Zeit Nervenheilk* 6:137–49.

______. 1903. Über die spastische und die syphilitische Spinalparalyse und ihre Existenzberchtigung. *Dtsch Zeit Nervenheilk* 23:347–77.

Erb, W., and F. Schultze. 1879. Ein Fall von progressiver Muskelatrophie mit Erkrankung der grauen Vordersaulen des Ruckenmarks. *Arch Psych Nervenkrankh* (Berlin) 9:369–88.

Kuh, S. 1922. Wilhelm Erb, 1840–1921. *Arch Neur Psych* 7:250–51.

McHenry, L. C. 1969. *Garrison's History of Neurology*, 298–99. Springfield, IL: Charles C Thomas.

Viets, H. R. 1953. Heinrich Erb (1840–1921). In *The Founders of Neurology*, 435–38. Ed. W. Haymaker and F. Schiller. Springfield, IL.: Charles C Thomas.

Westphal, C. E. 1875. Über einige durch mechanische Einwirkung auf Sehnen und Muskeln hervorgebrachte Bewegungserscheinungen. *Arch Psych Nervenkrankh* 5:803–34.

SIGMUND FREUD

SIGMUND FREUD'S life has been the subject of several well-known biographies as well as a brief autobiography (Clark, 1980; Gay, 1988; Jones, 1961; Freud, 1935). Although his productive career in neurology has been eclipsed by the magnitude of his contributions to psychiatry (Jelliffe, 1937), Freud's neurological training and discoveries are well recognized and his work on cerebral palsy has recently been briefly presented in American pediatric literature (Accardo, 1982).

Freud (1856–1939) (figure 1) was born in Moravia (later a part of Czechoslovakia) and moved to Vienna with his family at the age of four. He was at the top of his class at the *gymnasium* for seven years and, by his own account, enjoyed special privileges there (Freud, 1935). His father, Jacob Freud, also seemed to have recognized his son's brilliance; Ronald Clark relates that the musical interests of Freud's sisters were sacrificed to preserve the quiet environment that the young Freud required for his studies (Clark, 1980). In addition, Freud's father allowed him to choose a profession on the basis of his own inclinations. Although initially attracted to law, Freud was drawn toward natural science by the then recent theories of Darwin and decided to become a medical student "after hearing Goethe's beautiful essay on Nature read aloud at a popular lecture" (Freud, 1935). Although Freud registered in the University of Vienna's medical department in 1873, he initially pursued a broad curriculum with a particular interest in philosophy. In part because of the breadth of his interests, he required eight instead of the usual five years to graduate. In 1877, under the tutelage of the comparative anatomist Carl Claus, Freud presented a paper on the reproductive physiology of the eel (Clark, 1980).

Between 1877 and 1883, Freud worked in Ernst Brucke's Institute of Physiology. Brucke was one of the founders of a movement which began in the 1840s and has been designated the Helmholz School of Medicine. The other founders of this movement were Emil du Bois-Reymond, Carl Ludwig, and Hermann Helmholz. These four men and their students dominated German

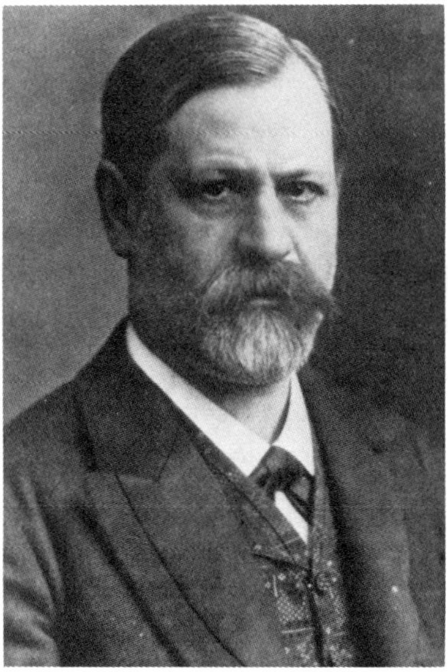

Figure 1. Sigmund Freud (1856–1939).

physiology during the last half of the nineteenth century (Amacher, 1965). While at the Institute, Freud devoted his attention to the phylogenetic evolution of the nervous system of the lamprey eel and crayfish, a subject in which interest had been spurred by the controversy surrounding the recent publication of Darwin's *The Origin of Species* (Clark, 1980). He developed a technique for staining nervous tissue with gold chloride; this led to a publication in the German medical literature as well as one in the journal *Brain* (Jones, 1961).

Freud's neuropathological interests subsequently shifted to the medulla oblongata. His methods of studying the medulla made use of a recent discovery by Paul Flechsig: various tracts in the central nervous system have independent timetables of myelination. By studying serial sections of fetal brains, he was able to make observations on the course of tracts that would have been lost in the "inextricable pictures of cross sections, which permit hardly more than a superficial topographical survey" when comparable adult material was examined (Jones, 1961, 137). Freud's investigations utilized the brains of experimental animals and also included human material. It seems likely that this early work, which led to three publications, contributed to his interest in cerebral palsy and was in part responsible for the emphasis that he placed on prenatal factors in its genesis.

During the time he worked with Brucke, Freud was "decidedly negligent" in pursuing his medical studies and did not receive his degree as Doctor of Medicine until 1881. He states in his autobiography that "the various branches of medicine proper, apart from psychiatry, had no attraction for me" (Freud, 1935). Although Freud enjoyed success in the laboratory and was designated for promotion when a suitable position became available, Brucke urged him to pursue a career in clinical medicine in order to better his financial situation (Freud, 1935). Freud spent his next three years at the Vienna General Hospital, rotating through the surgical services and later through the medicine department of Dr. Hermann Nothnagel, who was to become the editor of the *Handbuch* to which Freud contributed his monograph on infantile cerebral paralyses approximately fifteen years later. His experience in the Vienna General Hospital included five months in Theodore Meynert's department of psychiatry (Clark, 1980).

Freud transferred to the department of nervous diseases in 1884. Over the next few years he published a number of clinical reports. Freud observed that

the fame of my diagnoses and of their post mortem confirmation brought me an influx of American physicians, to whom I lectured upon the patients in my department in a sort of pidgin-English. I was able to localize the site of a lesion in the medulla oblongata so accurately that the pathological anatomist had no further information to add; I was the first person in Vienna to send a case for autopsy with a diagnosis of polyneuritis acuta (Freud, 1935, 20).

Freud read the account of Theodor Aschenbrandt on the stimulation effects of cocaine and began to experiment with the drug and encourage its use by friends in other branches of medicine. Although Freud made the observation that cocaine had anesthetic properties and wrote a monograph on the history of cocaine and its potential applications in medicine, "the decisive experiments upon animals' eyes" were made by his friend Carl Koller to whom Freud had introduced the drug (Freud, 1935; Jones, 1961).

In 1885 Freud received an appointment as *privatdozent* (university lecturer) for neuropathology, and this enabled him to secure a travelling fellowship to Paris, where he worked under Jean Martin Charcot for six months. The main result of this segment of Freud's education was to stimulate an interest in hysteria, which would ultimately lead to the methods and theory of psychoanalysis. Freud planned to carry out pathological studies of children's brains while at the Salpêtrière. However, his letters indicate that he abandoned his plans to pursue laboratory work during his sojourn in Paris (Clark, 1980).

On his return trip to Vienna, Freud "stopped for a few weeks in Berlin, in order to gain a little knowledge of the general disorders of childhood" in the clinic of Adolf Baginsky (Freud, 1935, 24). In a letter to his fiancée, he described his reaction to pediatric practice: "As long as their brains are free of disease, these little creatures are really charming and so touching when they suffer . . . I think I would find my way about in a children's practice in no time" (Clark, 1980, 76). Over the next several years, as the result of work done at the Kassowitz Institute in Vienna, he published several monographs dealing with unilateral and bilateral cerebral paralyses in children.

Freud had resigned his position at the Vienna General Hospital prior to leaving for his fellowship in Paris. On his return to Vienna in 1886, he entered practice as a specialist in nervous diseases. His views on hysteria brought him into conflict with Meynert, led to his exclusion from the Laboratory of Cerebral Anatomy, and perhaps accelerated the development of an independent approach to mental illness (Freud, 1935). Freud's major neurological publications after 1890 came at a time when he was already laying the foundations of modern psychiatry. *Studies on Hysteria*, which was written in collaboration with Josef Breuer, was published in 1895 and *The Interpretation of Dreams* in 1900.

His monograph on aphasia, *Zur Auffassung der Aphasien, eine Kritische Studie* (*On Aphasia: A Critical Study*), published in 1891 as the result of an invitation to contribute to a medical encyclopedia, reflected a mastery of the theories of Carl Wernicke and Ludwig Lichtheim as well as a broad understanding of neurology and neurophysiology. Freud meticulously reviewed the accepted categories of aphasia, revealed the limitations of current classifications, and also suggested that attempts to localize various aspects of language function appear inadequate to explain some forms of aphasia. Recognition that anatomic distribution of cerebral lesions does not always correlate predictably with clinical manifestations is also a theme to which Freud returned to in his book *Die Infantile Cerebrallähmung*. In his book *On Aphasia*, Freud introduced the term agnosia to neurology and proposed the category of agnostic aphasia in which the language disturbance resulted from failure of object recognition. He redefined the term asymbolia, which had previously been used by Karl Finkelnburg, to mean a disturbance in the association between word concept and object concept. Freud traced his own views of language to the writings of John Stuart Mill, which he had translated years earlier (Freud, 1953).

Freud's writings on cerebral palsy spanned a ten-year period beginning in 1889 when he was the first to report on the presences of visual field deficits in children with cerebral palsy (Freud, 1889). One of his best known works, in collaboration with Oscar Rie, was a 220-page monograph entitled *Klinische Studie über die halbseitige Cerebrallähmung der Kinder* (*Clinical Study on the Unilateral Cerebral Paralysis of Children*), which was printed in 1891. This extensive study of the literature and collection of case reports was of interest because Freud was the first to focus on the occurence of hemiatrophy on the affected paralysed side and also helped establish the choreoathetotic form of cerebral palsy as a distinct subtype of this disorder. Two years later a shorter monograph, further elaborating on the clinicopathological aspects of cerebral palsy, particularly in relation to Little's disease, was published. Freud also wrote a paper on the same subject, which appeared in the *Revue neurologique* (1893b). During the next four years Freud consolidated and revised these efforts into one of the most important works ever written on this subject, *Die Infantile Cerebrallähmung*.

Freud's *Die Infantile Cerebrallähmung* (*Infantile Cerebral Paralysis*) was published in 1897 for Nothnagel's *Handbuch der Allgemeinen und Speziellen Therapie*. In his letters, Freud expressed some frustration over the necessity of producing this work on cerebral paralysis at a time when he was already preoccupied with the neuroses: "I am fully occupied with the children's paralyses, in which I am not the least interested" (Accardo, 1982, 453).

Infantile Cerebral Paralysis was an exhaustive work divided into eleven chapters. The first seven chapters include a discussion of nosological considerations, an extensive review of the literature, detailed discussions of diplegic and hemiplegic forms, and an exhaustive compilation of the pathological anatomy of the disorder. The eighth chapter deals with the classification of various types of cerebral paralysis on the basis of their underlying pathology and etiological factors. In the chapter on pathological physiology, Freud focuses on the relationship between the distribution of pathological changes and clinical symptomatology. Chapter Nine reviews familial and hereditary forms of infantile cerebral paralysis while the following chapter examines the relation of epilepsy and mental impairment ("idiocy") to the other symptoms of the disorder. The brief final chapter discusses differential diagnosis and therapy.

Freud began with a pathological rather than a clinical definition of the disorder:

I actually advocate that this term be applied even to cases in which paralysis is completely absent or where the disease consists merely of a periodic recurrence of convulsions (epilepsy). This infantile cerebral paralysis is merely a contrived term of our nosographic classification, a label referring to a group of pathological cases. . . It would be desirable to replace this term by another not conveying such a definite, inadequate image. (Freud, 1968, 17)

Throughout his text, Freud's use of the general term "infantile cerebral paralysis" approximates the modern pediatric neurologist's phrase "nonprogressive encephalopathy." Freud amply justifies his desire for a looser interpretation by frequently pointing out the variability of clinical and pathological manifestations in patients with childhood encephalopathies and the lack of a predictable relation between pathologic features and clinical manifestations.

Freud was confronted with the task not only of cogently presenting his own schema of classification but also of justifying his departure from the classifications proposed by many who preceded him. Several themes recur throughout his work. He demonstrated transitional forms between types of cerebral paralysis, considered by other authors to be distinct in their clinical presentation; showed the lack of an exclusive relation between etiological factors and the type of deficit; and illustrated that the recognized deficit may evolve, diminish, appear, or disappear as a function of the patient's age. He made many pertinent observations concerning the relation of certain forms of motor deficit to other manifestations such as mental impairment ("idiocy"), aphasia, and visual disturbance. He appeared to achieve the balanced goal of arguing forcefully for his own views without engaging in excessive criticism of those propounded by previous authors.

Freud accorded particular importance to the views of William Little concerning the importance of various parturitional factors including premature birth. He disputed in several places the controversial view of Adolf Strümpell that encephalitis is the major factor responsible for infantile cerebral paralysis (Freud, 1968). Freud acknowledged that about one-half of all "noncongenital forms" of hemiplegic infantile cerebral paralysis are of unknown etiology and later stated that in his own case material, an etiology could not be identified in 34 percent of patients with cerebral diplegia (Freud, 1968). While accepting the term "Little's Disease," he did so with reservation and not as a synonym for "infantile cerebral paralysis." Rather, he restricted its use to diplegic cases in which factors related to delivery appeared to be of predominant importance. He suggested that a broader use of the term "would only serve to obscure Little's contribution in regard to the etiology of birth paralysis" (Freud, 1968, 260). He dealt at some length with the troublesome observation that many children experiencing obstetric difficulties did not develop infantile cerebral paralysis and surmised that

Little's etiology cannot in all cases exist without the simultaneous effects of congenital factors. Furthermore, one has to consider that the anomaly of the birth process, rather than being the causal etiological factor, may itself be the consequence of the real prenatal etiology. (Freud, 1968, 142)

Freud individually discussed various manifestations of nonprogressive encephalopathy. A recurring theme is that the severity of one neurological manifestation did not reliably predict the severity or even the existence of another. However, he did note that "one should add to the peculiarities of choreatic paresis the rarity of occurrence of aphasia, atrophy, epilepsy and slight degree of mental impairment" (Freud, 1897). He explained these observations by reference to a single autopsied case, reported by Louis Landouzy, who demonstrated a calcified lenticular lesion (Freud, 1968, 109).

Freud did not feel compelled to explain the pathologic or physiologic basis for certain manifestations of cerebral paralysis. In some cases, he examined the hypotheses that had been propounded, found them deficient, and acknowledged that a satisfactory alternative is not apparent:

The explanation of such trophic disturbances (growth arrest) following cerebral affections with a complete absence or only a trace of paralytic symptoms has not been made so far. The assumption of "trophic centers" in the cortex has merely the value of prejudiced circumvention of facts. (Freud, 1968, 120)

Freud noted that he was the first to report the association of homonymous hemianopsia with hemiplegic cerebral palsy (Freud, 1889; 1897, 89). He elaborated on the difficulty of detecting visual field defects in children. In reviewing the relative concomitants of "infantile cerebral paralysis", he made a forceful argument for the extension of the term to include a broad range of neurological deficits:

Such symptoms as hemianesthesia and hemianopsia are decisive in the interpretation of the concept of "hemiplegic cerebral paralysis" by forcing us to go beyond the literal meaning of the term and to eliminate the last possibility of considering this frequently occurring disorder a systematic disease limited to the gray motor cortex. The localization of the lesion cannot be the essential factor of infantile cerebral palsy. This is further confirmed by pathological anatomy, which exhibits in hemiplegic cerebral paralysis the same lesions in various other parts of the cortex or of the brain that, if they occurred in the motor regions, would also create hemiplegia. Consequently, it would be quite correct to attribute isolated hemianopsia to hemiplegic cerebral paralysis as long as the other clinical instances (etiology, course of disease, complications) show conformity. (Freud, 1968, 92)

In *Infantile Cerebral Paralysis*, Freud dealt with practical considerations in childhood language disorders but made little reference to the concepts in his earlier monograph, *On Aphasia*. He distinguished between acquired aphasia ("as a disturbance of already acquired speaking ability") and developmental language delay (in which "we are not justified to look at the disturbance as a focal symptom because delayed development of speech of children does occur so frequently as a symptom of poor cerebral development") (Freud, 1968, 92). He supported the views of previous authors, including Jean Louis Cotard, that aphasia in patients with hemiplegic cerebral palsy is not "a permanent symptom" and noted that aphasic disturbances in children are not uncommonly associated with left rather than right hemiparesis (Freud, 1968, 94). He summarized the conclusions of Max Bernhardt concerning aphasia in association with cerebral paralysis and expressed his agreement with the following conclusions that are generally accepted today: (1) Aphasia appears often at an early age; (2) The right hemisphere is often able to substitute for the left in language function; (3) Motor (expressive) aphasia is the most common type in childhood (Freud, 1968, 95).

Freud's chapter on familial and hereditary forms of infantile cerebral palsy included a detailed description of several degenerative disorders, including Pelizaeus-Merzbacher disease. On the one hand he appeared willing to include such conditions under the umbrella of cerebral paralyses, but he implied acceptance of the view that the great majority of cases of cerebral paralysis in childhood have a nonprogressive etiology: "It is, therefore, more probable that the forms of infantile cerebral paralysis we are considering actually are diseases with accidental etiology" (Freud, 1968, 318). In this context, Freud appears to use the term "accidental" in a broad sense to refer to disease processes that are not of genetic origin.

Freud's discussion of the pathology of infantile cerebral paralysis reviewed numerous entities that he divided into three categories: intrauterine forms, birth paralyses, and forms acquired postnatally (Freud, 1968, 159). He noted that neurological deficit may derive not only from injury to a portion of the nervous system already under development but also from injury at an earlier stage when development of a portion of the brain may "fail to materialize" (Freud, 1968, 175).

Freud brought coherence to the classification of infantile cerebral paralysis. He recognized that a broad range of etiological and pathological factors were associated with cerebral palsy and emphasized that lesions outside the motor system but otherwise identical to those which produce paralysis may cause disturbance of language and sensory function. He acknowledged that in a substantial proportion of patients, the etiology remained obscure even after careful evaluation. He recognized that obstetric factors did not account for all cases of infantile cerebral paralysis and accepted the term "Little's Disease" as appropriate for only one subgroup of infantile cerebral diplegia.

Freud's transition from the world of neurology to that of psychiatry is perhaps reflected in one of the last passages in the chapter devoted to "Epilepsy and Idiocy":

The condition underlying idiocy must be more specific. It must be related to a localized disturbance, although localization must not be used here in the usual sense, such as pertaining to a definite anatomical region or a histological layer of the brain, but in the sense that the injury affects one or the other of the complex apparatuses [sic] *that subserve mental functions. Any more definite conditions are completely unknown, just as we are completely in the dark in regard to the structure of the mental apparatus.* (Freud, 1968, 339)

Michael A. Pollack
ORLANDO, FLORIDA

REFERENCES

Accardo, P. J. 1982. Freud on Diplegia: Commentary and Translation. *Am J Dis Child* 136:452–56.

Amacher, P. 1965. Freud's Neurological Education and its Influence on Psychoanalytic Theory. *Psych Issues* Vol. 4, No. 4.

Clark, R. W. 1980. *Freud: The Man and the Cause, A Biography*. New York: Random House.

Freud, S. 1889. Ueber Hemianopsie in Fruhesten Kindesalter. *Wien med Wschr* 38:1081–86, 1116–21.

______. 1891. *Zur Auffassung der Aphasien, eine Kritsche Studie.* Leipzig: Deuticke.

______. 1893a. *Zur Kenntnis der cerebralen Diplegien des Kindesalters (im Anschlusse an die Little'sche Krankheit*). Wien: M. Perles.

______. 1893b. Les diplégies cérébrales infantiles. *Rev neur* 8:177–83.

______. 1897. *Die Infantile Cerebrällahmung*. Wien: Holder.

______. 1935. *An Autobiographical Study*. Authorized translation by James Strachey, 1935. New York: W. W. Norton & Co., Inc.

______. 1953. *On Aphasia: A Critical Study*. Translated by E. Stengel. London: Imago Publishing Co., Ltd.

______. 1968. *Infantile Cerebral Paralysis*. Translated by Lester A. Russin. Coral Gables: University of Miami Press.

Freud, S., and O. Rie. 1891. *Klinische Studie über die halbseitige Cerebrallähmung der Kinder*. Wien: M. Perles.

Gay, P. 1988. *Freud: A Life for Our Time.* New York: W. W. Norton Co., Inc.

Jelliffe, S. E. 1937. Sigmund Freud as a Neurologist. *J Nerv Ment Dis* 85:696–711.

Jones, E. 1961. *The Life and Work of Sigmund Freud.* Ed. Lionel Trilling and Steven Marcus. New York: Basic Books, Inc./Harper Colophon Books.

NIKOLAUS FRIEDREICH

NIKOLAUS FRIEDREICH (figure 1) was born into a medical family in Würzburg, Germany, on July 31, 1825. His father had been Professor of General Pathology at Würzburg. His grandfather, Nikolaus Anton Friedreich, was a director of the medicine clinic at Würzburg and was apparently interested in the nervous system, having described acute unilateral facial palsy in 1798, twenty-three years before Bell's description (Bird, 1979). Friedreich's education began in 1832. He obtained most of his undergraduate and medical training in Würzburg and worked initially with Carl Friedrich von Marcus, a blind clinician, and then with Rudolf Albert von Kolliker (1817–1905) in 1847 and 1848 (Clarke and O'Malley, 1968). However, his major mentor was Rudolph Virchow who held the chair of pathological anatomy in Würzburg and was a political activist for a time at the barricades during the revolution of 1848. In 1849 Friedreich joined the faculty in Würzburg. He presented his first paper on November 1, 1851, describing a case of lymphangiectasia of the penis. In 1853 he completed his private docent thesis on "Contributions to the Study of Intracranial Tumors." In 1854 he presented a series of papers on pneumothorax, emphysema, and typhus. In the autumn of 1856, Virchow was called to Berlin and Friedreich succeeded to his chair in 1857 at the age of thirty-one. Virchow's training provided Friedreich with a skill, which was developing in medicine at the time, of applying pathology to clinical disorders. Friedreich was a consummate clinician, especially interested in physical diagnosis. After only a year in Virchow's chair, Friedreich became director of the medical clinics at Germany's oldest university at Heidelberg. At the time, this school was rivaled only by those in Berlin and Vienna.

Friedreich was proficient in all areas of medicine, but his main interest was the nervous system. Many of his important contributions involved pediatric patients, most notably those with muscle disease and ataxia. He wrote an elaborate monograph on progressive muscular atrophy (Friederich, 1873). This work, regarded by contemporaries as his greatest ("Nikolaus Friedreich," 1882), was

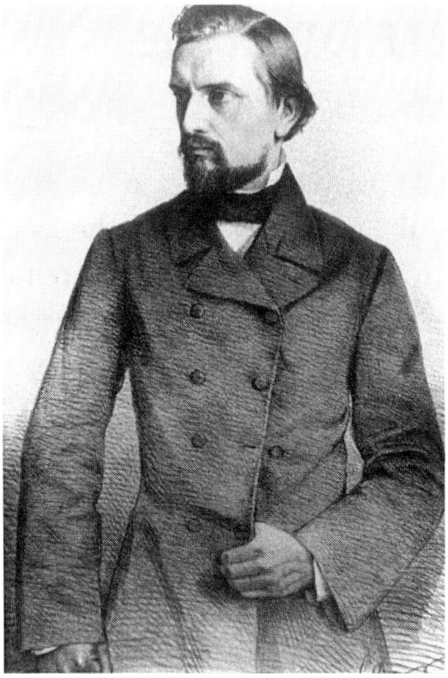

Figure 1. Nikolaus Friedreich (1825–1882).

helpful in the early understanding of muscular dystrophy, but it failed to distinguish atrophy from nonmuscular disorders. He published a total of eight monographs and fifty-one papers ("Nikolaus Friedreich," 1882).

Friedreich's most enduring contributions were his classic descriptions of the ataxia that now bears his name. This disorder begins in childhood and is characterized by progressive ataxia, scoliosis, and a cardiomyopathy. He published a large, three-part article in 1863 (Friedreich 1863a, b, c) and two follow-up articles (Friedreich, 1876, 1877). It is remarkable that he was able to distinguish these patients so clearly because there was, at the time of the initial report, no description of the deep tendon reflex or multiple sclerosis, and tabes dorsalis was a general descriptor of multiple conditions. Into this arena, somewhat euphorically, Friedreich entered with his first report. He might have seemed arrogant to contemporaries, but to us he appears prophetic:

Now at hand is the indispensable microscope to aid in research of the spinal cord. . . . the point in time may not lie too far away in which continued research, together with pathologic-anatomic clinical observations will clarify the vague subject of tabes dorsalis and the separate individual forms that are distinguishable. . . . My own clinical observations, made here at the convergence of two enchanting rivers in the middle of the beautifully landscaped banks . . . [*and*] *my position as head of the clinic has given me the opportunity to observe so many different variations of these illnesses that I feel well qualified to submit this report. My observations on these following specific spinal diseases have been so complete both symptomatically and etiologically that, if you will permit me, I will describe the strong characteristics that segregate these forms of spinal degeneration from the collective concept of Tabes Dorsalis.* (Friedreich, 1863a)

Friedreich described cardiac disease and pathology in his patients, but regarded this as an incidental complication, unrelated to the remainder of the clinical syndrome (Thoren, 1964; Tyrer, 1975). Friedreich also delineated the foot and spine deformities. He reported many of the critical neuropathologic changes: posterior column degeneration, loss of Clarke's column neurons, and possible lateral column involvement (Tyrer, 1975). He did not examine the dorsal root ganglion. In one paper he discussed the features that differentiated his patients from those with more common forms of tabes. In his last paper he noted his inability to obtain the deep tendon reflex, which was just then being developed as a clinical test. After reviewing nine case histories from the Lotsch, Süss, and Schultz families, he summarized his observations:

> *One recognizes the close agreement in these three (Schultz) cases and the examples of ataxic illness from my former dissertations. No essential differences obtain in the manner of development, the form of the ataxic symptoms or the course of the illness. All accounts indicate a hereditary predisposition with a predominance of female victims. The first symptoms occurred in the years preceding or just shortly before the completion of puberty. All had the same type of ataxic disturbances in the articular movements of the tongue, the characteristic nystagmus, the tendency towards many years of relative stability and the eminent chronic course of suffering. . . . Imperfect sensory perception ensues after many years of suffering. When I consider all these essential points of the clinical picture, in agreement in each of the Schultz sisters as well as my previously described patients, three of whom were autopsied, then I believe a distinctive picture emerges and that a diagnosis of a degenerative disorder of the dorsal white matter of the spinal cord should be considered.* (Friedreich, 1876)

Friedreich's descriptions were not immediately appreciated. Indeed, his obituaries in German do not even mention his papers on familial ataxia. However, Wilhelm Erb (1878) had written about the "Friedreich'sche Form der Tabes" and Gowers spoke before the Clinical Society of London in 1880 about Friedreich's contribution (Keppel-Hesselink, 1986). A. Brousse in France wrote about the "Maladie de Friedreich" (1882) and by 1886 J. S. Bury produced his treatise pointing out particularly the pediatric issues in "Friedreich's Disease" (Bury, 1886; Keppel-Hesselink, 1986). The president of the American Neurological Association on June 23, 1882, attacked Friedreich, although failing to notice Friedreich's efforts to distinguish his patients from others with tabes:

Twenty years ago, when doubt existed relative to the seat and nature of the lesion constituting the disease now generally known as locomotor ataxia, Friedreich, of Heidelberg, published an elaborate essay, of which the title, "On Degenerative Atrophy of the Posterior Columns of the Spinal Cord," indicated the view which he entertained of its morbid anatomy. . . . All writers on the subject, so far as my knowledge extends, have accepted, without question, Friedreich's view of their character, while no one has thought it worthwhile to study them in the light of our present knowledge. . . . As to the microscopic examination, it is almost valueless, owing to the imperfection of the methods for preparation . . . no neurologist of the present day, after a full consideration of these cases, would regard them as instances of locomotor ataxia.
(Hammond, 1882)

Friedreich was also initially misunderstood by Charcot's school, who considered his cases examples of multiple sclerosis. Friedreich was indignant, but soon the French were convinced. (Andermann, 1976) However, the confusion continued for many years, with multiple types of ataxia included in Friedreich's category. The confusion was so significant that progress was delayed. Thoren (1964) and the Quebec Cooperative Study Group (Geoffroy et al, 1976) can be credited with restoring our concept of Friedreich's disease to its historic (and current) meaning.

Friedreich's other enduring contribution was the introduction of the term *myoclonus*. In 1878 he evaluated the patient Ludwig Beierlein, later reporting his condition as "paramyoklonusmultiplex". (Friedreich, 1881) "Klonus" referred to the quick movements, "myo" was added to distinguish the movement from cerebral causes, and "para" to indicate its symmetry (Hallet et al, 1982; Hallet, 1986).

Richard Richter described the personal side of Friedreich. (Richter, 1970) His life was devoted largely to medicine. He spent most of his time administering to his clinic and university and running a very large consultative practice. His family was apparently his only diversion. In personality, he was loyal to many friends, but mistrustful of others and bitterly vindictive to enemies. He had a tremendous drive for work.

However, Friedreich perhaps had some diversions, for on excursions to the sea and a mountain climbing excursion in the fall of 1863 at the age of thirty-eight, he first complained of vertigo. By age fifty-seven, after keeping a calendar of his symptoms, he was able to self-diagnose the cause of this as well as his chest pain. Virchow, visiting him in his last autumn in Heidelberg, described him as serene and content; Friedreich knew his fate. He died suddenly on July 6, 1882, from an aortic aneurysm. (Virchow, 1882) Working until the end, his last paper on hysteria was published just after his obituary, which was authored by Virchow (1882). He died too young to be Herr Geheimrat ("The" Professor), but he left a lasting legacy. Virchow implored: "May the memory of this model in German medicine always be unforgotten!" Judson S. Bury summarized his contribution to pediatrics, noting that "our knowledge of affections of the posterior columns in children . . . is mainly founded on the observations of Friedreich" (Bury, 1886).

Friedreich was also, of course, a teacher. Among his mentors were Adlolf Kussmaul and Max Schultze. Most notable, however, was Friedreich's successor at Heidelberg, Wilhelm Heinrich Erb (1840–1921), who was to become Herr Geheimrat. Erb was also the father of German neurology and perhaps of world neurology because of his political zealousness for neurology as a separate specialty. Friedreich is then, as the prime force behind Erb's career direction, the Grandfather of Neurology. Erb, in one of his 273 publications, first established statistically in 1892, the syphilitic origin of tabes dorsalis; his mentor would have been proud.

David A. Stumpf
EVANSTON, ILLINOIS

ACKNOWLEDGMENTS

The author is grateful to Mr. Blair K. Bassler of Orange, California, whose Friedreich's disease was his stimulus to translate the original descriptions by Friedreich; the translation is available in the Waring Room of the Denison Library at the University of Colorado Health Sciences Center, Denver (call letters WZ 265 F9113b, 1976).

REFERENCES

Andermann, F. 1976. Nikolaus Friedreich and Degenerative Atrophy of the Posterior Columns of the Spinal Cord. *Can J Neur Sci* 3:275–77.

Bird, T. D. 1979. Nikolaus A. Friedreich's Description of Peripheral Facial Paralysis in 1798. *J Neur Neurosurg Psych* 42:56–58.

Brousse, A. 1882. *De l'ataxie héréditaire (maladie de Friedreich).* Montpellier: Boehn.

Bury, J. S. 1886. A Contribution to the Symptomatology of Friedreich's Disease. *Brain* 9:145–77.

Clarke, E., and C. D. O'Malley. 1968. *The Human Brain and Spinal Cord. A Historical Study Illustrated by Writings from Antiquity to the Twentieth Century*, 61–66. Berkeley: University of California Press.

Erb, W. 1878. *Handbuch der Krankheiten des Nervensystems.* Vol. 1. Leipzig: Vogel.

Friedreich, N. 1863a. Über degenerative Atrophie der spinalen Hinterstrange. *Virchows Arch path Anat* 26:391–419

______. 1863b. Über degenerative Atrophie der spinalen Hinterstrange. *Virchows Arch path Anat* 26:433–59

______. 1863c. Über degenerative Atrophie der spinalen Hinterstrange. *Virchows Arch path Anat* 27:1–26.

______. 1873. *Über progressive Muskelatrophie, Über wahre und falsche Muskelhypertrophie.* Berlin: A. Hirschwald.

______. 1876. Über Ataxia mit besonderer Berücksichtigung derhereditären Formen. *Virchows Arch path Anat* 68:145–245.

______. 1877. Über Ataxia mit besonderer Berücksichtigung derhereditären Formen. *Virchows Arch path Anat* 70:140–52.

______. 1881. Neuropathologische Beobachtung beim paramyoklonusmultiplex. *Virchows Arch path Anat* 86:421–34.

Geoffroy, G. et al. 1976. Clinical Description and Roentgenologic Evaluation of Patients with Friedreich's Ataxia. *Can J Neur Sci* 3:279–86.

Hallet, M. 1986. Early History of Myoclonus. In *Advances in Neurology*. Vol 43: Myoclonus, 7–10. Ed. S. Fahn et al. New York: Raven Press.

Hallet, M., C. D. Marsden, and S. Fahn. 1982. Origins of the Term Myoclonus. *Neurology* 32:A231.

Hammond, W. A. 1882. On the So-called Family or Hereditary Form of Locomotor Ataxia. *J Nerv Ment Dis* 9:485–500.

Keppel-Hesselink, J. M. 1986. Een discussie uit de vorige eeuw: Multipelesclerose of tabes dorsalis; of ziekte van Friedreich? *Ned Tijdschr Geneesd* 130:2353–56.

______. 1882. Nikolaus Friedreich. *Zeit klin Med* (Berlin) 5:281–84.

Richter, R. B. 1970. Nikolaus Friedreich (1825–1882). In *The Founders of Neurology*, 439–41. Ed. W. Haymaker and F. Schiller. 2d ed. Springfield: Charles C Thomas.

Schoenberg, D. G., and B. S. Schoenberg. 1977. Eponym: Nikolaus Friedreich and Ataxia: Tabes or not Tabes? *South Med J* 70:749.

Thoren, C. 1964. Cardiomyopathy in Friedreich's Ataxia. *Acta Paed Scand* 53 (Suppl. 153):1.

Tyrer, J. H. 1975. Friedreich's Ataxia. In *Handbook of Clinical Neurology*, vol. 21, 319–64. Ed. P. J. Vinken and G. W. Bruyn. Amsterdam: North Holland Publishing Co.

Virchow, R. 1882. Zur Erinneurung an Nicolaus Friedreich. *Virchows Arch path Anat* 90:215–20.

PHILLIPE GAUCHER

ALTHOUGH PHILLIPE CHARLES ERNEST GAUCHER (1854–1918) (figure 1) is best known to child neurologists for his description of what came to be known as Gaucher's Disease, his contemporaries knew him as an excellent clinician and pugnacious defender of his ideals. He was best known as a syphilographer, dermatologist, and French patriot (Sergent, 1918).

Gaucher was born July 26 at Champfleury Nievie, France. He was an intern of the Paris Hospitals beginning in 1877 and studied under Jules de Bucquoy, Pierre-Carl Potain, Charles Bouchard, Louis Landouzy, and Jean-Baptiste Hillairet. While studying in the histology laboratory of Charles Robin, he described the disorder that bears his name.

In his doctoral thesis, Gaucher described a disorder that he labelled "l'epithélioma primitif de la rate, hypertrophie idiopathique de la rate, sans leucémie" (Gaucher, 1882). He described one patient and briefly mentioned two others. His patient was a 22-year-old woman who developed splenomegaly at age seven following an episode of typhoid fever. At age twenty, she became ill with multiple episodes of epistaxis, jaundice, progressive massive splenomegaly, cramping abdominal pains, purpura, and diarrhea. She finally died from pneumonia, complicated by splenic compression of the diaphragm. At autopsy, the spleen was enormous and the

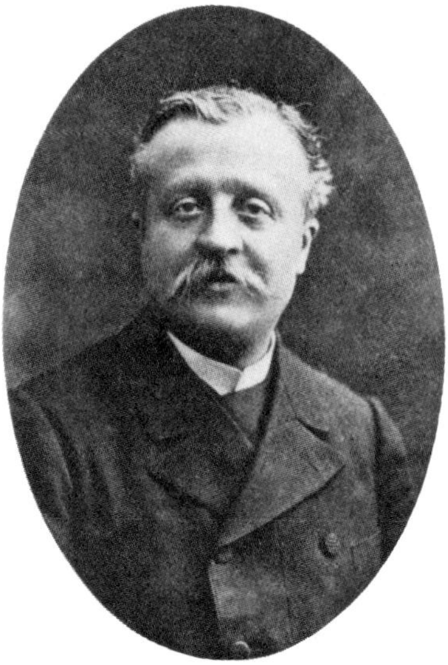

Figure 1. Phillipe Charles Ernest Gaucher (1854–1918).

liver cirrhotic. The brain was not examined because the patient apparently had no neurologic symptoms. Microscopic examination revealed patchy replacement of the normal splenic architecture by round or polyhedral shaped "plain" or epithelial cells. Gaucher speculated that these changes were due to abnormal hematopoiesis. He may have actually described a myeloproliferative syndrome (Miale, 1971). The disorder was characterized by gradually progressive, nearly painless splenomegaly with later epistaxis, purpura, pedal edema, and eventual cachexia. Neither mental status nor neurologic abnormalities were described in any of Gaucher's patients. This disorder soon became known as "maladie de Gaucher" (Gougerot, 1918), or Gaucher's Disease.

Despite Gaucher's early description, his disorder awaited later investigation before its systemic character and neurologic involvement were understood. James Collier, in 1895, and Louis Picon and André Raymond in 1896, described lymph node involvement. Nathan Brill, who noted familial inheritance in 1901, found bone marrow involvement in 1904. It was not until 1921 that C. L. Rusca reported an eleven-month-old infant with neurologic involvement. However, the section dealing with neuropathology was brief and actually mentioned no alterations in the brain or spinal cord other than "ischemic" changes in the neurons with some reduction in the number of pyramidal cells. The classic clinical and pathologic account of neurologic involvement in Gaucher's Disease was that of Charles Oberling and Pierre Woringer (1927). They reported the occurrence of the disease in four members of one family, each showing head retraction with neck rigidity, opisthotonus, spasticity, laryngeal spasm, dysphagia, trismus, strabismus, and tonic posturing. The neuropathology of two of these infants was limited to the cortical neurons. The cell bodies were shrunken and many cells contained single large or multiple vacuoles within the cytoplasm. Arturo Aballi and Katsuji Kato in their review of seventeen cases (1938) recognized that neurologic involvement developed when the disease began within the first six months of life. Since then there have been further careful neuropathologic investigations (Barlow, 1957; Banker, Miller and Crocker, 1962) and numerous biochemical investigations that have delineated the defect in glucosecerebroside metabolism that is characteristic of this disease.

Gaucher received his medical degree in 1882 and practiced in a clinic while he continued his pathologic studies at the University of Paris. He investigated Bright's Disease and the pathology of diphtheritic paralysis. In 1886 he was appointed physician of the Paris Hospitals and physician and Professor agrégé of the Hospital Saint Louis in 1892. He was a protegee of Alfred Fournier and devoted his time to cutaneous diseases and syphilology.

As a dermatologist, Gaucher studied tuberculosis and pellagra, and proposed an auto-immune mechanism he termed "auto-toxique" for eczema and arthritic diseases. He described serodiagnostic tests for leprosy and fungal diseases. However, he was primarily concerned with syphilis and its protean manifestations.

In 1902 he succeeded Alfred Fournier as Professor of Cutaneous Diseases and Syphilography of the Faculty of Medicine of the University of Paris. He extensively studied the histology of syphilitic lesions and described dental manifestations of syphilis. He also wrote of its nasal, ocular, and cutaneous manifestations. He thought separation of the median incisors was a manifestation of syphilis. He blamed many disorders on this disease, including appendicitis, Raynaud's disease, infantile paralysis, and tonsillitis (Gougerot, 1918). He championed treatment of syphilis with mercury. He was, however, thought by some contemporaries to be erratic and rash.

Gaucher was a leader of French medicine. He founded *Annales des maladies vénériennes* in 1906 (J. E. L., 1918). He was vice president of the French Society of Dermatology and Syphilography, president of the Medical Society of the Hospitals of Paris, and president of the General Association of French Physicians. In this capacity, he attempted to curb prostitution so as to prevent the spread of syphilis. He was elected to the Academy of Medicine in 1910 (J. E. L., 1918).

As a teenager, Gaucher grew up in the midst of the Franco-Prussian War. In 1914, with the start of the First World War, he was too old to enlist, and so relinquished his high position to organize and run the military Villemin Hospital. While serving in this capacity, he died of obliterating thrombotic aortitis on January 25, 1918, at the age of sixty-four.

Fred Haruda
SALINAS, CALIFORNIA

REFERENCES

Aballi, A. J., and K. Kato. 1938. Gaucher's Disease in Early Infancy. *J Ped* 13:364–80.

Banker, B. Q., J. Q. Miller, and A. C. Crocker. 1962. The Cerebral Pathology of Infantile Gaucher's Disease. In *Cerebral Sphingolipidoses, A Symposium on Tay-Sach's Disease and Allied Disorders*, 73–99. Ed. S. M. Aronson and B. W. Volk. New York: Academic Press.

Barlow, C. F. 1957. Neuropathologic Findings in a Case of Infantile Gaucher's Disease. J Neuropath Exp Neur 16:238–50.

Birch, C. A. 1973. Phillipe Charles Ernest Gaucher, M.D.: Gaucher's Disease. *Practitioner* 210:580.

Gaucher, P. C. E. 1882. De l'Epithélioma primitif de la rate hypertrophie idiopathique de la rate, sans leucémie. Paris: Faculté de Médicine.

Gougerot, H. 1918. P. C. E. Gaucher, M.D. *Ann mal vénér* 13:129–39.

J. E. L. 1918. Ernest Gaucher. *J Cutaneous Dis* 36:493–94.

Miali, J. 1971. Hematopoetic System: Reticuloendothelium, Spleen, Lymph Nodes, Blood and Bone Marrow. In *Pathology*, 1297–1386. Ed. W. A. B. Anderson. St. Louis: C.V. Mosby.

Oberling, C., and P. Woringer. 1927. La Maladie de Gaucher chez le nourisson. *Rev franc péd* 3:475–532.

Rusca, C. L. 1921. Sul morbo de Gaucher. *Haematologica* 2:441–509.

Sergent, E. 1918. Mort du Professeur Gaucher. *J méd* 89:153–55.

GEORGES GILLES DE LA TOURETTE

GEORGES GILLES DE LA TOURETTE (1857–1904) (figure 1), one of Jean Martin Charcot's favorite pupils and his self-appointed amanuensis, contributed substantially to child and adult neurology, psychiatry, and forensic medicine; distinguished himself as a champion of the disadvantaged; and managed to have a disease named after him. But in spite of his impressive achievements in medicine, social reform, and literature, he has been neglected by historians. Only a brief, incomplete biography by his colleague, Paul LeGendre (1904), and other more recent reports (Stevens, 1971; Guilly, 1981) attest to the resourcefulness and lasting accomplishments of this colorful and versatile neurologist and psychiatrist. He is known today by the eponym that Charcot magnanimously bestowed on the disease "tic convulsif," an entity that typically first appears in children and is characterized by frequent and involuntary movements of the head and trunk accompanied, on occasion, by vocal tics and, in rare cases, by coprolalia.

Besides his numerous works on neurology and psychiatry, Tourette also wrote on several historical subjects. These include an authoritative documentation and analysis of the trial and immolation of Father Grandier, who was found guilty in 1634 of demonically possessing a whole convent of nuns, including the Mother Superior, Soeur Jeanne des Anges, in Loudun, Gilles de la Tourette's hometown. He also wrote a retrospective investigation of the death of Charles I, a comprehensive biography of Théophraste Renaudot, the famous seventeenth-century physician, and numerous articles on the theater and drama.

Tourette's book (written with Dr. Gabriel Legue), *Soeur Jeanne des Anges*, provided material for such works as John Whiting's play, *The Devils*, an adaptation of Aldous Huxley's *The Devils of Loudun*, and Arthur Miller's *The Crucible*. The central figure in this historical incident was Soeur Jeanne des Anges, the 28-year-old Mother Superior of a small nunnery, who invited the handsome and brilliant local priest, Urbain Grandier, to be spiritual advisor to the convent.

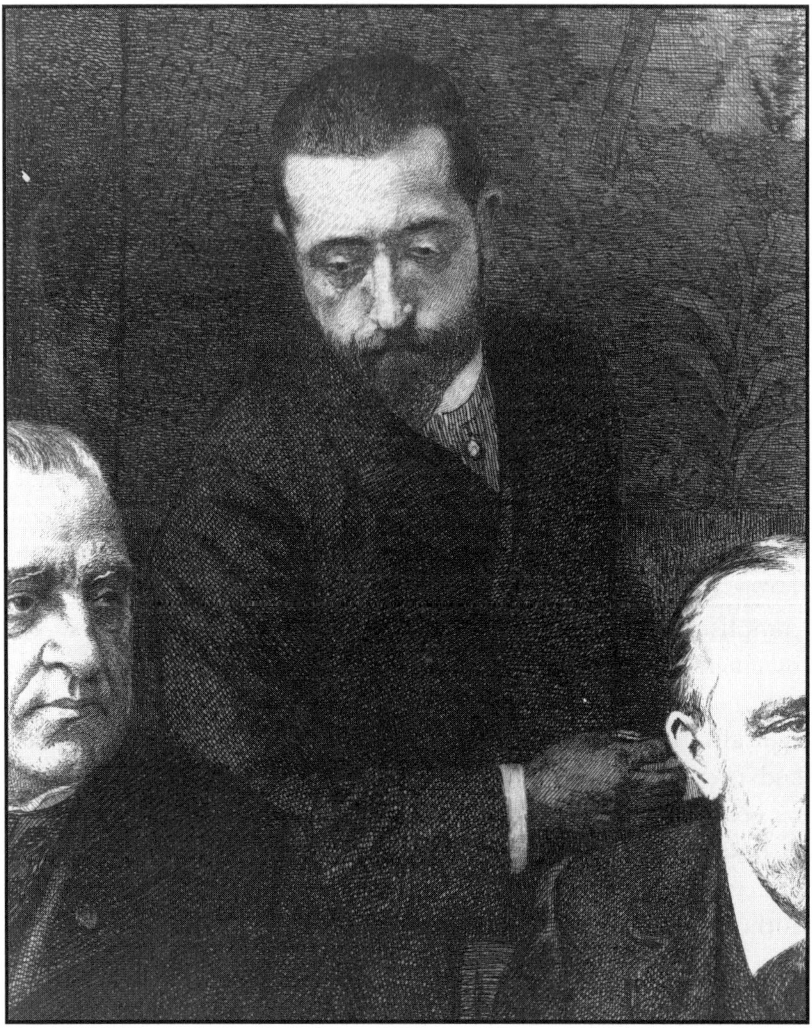

Figure 1. Portrait of Georges Gilles de la Tourette (1857–1904). Charcot is seated on Tourette's right.

When he arrogantly rejected her offer, she accused him of conspiring with the devil to possess her and subsequently her entire convent of nuns, causing them to utter obscenities and engage in lewd and depraved behavior. Investigation by high church authorities confirmed the charge and exorcism was prescribed. These proceedings attracted a prurient audience from all over France, and the sleepy town of Loudun temporarily prospered. Father Grandier steadfastly refused to confess the alleged collusion with the devil. The influential townspeople whom he had antagonized, the political forces that he opposed, the fellow clerics who envied his talents, and especially Cardinal Richelieu, whom he had affronted, prevailed. He was burned alive. Gilles de la Tourette's annotation and analysis of this incident of mass hysteria is searching and comprehensive; it reflects his and his contemporaries' extensive experience and preoccupation with hysteria in Charcot's clinic.

A man's character is his destiny and Gilles de la Tourette undoubtedly was stamped from the same template as his hero, Renaudot. Both suffered tragedy. The small-town milieu of Loudun with its parochial prejudice and values was common background, although Tourette left Loudun in his youth. Paul LeGendre described him as unruly but usually the first pupil in his class, finishing two preparatory years of study in one so that he was able to start his medical studies at the age of sixteen. His mother considered him too young to be left alone at this age in the Latin Quarter of Paris and sent him to Poitiers, where he remained for about four years.

His colleague, LeGendre, offered the opinion that had he gone to Paris he would easily have fallen prey to the easy life of the brasseries of the Boulevard St. Michel; since he was inordinately fond of history and literature he might have left his medical studies to pursue these subjects. Fortunately for neurology, and thanks to the inspiration of Charcot, Gilles de la Tourette did not defect.

As with his fellow neurologists and psychiatrists, the deepest imprint on his professional and personal life was made by the inspiring teacher, Charcot. In the foreword to Tourette's three-volume work on hysteria, Charcot praised his apt student for his clinical perspicacity and graciously credited him with careful observation and careful recording of facts, and also for judiciously enlarging on Charcot's own observation.

The imperious, aloof Charcot, who was dubbed the "Caesar" of the Salpêtrière, showed other evidences of generosity and subtle kindness in his relationship with Tourette and permitted him to apply his name to the "tic convulsif." This syndrome characteristically occurs in boys between the ages of seven and fifteen. It begins with facial tics and grimacing, which increase in frequency and extent. These brief, explosive, involuntary movements spread and implicate the neck, shoulders, trunk, and legs in a paroxysmal, stereotyped, vigorous movement that in some instances is sufficiently violent to catapult the patient from a chair. These spasmodic movements are often accompanied by a loud expiratory grunt or, most often, a sharp bark. In addition, coprolalia, echolalia, and different forms of obsessive and compulsive disturbances may occur. Jean Itard is usually given credit for describing the first case in 1825. The victim was the Marquise de Dampierre, whose symptoms began at the age of seven and persisted until her death at the age of eighty-five. The coprolalia and barking forced her to become a recluse. There was actually an earlier instance of this disease that was not reported in medical journals. Prince Conde was the victim, and he was compelled to stuff his mouth with any nearby object, including a curtain, to suppress an involuntary bark in the presence of Louis XIV. The famous case report of Itard's was alluded to by many neurologists in the nineteenth century, including Vladimir Roth, Claude Sandras, Tourette, LeGendre, and Charcot (Stevens, 1971). The usually impeccable William Osler also erroneously referred to this case as being the first recorded instance (Osler, 1890).

The evolution of this disorder as an entity is a fascinating historical vignette. It began with the American neurologist, George Beard, who described in 1880 an even more bizarre syndrome in a paper entitled "Experiments with the Jumpers or Jumping Frenchmen of Maine," which was based on his observations of fifty cases, including fourteen cases in four families. He found that the disorder began in childhood, was familial, rarely affected females, persisted throughout life, and was characterized by a bark and loud jump in response to a sudden noise or startling event. In addition, some of the patients showed echolalia and some responded automatically to a quick loud command by repeating the command and executing the act even if it were dangerous or humiliating to them. After Beards' article, this syndrome strangely disappeared from the literature until two cases were reported in June 1965 (Stevens, 1965).

Tourette translated Beard's article in 1881 and later described similar instances that occurred in France and Russia. William Hammond, one of the major figures in American neurology at that time, had reported a case of a jumping Frenchman in Russia, whom he did not actually observe. His article was severely criticized. These reports motivated Charcot to direct Tourette to study these strange disorders; he later permitted Tourette to attach his name to the disease ("tic convulsif"). This historical event occurred at a clinical meeting in 1885 when Tourette was twenty-seven. Even in 1885, when diseases to give away were plentiful, this was something to write about and Paul Le Gendre did so:

Not every one gets to go to Corinth; still fewer get a disease named for them. We do not know if our friend had the first of these good fortunes. Charcot who certainly is the best judge in such matters declared this year at a clinical meeting that the neurological disease of Gilles de la Tourette is an entity of sufficient special characteristics to be named for our friend. (LeGendre, 1904)

Tourette had taken the first step in that direction in 1881, three years before he joined Charcot's staff at the Salpêtrière, when he translated Beard's article, which he simply signed without comment. In 1884 he joined Charcot at the Salpêtrière and in July of that year published his article "Jumping, Latah and Myriachit"; he believed that all three conditions were the same. The following year, "Etude sur une affection nerveuse caracterisée par de l'incoordination motrice accompagnée de écholalie et de coprolalie" (Study of a Neurologic Condition Characterized by Motor Incoordination Accompanied by Echolalia and Coprolalia) was published. In this two-part paper, Tourette reviewed and contrasted the previous case reports with the clinical features of nine patients seen at the Salpêtrière.

The condition which we will describe generally starts at a young age. In our nine cases, it began once at age 6, twice at 7, three times at 8, once at 9, once at 14, and once at 16. Beard described having seen children from 4 to 7 years of age who were afflicted with the jumping disease. It begins thus during childhood or at the latest during adolescence. It seems to affect males more often, although we observed two women and O'Brien also noted affected Malaysian women. Nevertheless, in all groups, men constitute the majority of cases. Among the various cases hypothesized to be important are high-strung emotions and fear. However, the true basis of these conditions, as in all nervous diseases, is clearly hereditary. "These tics are often hereditary" wrote Trousseau. "This condition," writes Beard, "is hereditary as is madness or epilepsy . . . in a family whom I examined, there were four jumpers; the father, the son and two young lads age 4 to 7. In another, three brothers were affected." (Goetz and Klawans, 1982, 4)

Besides including several interesting case histories, he delineated the natural evolution of this disorder in children as is noted in these observations:

The mode of onset (at least in the cases we have observed, which are the only ones on which we have complete information) is practically identical. Motor incoordination is the first indication of disease. These twitches or uncoordinated movements present insidiously without affecting the general health of the subject. They start most often in the face or upper extremities, and in the latter case, one arm is involved before the other, although eventually both show abnormalities. In school and at home, teachers and parents notice arms that shake, fingers that extend and flex, and shoulders that flinch, making work difficult. Almost at the same time (the intervals varying from subject to subject) facial movements appear. These latter movements may in some cases precede the extremity incoordination. They most often consist of eye squints, facial grimaces, or teeth grinding due to masseter contraction. The tongue projects out of the mouth and is sometimes bitten as a result of masseter contractions. The neck muscles may flinch, the head may be alternately extended or flexed, and the sternocleidomastoids may fling the head from one side to the other. (Goetz and Klawans, 1982, 4)

In part two of this paper, Tourette included several quotations from his own patients, as well as those from earlier papers, which exemplify the psychological stress from which patients with this disorder suffer.

In listening to a discussion I was seized by the almost irresistible need to repeat a word or the end of a sentence. I needed all my strength and sense of propriety to hold back from repeating this word out loud; as I could only restrain myself part way, I saw on different occasions how people around me clearly heard my noises. . . . Furthermore, every intellectual faculty for the moment is absorbed by the word or sentence that is being repeated so that my train of thought is usually lost. The word heard or read rises to one's lips to be repeated at varying intervals, but always coincident with or at the end of the tormenting muscle jerks. (Goetz and Klawans, 1982, 7)

Later Tourette summarized the major features of this syndrome in a succinct and clear-cut fashion, displaying the qualities of his intellect for which he was regarded by his colleagues and which were appreciated by his mentor, Charcot:

Let us recall first some of the fundamental symptoms: (1) this illness is hereditary; it is characterized by motor incoordination in the form of abrupt muscular jerks that are often severe enough to make the patient jump; (2) the incoordination can be accompanied by articulated or unarticulated sounds. When articulated, the words are often repetitions of words which the patient may have just heard. Such vocal imitation (echolalia) may have a physical corollary whereby the subject imitates an act or gesture that he has just seen; (3) among the expressions which the patient may repeatedly utter during one of his convulsions, some have the special character of being obscene (coprolalia); (4) the physical and mental health of these patients is otherwise basically normal. The condition seems incurable and life long, with onset in childhood. (Goetz and Klawans, 1982, 10)

Two years after this publication, on December 13, 1887, Charcot, in one of the Tuesday Lessons at the Salpêtrière, presented the case history of a twelve-year-old boy with "tic convulsif," further commenting on this condition and, in later lectures, clearly separating it from the choreiform disorders (Goetz, 1987).

As Charcot advanced in age, he became more dependent on Tourette and subsequently bestowed on him the honor and heavy task of compiling Charcot's major studies on hysteria, *Traité clinique et thérapeutique de l'hystérie d'après l'enseignement de la Salpêtrière*. The first of these volumes appeared in 1891; the third and last, totalling 1,800 pages, in 1895 (Guilly, 1981). In 1893, in the midst of this work, Tourette lost his son and was victimized by a young woman whose paranoid projections were reminiscent of those of Soeur Jeanne des Anges against Father Grandier. She believed she was under the hypnotic influence of Tourette and shot him three times as he sat in his office. One bullet hit him in the occipital region but was removed and he recovered.

Tourette's subsequent works are considered somewhat erratic and puzzling (Guilly, 1981). In between periods of depression and hypomania, he published a well-written and clear monograph *Traité pratique de l'épilepsie* (1900) but, by 1902, his behavior was becoming more disturbed and he was placed on indefinite health leave from his position at the Sainte Antoine Hospital. His family admitted him to a health clinic in Lausanne where he died in

1904, presumably of syphilitic cerebral involvement. A serendipitous syndrome and its eponym is probably the most lasting monument to this talented neurologist and psychiatrist whose contribution to child neurology is becoming increasingly appreciated as more children with subtler variations of this complex and bewildering disorder are recognized.

Harold Stevens
WASHINGTON, D.C.

Stephen Ashwal
LOMA LINDA, CALIFORNIA

REFERENCES

Beard, G. M. 1880. Experiments with "Jumpers" or "Jumping Frenchmen" of Maine. *Pop Sci Month* 18:170–78.

Gilles de la Tourette, G. 1883. *Théophraste Renaudot d'après des documents inédits.* Paris: Plon et Cie.

______. 1884. Jumping, latah, myriachit. *Arch neur* (Paris) 8:68–74.

______. 1885. Étude sur une affection nerveuse caracterisée par de l'incoordination motrice accompagnée de écholalie et de coprolalie. *Arch neur* (Paris) 9:19–42, 158–200.

Goetz, C. G. 1987. *Charcot the Clinician. The Tuesday Lessons: Excerpts from Nine Case Presentations on General Neurology Delivered at the Salpêtrière Hospital in 1887–88, by Jean-Martin Charcot.* Translated with commentary by Christopher G. Goetz. New York: Raven Press.

Goetz, C. G., and H. L. Klawans 1982. Gilles de la Tourette on Tourette Syndrome. In *Gilles de la Tourette Syndrome*, 1–16. Ed. A. J. Friedhoff and T. N. Chase. New York: Raven Press.

Guilly, P. 1981. Gilles de la Tourette. In *Historical Aspects of the Neurosciences: A Festschrift for Macdonald Chritchley*, 397–413. Ed. F. C. Rose and W. F. Bynum. New York: Raven Press.

Hammond, W. A. 1884. Myriachit: Newly Described Disease of the Nervous System and its Analogues. *NY Med J* 39:191–92.

Itard, J. M. G. 1825. Mémoire sur quelques fonctions involontaires des appareils de la locomotion, de la préhension et de la voix. *Arch méd gén* (Paris) 8:385–407.

LeGendre, P. 1904. *Gilles de la Tourette.* Paris: Typographie Plon-Norrit.

Legue, G., and G. Gilles de la Tourette, editors. 1886. *Soeur Jeanne des Anges: Autobiographie d'une hystérique possédée.* Paris: Charpentier et Cie.

Osler, W. 1890. On the Form of Convulsive Tic Associated with Coprolalia. *Med News Phila* 57:645–47.

Stevens, H. 1965. Jumping Frenchmen of Maine. *Arch Neur* 12:311–14.

______. 1971. Gilles de la Tourette and his Syndrome by Serendipity. *Am J Psych* 128:489–92.

SIR WILLIAM GOWERS

WILLIAM RICHARD GOWERS (1845–1915) (figure 1) was born in Hackney, a village north of the City of London. His father was a shoemaker and died when he was eleven. His mother took him back to her relatives in Oxford, where he was fortunate to get a scholarship to Christ Church College School. He remained there until 1860, then worked on a farm in Yorkshire. Shortly afterward he went to live with relatives in Essex and was offered an apprenticeship with Dr. Thomas Simpson.

Gowers was a well-disciplined young man who had taught himself shorthand and kept a careful diary. He obtained the London Matriculation Certificate in 1863 and in September of that year entered the University College Hospital as a medical student. By 1867, he was working as an assistant to Sir William Jenner, physician to Queen Victoria. At that time he came in contact with Sir John Russell Reynolds, one of the founders, in 1860, of the National Hospital for the Paralyzed and Epileptic at Queen's Square, London. Gowers went on to get an M.B. in London in 1869 and an M.D. in 1870.

It was in that year that he became a medical registrar at Queen's Square, which by 1868 could accommodate sixty-four patients. Two years later Gowers became an assistant physician and, in 1879, a fellow of the Royal College of Physicians. Pediatric neurological cases at the Hospital for Sick Children, located around the corner from Queen's Square, were brought there for consultations with Dr. Gowers and others at the end of the nineteenth century.

Gowers's first papers in 1874 were on traumatic epilepsy. In

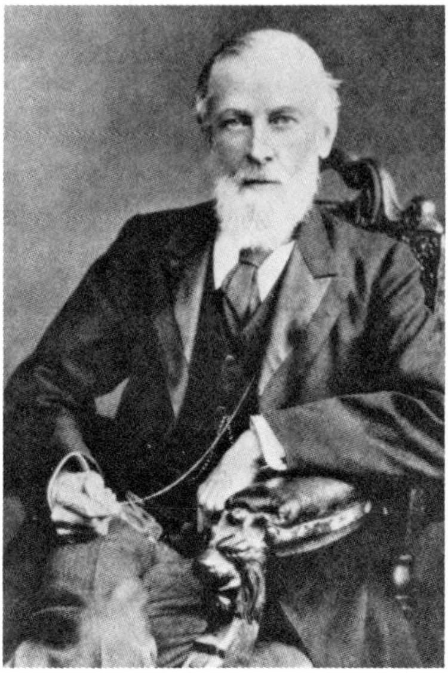

Figure 1. Portrait of Sir William Gowers (1845–1915).

1880, he was invited to give the Gulstonian Lectures in which he discussed epilepsy, using a series of 1,450 personally observed cases. In 1879 he published a monograph called *An Atlas of Medical Ophthalmoscopy*. This is a remarkable book with numerous colored drawings of fundi, extensive clinical details, and pathological drawings of many of the cases presented.

One of Gowers's first contributions to child neurology was his treatise on pseudohypertrophic paralysis, also published in 1879 and based on his studies of twenty patients, including one autopsy. He summed up the disease as follows:

The disease is one of the most interesting and at the same time most sad, of all those with which we have to deal: interesting on account of its peculiar features and mysterious nature; sad on account of our powerlessness to influence its course, except in a very slight degree, and on account of the degree, and on account of the conditions in which it occurs. It is a disease of early life and early growth, manifesting itself commonly at the transition from infancy to childhood, it develops with the child's development, grows with his growth, so that every increase in stature means a decrease in weakness and each year takes him a step forward on the road to helpless infirmity and in most cases to an early inevitable death. (Gowers, 1879b, 1)

It was at this time that he described the maneuver, now called the Gowers Sign, whereby a child with proximal weakness in the lower extremities uses the upper extremities placed on the knees and thighs to get himself upright (figure 2).

In 1886 volume 1 of the *Manual of Diseases of the Nervous System* appeared. This book dealt with diseases of the spinal cord and peripheral nerves; two years later, volume 2, which dealt with cerebral disorders, was published. It is interesting to note that most of the etchings in these books were done by Dr. Gowers himself.

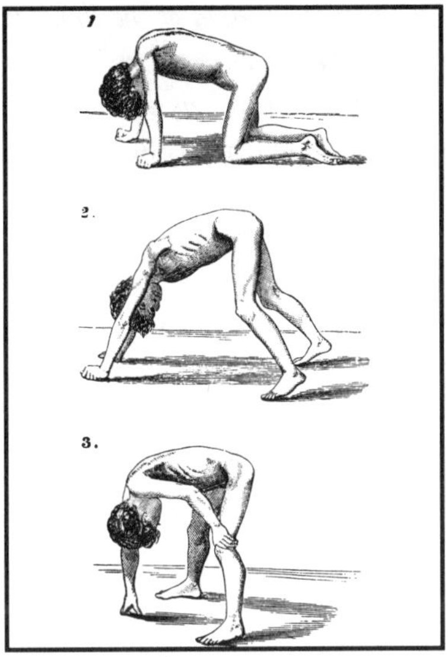

Figure 2. Etching of the Gowers Maneuver (Gowers, 1886).

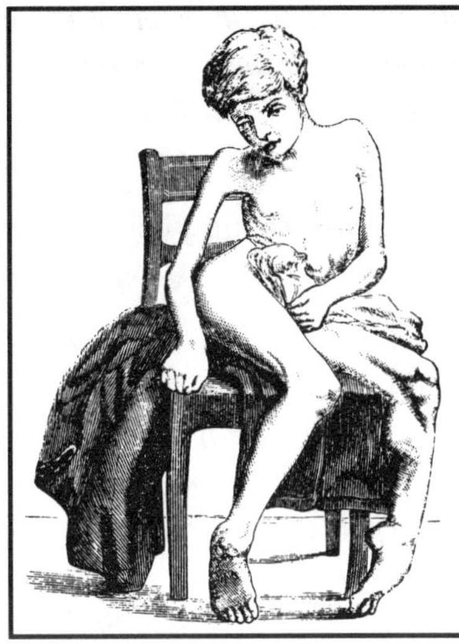

Figure 3. Etching of an older child in the late stage of pseudohypertrophic paralysis (Gowers, 1886).

A review in the *British Medical Journal* at the time said, "No better manual on nervous diseases has been presented to the medical profession." These books had a major impact on the study and practice of neurology in Europe and North America. They were translated into many languages and were referred to as "the Bible of Neurology." By 1892 William Osler, in his *Principles and Practice of Medicine*, referred to Dr. Gowers's maneuver as "so well known through Gowers's figures."

Pediatric neurological topics covered in these manuals included discussions on infantile meningeal hemorrhage (cerebral birth palsy); infantile convulsions: infantile eclampsia; congenital ptosis; hydrocephalus; seizures associated with hemiplegia; acute meningitis; tuberculoma of the cerebellum in a child; lead poisoning; diphtheric paralysis; acute poliomyelitis and a long discourse on pseudohypertrophic paralysis (figure 3). On fixed wry neck: congenital torticollis, he wrote:

The condition is met with chiefly in children and is thought to depend, in some cases, upon injury to the muscle from traction on the neck that occurs during birth. In other cases, it is supposed to be due to developmental shorten-

ing of the muscle, the result of the inclined position of the head of the child in the pelvis. It is much more frequent on the right side . . . . since in 70 cases out of 100 the head is in the first position which entails an inclination such as would permit the right sterno-mastoid to shorten. (Gowers, 1886, 610)

When discussing habit spasms, he said:

When it commences in childhood, the affection commonly ceases after a few months or years, but occasionally goes on to middle life or even longer. It usually begins between the ages of 6 and 14; I have known it to commence as early as 4. In cases in which something like direct inheritance can be traced it is probable that this influence has been at work. The most common is blinking of the eyelids. . . . Another is moving the angles of the mouth first to one side and then to the other. . . . The deterring influence of strangers is often very marked. (Gowers, 1886, 586)

Gowers's descriptions of childhood Sydenham Chorea in the second edition of the *Manual* published in 1893 are of interest.
He wrote:

The mental state may be normal, but in severe cases there is usually some irritability and often distinct mental dullness. In other cases, irritability may pass into excitement . . . and there is excited delirium, which in its restlessness may resemble mania. . . .

The movements are always increased by excitement and by attempts at voluntary movement and are lessened by repose, physical and mental. They invariably cease during sleep, natural or induced, but their severity may prevent sleep for days together. . . .

Thus, objects which are being carried are suddenly dropped and in one lad the first indication of the commencing disease was that in throwing a cricket ball the fingers relaxed their grip too late and the ball simply fell to the ground.

It may be limited to one side (hemichorea) or it may affect one side first and afterwards the other. (Gowers, 1893, 546)

In 1888 Gowers also published a two-part series of articles in the *Lancet* entitled "Clinical Lecture on Birth Palsies," which was based on a lecture given at University College Hospital in June, 1886. The following three extracts from this paper demonstrate Gowers's resources as a meticulous neurologist who incorporated clinicial with pathological concepts, who was one of the first to use the term "cerebral palsy," and who realized then that not all such cerebral disorders were due to obstetrical mishap:

Children are sometimes born with morbid states that do not exist at the commencement of the short but perilous journey by which they enter the world. These morbid states are the results of injuries received during the process of birth. The forms of palsy that result from such injury constitute our subject today. "Obstetrical paralyses" they have been sometimes termed, but "obstetrical" is that which relates to "obstetrics", and "obstetrics", as you know, is a science and an art, and it is hardly fair to associate these diseases too closely with it. We will therefore term them simply "birth palsies." (Gowers, 1888a, 709)

If the injury to the brain is chiefly one-sided, the resulting symptoms may resemble those of the "acquired" hemiplegia that occasionally results from a sudden lesion during infancy. But such a lesion has been attended with acute symptoms at the time of the onset, and of these there generally is a clear history. Moreover, birth palsy is scarcely ever strictly unilateral; one side may be much more affected than the other; but if you examine the limbs that seem to be normal, you will find that they present slight disturbance of the same kind as that which is so marked on the other side. A greater difficulty is presented by the cases in which the legs suffer much more than the arms, and in which the spastic paralysis of the legs resembles very closely that which is produced by disease of the spinal cord. Here also, however, you will find traces of the disorder in the parts that appear at first sight to be free. The movements of the hands are distinctly awkward, and differ from those of a healthy child, although the parents often have not recognized the abnormality. Even without this, you will be justified in suspecting that the case is one of birth palsy if there is no history of a definite onset — if the child, for instance, has never been able to walk. (Gowers, 1888a, 759)

When the weakness of the legs is slight, so that the child is able to walk but in an awkward manner, the condition is occasionally mistaken for pseudo-hypertrophic paralysis. . . . Lastly, there is one test which alone decides the question — the state of reflex action in the legs. In birth palsy the knee jerk is excessive, and a cutaneous stimulus excites reflex spasm. In the muscular disease the knee jerk is never increased; it may be normal, but it is often diminished or lost, and you cannot, by any peripheral impression, produce the extensor spasm so characteristic of birth palsy. (Gowers, 1888a, 760)

Gowers was a keen and accurate diagnostician. When he visited his wards, he would carefully read the case notes made by his assistants. He would go over points in the history and then do a detailed examination. He was a brilliant teacher and his clinic was crowded with physicians from all over the world. He would think aloud as he took the history, examined the patient and discussed the differential diagnosis, prognosis and treatment.

Gowers had a frail build, but a distinguished appearance with a square-shaped grey beard and rather long hair. He had ice-blue eyes and tended to be somewhat aloof from his colleagues and assistants. His voice was strident and his gait somewhat awkward. He has often been contrasted, unfavorably, with his older colleague, Hughlings Jackson, who was easy-going and personable (Critchley, 1949, 89). Dr. Gowers was also somewhat intolerant, particularly, it seems, of women doctors.

Gowers formed the Society of Medical Phonographers, devoted to the use of shorthand, in 1894. There were sixty active members, but over time numbers dwindled and the Society was dissolved in 1912. In 1897 he was knighted. Gowers had married a relative of Sir John Russell Reynolds in 1875 and lived at 50 Queen Anne St. in London, where he raised four children and conducted a practice as a consultant neurologist until his retirement. He was a devoted husband and father and enjoyed playing chess, billiards, and table tennis after dinner with his children. He was also an artist. He enjoyed doing etchings, engravings, and pencil drawings. One of his etchings was exhibited at the Royal Academy.

In 1894 Gowers had a painful bout of sciatica. This led to a breakdown, followed by a recuperative voyage to South Africa. He began to look older than his years and by the age of sixty-two, began to retire. His wife died of pneumonia in 1914 and he died in May of 1915.

One of Gowers's most lasting contributions was *Epilepsy and Other Chronic Convulsive Diseases*, the first edition of which was published in 1881 and the second, more expanded, edition in 1901. He discussed 3,000 cases of epilepsy that he had dealt with, of which 27.5 percent were under the age of 10 and a further 46.5 percent between the ages of 10 and 19. Of all his cases, 155 were under the age of 1 and 93 were between 1 and 2 years. In dealing with prognosis of epilepsy he wrote, "The tendency of the disease is to self-perpetuation; each attack facilitates the occurrence of another, by increasing the instability of the nerve elements" (Critchley, 1949).

In another great treatise, the *Borderland of Epilepsy: Faints, Vagal Attacks, Vertigo, Migraine, Sleep Symptoms and Their Treatment*, published in 1907, he expounded upon the differential diagnosis of seizures, including pseudoseizures. Of great note were his observations of migraine and the differentiating points between migraine and epilepsy. For instance, the premonition of migraine always lasted many minutes as opposed to an epileptic aura that lasted only a few seconds; furthermore, a sensory disturbance in migraine may affect both hands, but this was never the case in focal epilepsy. He also discussed vertigo as part of a migraine syndrome.

Many of these descriptions are valid in their entirety to this day. It is of interest that Sir William Gowers was primarily an adult neurologist but his numerous contributions concerning childhood neurological diseases such as epilepsy, migraine and, of course, Duchenne Dystrophy, were seminal to pediatric neurology in his day and are an integral part of the present-day knowledge and practice of pediatric neurology.

Israel F. Abroms
WORCESTER, MASSACHUSETTS

REFERENCES

Critchley, M. 1949. *Sir William Gowers 1845–1915: A Biographical Appreciation.* London: Heinemann.

Gowers, W. R. 1879a. *A Manual and Atlas of Medical Ophthalmoscopy.* London: J. & A. Churchill.

______. 1879b. Pseudohypertrophic Muscular Paralysis. *Lancet* (July 5) 2:1–2; (July 12) 2:37–39; (July 19) 2:73–75; (July 26) 2:113–16.

______. 1879c. *Pseudohypertrophic Muscular Paralysis.* London: J. & A. Churchill.

______. 1881. *Epilepsy and Other Chronic Convulsive Diseases: Their Causes, Symptoms and Treatment.* London: J. & A. Churchill.

______. 1886. *A Manual of Diseases of the Nervous System.* Vol. 1: *Diseases of the Nerves and Spinal Cord.* London: J. & A. Churchill .

______. 1888a. Clinical Lecture on Birth Palsies. Delivered at University College Hospital, June, 15, 1886. *Lancet* (April 14) 1:709–11; (April 21) 1:759–60.

———. 1888b. *A Manual of Diseases of the Nervous System.* Vol. 2: *Diseases of the Brain and Cranial Nerves; General and Functional Diseases of the Nervous System.* London: J. & A. Churchill.

———. 1892. *A Manual of Diseases of the Nervous System.* Vol. 1: *Diseases of the Nerves and Spinal Cord.* 2d ed. London: J. & A. Churchill.

———. 1893. *A Manual of Diseases of the Nervous System.* Vol. 2: *Diseases of the Brain and Cranial Nerves: General and Functional Diseases of the Nervous System.* 2d ed. London: J. & A. Churchill.

———. 1899. *A Manual of Diseases of the Nervous System.* Vol. 1. 3d ed. Ed. W. R. Gowers and J. Taylor. London: J. & A. Churchill.

———. 1901. *Epilepsy and Other Chronic Convulsive Diseases: Their Causes, Symptoms and Treatment.* 2d ed. London: J. & A. Churchill.

———. 1907. *The Borderland of Epilepsy: Faints, Vagal Attacks, Vertigo, Migraine, Sleep Symptoms and Their Treatment.* London: J. & A. Churchill.

McHenry, L. C. 1969. *Garrison's History of Neurology.* Springfield, IL: Charles C Thomas.

Osler, William. 1892. *The Principles and Practice of Medicine*, 997. New York: D. Appleton & Co.

Pepper, William, editor. 1893. *A Text Book of the Theory and Practice of Medicine by American Teachers.* Vol. 1, 854. Philadelphia: W. B. Saunders.

JOHANN HOFFMANN

AT THE TURN OF the twentieth century, clinical neurology was emerging as an exciting and demanding specialty. Many neurological disorders had been described in the preceding fifty years but in Germany, neurology was considered a subspecialty of medicine rather than psychiatry. At this time, Nikolaus Friedreich and Wilhelm Erb were active at the University of Heidelberg, one of the most prestigious medical schools in Europe. Erb was considered the model and mentor of this German school of neurologists. Johann Hoffmann (1857–1919) (figure 1) was probably the youngest of those who assembled at Erb's clinic in Heidelberg. As his assistant, Hoffmann was held in the highest esteem by Erb, who would outlive him to write a long tribute to his student (Erb, 1920). Hoffmann spent almost his entire career at the University of Heidelberg. His academic appointment spanned over thirty years, during which he participated in the growth of this clinical discipline and emphasized the importance of correlating neuropathological findings with physical signs. Hoffmann was the epitome of the German neurology professor, beloved by colleagues and students alike (Schonfeld, 1962).

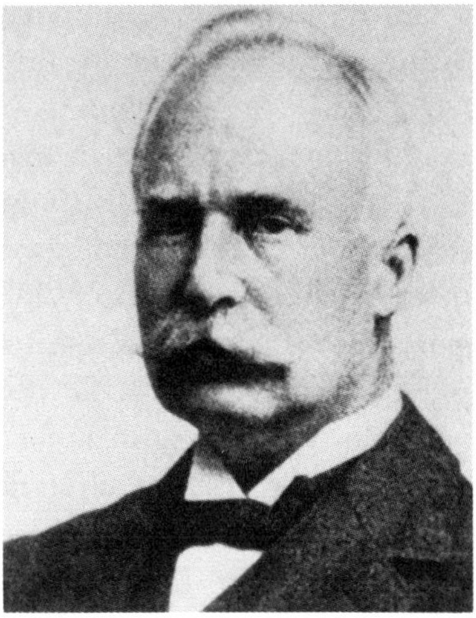

Figure 1. Official portrait of Dr. Johann Hoffmann (1857–1919).

Johann Hoffmann was born on March 28, 1857, in Rheinhessen in the state of Hessen, presently located in West Germany. He was the son of a farmer, the mayor of Hahnheim. Adolf Strümpell (1920) surmised that Hoffmann attended gymnasium in Mainz, while Erb (1920) stated that he received his early education at home through private tutors and then attended gymnasium at Worms. He studied medicine at universities in Heidelberg, Strassburg, and Berlin. Little is known about his performance other than the fact that he passed his final state exams during the winter of 1882–83 with a grade of superior. Soon after he received his degree. His doctoral dissertation entitled "Ein Fall von Acuter Aufsteiger Paralyse ("A Case of Acute Ascending Paralysis") was published in Berlin in 1884. This clearly described a patient with Guillain-Barré syndrome, or postinfectious polyradiculitis, and suggested that Hoffmann's early association with Erb influenced his choice of specialty.

While a student at the University of Heidelberg, Hoffmann worked as an assistant to Friedreich at the medical clinic. After Friedreich's death in the winter semester of 1882–83, Professor Adolf Weil assumed the role of acting director of the medical clinic and, like Friedreich, held Hoffmann in high esteem. Erb returned from Leipzig later that spring to become the director of the clinic. Both Erb and Hoffmann felt strongly that thorough knowledge of internal medicine was a prerequisite for the proper practice of neurology. Hoffmann was highly respected as a "consolarius," an expert consultant in all branches of internal medicine. Strümpell stated, "From Erb, Hoffmann learned the attributes which made him famous — meticulous clinical and anatomical examination, great care in making decisions, and an incorruptible love for the truth" (Strümpell, 1920). With Erb, Hoffmann studied both neuropathology and electrotherapy, the forerunner of modern clinical electrophysiology, in which Hoffmann continued working, teaching, and researching even after Erb's retirement.

Hoffmann became a faculty member and lecturer at the University of Heidelberg in January of 1888. Just prior to this, he had written "Über das Verhalten der Sensiblen Nerven bei der Tetanie" ("Disturbances in Sensation During Tetany," 1887) and "Zur Lehre von der Tetanie" ("Concerning Tetany," 1888a). During his academic career, he published a total of thirty-six original papers, including several classics of clinical neurology. As an academic neurologist in the nineteenth century, Hoffmann saw patients of all ages, with a wide variety of diseases and states. His papers, like those of his contemporaries, included many single case reports. However, these reports describe in expert detail previously unappreciated clinical syndromes, such as brachial plexopathy (Hoffmann, 1888b). He pointed out the perplexing association of early onset cataracts and myotonic dystrophy (Hoffmann, 1912), something most neurology residents now recite without thinking. Taken as a whole, his works show his clinical skill and his particular interest in motor problems that could be localized to the spinal cord or the peripheral nervous system. He pointed out that myotonia seemed to be related to denervation (1896a) and that myotonia congenita may occur in a second "atrophic or dystrophic" form (1896b, 1903). His mentor, Erb, had noted some time earlier the heterogeneity among patients with "Thomsen's disease." The fact that Hoffmann performed and studied muscle biopsies ("extirpations of muscle pieces") on many of his patients shows the importance of pathology in the practice of clinical medicine a century ago (Hoffmann, 1903). Much of the man's astuteness may be attributed to his appreciation for the neuroanatomical and pathological correlates to his clinical observations. Thus, he concluded that patients with myotonia (electrical "tetany") and dystrophic muscle had a disease that was different from Thomsen's myotonia congenita, wherein the muscle biopsy was generally unremarkable. "Myotonia atrophica" was not recognized as an entity by others until 1909 (Batten and Gibb, 1909).

Hoffmann's writings on progressive infantile spinal muscular atrophy are his most famous. Hoffmann described the disease in a series of meticulously detailed papers. In 1892, while at Erb's clinic in Heidelberg, he published his first paper on the subject: "Über familiare progressive spinale Muskelatrophie" ("Familial Progressive Spinal Muscular Atrophy"). He credited Guido Werdnig with having published two cases the previous year and placed himself in full agreement with Werdnig's conclusions regarding the familial and progressive nature of the disease. "Über chronische spinale Muskelatrophie im Kindesalter auf familiärer Basis" ("Concerning Chronic Spinal Muscular Atrophy in Children, on a Familial Basis") appeared in 1893 (figure 2), another paper on the matter in 1897, and two more in 1900. Altogether, he described seven cases in four families with twenty affected members. The children were normal at birth but developed severe hypotonia in the latter part of the first year of life and died between fourteen months and five years of age. Hoffmann presented autopsy findings in several of the cases, demonstrating degeneration of the anterior horn cells of the spinal cord and extensive atrophy of skeletal muscle. His case reports, along with those of Werdnig (1891) from the Institute of Pathology at the University of Graz, were not only the first to recognize spinal muscular atrophy as a single entity in children, but probably the first to suggest a pathogenesis. In comparison, amyotrophic lateral sclerosis had been recognized for several decades as an acquired disease in adults. Later work by Joseph Godwin Greenfield (Greenfield and Stern, 1927), Sven

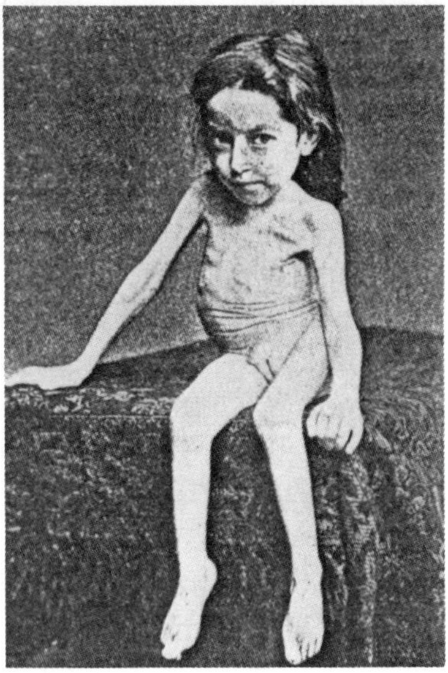

Figure 2. A four-year-eleven-month-old girl with spinal muscular atropy, from Hoffmann's paper "Ueber chronische spinale Muskelatrophie im Kindesalter auf familiärer Basis" (1892–93).

Brandt (1950), and Randolph Byers and Betty Banker (1961), would establish "Werdnig-Hoffmann disease" as a primary, genetic disorder of the motor neuron.

Another contribution to neurology for which Hoffmann is remembered is the digital reflex known as "Hoffmann's sign." Although it was originally described in the literature by Hans Curschmann in 1911, it is thought that Hoffmann discovered this sign in 1904. Curschmann was assistant to Hoffmann at the medical clinic in Heidelberg from 1901 to 1904. According to Curschmann, Hoffmann demonstrated this digital reflex in his lectures and clinics; Curschmann labeled the reflex "Hoffmann's sign" (Bendheim, 1937). In 1933 Temple Faye and Henry Gotten's review of the literature on this subject could reveal no published reference by Hoffmann describing the sign.

In 1891 Hoffmann was appointed to the position "Ausserordentlicher Professor" — the equivalent of Associate Professor. In 1892–93, he took a sabbatical, during which he travelled to both Paris and London. While in London, he studied with the British neurologist, Victor Horsley, with whom he maintained close correspondence after returning to Heidelberg. Hoffmann received a full professorship in neurology and electrotherapy in the spring of 1907 while he was director of the Department of Neurologic Patients at the clinic at Heidelberg. He then became director of the outpatient department for neurology and electrotherapy.

Not much seems to have been written about the private life of this modest man. He married Fanny Luise J. (Clemm) Giulini in 1902 at the age of forty-five (Schonfeld, 1962). There were no children from this union, although she may have had children from a previous marriage. Erb obviously regarded Hoffmann as a close friend and Strümpell described Hoffmann as a "happy family man, active and industrious" (Strümpell, 1920).

In 1910 Hoffmann became an "Ordentlicher Honorarprofessor", (full professor) and in 1914, he received "Etatmaessiger Professor" (full tenure). When Erb retired, Professor Kehl took over as director of the Medical Polyclinic in Heidelberg. With the outbreak of World War I, Kehl served as consulting Surgeon General for internal medicine and was frequently called to the battlefield.

During Kehl's absence, Hoffmann was entrusted with directing the medical clinic at Heidelberg, in addition to directing the education department. His last academic honor was appointment to Professor Ordinarius for neuropathology in 1919. "He carried out his duties without regard to his own health", Erb said (1920). Hoffmann developed an abscess of the maxilla, which had been ignored and led to sepsis, and his health never returned to its previous state. On the morning of November 1, 1919, Johann Hoffmann died at the age of sixty-two, having been in bed for fifteen weeks. "In a most selfless manner, he had made arrangements for the events of his death, showing his true character and pure disposition in every way" (Erb, 1920).

Susan T. Iannaccone

Onasis Caneris

CINCINNATI, OHIO

ACKNOWLEDGMENTS

Thanks go to Dr. Franz Nave for his generous translations, to Stephanie Gates for her tireless duty at the photocopier, and to the library of the University of Heidelberg (Universitatsbibliothek D 69 Heidelberg) for sending me copies of original papers and photographs.

REFERENCES

Batten, F. E., and H. P. Gibb. 1909. Myotonia Atrophica. *Brain* 32:187–205.

Bendheim, O. 1937. On the History of Hoffmann's Sign. *Bull Hist Med* 5:684–86.

Brandt, S. 1950. *Werdnig-Hoffmann's Infantile Progressive Muscular Atrophy: Clinical Aspects, Pathology, Heredity and Relation to Oppenheim's Amyotonia Congenita and Other Morbid Conditions with Laxity of Joints or Muscles in Infants.* Copenhagen: Ejnar Munksgaard Forlag.

Byers, R. K., and B. Q. Banker. 1961. Infantile Muscular Atrophy. *Arch Neur* 5:140–64.

Curschmann, H. 1911. Über die diagnostische Bedeutung des babinskischen Phaenomens im praeuraemischen Zustand. *Münch med Wschr* 39:2054–57.

Erb, W. 1920. Johann Hoffmann. *Dtsch Zeit Nervenheilk* 65:1–24.

Fay, T. and H. B. Gotten. 1933. Clinical Observations on the Value of the Hoffmann Sign. *J Nerv Ment Dis* 77:594–600.

Greenfield, J. G. and R. L. Stern. 1927. The Anatomical Identity of the Werdnig-Hoffmann and Oppenheim Forms of Infantile Muscular Atrophy. *Brain* 50:652–86.

Hoffmann, J. 1884. Ein Fall von acuter aufsteiger Paralyse. *Arch Psych* (Berlin) 15:140–50.

______. 1887. Über das Verhalten der sensiblen Nerven bei der Tetanie. *Neur Centralbl* (Leipzig) 6:169–72.

______. 1888a. Zur Lehre von der Tetanie. *Dtsch Arch klin Med* (Leipzig) 43:53–119.

______. 1888b. Isolirte peripherische Lahmung des Nervus suprascapularis sinister. *Neur Centralbl* (Leipzig) 7:254–57.

______. 1892. Ueber familiäre progressive spinale Muskelatrophie. *Arch Psych* (Berlin) 24:664–46.

______. 1892–93. Ueber chronische spinale Muskelatrophie im Kindesalter auf familiärer Basis. *Dtsch Zeit Nervenheilk* 3:427–70.

______. 1896a. Weiterer Beitrag zur Lehre von der Tetanie. *Dtsch Zeit Nervenheilk* (Leipzig) 9:278–90.

______. 1896b. Ein Fall von Thomsen'scher Krankheit, complieirt durch neuritis multiplex. *Dtsch Zeit Nervenheilk* (Leipzig) 9:278–90.

______. 1896–97. Weiterer Beitrag zur Lehre von der Hereditaren progressiven spinalen Muskelatrophie im Kindesalter nebst Bemerkungen über den fortschreitenden Muskelschwund im Allgemeinen. *Dtsch Zeit Nervenheilk* (Leipzig) 10:292–320.

______. 1900a. Über die hereditäre progressive spinale Muskelatrophie im Kindesalter. *Münch med Wschr* 47:1649–51.

______. 1900b. Dritter Beitrag zur Lehre von der hereditaren progressiven spinalen Muskelatrophie im Kindesalter. Dtsch Zeit Nervenheilk 18:217–24.

______. 1903. Zur Lehre von der Thomsen'schen Krankheit. *Arch Psych* (Berlin) 37:668.

______. 1912. Katarakt bei und neben "Atrophischer Myotonie." *Arch Ophthal* (Leipzig) 81:512–17.

Schonfeld, W. 1962. Johann Hoffmann (1857–1919), der Heidelberger Neurologe, Schuler und Freund Wilhelm Erb's. Ruperto-Carola: Mitteilungen des Veseiningung des Freunde des Studentenschraft des Universitat Heidelberg.

Strümpell. A. 1920. Johannes Hoffmann. *Med Klin* 16:53–54.

Werdnig, G. 1891. Zwei hereditäre frühinfantile Fälle von progressiver muskelatrophie unter dem Bilde der Dystrophie aber auf neurotischer Grujndlage. Arch Psych Nervenkrankh 22:437–80.

JOHN HUGHLINGS JACKSON

AN APPRECIATION OF John Hughlings Jackson (1835–1911) (figure 1) from the perspective of a child neurologist is fraught with a central irony of character. He was by all accounts an austere, remote man, shy, serious, dignified, and a contemplative philosopher by nature. Yet, by profession, he was thrust among the most vulnerable of society, among whom he exercised sympathetic and meticulous clinical scrutiny, a scrutiny that was the foundation for the greatness of his conceptual analyses.

During his most productive period, John Hughlings Jackson married his cousin in 1865. After years of "Jacksonian" seizures, she died of cerebral thrombosis in 1876. He lived the last thirty-five years of his life inconsolable, childless, and alone (Jackson, 1925; Critchley, 1960a). This solitary figure, this grave countenance, emanated a gentle melancholy. Yet his associates described him as having a keen sense of humor and an unpredictable fancifulness. His solicitous interest in the lives of his students and their families was reciprocated by warmth and affection from his contemporaries and his disciples. Although without children, he liked their companionship. He was "at home with children" for they recognized his simplicity of nature (Obituary, 1911).

Hughlings Jackson's unparalleled ability to generalize from the detailed observations of a single patient produced an integrated design of the central nervous system and resulted in the intellectual basis for twentieth century neurology (Buzzard, 1934). In particular, he took an ancient malady, epilepsy, which was encumbered by prejudice and despair, and exposed the child and adult manifestations to detailed clinical attention and powerful logic.

Called the "Master" by contemporaries and successors, Hughlings Jackson rewrote the principles of neurology in the latter half of the nineteenth century, now called the "Age of Hughlings Jackson" (Jackson, 1931). What manner of man and intellect was Hughlings Jackson? Being the youngest of five children might explain his reasonable and affectionate nature. His Yorkshire father may have left him a legacy of energy, courage, and receptivity to new ideas and friends; and his Welsh mother gave him the cap-

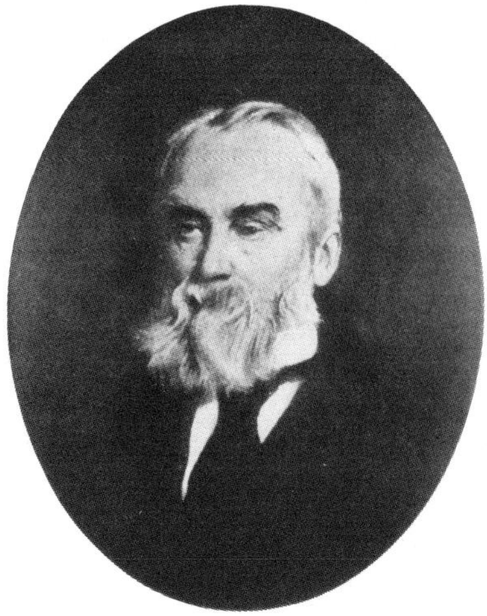

Figure 1. John Hughlings Jackson. (1835–1911). Photograph taken from a painting at the National Hospital in Queen's Square.

acity for tenderness, loyalty, and ever staunchness toward the elderly (Buzzard, 1911). Today's writers describe him as a "loved" man, "modest, kindly, warm hearted" with a "roguish sense of humor" (Critchley, 1986). Examples of the latter range from the gentle desire for a ". . . slight dash betwixt my two names. . . ." (Swash, 1986) to the remarkable ripostes of occasional necessity: "An eminent physician . . . described my aim as being to prove two things . . . that a motor centre does and also that it does not represent movements. I never consciously attempted that very marvelous feat" (Jackson, 1890).

Born in Yorkshire in 1835, Hughlings Jackson died in London in 1911. He trained at the soon-to-vanish York Medical School under Thomas Laycock of reflex physiology fame. This training was followed by a year at St. Bartholomew's in London. He eventually was positioned as assistant physician (1862), then physician (1867) to the National Hospital, Queen's Square, until his retirement in 1906. He was a founder of the journal *Brain* in 1878, and a year later was elected Fellow of the Royal Society, Great Britain's most august scientific organization. His conceptual ascendency among his contemporaries was swift, resulting from the publication of over three hundred papers. A third were written in the decade of the 1860's. Hughlings Jackson was universally regarded as one of the greatest neurologists of the nineteenth century, and his genius consisted of deriving general truths from his clinical practice and the autopsy room. This genius was not fully appreciated until his intellectual generalizations from specific patient observations were submitted to the crucible of twentieth-century experimental neurophysiology.

Not only is Hughlings Jackson the father of modern neurology but also the progenitor of many central concepts in child neurology. These include: a hierarchical concept of central nervous system anatomy and function; the bilaterality of speech and other functions in the developing brain with increasing localization upon maturation (Head, 1915); cortical inhibition in which the most recently developed central nervous system (CNS) inhibits and controls the earlier developed CNS; focal seizures as a cortical phenomenon that first manifest in the child with various subtypes, including Uncinate (temporal lobe) epilepsy and Rolandic (Jacksonian focal motor) seizures; a transition of seizure morphology with CNS maturation; inherited transmission of some generalized seizures; the "greater prevalence of convulsive diseases in young children" due to "greater instability" of neurons (Jackson, 1931, 222); childhood chorea and its localization to the basal ganglia, presaging modern neurochemistry of extrapyramidal disease; hysteria and malingering as a common cause of opisthotonos in adolescent boys (Jackson, 1931, 362); mirror or adventitious movements structurally minor but functionally important in the organic brain syndromes of learning disabled children (Jackson, 1931, 364); vertigo as it relates to migraine or seizures in children; importance of bilateral papilledema as a premonitory sign of sudden death as had been seen in childhood cerebellar tumors; and the anatomical analysis of "positive" and "negative" signs as they relate to the developing central nervous system.

Hughlings Jackson outlined a hierarchy of the CNS at three levels of evolution (Jackson, 1884; Jackson, 1886; Jackson, 1890; Jackson, 1898). The lowest sensorimotor, the cord, medulla and pons, "represents" the simplest movements of all parts of the body. The middle level, the Rolandic and possibly Striatal regions, "re-represents" more complex movements of all parts. The highest, the "Prae Frontal" lobes, the "organ of mind" "re-re-represents" all parts in their most complex function, the "acme of the evolution." This was a dynamic evolution of control from the most automatic to the most purposeful movements, from the most to the least organized, from the simplest to the most complex of sensorimotor integration (Jackson, 1898). Hughlings Jackson's hierarchical concept of the central nervous system has been central over the past one hundred years to our understanding of the child's developing brain. It has predicted our current notions of fetal and postpartum CNS development.

Hughlings Jackson argued that brainstem anatomy subserves

sounds, the subcortex words, and the cortex the language of ideas. The "cortex has a memory only for tunes, never for notes." That different parts of the neuraxis hierarchy have memory for different characters of movement not muscle (Jackson, 1931, 37) was experimentally validated by Charles Sherrington and Derek Denny-Brown in the two succeeding generations of neurophysiologists. Hughlings Jackson was the first to argue cogently that it is "absolutely impossible to have functional change . . . without a corresponding structural change." The fact that functional change cannot "exist by itself" has fueled the present generation of neurophysiologists to seek these structural changes in the molecules of biochemistry, however "imperfectly" appreciated (Martin, 1975).

Hughlings Jackson conceptualized that CNS function and anatomy become more complex as we ascend the evolutionary scale by species (phylogeny) and by the individual (ontogeny). The organization of the central nervous system progresses from a highly organized, functionally simple organ of the newborn to a lesser organized, but more complex, performing organ in the adult. He drew a distinction between the "highly organized state" of an infant's brain and the "complexity" of an adult's brain. This raises two additional concepts of Hughlings Jackson that are central to child neurology: Cortical inhibition and cerebral localization.

Cortical inhibition increases with maturation and prevents excessive discharges from lower centers (Jackson, 1898). The "most lately developed level controls and inhibits the lower levels" (Jackson, 1931, xiii). This concept is the direct antecedent of reigning neuroanatomy and neurophysiology in which the cerebral cortex becomes more complex in its axodendritic and axoaxonal synapses, hence exerting increasingly greater control over the subcortex as the infant's brain matures. Conversely, with "dissolution" (disease) of the cortex, there is loss of cortical inhibition and wasting of sophisticated higher function, such as language, cognition, perceptual, motor, and affective function. The lower centers, or the subcortex, are free to reexert their more simple functions. Like the diseased senile brain that has lost cortical inhibition, the neonate, who has yet to gain cortical inhibition, exhibits a variety of subcortical activities or release reflexes such as the Moro, suck, root, glabellar, grasp, tonic neck, stepping, and placing reflexes. Additionally, the immature brain, like the diseased CNS, evinces incomplete higher cortical function.

Hughlings Jackson's cerebral localization was a synthesis of the biological conception of brain localization for mental faculties, Franz Joseph Gall's theory of the preceding generation; the concept of biological evolution of his contemporary, Herbert Spencer; and nineteenth-century associative psychology. Cerebral localization was a pragmatic resolution of the "mind-body" relationship that had beset metaphysics for 2500 years. He combined psychological and physiological events, using biological concepts such as integration and representation, not to simply accumulate facts and verify concepts, but to comprehend the "underlying significance of phenomena" (Broadbent, 1903). "Mind" was not a faculty residing somewhere in the central nervous system. Rather, the "mind" was the result of the process of CNS activity. It could not be analyzed physiologically any more than the brain was subject to metaphysics. In repudiating the notion of "abrupt geographic localizations," or cortical mosaicism, he resisted topography in the interests of phenomenology.

The phenomena of thought, speech, and movement were a constellation of brain activity of specific parts and levels, singular yet integrated. The brain was "an organ for the coordination of impressions and movements" (Jackson, 1931). "Mental states arose during but not from the activity of brain." "The cortex represents processes and not structures" (Walshe, 1961). To understand Hughlings Jackson's science of neurology was to understand the organic evolution of brain from the lowest form of life to the human species and to fathom the maturational changes from neonate to adult.

Early in Hughlings Jackson's professional life there was a consensus that the "seat of epilepsy" was in the medulla oblongata (Jackson, 1886). Fits were considered reflex in origin, due to a physical stimulus that ultimately produced vascular spasm and hence reduction in blood flow to the brain. Based upon clinical observation and pathological correlation, Hughlings Jackson demonstrated that the cerebral hemispheres, not the medulla, produced unilateral seizures (Jackson, 1863; Jackson, 1864). He shifted the anatomical substrate of epilepsy to the efferent system that controlled voluntary movement: the corpus striatum, the Rolandic region, and the "Prae Frontal lobe." This was based upon the postmortems of individual patients who had suffered from hemiplegia, aphasia, and seizures (Jackson, 1870). Aphasia and plegia were caused by destroyed neural tissue in the left cerebral hemisphere, seizures by the instability of surrounding gray cells. This was soon confirmed by David Ferrier's ablation and stimulation studies of "destroying and discharging lesions" (Ferrier, 1873).

Ferrier's studies led to Hughlings Jackson's revolutionary theory that seizures were based upon neuronal dysfunction. "Epilepsy is the name for occasional sudden excessive rapid and local discharges of gray matter" (Jackson, 1873; Jackson, 1890). This neuronal theory, derived from the bedside and the autopsy room, permeates the science of modern child neurology. Excessive gray matter discharge followed by exhaustion, "comparatively slight instability" (Jackson, 1890) predicts the electrochemical membrane physiology of depolarization, followed by hyperpolarization due to the sodium, potassium, and calcium chemical shifts. His notion of "morbid nutrition" as the cause of excessive discharges of nerve cells "high instability" (Jackson, 1890) fuels research in cellular metabolism during seizures using the modern probes of positron emission and magnetic resonance spectroscopy. Hughlings Jackson's focus on the tissue-organ-function triad represents a twentieth-century perspective and differed sharply from the undifferentiated vascular and humoral theories of his predecessors and coevals (Jackson, 1898).

A second major contribution to the study of epilepsy was Hughlings Jackson's analysis of the "three kinds of fits corresponding to the three evolutionary levels" (Jackson, 1890). These included: the "Pontobulbar" fits of cord, medullary, and pontine origin; the "epileptiform" seizures of Rolandic (motor cortex) and corpus striatum origin; and "epilepsy proper" of "Prae Frontal lobe" ("acme of the evolution") origin. He used the term *fit* to include "convulsive paroxysms of all kinds dependent on excessive discharges beginning in . . . any one of the three levels." He successfully conceptualized the nature of epilepsy, thus superseding the endless nosologic classifications of his day.

Hughlings Jackson recognized that the morphology of seizures depended upon the maturation of the developing central nervous system. Seizure types were age dependent. "Rigor" or "inward fits," "lowest level fits," rarely occurred under six months of age due to brainstem immaturity (Jackson; 1886; Jackson; 1898). They become the dominant seizure type for infants from between two to six months to two years. Seizures of this type were due to rickets, catarrhal laryngitis, congenital heart disease, and pertussis. They showed in common the net effect of hypoxia-ischemia. "Such attacks are chiefly observed in little children during the first year of life" when "cyanosis rapidly reaches its highest grade" followed by the "accumulation of . . . acid in the blood" (Jackson, 1886). The mechanism was the same, reduced circulation to brain tissue whether due to tumor, infection (syphilis), or arterial occlusion (Jackson, 1870).

After two years of age, akinetic seizures with afferent stimulation as a provocateur became a common type (Jackson, 1931, 363). The emergence of focal seizures of cerebral hemisphere origin occurred in mid childhood and adolescence. These seizures included the two extensively studied by Hughlings Jackson: the focal motor, later called Jacksonian, seizure of Rolandic origin, and the temporal lobe seizure of Uncinate origin (Jackson and Colman, 1898). Both are now called partial seizures, the former simple, the latter complex.

Hughlings Jackson vividly describes temporal lobe fits as "dreamy states" or "intellectual auras." These were characterized by visual or olfactory hallucinations, absence, anxiety, fear, horror, rapture, "mental diplopia," and a semiconscious wakefulness. There was incomplete voluntary control with a "time gap" (amnesia) and a "deathly pale or livid countenance." These "auras" and "states" presaged Uncinate fits. Linking of dreamy states and special sensory auras with an Uncal lesion reflected the assiduous character of his patient follow-through, a willingness to wait seventeen years to confirm a clinical pathological correlation from which he could then generalize (Jackson and Colman, 1898). The analysis of these seizure types illuminates Hughlings Jackson's methods. Unilateral signs such as focal seizures, hemiplegia, and visual and speech disorders were systematically related to an anatomical substrate (Jackson, 1882; Jackson, 1931, 37).

Seen by Hughlings Jackson in all ages from mid childhood onwards, focal motor fits were generated by an "excessively and rapidly discharging" lesion and the convulsive outburst was "simply a brutish development of many of the patient's ordinary movements."

This often resulted in "the perfect paralysis." This was due, as Hughlings Jackson quotes Robert Todd's 1854 opinion with approval, to "exhaustion of nerve fibres by the excessive discharge in the paroxysm" (Jackson, 1882).

His break with all prior authority strikes home with any child-care physician. His preoccupation with the relation between seizure types and maturational age laid the foundation for the eventual emergence of child neurology as a separate specialty.

An interesting footnote to Hughlings Jackson's career is his return to "eccentric factors." By this he meant afferent peripheral stimuli such as emotional stress, physical sickness, and fever. Thought by his predecessors to be the prime cause of seizures, these conditions were viewed by Hughlings Jackson as provocateurs of fits because they upset the equilibrium of a preexisting "unstable patch." This is the direct precedent for our current notions of seizure breakthroughs in children, from simple febrile seizures to partial complex of any structural cause.

A central theoretical discovery, crucial to our present understanding of the developing child's brain, was his analysis of "positive and negative symptoms" (Jackson, 1884). He insisted upon the "impossibility of positive symptoms from negative lesions" (Martin, 1975). "Positive symptoms" such as hallucinations, garbled speech, chorea, and seizures, are subserved by "nervous elements untouched by any pathologic process." That "they arise during activity on the lower level of evolution" reflected his views on hierarchal CNS function and cortical inhibition (Jackson, 1884).

Conversely, "negative symptoms," such as plegia, are due to destructive lesions. Positive symptoms occurring with destructive lesions emanate from uncontrolled activity of remaining normal anatomy. This concept revolutionized neurophysiology, and only beginning with the experimental genius of Sherrington at the turn of the twentieth century did neurologists begin to understand the significance of a negative lesion enabling a positive symptom to occur through the jettison of normal inhibition. Hughlings Jackson recognized this not only for neurologic disease but also for maturation of the developing brain.

Nowhere is this concept better illustrated than in the infant's brain, whereby during the first year of life the elaboration of cortical synapses and subcortical myelination results in increasing cortical inhibition. This results in loss of motor automatisms of subcortical, or brainstem, origin, such as the suck, root, grasp, Moro, glabellar, tonic neck, stepping, and placing functions, and the development of voluntary motor function. In disease, the remaining healthy but uninhibited brain demonstrates new manifestations. These were Hughlings Jackson's "positive symptoms." His particular genius, and upon which modern neurophysiology and chemistry are based, was the ability to interpret "disorders in terms of normal function 'What can symptoms tell us of normal functions?'" (Walshe, 1961). Every modern neuroprobe uses this principle. For example, the positron emission tomographic demonstration of glucose utilization during seizures is used as the basis for neurosurgical extirpation.

A review of Hughlings Jackson's views on speech disorders, although never mentioned in relation to children, is important because his ideas contributed to our understanding of how speech develops during childhood (Head, 1915; Critchley, 1960b; Walshe, 1961). He set about to explain the phenomenology of normal speech by attempting to elucidate the anatomical and physiological basis of disordered speech. His singular vision was the concept that "to locate the damage which destroys speech and to locate speech are two different things" (Jackson, 1915a). The cerebral localization of normal speech was quite different from the localization of a lesion producing a speech disorder.

The first to explicate the syndrome of left middle cerebral artery occlusion, Hughlings Jackson deduced from his of patients with right hemiplegia, aphasia, and right focal motor seizures that the left hemisphere was for the ". . . voluntary use of words . . . into speech." The right hemisphere was for the "most automatic use of words" (Jackson, 1915a). Thus he acknowledged both the "duality of the brain," its equipotential nature, and its localizing character, a process that occurred with maturation. This is our present view of cognitive and language evolution from the newborn to the adult.

As a neurologist, Hughlings Jackson attempted to dissect language disorders as a reflection of cerebral localization; as a philosopher he saw the disorders in the context of a wholly integrated circuit encompassing the whole of the central nervous system.

Although left middle cerebral artery occlusion resulted in loss of verbal language, it did not destroy all language function. "Speech is a *part* of thought . . . which we may or may not exteriorize. . . . Speechlessness does not imply wordlessness" (Jackson, 1915a). In modern terms, an expressive aphasia does not imply the inability to think or understand words. Rather, it is the inability to form or to express a proposition in words. The auditory and visual word-mental images may be intact.

In dissolution (disease), one often retains understanding even as one can no longer speak. In evolution (maturation), a child first understands before he can speak. Furthermore, and directly antecedent to our present theory of cognitive development, Hughlings Jackson elucidated two modes of expression: emotional and intellectual (Jackson, 1915b). Emotional speech is automatic and used to exhibit feelings. Emotional words are "symbols of emotions" (Jackson, 1915c). Intellectual speech, used to convey propositions, is "voluntary and propositional" or "symbols of ideas." Disease may separate the two forms of speech, just as maturation unites them. In the developing child, internal speech leads to the utterance of articulated words, or external speech. Nothing today in our understanding of language development was unanticipated by the conceptual genius of Hughlings Jackson.

Hughlings Jackson invested his time and interests in many other topics of clinical importance to the practitioner of child neurology. The use of the ophthalmoscope was an example. Since the optic nerve is a "fragment" of the central nervous system, "you cannot investigate cases of cerebral disease methodically unless you use the ophthalmoscope" (Jackson, 1958, 251). Thus, Hughlings Jackson was instrumental in promoting the use of this device by subsequent generations of neurologists who unfailingly carry around one of the two prime tools of labor: the ophthalmoscope. He was the first to use this instrument, ten years after its invention by Hermann Helmholtz, in order to diagnose CNS disease. Tumors of the cerebellum were first recognized by Hughlings Jackson to produce double optic neuritis in children without loss of vision (Jackson, 1958, 329). He was the first to comprehensively describe the cerebellar tumor syndrome in children. "There is a vast increase of fluid in the lateral ventricles . . . the head enlarges . . . [there is a] great hebetude of mind . . . [and] a slow failure of mental faculties" (Jackson, 1958, 333). "Reeling" (ataxia), "rigidity

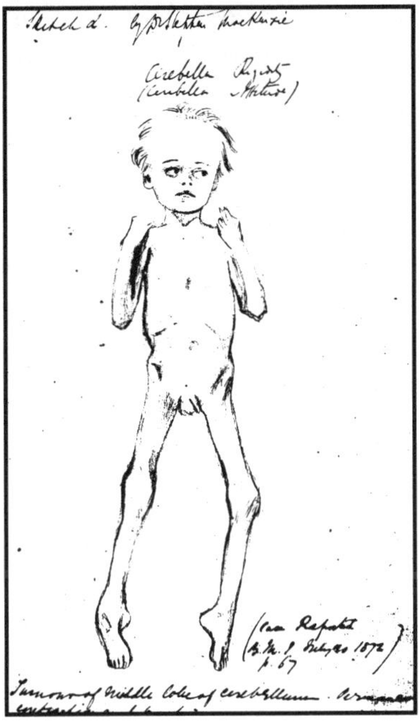

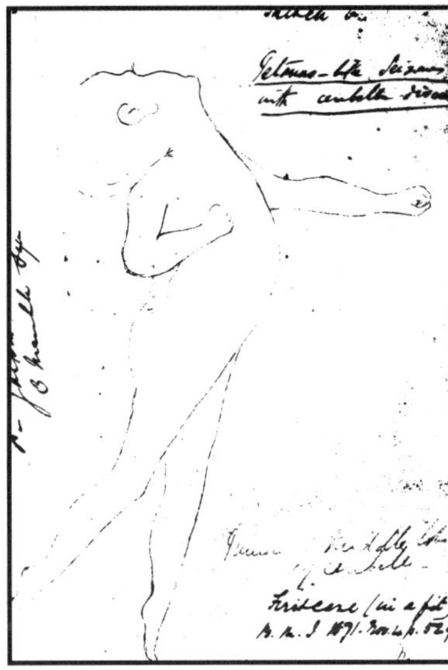

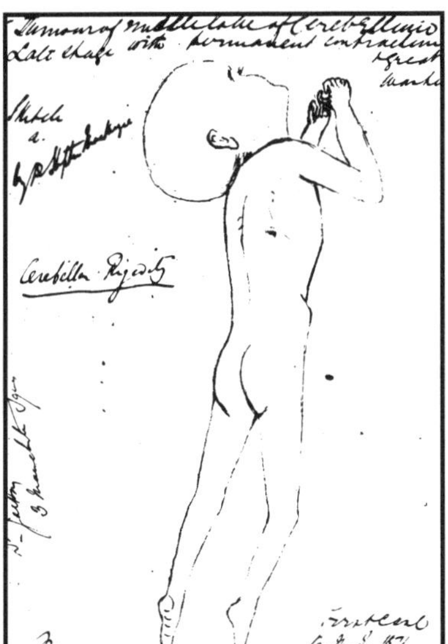

Figures 2a, b, c. Hughlings Jackson's interest in posterior fossa tumors of childhood is reflected in these three drawings with his annotations: A. A description of cerebellar rigidity from his own papers. B and C were also drawn by Dr. Stephen MacKenzie and annotated by Hughlings Jackson. The originals hang in the National Hospital Library, Queen's Square.

or opisthotonos," and "tetanus-like seizures" (decerebration) constituted the motor hallmarks figures 2a, b, c). This, together with double optic neuritis, were premonitory signs of sudden death in the child. Rigidity or opisthotonos may also occur in adolescence as a consequence of hysteria and malingering (Jackson, 1931, 362; Riese and Goody, 1955).

Vertigo as a symptom of seizures or migraine in children was first conceptualized by Hughlings Jackson following his observations in adults (Jackson, 1880). This study illustrates the flow of his inductive method: his mastery of the empirical method from which sprang his logical generalizations. It also accents another facet of his existence. His writings have suggested to some commentators a lack of concern for the patient as a person and for his treatment (Lennox, 1970). This is false. He described his successful treatment of a 22-year-old soldier with "auditory vertigo" who "left the hospital in a state of intense gratitude" (Jackson, 1880).

The central irony of Hughlings Jackson's character was one of appearances. The world of reality gave us a man of unsurpassing clarity of thought and vision, representing the foundation of modern neuroscience. He was also a man of warmth and simplicity who was "at home with children."

Ronald S. Gabriel
LOS ANGELES, CALIFORNIA

REFERENCES

Broadbent, W. 1903. Hughlings Jackson as Pioneer in Nervous Physiology and Pathology. *Brain* 26:305–82.

Buzzard, E. F. 1934. Hughlings Jackson and His Influence on Neurology. *Lancet* 2:909–13.

Buzzard, T. 1911. Obituary. John Hughlings Jackson. *Brit Med J* 2:952–53.

Critchley, M. 1960a. Hughlings Jackson The Man and the Early Days of the National Hospital. *Proc Roy Soc Med* 53:613–18.

______. 1960b. The Contributions of John Hughlings Jackson to Neurology. *Cereb Palsy Bull* 2:79.

______. 1986. Hughlings Jackson: The Man and His Time. *Arch Neur* 43:435–37.

Ferrier, D. 1873. Experimental Researches in Cerebral Physiology & Pathology. *West Riding Lunatic Asylum Medical Reports* 3:30–96.

Head, H. 1915. Hughlings Jackson on Aphasia and Kindred Affections of Speech. *Brain* 38:127.

Jackson, J. H. 1863. Syphilis Followed by Unilateral Convulsions Four Months Afterwards — Temporary Hemiplegia — Paralysis of Sixth Nerve on the Same Side — Recovery. *Med Times Gaz* 1:3.

______. 1864. Loss of Speech with Hemiplegia on the Left Side — Valvular Disease — Epileptiform Seizures Affecting the Side Paralyzed. *Med Times Gaz* 2:166–67.

______. 1870. A Study of Convulsions. *St. Andrew's Med Grad Assoc Trans* 3:162–204.

______. 1873. On the Anatomical, Physiological, & Pathological Investigation of Epilepsies. *West Riding Lunatic Asylum Medical Reports* 3:315.

______. 1880. Lecture on Auditory Vertigo. *Lancet* 2:525–28.

______. 1882. Localized Convulsions From Tumour of the Brain. *Brain* 5:364–74.

______. 1884. Croonian Lectures on Evolution and Dissolution of the Nervous System. *Brit Med J* 1:591, 660, 703 et seq.

______. 1886. A Contribution to the Comparative Study of Convulsions. *Brain* 9:123.

______. 1890. The Lumleian Lectures on Convulsive Seizures. *Brit Med J* 1:703–07.

______. 1898. The Hughlings Jackson Lecture on the Relations of Different Divisions of the Central Nervous System to One Another and to Parts of the Body. *Lancet* 1:79–87.

______. 1915a. On the Nature of the Duality of the Brain. *Brain* 38:801–03.

______. 1915b. Notes on the Physiology and Pathology of Language. *Brain* 38:48–58.

______. 1915c. Words and Other Symbols in Mentation. *Brain* 38:175–86.

______. 1925. *Neurological Fragments, with Biographical Memoir by James Taylor and Including the* Recollections *of Jonathan Hutchinson and Charles Mercier*. Oxford: Oxford Medical Publications.

______. 1931. *Selected Writings of John Hughlings Jackson*. Edited for the Guarantors of *Brain* by James Taylor with the advice and assistance of Gordon Holmes and F. M. R. Walshe. London: Hodder & Stoughton, Ltd.

______. 1958. *Selected Writings of John Hughlings Jackson*. Reprint of 1931 edition. Vol. 2 Ed. Taylor, Holmes, and Walshe. New York: Basic Books, Inc.

Jackson, J. H., and W. S. Colman. 1898. Case of Epilepsy with Tasting Movements and Dreamy State — Very Small Patch of Softening in the Left Uncinate Gyrus. *Brain* 21:580–90.

Lennox, W. 1970. Hughlings Jackson. *Founders of Neurology*, Ed. W. Haymaker and F. Schiller. Springfield: Charles C Thomas.

Martin, J. P. 1975. Kinnier Wilson's Notes of Conversations with Hughlings Jackson. *J Neur Neurosurg Psych* 38:313–16.

Obituary. 1911. John Hughlings Jackson. *Brit Med J* 2:950–54.

Riese, W. and W. Gooddy 1955. An Original Clinical Record of Hughlings Jackson with an Interpretation. *Bull Hist Med* 29:230–38.

Swash, M. 1986. John Hughlings Jackson: A Sesquicentennial Tribute. *J Neur Neurosurg Psych* 49:981–85.

Walshe, F. M. R. 1961. Contributions of John Hughlings Jackson to Neurology. *Arch Neur* 5:119–31

WILLIAM JOHN LITTLE

AMONG THE HONORABLE company of surgeons who have made fundamental contributions to child neurology, a British orthopedic surgeon, William John Little (1810–1894) (figure 1), is preeminent. As one reads both the body of his work and what is written about him, what stands out is the integration of his personal and professional life — a synthesis of the microscopic and the macroscopic, of the particular experience and the broad reflective view of a nineteenth-century naturalist. He sought a remedy for his own affliction of club foot and, having found it, extended it energetically to others. He is credited with propagation and acceptance of Louis Stromeyer's innovative surgery for this problem, and with the establishment of the Charitable Hospital for the Cure of Deformities, which became the Royal Orthopaedic Hospital. But it is to his powers of observation, description, and documentation that we owe his central contribution to child neurology. He identified a link between prematurity, asphyxia of the neonate, and motor and mental impairment on a neurologic basis (Accardo, 1989).

William John Little was born on August 7, 1810, in London. The nation had been impoverished by the long war with France, but his parents, who kept the Red Lion Inn and quartered the Tenth Hussars, were prosperous enough to afford medical care and an excellent education for their son. It is thought that his life was saved when, as a sickly child not really expected to live, he was sent to the country in a last effort to recover his health, infantile paralysis having been indicated as the cause of the weakness and deformity of his left foot (Jones, 1949). He received his elementary education in private London schools and at six and a half years of age was sent to school at St. Margaret's. Thereafter, he studied languages and mathematics at the Royal College of St. Omer's in France. Returning to England at fifteen, he first apprenticed himself to an apothecary and three years later entered the London Hospital where he studied anatomy, medicine, and surgery, and spent a year as a resident "dresser" (Little, 1837). He was admitted to the College of Surgeons at the age of twenty-three, continued his studies in comparative anatomy, zoology, and physiology, and briefly was in private surgical practice. Wishing, however, to obtain a hospital appointment according to a contemporary biographer, he went to Germany to complete the necessary studies (Biographical sketch, 1854). Upon his return, at the age of twenty-seven, he was licensed by the Royal College of Physicians and was subsequently appointed to the London Hospital where, at thirty-four, he was appointed the sole professor of medicine (Brown, 1935).

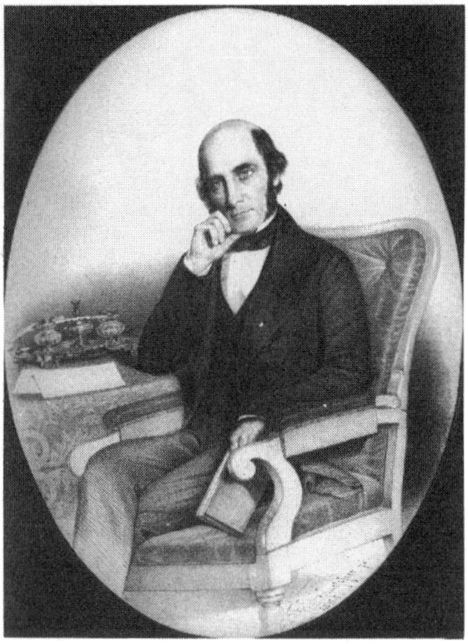

Figure 1. William John Little (1810–1894). Lithograph portrait by F. Schapper, 1854.

Little got on well with his colleagues and his early professional relationships became enduring friendships, but a less happy, more personal subtext affected his activities. In the preface to his 1839 publication of *A Treatise on the Nature of Clubfoot and Analogous Distortions*, he wrote:

At an early period of my medical studies, I devoted much attention to the nature of these distortions, from the circumstances of my being afflicted with Talipes in the left foot and, although I consulted the most approved surgical authorities and many members of the profession in the metropolis, from none did I receive the slightest prospect of cure . . . only the most discouraging opinions: the affection having invariably been attributed to malformation and ankylosis of the individual bones of the tarsus, the muscular contraction having been regarded as secondary. (Little, 1839, vii–viii)

Reading in the French and German literature, however, he learned of the operation of sectioning the Achilles tendon that had been proposed and initiated by Jacques Delpech in 1823 and subsequently developed by Stromeyer some ten years later. Continuing his inquiries in Leyden, Dresden, Berlin and Hanover, and satisfying himself of the rationality of the procedure and the soundness of the surgeon (for Dr. Little was always a deliberate and methodical man), "I determined on placing myself under the care of Dr. Stromeyer; and to his skill and kindness I am indebted for the restoration of my foot" (Little, 1839, x). Little's sense of gratitude was unending and apostolic. He wrote his required dissertation and entitled it "Sympolae ad talipedem varum cognoscendum" ("Contribution to the Knowledge of Club Foot"), in which he reviewed the anatomy, pathology, and historically held theories of causation and promoted Stromeyer's operation (Little, 1837). The thesis was dedicated to Stromeyer. He gained operative experience abroad and established the operation in England (he was not the first to perform a tenotomy there, but was its most effective advocate), and continued always to champion the victims of orthopedic deformities. He gave Stromeyer's name to his third son. Years later, when Stromeyer was being fêted by an international community celebrating the jubilee of his doctorate, he exclaimed to Little, "I owe all this to you" (Obituary, 1894).

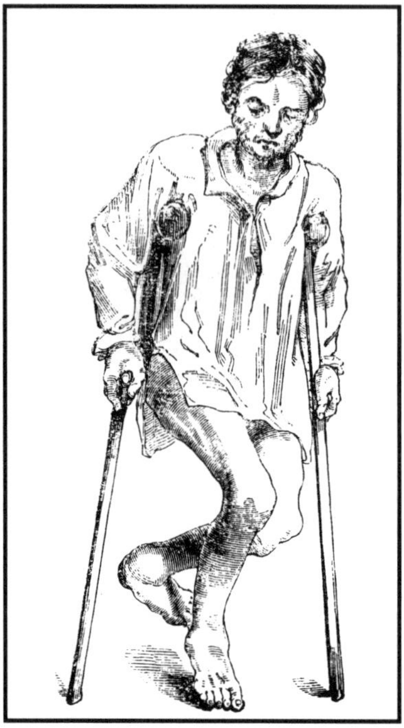

Figure 2. A drawing of one of Little's patients with "spastic contractures of the lower extremities" who he felt was a good candidate for release of the "adductors of the thighs, the hamstrings, gastrocnemii and adductors of the feet." From "Course of Lectures on the Deformities of the Human Frame," originally *Lancet* 1 (1843): 351, figure 14.

Little's tremendous clinical experience with orthopedic patients provided a generous bank of data for his observations and, certainly, it was not uncommon in his time for physicians, including obstetricians, to keep track of their experiences. In the first volume of the *Transactions of the Obstetrical Society of London* we find two such reports, one describing 4,049 patients, the experience of twenty years (Dunn, 1859); and one on 6,465 births, the experience of fifty years (Bailey, 1859). But obstetricians of the time appeared to recognize only two outcomes of parturition, apart from maternal health — a living infant, or a dead one. Even in those days some very premature babies, the products of seven months gestation, survived. Little records that some of these babies weighed only about forty ounces (Little, 1853). Beyond the phenomenon of survival, however, there appears to have been no special interest in the outcome. In similar fashion, some extraordinary resuscitations took place and were duly reported as curiosities. The obstetrician, arriving to find an infant delivered and discarded as dead half an hour before, might set straight to work on the apparent stillborn and, following principles of resuscitation outlined by Marshall Hall, be successful. At a time when the moral propriety of the induction of labor was debated, there seemed to be no question about the rightness of this action, surely in part at least because the outcomes were not pursued. The history of the neonate was not linked to the outcome of the child, and obstetricians were focused almost exclusively on the mother.

This passage from volume one of the *Transactions of the Obstetrical Society of London* is revealing:

It may be that I have erred, in avoiding at times the use of forceps, and that their timely application, in some few instances, might have saved the life of the child. . . . But, still, I quite concur in the belief of Dr. Collins, "that where the patient has been properly treated from the commencement of her labour . . . the death of the child takes place in laborious and difficult labours before the symptoms become so alarming as to cause any experienced physician to lessen the head." The stethoscope, indeed, seems to have placed this matter beyond dispute. But, once satisfied of the death of the child, I have not hesitated . . . to have recourse . . . to craniotomy. . . . The use of the stethoscope in such cases is of the last importance. (Dunn, 1859, 279)

I believe Little's mind was uniquely prepared to consider such historical relationships for several reasons. First, he saw his patients at a later period in their lives. He followed them for years and could appreciate the evolving declaration of pathological states, such as mental deficiency and spasticity, which were not necessarily evident at birth yet which had no more proximate cause (figure 2). Second, Darwinism was in the air. The comparative, inductive reasoning that *On the Origin of Species* would crystallize was implicit in the natural sciences that Little studied. Thus considered, comparative anatomy is a branch of natural history that teaches us that forms are not *sui generis*, but rather evolve obedient to discernible principles of determination. Third, and perhaps most important, Little knew from personal experience that deformity, in order to be conquered, must first be made a part of the natural world. To the extent that deformity was perceived as monstrous, something outside of nature, it was perceived as immutable and impossible to remediate. That was the attitude with which he had met when he sought advice about his own deformity, and against which he argued in his lectures. "Many malformations . . . are termed monstrosities, and nothing of practical value can be said concerning them. I shall dismiss the subject" (Little, 1843–44, 749). It was also necessary for him to argue the case with his colleagues and students, that malformations were not produced by frightening impressions made on pregnant women.

Instead of clubfoot, for example, being considered what it really is, a mere distortion of parts originally well formed, the popular notion is, that it depends on a deficiency of some of the parts of the limb; that is, is a malformation, a monstrosity, a lusus naturae, or an arrêt de développement. This, like other almost equally obsolete opinions of the medical profession, has obtained a firm hold of the minds of the public, and will retain it for generations after the advance of science has introduced other explanations of the nature of the disease. Believing, also, that it is solely a misfortune afflicting the infant anterior to birth, its production has been attributed, like that of other so-called malformations, to some occult maternal influence acting on the embryo — to the strange ideas and freaks of imagination which occasionally affect pregnant women. (Little, 1843–44, 682)

Then what was the cause?

One of the most striking facts elicited from comparison of non-congenital with congenital deformities is, that certain deformities which are slowly acquired in extra-uterine existence. . . are faithfully represented in certain deformities which originate during intrauterine life. This fact is no sooner seized than the mind of the observer is at once led to the inference that the causes which have produced these identical phenomena must have been identical. (Little, 1843–44, 680)

His pathological material had convinced him that the same deformity might arise from multiple causes and he showed to his students apparently identical specimens arising from diverse etiologies. Extending his original dissertation in his lectures, Little had outlined a general classification which, although anatomical rather than etiological, had sorted out inflammatory, structural, and neurologic causes; distinguishing among the latter paralytic, what we would call lower motor neuron, and spastic, or upper motor neuron, types. And as his work progressed, he argued that these causes might be present before, as well as after, birth. But this thinking was as much mechanical as etiological, and up to a certain point he had considered only the two states, before and after birth, much as his obstetrical colleagues had considered two states of the infant, dead and alive. This scheme could not satisfy the many cases in which the child had been born without deformity, but had acquired it over time without convincing intervening illness or accident. As case after case accumulated in which prematurity or asphyxia neonatorum figured in the history, his attention became drawn to parturition, the time between two states of being (before and after birth), until at last he carried his conviction to the obstetricians, laid it before them, and charged them (in his responsible, scholarly, and well-mannered fashion) with the assumption of their obligations as historians of that portion of the natural world that they were uniquely situated to observe:

I believe I am now enabled to form an opinion of the nature of the anatomical lesions and the particular abnormal event at birth on which the symptoms depend. Moreover, as the study of the proximate cause of the affections which I shall describe requires the light of such facts as the members of this Society have peculiar opportunities of supplying, I make no further apology for occupying the Society's time. (Little, 1861a, 295)

The paper read before the Obstetrical Society of London on October 2, 1861, and printed in their *Transactions* (Little, 1861a), was summarized in the *Lancet* as follows:

The author introduced his subject by stating that pathology had gradually taught that the foetus in utero was subject to diseases similar to those which affect the economy at later periods of existence, and that this was particularly true as regards deformities. Thus we had congenital and non-congenital club-foot, rickets, degeneration of muscles, and amputations in utero. But there was another epoch of existence, namely, the period of birth. . . . He said that the object of his communication was to show that the act of birth did occasionally imprint upon the nervous and muscular systems of the nascent organism very serious and peculiar evils. His opinion was that asphyxia neonatorum through injury to nervous centres was the cause of the contractions which originate at birth — more or less general spastic rigidity, and sometimes of paralytic contraction . . . varying in effect from the slightest impairment to complete imbecility of mind and body. (Lancet, 1861b, 378)

What linked together prematurity and asphyxia at term was acidosis and respiratory failure. Ischemia was also important.

The state of things in the foetus at the moment of birth — at the moment of entire withdrawal of placental or maternal circulatory influence — was one of the imminent failure in decarbonization of the blood. If pulmonary respiration were not immediately established . . . asphyxia neonatorum took place . . . .

He remarked that asphyxia neonatorum was very apt to be accompanied and followed by convulsions, as convulsions at or subsequent to birth were only a symptom of lesions of nervous centres, though they might act on those centres, and thus probably aggravate the disorder.

He stated one fact as common to all the forty-seven cases of persistent spastic rigidity appended to his paper — namely, that some abnormal circumstance had attended the act of parturition, or rather the several processes concerned in separating the foetus from the parents. (Little, 1861b, 379)

For more than a century after the publication of this paper, the silence concerning it was almost palpable. It seemed no one was able to believe or accept Little's ideas. Finally, Dr. Barnes, a member of the Society, broke this silence: "The difficulty there appeared to be in discussing this excellent paper arose, no doubt, from the entire novelty and originality of the subject. Dr. Little had brought before the obstetrical world new matter for inquiry of the highest interest" (Little, 1861a, 341). Dr. Tyler Smith, president of the Society, said that he thought teething was responsible for most cases of paraplegia and hemiplegia in children. And there it lay, more or less, for over twenty years, despite Little's reference to over two hundred cases of brain injury due to birth injury (figure 3) and his presentation and detailed documentation of sixty-three cases for the Society. And how well he described them! Who in pediatrics or child neurology would not recognize these children?

Sometimes the affection of one limb only is observed by the parent, but examination usually shows a smaller degree of affection in the limb supposed to be sound. . . . In most cases, after time . . . the thighs cannot be completely abducted or extended, the knees cannot be straightened, nor can the heels be properly applied to the ground. . . . Sometimes articulation is only slow and difficult, like other acts of volition. . . . Sometimes the speech is nervous, impulsive, or stuttering. Often during the earliest months of life deglutition is impaired, and the power of carrying saliva into the fauces is not acquired until late. The intellectual functions are sometimes quite unaffected, but in the majority of cases the intellect suffers from the slightest impairment which the parent unwillingly acknowledges or fails to perceive up to entire imbecility. . . .

In other cases, where intellectual powers are good, a preternatural impulsive nervous condition of mind exists, combined with an agitated, eager, anxious mode of performing acts of volition. (Little, 1861a, 301–2, 304)

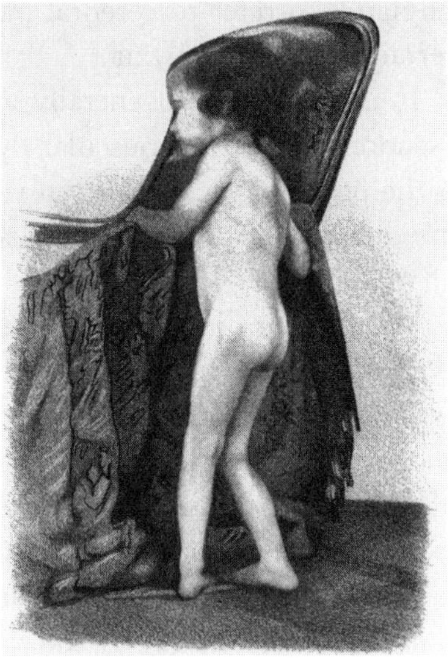

Figure 3. A young girl with spastic cerebral palsy. The legend by Little noted "Contractures of adductors and flexors of lower extremities. Left hand weak. Both hands awkward. More paralytic than spastic. Born with navel-string around neck. Asphyxia neonatorum one hour." From "On the Influence of Abnormal Parturition . . . ." *Trans Obstet Soc Lond* 3(1861a): 344, plate 7.

When Little died in 1894 after ten years of retirement, no mention was made of this aspect of his work in any obituary. According to James Collier, the name "Little's Disease" for spastic diplegia was first suggested in 1888 by Theodorus Rupprecht (Collier, 1899, 396). In the nineteenth century, as now, people argued against the importance of the birth history, assigning it a secondary place in terms of causality. Little himself did not ascribe all instances of abnormality to this process, recognizing mechanical injury or other factors innate to the mother or child as also being pertinent. The majority of the children he described with spastic rigidity evident at birth probably fall into the latter category, and it was proposed by some to limit the term "Little's Disease" to this group (Collier, 1899, 407; 1924). It has, however, more generally been used, especially in

England, to refer to cerebral palsies of diverse etiologies including, certainly, birth asphyxia.

It is perhaps not generally appreciated that Little also described pseudohypertrophic muscular dystrophy and its characteristic muscle pathology some ten to fifteen years before Duchenne. He also recognized myotonia, which he related to writer's cramp (Little, 1853, 14–16, 186–87).

We do not know much more about Little himself. Everyone, even obstetricians, seemed to like him, and he was much praised as a teacher and practical clinician. Orthopedics in one way or another pervaded even his domestic life. He married the daughter of an orthopedic surgeon and they had eleven children, of whom two of the four sons became orthopedic surgeons. The man who looks at us from his portraits seems wise and kind. He would have conducted his rounds as the visiting physician to the Asylum for Idiots at Earlswood and the Royal Hospital for Incurables without any of the political meanness of spirit or sadistic voyeurism that certainly occurred at the Salpêtrière from time to time. One can see in him the man who interrupted a lecture on club foot with a digression on its psychological impact (Little, 1843–44, 40), a man who could sympathize even with Richard III (born premature with feet first) for his deformities of body and spirit (Little, 1861a, 343). A good man, he completed the transition from sorrow caused by personal affliction to compassion, giving his energies to the present needs of others and his observations and insights to the future. We are reminded of Robert Frost's words:

Only where love and need are one
And the work is play for mortal stakes,
Is the deed ever really done
For Heaven and the future's sakes.

Mary Anne Whelan
COOPERSTOWN, NEW YORK

REFERENCES

Accardo, P. 1989. William John Little and Cerebral Palsy in the Nineteenth Century. *J Hist Med* 44:56–71.

1854. Biographical sketch of William John Little, M.D. *Lancet* 2:16–22.

Bailey, W. H. 1859. Statistics of Midwifery, from July, 1808 to December, 1858 in the Practice of W. H. Bailey, Esq., F.E.C.S., of Thetford. *Trans Obstet Soc Lond* 299–307.

Brown, G. H. (compiler). 1935. *Lives of the Fellows of the Royal College of Physicians of London, 1826–1925.* London: Royal College of Physicians.

Collier, J. S. 1899. Cerebral Diplegia. *Brain* 22:373–441.

______. 1924. The Pathogenesis of Cerebral Diplegia. Brain 47:1–21.

Dunn, R. 1859. On the Statistics of Midwifery, from the Records of Private Practice. Trans Obstet Soc Lond 1:279–97.

Frost, R. 1969. Two Tramps in Mud Time. In *The Poetry of Robert Frost*, 277. Ed. E. C. Lathem. New York: Rhineholt-Winston.

Jones, A. R. 1949. William John Little. J Bone Joint Surg 31B:122–26.

Little, W. J. 1837. *Symbolae ad talipedem varum cognoscendum.* Thesis. Berlin.

______. 1839. *A Treatise on the Nature of Clubfoot and Analogous Distortions; Including Their Treatment Both with and without Surgical Operation.* London: Jetts.

______. 1843–44. Course of Lectures on the Deformities of the Human Frame. *Lancet* 1:5–7, 38–44, 70–74, 209–12, 230–33, 257–60, 290–93, 318–20, 346–49.

______. 1853. *On the Nature and Treatment of the Deformities of the Human Frame: Being a Course of Lectures Delivered at the Royal Orthopaedic Hospital in 1843, With Numerous Notes and Additions to the Present Time.* London: Longman, Brown, Greene, and Longmans.

______. 1861a. On the Influence of Abnormal Parturition, Difficult Labor, Premature Birth, and Asphyxia Neonatorum, on the Mental and Physical Condition of the Child, Especially in Relation to Deformities. *Trans Obstet Soc Lond* 3:293–344.

______. 1861b. On the Influence of Abnormal Parturition, Difficult Labor, Premature Birth, and Asphyxia Neonatorum, on the Mental and Physical Condition of the Child, Especially in Relation to Deformities. *Lancet* 2:378–80. (This is a summary of the paper read before the Obstetrical Society of London.)

McHenry, L. C. 1969. Garrison's History of Neurology. Springfield, IL: Charles C Thomas.

Obituary. 1894. William John Little, M.D. *Lancet* 2:168–69.

WILLIAM MACEWEN

WILLIAM MACEWEN (1848–1924) (figure 1) left an impressive legacy to modern-day medicine. He was a pioneer in the development of neurology and significantly contributed to the fields of pediatric neurology, anesthesia, and orthopedic and general surgery. Macewen made his mark as a strongly individualistic, inventive, and combative man. His contributions, however, are so varied and of such high quality that he is regarded as one of the greatest surgeons of all time (Jones, 1952).

Macewen was the twelfth and youngest child born to a seafaring father who was a marine trader and ferry captain. He was born on the Scottish island of Bute, not far by boat from Glasgow, on June 22, 1848. He spent his boyhood half on his family's farm and half on fishing boats, which was the major occupation of the island's inhabitants. In fact, he felt the call of the sea all his life, returning to it whenever he could. He owned a small estate on the coast of Bute where he engaged in farming and yachting. As an old man, people said he reminded them of a Viking from a Norwegian saga (Williams, 1946).

Macewen was a rather tall boy who attended the Collegiate School in Glasgow. He seemed quite bright and lively but appeared to excel more on the athletic field than in the classroom (Jones, 1952). There had been no doctors in his family; nonetheless, he went on to Glasgow University in 1865, in order to pursue a career in medicine. When he entered the university, he seemed almost immediately to come under the influence of Joseph Lister. This was at precisely the same era that Lister began to apply carbolic acid to compound fracture wounds in order to kill microbes and promote wound healing. For four years he observed the evolution of the system of antisepsis, serving as Lister's dresser for part of that time.

Macewen graduated as Bachelor of Medicine and Master of Surgery in 1869 and, at the same time, Lister left Glasgow to move to Edinburgh. Macewen quickly qualified and served as house physician and house surgeon. Shortly thereafter, he was appointed superintendent of the Glasgow Fever Hospital at Belvedere. This post became quite notable because he realized, early in his career, the need to separate infectious diseases from other illnesses.

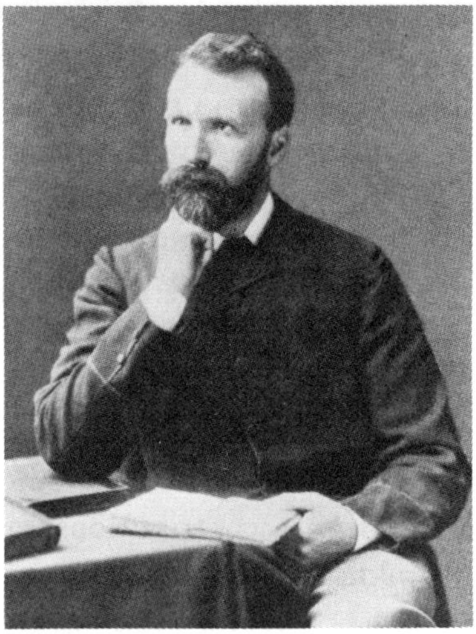

Figure 1. William Macewen (1848–1924).

In 1871 Macewen was chosen casualty surgeon to the Central Police Division of Glasgow. Based on his experience with the police, Macewen published an important paper entitled "A Consideration of the Means We Possess for Distinguishing Between Coma Arising from Alcoholic Intoxication and That Produced by Apoplexy, Fracture of the Base of the Skull and Other Causes" (1879a). Macewen observed that the pupil of the eye in such a state remained contracted as long as the individual was undisturbed. However, when there was a stimulus, such as passive movement of a limb, which did not awaken the patient, the pupil dilated briefly and then contracted as soon as the stimulus ceased. In this way, he was able to differentiate between someone who was drunk and one with a serious head injury. This sign is sometimes known as a "Macewen pupil" (Jones, 1952).

Macewen was appointed full surgeon to the Glasgow Royal Infirmary in 1876, at the age of only twenty-eight. He spent sixteen immensely productive and innovative years in this post. It was here that he introduced endotracheal intubation instead of tracheostomy, a new radical cure for hernia, and the introduction of catgut, which he personally and meticulously prepared until the end of his career (Jennett, 1976). He soaked this ligature in chromic acid, which not only sterilized it but subjected it to a kind of tanning process so it would last longer before being absorbed by the tissue on which it was used (Williams, 1946).

Before discussing Macewen's contributions to the surgery of the brain and spine, mention must be made of some of his other innovations. While at the Royal Infirmary, Macewen became a leader in the move from antiseptic to aseptic surgery, abandoning wooden and bone-handled instruments in favor of metal ones. He had an operating table that he had designed and constructed to his requirements. He dressed in a gown that could be sterilized, which made him an object of ridicule.

Macewen presented an historic paper to the Royal Society in 1891 on the transplantation of bone. This concerned transplantation between animal species, between patients, and from one bone to another in the same patient. Until Macewen proved otherwise, it was generally accepted that bone grew from periosteum. He proved, however, that bone was reproduced only from bone cells or osteoblasts, and that the periosteum was merely a limiting membrane of fibrous tissue (Duguid, 1957).

Macewen's contributions to neurology, and ultimately to child neurology, began in 1876 with his "Case in Which the Symptoms of Focal Cerebral Disease Led to the Diagnosis of a Lesion in Broca's Lobe" (Macewen, 1893a, 189). The case involved a boy with a skull fracture and infected forehead wound. The patient had a convulsion that started on the right side, subsequently became generalized, and was followed by temporary hemiplegia and aphasia. Macewen applied the newly emerging principles set forth by Hermann von Helmholtz (the inventor of the ophthalmoscope, 1849), Paul Broca (1861), John Hughlings Jackson (1869), and David Ferrier (1873), regarding localization and function in the brain. He correctly surmised that the lesion was near Broca's area (Young, 1926). He also made it clear that, if a surgeon were guided by the location of the scar on the boy's forehead and an operation were performed, an abscess would have been found. The boy's family refused to allow an operation and the boy died. The family then permitted him to trephine the skull and he found an abscess in Broca's area, just as he had expected (Jennett, 1976).

Three years later, in 1879, he finally had his chance. A boy fell on his face, bruising it badly. Six days later, he developed twitching of the left side of his face, gradually involving the left arm, and eventually the left leg with preservation of consciousness. Macewen wrote in his paper (Macewen, 1879b) that "it was therefore resolved to expose that portion of the brain," which he did. He removed a subdural hematoma over the right motor strip and the child recovered fully (Jefferson, 1950). Macewen continued to apply the principles of cerebral localization and successfully operated on five more patients with brain disease, including two tumors, between 1879 and 1883. Because several of Macewen's early operations were for abscess, he published his most famous work *Pyogenic Diseases of the Brain and Spinal Cord* (Macewen, 1893a). His *Atlas of Head Sections* was published in 1893, which included illustrations of sections of the entire head (Macewen, 1893b). In both these monumental works, Macewen himself drew all the illustrations.

Pyogenic Diseases of the Brain and Spinal Cord was a substantial work of 350 pages and 60 illustrations. It began with 50 pages on the anatomy of the temporal bone and the venous drainage of the head, based on the dissection of 450 skulls. There are chapters on the pathology and symptoms of brain abscess and meningitis, as well as on thrombosis of intracranial sinuses. The two final chapters address treatment and results, emphasizing that proper early management could often prevent intracranial infection. He concluded his book with a fascinating tabulation of his results.

Of twenty-four patients operated on with intracranial abscess, including four in the cerebellum, only one patient died. It is no wonder then that he concluded "in uncomplicated abscess of the brain, operated on at a fairly early period, recovery ought to be the rule" (Macewen, 1974).

Another of Macewen's outstanding contributions to medicine, with particular application to pediatric neurology, has become known as the "cracked pot" sign or Macewen's sign (Macewen, 1893a, 146). Using his cogent powers of observation, Macewen noted a differential percussion note that was elicited through the vibrations set up in the cranial wall when this was percussed by the finger. This note was modified by the consistency and volume of the cranial contents at any particular time and by their relation to the bones of the skull. In healthy individuals, especially children (in whom the fontanelles have closed), the percussion note was a dull sound with a nearly constant pitch over the entire skull vault. In the presence of disease, especially a process producing hydrocephalus, the resonance of the note was greatly increased (the "cracked pot" sound) and might vary according to the position of the head. This sign remains an often forgotten, but interesting, clinical tool in the evaluation of children with neurologic disease.

In 1889 Macewen was invited to become the first professor of surgery at the newly founded Johns Hopkins Hospital in Baltimore, at any salary which he might choose. He declined this offer. It had been postulated that he refused because he was unable to get the assurance that the training and supervision of the nurses would be under his direct control (Jennett, 1976). In 1892, at the age of forty-four, Macewen was appointed Regius Professor of Surgery at the University Medical School in Glasgow, the post which he held until his death in 1924 (Comrie, 1932). Macewen was knighted in 1902 and remained busy with teaching, practice, and travel until the outbreak of World War I, when he was appointed Surgeon Rear Admiral in charge of naval medical services in Scotland. Macewen left behind some seventy published papers, lectures, and addresses (Bowman, 1942; Bett, 1948) and was a major influence in modern medicine, especially child neurology and neurosurgery.

William Macewen was never known as a team player or collaborator — this was his major shortcoming. His attitude toward his opponents was one of majestic indifference, punctuated by powerful denunciations. Once, when he had described an antagonist as "no better in reasoning power than a cabbage" and was asked to apologize, Macewen answered "Yes, we apologize — to the cabbage." In speaking of himself, he always used the royal "we." Lloyd George summoned Surgeon Rear Admiral Macewen to London in order to peform an urgent operation, and the great man replied by telegram: "We are in Glasgow if you wish to consult" (Williams, 1946).

David M. Kaufman
NEW YORK, NEW YORK

REFERENCES

Bett, W. R. 1948. Sir William Macewen (1984–1924). An Eponymic Centennial Note. *J Bone Joint Surg* 30B:376.

Bowman, A. K. 1942. *The Life and Teaching of Sir William Macewen*. London, Edinburgh, Glasgow: William Hodge and Co., Ltd.

Comrie, J. D. 1932. *History of Scottish Medicine*. Vol. 2. London: Bailliere, Tindall and Cox. Published for the Wellcome Historical Medical Museum.

Duguid, C. 1957. Macewen of Glascow: A Recollection of the Chief. Edinburgh: Oliver and Boyd.

Hamilton, D. 1981. *The Healers: A History of Medicine in Scotland.* Edinburgh: Canongate.

Jefferson, G. 1950. *Sir William Macewen's Contribution to Neuro-Surgery and its Sequels. Glasgow: Jackson, Son and Co.*

Jennett, B. 1976. Sir William Macewen 1848–1924. Pioneer Scottish Neurosurgeon. Surg Neur 6:57–60.

Jones, A. R. 1952. Sir William Macewen. *J Bone Joint Surg* 34B:123–28.

Macewen, H. A. 1974. *The Man in the White Coat.* Glasgow: John Smith and Son, Ltd.

Macewen, W. 1879a. A Consideration of the Means We Possess for Distinguishing between Coma Arising from Alcoholic Intoxication and That Produced by Apoplexy, Fracture of the Base of the Skull, and Other Causes. Glasgow Med J 1879, 2:1.

Macewen, W. 1879b. Demonstration by Operation of Subdural Haemorrhage, Located by a Consideration of the Physical Signs. *Brit Med J* 2:1022.

______. 1893a. *Pyogenic Infective Diseases of the Brain and Spinal Cord; Meningitis, Abscess of Brain, Infective Sinus Thrombosis.* Glasgow: James MacLehose and Sons.

______. 1893b. *Atlas of Head Sections.* Glasgow: James MacLehose and Sons.

Williams, H. 1946. *Doctors Differ: Five Studies in Contrast.* London: Jonathan Cape.

Young, A. 1926. *Sir William Macewen. An Oration.* Glasgow: Jackson, Wylie and Co.

PIERRE MARIE

PIERRE MARIE (figure 1) was born in Paris in 1853 and died in 1940, shortly after the onset of World War II. His parents were wealthy and he had a classical undergraduate education in a private boarding school. After securing his baccalaureate, he proposed his plan for a medical career to his father, who rejected it and insisted he study law. Three years later Marie passed his bar examination in Paris and then had his way and entered medical school. He was successful in the highly competitive public concourse for

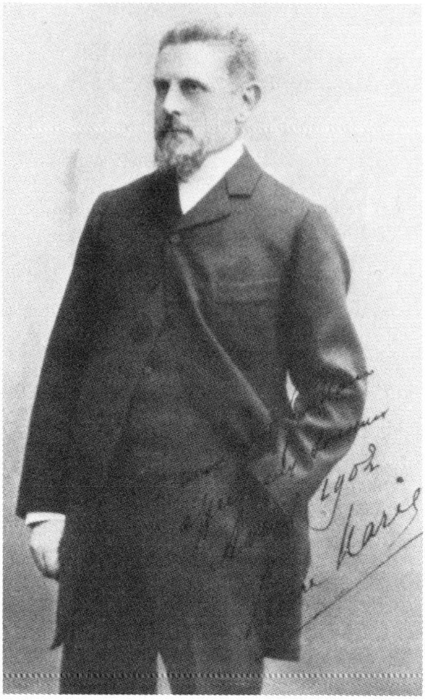

Figure 1. Pierre Marie (1853–1940).

internship in the hospitals of Paris. His most influential mentors during this time were Jean Martin Charcot and Abel Bouchard. Charcot was impressed by Marie's intellect as well as his depth of knowledge in the arts and humanities. Marie possessed the ability to make observations that others had overlooked or ignored. He was often able to arrive at a diagnosis from the appearance of a patient (Behague 1952, 734). Charcot appointed him successively as his *chef de clinique*, *chef de laboratoire* and personal secretary. At the Salpêtrière Marie was the contemporary of an illustrious group of former and current students of Charcot that included Fulgence Raymond, Edouard Brissaud, Joseph Babinski and Georges Gilles de la Tourette. Sigmund Freud spent several months in Paris in 1885 and 1886 where he met Marie. Marie proposed a paper on hysteria but, for unknown reasons, withdrew from the plan (Jones, 1953). Freud ultimately published his own paper on this subject. In 1889 through another demanding concourse, Marie achieved the top rung of academic medicine and became *professeur agrégé.*

His contributions to child neurology began with his publication with Charcot concerning an often familial form of progressive muscular atrophy, later known as Charcot-Marie-Tooth disease, and now classified as hereditary motor sensory neuropathy Type I (Charcot and Marie, 1886). They described five personal observations and reviewed the reports of nineteen other cases. They stressed that this particular form of atrophy had its onset in childhood or adolescence. The atrophy characteristically began in the lower limbs. The extensor of the great toe was most frequently involved. Two to three years later, atrophy of the hands and forearms followed (figure 2). Only two of their five patients had a family history; however, a strong familial occurrence had been stressed by others. In his professorial lectures on diseases of the spinal cord, he focused on the infectious etiology of poliomyelitis and stressed the vasomotor changes associated with limb atrophy (Marie, 1895). Marie believed that infection played a role in infantile cerebral hemiplegia and was one of those who originally proposed a similar cause for multiple sclerosis (Guillain, 1952, 732). He also held that seizures which occurred in childhood were often secondary to infection (Marie, 1887). Freud, in his work *Die Infantile Cerebrallähmung*, made frequent reference to Marie's observations (Freud, 1897). Marie, in turn, was equally impressed by and supportive of Freud's work on this subject, which was published in the *Revue neurologique*, a journal founded by Brissaud and Marie in the same year (Marie, 1893). Marie and Paul Sainton reported their findings on cleidocranial dysostosis stressing the hereditary and musculoskeletal abnormalities (Marie and Sainton, 1898). He also reported his observations in achondroplasia (Marie, 1900). Another work was his fundamental description of acromegaly, regarded by many as one of the earliest clinical investigations in endocrinology (Marie, 1886). In addition, he described hypertrophic pulmonary osteoarthropathy (1890), ankylosing spondylitis (1898), and hereditary cerebellar ataxia (1893). For this latter problem, Marie offered no personal observations but attempted to clarify a mixed

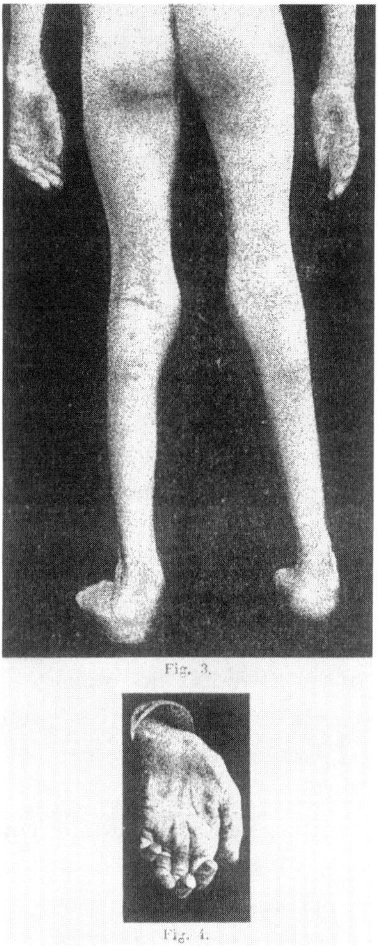

Figure 2. Second observation of Charcot and Marie illustrating atrophy in an 11½-year-old boy. Onset was at age three or four (Charcot and Marie, 1886).

group of clinical disorders previously reported by several authors (Greenfield, 1954). To some degree, he offered a classification of the ataxia disorders. In some cases, the ataxia began in childhood. In other families, it occurred in the third and fourth decades. An initial unsteadiness in walking heralded the onset of the illness. In some families, loss of vision was a prominent finding.

Marie's laboratory work was fundamentally neuropathological in scope. Like Charcot, he had little inclination or interest in experimental physiology. Marie is most known today for the unique position he took in his paper of 1906, stating that the "third left frontal convolution played no special role in the function of language." His position, which was contrary to long standing traditional views, resulted in a series of intense, often passionate, analytical discussions at the French Society of Neurology in 1908 (Cole and Cole, 1971). At this time neuropsychologic testing used by Marie became prominent in the study and measurement of cognition and language skills. Before the aphasia meetings Marie and Joseph Dejerine had heatedly disagreed about the role of the posterior roots in ataxia (Dejerine, 1893). Gustave Roussy described his teacher as proud, authoritative, uncompromising, and focused on converting others to his point of view (Roussy, 1940).

In his early years, Marie enjoyed fencing and golf. He was also an excellent marksman and travelled widely throughout Europe. He and his wife were intensely devoted to one another and to their son and daughter. He was a dedicated collector of art works, as was Charcot. He and his wife lived modestly and never entertained on a grand scale, unlike the Charcots. Dinner parties were usually reserved for close friends and students. Marie was disinclined to stimulants and shunned coffee, but he rolled his own cigarettes and was partial to small quantities of prune liquor (Behague, 1952). To those who were not his intimates, Marie presented a sense of reserve, superiority, and distance. The time he spent riding to work each day in his horsedrawn cab was spent reading and annotating a wide variety of journals which he would distribute to his students for future reference (Guillain, 1940).

Upon the death of Charcot in 1893, the sole chair for professor of diseases of the nervous system at the Faculty of Medicine had to be filled. Fulgence Raymond was senior to Marie and his appointment seemed logical (Satran, 1974). In 1907 Marie accepted the position as professor of pathologic anatomy and dedicated himself solely to teaching. When Raymond died in 1910, Dejerine succeeded to the chair. Macdonald Critchley has questioned the rationale of the Dejerine appointment, which filled a clinical chair with a man whose leading strengths were in neuroanatomy (1964). Marie's efforts in clinical neurology were restricted to injuries of the nervous system secondary to trauma. In World War I, the Salpêtrière was a center for nervous system wounds and, during this time, Marie was assisted by Henry Meige and Charles Foix. Marie was in his mid sixties and past his most productive years when he finally succeeded to the professorship after Dejerine's death in 1917.

Over a period of a few years, a series of tragedies, commencing with the death of his daughter and then of his wife and son, led to his isolation. Abruptly in 1923, without advance notice or ceremony, he relinquished his professorship and withdrew from the medical community. On the Côte d'Azur, he found solitude; nevertheless, he did not completely isolate himself because he still remained supportive to his former students and friends.

All of his life, Marie had been dedicated to the exploration of new concepts and challenging old ones. He disdained awards and honors. Some of his bitterness in later life is revealed in his comment "You see it's better to love nature and the arts, since contact with mankind is very often disillusioning; nature never deceives us" (Lhermitte, 1941).

Marie left a rich legacy in medicine and neurology. He trained many students from home and abroad. The most notable of these include Georges Guillain, Jean Lhermitte, André Leri, and Charles Foix. Kinnier Wilson, Georges Marinesco, Frederick Bremer, and Percival Bailey were a few of his students who also made their contributions to the growth and development of neurology and child neurology (Guillain, 1952, 733).

Richard Satran
ROCHESTER, NEW YORK

REFERENCES

Behague, P. 1952. Pierre Marie intime. *Rev neur* 82:733–39.

Charcot, J. M., and P. Marie. 1886. Sur une forme particulière d'atrophie musculaire progressive souvent familiale. *Rev méd* 6:97–138.

Cole, M. F., and M. Cole. 1971. *Pierre Marie's Papers on Speech Disorders*. New York: Hafner Publishing Co.

Critchley, M. 1964. Pierre Marie 1853–1940. In *The Black Hole and Other Essays*, 146–54. London: Pitman Med. Pub. Co. Ltd.

Dejerine, J. 1893. Du rôle joué par les lésions des racines postérieures dans le sclérose médullaire des ataxiques. *Prog méd* 18:1–2.

Freud, S. 1897. *Die Infantile Cerebrallähmung*. Wien: Holder.

______. 1968. *Infantile Cerebral Paralysis*. Translated by L. A. Russin. Coral Gables: University of Miami Press.

Greenfield, J. G. 1954. *The Spinocerebellar Degenerations*, 34–66. Springfield, IL: Charles C Thomas.

Guillain, G. 1940. Pierre Marie (1853–1940). *Bull Acad Med* 123:524–34.

______. 1952. Pierre Marie. Sa vie et son oeuvre scientifique. *Rev neur* 82:726–33.

Jones, E. 1953. *The Life and Work of Sigmund Freud*. Vol. 1, 210. New York: Basic Books, Inc.

Lhermitte, J. 1941. Pierre Marie 1853–1940. *Paris méd* 119: Annexe 11–12.

Marie, P. 1886. Sur deux cas d'acromégalie. (Hypertrophie singulière non congenitale des extrémitées supérieures, inférieures et céphalique). *Rev méd* 6:297–333.

______. 1887. Note sur l'étiologie de l'épilepsie. *Prog méd* 15:333–34.

______. 1890. De l'ostéo-arthropathie hypertrophante pneumique. *Rev méd* 10:1–36.

______. 1893. Sur l'hérédo-ataxie cérébelleuse. *Sem méd* 13:444–47.

______. 1895. *Lectures on Diseases of the Spinal Cord*. Translated by M. Lubback. London: New Sydenham Society.

______. 1898. Sur la spondylose rhizomélique. *Rev méd* 18:285–315.

______. 1900. L'achondroplaisie dans l'adolescence et l'âge adulte. *Presse méd* 2:17–23.

______. 1906. Révision de la question de l'aphasie: la troisième circonvolution frontale gauche ne joue aucun rôle special dans la fonction du language. *Sem méd* 26:241–47.

Marie, P., and P. Sainton. 1898. Sur la dystose cléidocranienne héréditaire. *Rev neur* 6:835–38.

Roussy, G. 1940. Pierre Marie. *Presse méd* 48(1):481–83.

Satran, R. 1974. Fulgence Raymond: The Successor of Charcot. *Bull NY Acad Med* 50:931–42.

HERMANN OPPENHEIM

HERMANN OPPENHEIM (1859–1919) (figure 1) entered the field of academic neurology when it was at its zenith in Germany. He was born in Warburg, Westfalen, and studied at nearby Göttingen, then Bonn and Berlin, completing his doctoral dissertation on urea metabolism in 1881 (Stern, 1959). Little is readily available regarding his early years, but he was considered something of a rising star in the academic community of the 1880's. Within fourteen years of his first clinical appointment at the Charité Hospital, he had written a two-volume textbook of neurology, the *Lehrbuch der Nervenkrankheiten* (1894), that was to reappear in seven editions, the last in 1923 (Stern, 1959). He was a popular teacher and lecturer in areas of both clinical neurology and psychiatry, two aspects of what was then considered one subspecialty. In Germany at that time psychiatry was quite strong and most physicians were "neuropsychiatrists" even if they were just interested in neurology. However, there was no specific term used. The strong influence of psychiatry has been felt by many to have impeded the growth of neurology in the early twentieth century. Despite his popularity and a vast bibliography (reportedly 220 original works; Stern, 1959), Oppenheim did not achieve the position of director of the Royal Polyclinical Institute in Berlin for which he was nominated in 1890 (Weil, 1953). Oppenheim was to follow in the footsteps of Moritz Heinrich Romberg (1786–1873), considered one of the founders of neurology, Wilhelm Griesinger (1817–1890), the famed psychiatrist, and Carl Westphal (1833–1890), well known to neurologists for his description of the Edinger-Westphal nucleus. Oppenheim was Westphal's favorite student. After Westphal's early death, Oppenheim was provisionally given this position and received full faculty support. He was apparently rejected for political reasons. This event may have been an omen; his writings after 1900 were vastly influenced by the politics of eastern Europe. Many of his papers consider the diagnosis and management of neurosis (Oppenheim, 1917a, b, c) and peripheral nerve injuries suffered in the line of duty during World War I.

When he was not granted a faculty chair in 1890, Oppenheim

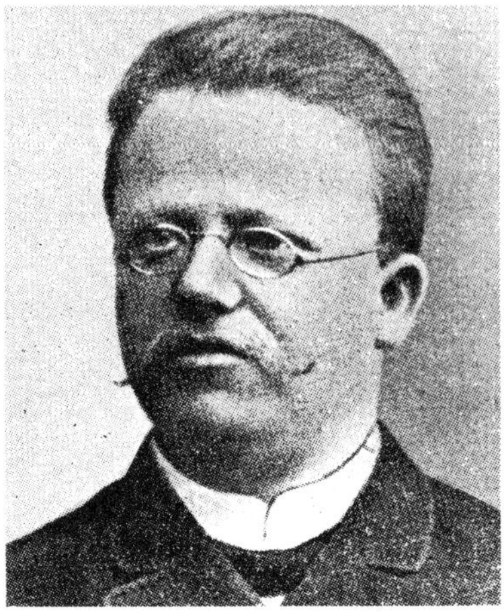

Figure 1. Hermann Oppenheim (1859–1919).

left academics and founded a private clinic for neurologic ("nervous") diseases. His reputation became widely known and he continued teaching and writing (Nonne, 1959; 1960). A sampling from Oppenheim's curriculum vitae shows that his interests included all types of neurologic disorders, from metastatic brain tumors (Oppenheim and Koehler, 1890; Oppenheim, 1919) to traumatic injuries of peripheral nerves (Oppenheim, 1917c). He may have been the first to describe post-traumatic neurosis, which he found rather common among veterans of World War I, but which was not well known until the post-Vietnam era (Oppenheim, 1889; 1917a).

Oppenheim is also credited with introducing the term *dystonia musculorum deformans* and recognized that this was an organic nervous-system disease, rather than a form of hysteria (Oppenheim, 1911). He observed that the cardinal symptom of the disease was motor involvement that consisted of alterations of tone between hypotonia and a tendency to tonic muscle contractions, which were induced or worsened by walking or standing. The occurrence of pronounced lordosis in many patients led him to suggest the term *dysbasia lordotica progressive* as an alternative to *dystonia muscularum deformans*.

Oppenheim's *Lehrbuch der Nervenkrankheiten* was considered one of the most clinically useful neurological texts of its time. Along with William Gowers's *A Manual of Diseases of the Nervous System* (1886–88), it provided an excellent section on the details of the bedside neurological examination. Oppenheim not only described the clinical examination of the patient with spasticity but was the first to recognize the close association between spasticity and hyperreflexia. He also observed that spastic muscles could be fully extended when slowly stretched, in contrast to rapid stretching, which would induce an abrupt increase in muscle tone. These observations formed the basis of portions of the neurological examination that are used today by all neurologists. Oppenheim was also aware of the work of Joseph Babinski (1857–1932) and his well-known extensor plantar reflex. He was among the first to recognize that patients with a positive Babinski sign usually had spasticity (McHenry, 1969, 352). The "Oppenheim reflex," also a component of the standard neurological examination as a manifestation of frontal lobe disease, was described in his *Lehrbuch*.

It is at once curious and ironic that perhaps the shortest and least impressive of Oppenheim's works led to a controversy among pediatric neurologists that lasted almost three quarters of a century. In 1900 he published a two-page article entitled "Über allgemeine und localisierte Atonie der muskulatur (Myatonie) im frühen Kindesalter" ("About Generalized and Localized Atonia of the Muscles (Myatonie) in Early Childhood") (Oppenheim, 1900). This is a direct translation of the title that led to the widespread use of the term *Oppenheim's amyotonia*. The confusion of the words *atonia* and *myatonie* or *myotonia* is immediately evident. Moreover, at this point in history, neurologists, including Oppenheim, were only beginning to use the galvanometer, a primitive form of the electromyograph machine, for diagnostic purposes. *Myotonia congenita* was a recognized entity, but it was still frequently confused with *myotonia dystrophica*; both diseases were associated with electrical *myotonia*, but there was also poor muscle tone or *atonia* in the latter. Thus, unwittingly, Oppenheim seems to have confused two words: *atonia* or *hypotonia* and *myatonie* or *myotonia*. The distinction may have been clear in his mind, but it became muddy in the minds of his English translators resulting in the still frequent use of the incorrect term *amyotonia* (Brandt, 1950; Walton, 1956).

In his short report, Oppenheim described children, from age one to two months up to two years, with severe atonia or paralysis. He did not state how many such patients he saw, but he was specific in stating that the lack of voluntary movement was different from "Little's disease," or congenital hemiparesis, presumably because the latter was asymmetric. He described "loose and soft" muscles in the infants — whom we now call "floppy infants" (Dubowitz, 1964). He was impressed by the patients' alertness and "perceptive functioning" and stated that the condition seemed to be congenital. He even speculated that the problem could be attributed to "disturbed development . . . in the anterior horn cells."

Probably the greatest confusion arose from his claim that he had observed improvement in some children, even "disappearance of symptoms." This claim was not supported with evidence. He finished his claim with this explanation: "At the present I am intensely occupied with other work . . . and plan to publish later a more extensive publication." He never did. Rather, in 1904 and again in 1912, he gave two brief abstracts that were read before German neurological and medical societies (Brandt, 1950, 5).

Johann Hoffmann and Guido Werdnig had independently described infantile spinal muscular atrophy, including the microscopic analysis of spinal cords from several patients, nearly ten years prior to Oppenheim's report (Hoffmann, 1891, 1892; Werdnig, 1891). All three men were still lecturing in Germany in 1900. Oppenheim's amyotonia became a clinical entity although the neuropathology of it was not clear, as he had not presented any neuropathology in his three case reports. In Oppenheim's first two reports, he asserted that he was unaware of any other writer describing this type of weakness, but this probably was the same weakness that had been described by Werdnig and Hoffmann, as well as by John Thompson and Alexander Bruce (Buchanan, 1958). Oppenheim must have been aware of these reports and it is somewhat remarkable that they were not mentioned, even to assert the fact that they referred to a different disease. The confusion in the neurological literature over the next twenty years is reflected by there being more publications on Oppenheim's amyotonia than on the more important Werdnig-Hoffmann disease. The report of William Spiller supposedly lent confirmatory support to Oppenheim's concept, as the patient who died at age two years had normal anterior horn cells in the spinal cord but atrophic muscle (Spiller, 1905). However, the child also had optic atrophy, impaired vision and other delayed developmental parameters (Buchanan, 1958). The majority of writers at that time agreed that there were two distinct disorders and, to minimize the eponymic confusion, James Collier and S. Kinnier Wilson suggested the term *amyotonia congenita* for Oppenheim's disease (Collier and Wilson, 1908).

The controversy was actually settled by J. Godwin Greenfield and Ruby Stern in 1927 with a treatise in which they compared the pathology of patients described by Hoffmann, Werdnig, and

Oppenheim. They showed that the neuropathologic lesions were identical in all the children described with this clinical syndrome of severe hypotonia and weakness (Greenfield and Stern, 1927). Their conclusion was that Oppenheim's "amyotonia" was, in fact, infantile spinal muscular atrophy, the familial disorder of anterior horn cells described by Werdnig and Hoffmann. It took another twenty-five years for the dissenters to win. The studies of Sven Brandt, John Walton, and Randolph Byers and Betty Banker, further laid to rest any confusion about these disorders (Brandt, 1950; Walton, 1956; Byers and Banker, 1961). John Walton's 1956 review of 109 patients diagnosed as *amyotonia congenita* observed that fifty-five of the fifty-six patients who died had anterior horn cell disease. Walton, in this paper, proposed the term *benign hypotonia* and the following year, the term *benign congenital hypotonia* referring to those children who seemed to resemble those few patients of Oppenheim's who had recovered. Whether there are cases of spinal muscular atrophy in which progression plateaus or reverses remains under study today (Russman, Melchreit, Drennan, 1983), and pediatric neurologists still argue over the existence of *benign congenital hypotonia*. Upon his untimely death from a heart attack at the age of sixty, Oppenheim was eulogized as a great clinical neurologist (Saenger, 1919). He will perhaps be remembered best as one of the great German neurologists at the turn of the twentieth century, carrying on the tradition of Moritz Romberg at a time when neurology was a less influential discipline than psychiatry. He should be best remembered by child neurologists for his bringing to our attention the disabling condition of *dystonia musculorum deformans* and for his *Lehrbuch,* which strongly influenced the next generation of neurologists, such as Ludwig Bruns, who began to write in depth about childhood neurological disorders.

Susan T. Iannaccone
CINCINNATI, OHIO

ACKNOWLEDGMENTS

I wish to thank Dr. Franz Nave for his generous translations, and Stephanie Gates for her tireless efforts at the photocopier.

Brandt, S. 1950. *Werdnig-Hoffmann's Infantile Progressive Muscular Atrophy.* Copenhagen: Ejnar Municksgard.

Buchanan, D. 1958. Spinal Nuclear Amyotrophy and Other Causes of Flaccidity in Infancy. In *Clinical Neurosurgery (Proc. Neurosurgery Meetings).* Vol. 3, 177–89. Ed. R. G. Fisher. Baltimore: Williams and Wilkins Company.

Byers, R. K., and B. Q. Banker. 1961. Infantile Muscular Atrophy. *Arch Neur* 5:140–64.

Collier, J., and S. A. K. Wilson. 1908. Amyotonia congenita. *Brain* 31:1.

Dubowitz, V. 1964. Infantile Muscular Atrophy. A Prospective Study with Particular Reference to a Slowly Progressive Variety. *Brain* 87:707–18.

Gowers, W. R. 1886–88. *A Manual of Diseases of the Nervous System.* London: J. & A. Churchill.

Greenfield, J. G., and R. O. Stern. 1927. The Anatomical Identity of the Werdnig-Hoffmann and Oppenheim Forms of Infantile Muscular Atrophy. *Brain* 50:652–86.

Hoffmann, J. 1891. Über chronische spinale Muskelatrophie im Kindesalter, auf familiärer Basis. *Dtsch Zeit Nervenheilk* 1:95.

______. 1892. Über familiäre progressive Spinale Muskelatrophie. *Arch Psych* (Berlin) 24:644–46.

McHenry, L. C. 1969. *Garrison's History of Neurology.* Springfield, IL: Charles C Thomas.

Nonne, M. 1959. In Memorium Hermann Oppenheim und Ludwig Bruns anläblich der Wiederkehr ihres 100. Geburtstages. *Zentral ges Neur Psych* 148:17.

______. 1960. Die letzte Vorlesung von Max Nonne. *Münch med Wschr* 102:989–94.

Oppenheim, H. 1889. *Die Traumatischen Neurosen.* Berlin: Verlag von August Hirschwald.

______. 1894. *Lehrbuch der Nervenkrankheiten.* Berlin: S. Karger.

______. 1900. Über allgemeine und localisierte Atonie der muskulatur (Myatonie) im frühen Kindesalter. *Mschr Psych Neur* 8:232–33.

______. 1911. Über eine eigenartige Krampfkrankheit des kindlichen und jugendlichen Alters (Dysbasia lordotica progressiva, Dystonia musculorum deformans). *Neur Centralbl* 30:1090.

______. 1917a. Stand der Lehre von den Kriegs und Unfallneurosen. *Berl klin Wschr* 54:1169–72.

______. 1917b. Zur Kenntnis der Veronalvergiftung und der Funktionellen formen der Sehstörung. *Dtsch Zeit Nervenheilk* 57:1–35.

______. 1917c. *Beiträge zur Kenntnis der Kriegsverletzungen des peripherischen Nervensystems.* Berlin: Verlag von s. Karger.

______. 1919. Fortlaufende Beiträge zur Lehre von den Hirngeschwülsten. *Dtsch Zeit Nervenheilk* 64:75–101.

Oppenheim, H., and R. Koehler. 1890. Casuistischer Beitrag zum Capitel der Hirnchirurgie. *Berl klin Wschr* 27:677–81.

Russman, B. S., R. Melchreit, and J. C. Drennan. 1983. Spinal Muscular Atrophy: The Natural Course of Disease. *Muscle & Nerve* 6:179–81.

Saenger. 1919. Zum Andenken an Hermann Oppenheim. *Dtsch med Wschr* 45:830.

Spiller, W. G. 1905. Generalized or Localized Hypotonia of the Muscles in Childhood (Myotonia congenita). Report of a Case with Necropsy. *Univ Penn Med Bull* 17:342.

Stern, A. 1959. Gedenktage, Hermann Oppenheim. *Dtsch med Wschr* 49:2207.

Walton, J. N. 1956. Amyotonia congenita. *Lancet* 1:1023.

______. 1957. The Limp Child. *J Neur Neurosurg Psych* 20:144–54.

Weil, A. 1953. Oppenheim, Hermann (1858–1919). In *Founders of Neurology*, 128–29. Ed. Webb-Haymaker. Springfield, IL: Charles C Thomas.

Werdnig, G. 1891. Zwei frühinfantile hereditäre Fälle von progressiver Muskelatrophie unter dem Bilde der Dystrophie aber auf neurotischer Grundlage. *Arch Psych Nervenkrankh* 22:437–80.

WILLIAM OSLER

THE NAME OF William Osler evokes an image of a dynamic, thoughtful, multifaceted, and disciplined individual who made extraordinary contributions to the development of medicine, in the United States and throughout the world. To these can be added Osler's contributions to the field of child neurology. For at the time he was active, the fields of pediatrics and neurology were just beginning to develop in the United States. Osler's bibliography includes over fourteen hundred papers, monographs, and notes exploring almost every subspecialty and, of these, it has been estimated that approximately two hundred works deal with neurology and over one hundred with pediatrics (Robbins and Cristie, 1963; Ebers, 1985). Osler's clinical research and writings in these areas concentrated on the field of child neurology, including such topics as cerebral palsy, chorea, tics, muscular dystrophy, and childhood migraine.

Born at Bond Head near Toronto, Canada, William Osler (1849–1919) (figure 1) was the eighth child in a family of nine children. He was described as a bright, athletic youngster, given to mischief and practical jokes (Cushing, 1925). He received his early education first at nearby grammar schools and later in boarding schools at Barrie and Weston. At the Trinity College School in Weston, he came under the influence of the school's founder, the Rev. William Johnson, an amateur naturalist who owned a microscope. Through Johnson, Osler developed an avid interest in the study of nature, which continued even after his decision to study medicine.

Osler entered Trinity College in Toronto in 1867 intent on following his father's footsteps into the ministry, but at the beginning of his second year decided to enter medical school. In 1870 he transferred from Toronto to McGill University in Montreal to take advantage of the excellent clinical facilities. Following his graduation from McGill in 1872, Osler spent two years studying in Great Britain and Europe, where he met William Macewen, Charles Darwin, Burdon Sanderson, Rudolf Virchow, and other eminent scientists.

Shortly after Osler's return to Canada in 1874, he was appointed lecturer in the Institutes of Medicine at McGill. During a decade on the McGill faculty, he began the extensive postmortem and histological studies that support his later writings. In 1884, due largely to the efforts of Silas Weir Mitchell and H. C. Wood, Osler was appointed Professor of Clinical Medicine at the University of Pennsylvania. Osler's reputation continued to grow and, in 1889, he began his new position as Chief of Medicine at the newly established Johns Hopkins Hospital in Baltimore. Here he wrote his classic *Principles and Practice of Medicine* (Osler, 1892) and described hereditary hemorrhagic telangiectasia (Osler, 1901a). From the time he left Johns Hopkins in 1905 until his death on December 29, 1919, Osler was Regius Professor of Medicine at Oxford University. This last move was dictated in part by his health and the ever-increasing burden of teaching, writing, and clinical duties.

Osler's many contributions to internal medicine and his fame as a teacher and clinician have largely obscured his contributions to neurology. Yet his bibliography reflects an interest in the nervous system that spanned both clinical and theoretical topics and was sustained throughout his career. Osler disproved the notion that the brains of criminals are anatomically distinct, and another early paper touched on the mind-brain question that was then being debated. His early interest in brain anatomy is evidenced by his study of the comparative neuroanatomy of the seal.

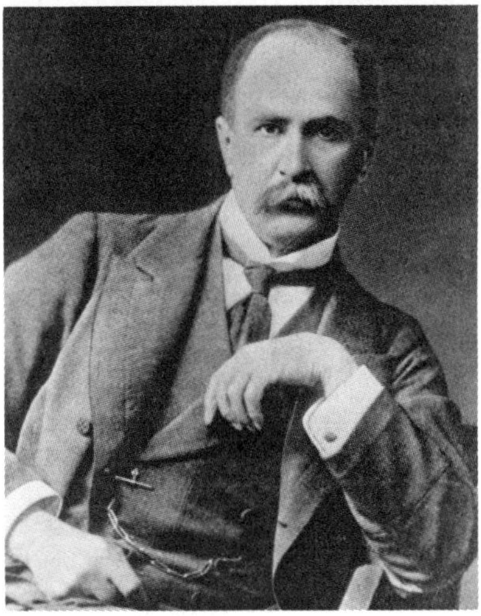

Figure 1. William Osler (1849–1919).

Osler published numerous papers on clinical neurology and neuropathology, including several on stroke, intracranial aneurysm, brain tumors, and spinal cord disorders (Abbott, 1939). Osler described the three forms of "muscular atrophy" known at the time: pseudohypertrophic muscular dystrophy, Erb's disease, and Duchenne's disease. He concluded:

We may regard these afflictions as different forms of one and the same disease, a primitive progressive myopathy, the lesion being an interstitial myositis with a variable production of adipose tissue and occasional hypertrophy of individual muscle fibers. Clinically they present certain differences by which the varieties may be recognized, but there are intermediate forms which serve to show the essentials of the disease. (Osler, 1885a, 681)

He also contributed to the growing literature on Friedreich's ataxia (Osler, 1888a) and facioscapulohumeral muscular dystrophy (Osler, 1889a), and he studied the significance of cranial bruits in children, concluding that the finding is usually of no significance (Osler, 1880). While a good many of these articles are routine case reports of little lasting significance, others, such as his paper on Jacksonian epilepsy and cerebral localization (based on a pathologic study of a girl with a glioma), were more important (Osler, 1885b). Osler also contributed numerous editorials and book reviews related to neurologic topics, as well as chapters on neurologic subjects in textbooks written by William Pepper and Francis X. Dercum.

In 1885 Osler was elected to membership in the Philadelphia Neurological Society, which had been founded the previous year. Silas Weir Mitchell was the first president of the society and remained president during Osler's stay in Philadelphia (Spiller, 1935). Osler regularly attended the Society's meetings and showed a keen interest in neurology (Mills, 1927). Soon after Osler's arrival in Philadelphia, he was appointed to the staff of the Philadelphia Orthopedic Hospital and Infirmary for Nervous Diseases. Here Osler initiated much of his work on the neurologic disorders of children, although some of his experience was not published until after leaving Philadelphia (McHenry, 1984). At the Infirmary, Osler worked closely with Mitchell; his son, John K. Mitchell; Morton Sinkler; and Morris J. Lewis (Rogers, 1959, 1970). Osler continued to perform numerous autopsies and gave special attention to the study of lesions of the brain, spinal cord, and the thoracic viscera (Mills, 1927; Middleton, 1976). In 1888 Osler was elected to the American Neurological Association.

Osler called attention to the association between acquired chorea and endocarditis, remarking that "there is no known disease in which endocarditis is so constantly found, as in chorea," and documented a cerebral embolus in a child with rheumatic heart disease (Osler, 1887a). Two additional articles detailed his accumulating experience with 410 cases of chorea at the Infirmary (Osler, 1887b), but the monograph summarizing this work on chorea was not completed until after his move to Baltimore. This book was dedicated to William Gowers (Osler, 1894).

Although Richard Bright had noted the association between heart disease and chorea, it was Osler, among others like Octavius Sturges, who solidly established it (Ebers, 1985). His work on chorea is still considered an excellent clinical epidemiologic study and his introductory historical comments are still worth reading. Osler criticized Sir Thomas Sydenham for using the term "chorea" which, he states, had been coined by Paracelsus to describe the "dancing mania" for the disorder Sydenham had observed. His implication was that Sydenham inadvertently added a certain degree of confusion to the understanding of this disorder by implying that it was related to the epidemics of mass hysteria that occurred in the middle ages. Osler's own clinical description of children with chorea minor is actually quite similar to Sydenham's original:

Although the disease may begin quite abruptly, as a rule the cases present premonitory symptoms, motor and psychical. The child is restless and unable to sit still, a condition well expressed by the term "fidgets" often used by mothers in describing the onset. The entire disposition may be changed, and the child becomes irritable, cross, and unmanageable. Emotional disturbances are common, the child crying on the least provocation. Night terrors have been noted in many instances. Punishment inflicted at this stage by thoughtless parents or teachers aggravates the mischief, or even precipitates the attack. The appetite may fail and anemia not infrequently develops. Headache is not an uncommon complaint. Less frequently there may be at this stage pains in the limbs, usually in the legs, or about the joints. After a week or more of these symptoms the restlessness increases, and the sudden involuntary movements characteristic of the disease begin. These are often first noticed at table, when the child spills a tumbler of water by a sudden jerk, or upsets a plate, or drops something. Beginning as a rule in the hands and arms, the brusque, involuntary movements give a very characteristic stamp to the muscular disorder. (Osler, 1894)

Osler also reported in detail two families with Huntington's chorea, including one autopsy in which he mentioned ventricular dilatation but not atrophy of the caudate nucleus (Osler, 1893).

A series of articles in *Medical News* (Osler, 1888b) on childhood cerebral palsy summarized Osler's experience with 120 children from the Infirmary. These articles formed the basis for his classic monograph on cerebral palsy, which was dedicated to Silas Weir Mitchell (Osler, 1889b). Osler's publications on cerebral palsy appeared about the same time as the work of Gowers and, like Gowers, Osler emphasized the diverse causes of childhood hemiplegia. Osler classified his patients with nonprogressive upper motor neuron dysfunction according to the distribution of their weakness (hemiplegia, diplegia, and paraplegia) and separated the children with congenital dysfunction from those whose weakness was acquired later in childhood (figure 2). The monograph contains numerous case descriptions and emphasizes signs, symptoms, and etiology. Osler also included some sketches of neuropathological material correlating the clinical and pathological findings (figure 3). Several of the children with acute weakness probably suffered cerebrovascular occlusions, although Osler rejected this diagnosis: "We should naturally think that embolic processes had much to do

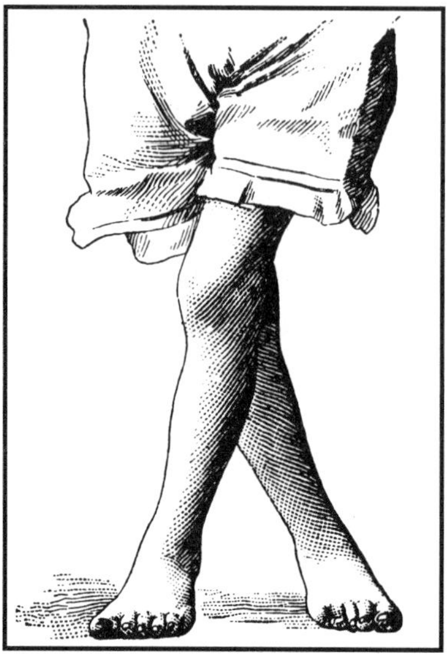

Figure 2. Drawing of a child (originally figure 4, p. 80) from *The Cerebral Palsies of Children* showing classical spastic diplegia.

with the production of hemiplegia in children, but neither in the literature nor in our records is there support for this view."

Several extracts from Osler's *The Cerebral Palsies of Children* will perhaps better exemplify Osler's acumen and his ability to elucidate and present clinically relevant material. On discussing the prognosis of children with hemiplegia, he has the following to say:

Prognosis. — Parents are naturally intensely anxious as to the prospects of a child attacked with hemiplegia. As a rule, the younger the subject the greater the liability to serious and permanent damage. The nature of the lesion doubtless has an important influence, vascular obstruction being more favorable than meningo-encephalitis, and the latter than tumour, but the diagnosis of the exact condition is by no means always easy. Of the bodily defect, about which the greatest uneasiness is displayed, we can almost invariably predict great improvement, particularly of the leg. Perfect recovery of the arm is rare, of the face more frequent. The development of post-hemiplegic movements is a bad omen, as such cases are more likely to have epilepsy, which constitutes one of the most serious sequences of the disease. Not only are the attacks dangerous in themselves, but they undoubtedly tend to aggravate existing mental defects. They may not develop for some years after the onset of the paralysis and may be deferred till the period of puberty. More distressing still to the relatives is the enfeebled mental state which so often follows infantile hemiplegia. (Osler, 1889b, 54)

On the subject of spastic quadriplegia or what was then termed "bilateral spastic hemiplegia," he noted the following in his introduction to this chapter:

In infantile hemiplegia a great majority of the cases occur within the first three years of life, and in only a limited number is the condition congenital,

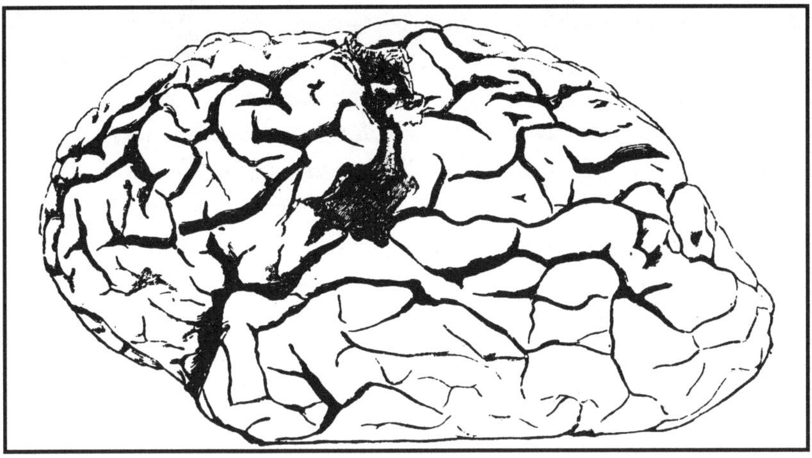

Figure 3. Drawing of the left hemisphere of a child with cerebral palsy showing sclerosis (originally figure 1, p. 45) from the same book on cerebral palsy.

either the result of intra-uterine disease or of accident during parturition. In bilateral hemiplegia and in paraplegia the reverse holds good; in a large proportion of the cases the trouble dates from birth, and is the result of injury to the child during its passage into the world. Hence the appropriateness of the term birth palsies, applied to these cases by Gowers. Strictly speaking, these cases should be considered together, as they depend on essentially similar conditions, and we may find the arms so slightly affected that it is difficult to say whether the case is one of diplegia or paraplegia; but there is a sufficient number of clearly defined cases in each group to make a division advisable, and there are questions relating to the spastic paraplegia of children which deserve separate consideration. (Osler, 1889b, 56)

Osler also had some interesting, and perhaps prophetic, comments about the surgical treatment of epilepsy in regard to patient selection:

An important question of practical moment has arisen in connection with the propriety of surgical interference in these cases. Jacksonian epilepsy has now its surgical aspects, and there have already been several successful cases of removal of tumors from the motor areas of the cortex. Infantile hemiplegia offers some of the most typical instances of cortical epilepsy, and it may be well to consider how far it is likely that surgical interference can here be successful. As we have seen, in the review of the morbid anatomy, the conditions to be dealt with are (1) apoplectic, embolic or thrombotic foci, which are as frequently in the territory of the central as of the cortical arteries; (2) sclerosis; and (3) porencephalus. I do not think that, in any of the cases which I have reviewed, the anatomical condition offered the slightest possibility of relief from surgical interference. I except the case of glioma of the paracentral lobule to which I referred. This girl had had Jacksonian epilepsy for many years and the tumor could have been readily removed. . . . When sclerosis exists the area is usually too large for removal; when porencephalus is present, we are not, as Dr. Morton Prince said in the discussion on Dr. Bullard's case, "likely to improve a pure paralysis due to a hole in the brain, by making the hole bigger." (Osler, 1889b, 101–2)

Osler wrote on numerous other topics of pediatric neurological interest. This included several papers on sporadic cretinism (Osler, 1897b, 1901b); neuritis in typhoid fever, which may actually have been an early description of Guillain-Barré syndrome; bacterial and tuberculous meningitis (1881–82, 1899, 1901c), and myotonia congenita (1886).

In late 1890 Osler published a detailed description of a thirteen-year-old girl with Tourette's syndrome, along with a review of the clinical manifestations of the disorder (Osler, 1890). Two other patients with Tourette's syndrome were described in Osler's book on chorea. These were among the first descriptions of the disease in English, and remain remarkably vivid and complete even a century later. Osler considered the condition uncommon and rejected the idea that it was merely a psychological condition. Several years later, he proposed a classification of the tic disorders and tried to eliminate the confusion surrounding terminology then in use (Osler, 1897a).

The first edition of Osler's *Principles and Practice of Medicine* made its debut in 1892 and contained about three hundred pages devoted to disorders of the nervous system (Osler, 1892). This emphasis reflects to a remarkable degree Osler's own interests, experience, and prior publications. There is a large section, for example, on chorea and tic disorders, as well as a separate section on hemiplegia and diplegia in children. He described 460 children with epilepsy, the majority of whom were seen during his sojourn in Philadelphia. The importance of migraine in children is emphasized: "Many attacks of severe headaches in children are of this type." Hydrocephalus, tumor, and various infections common in children are described in detail. The importance of Osler's textbook to the development of child neurology lies not so much in its originality of thought but rather in its dissemination of information. The book flourished through many editions and was no doubt the primary source of information on the neurologic disorders of children for many physicians.

Even after Osler's death in 1919, his association with the nervous system continued (Ebers, 1985). Because of his interest in the mind-brain problem, Osler left his brain to the Wistar Institute in Philadelphia for study. His brain, along with those of the scholars Granville Hall and Edward Morse, were studied by Henry Donaldson and Myrtle Canavan in great detail and compared with Canavan's previous studies of the brain of Ernest Southard, Bullard Professor of Neuropathology at Harvard (Donaldson and Canavan, 1928; Ebers, 1985).

William Osler played a considerable role in the development of child neurology through his original work on chorea, tic disorders, and cerebral palsy. His interest in neurologic disorders spans his entire career but was especially keen during his years in Philadelphia, where he was stimulated by some of the great neurologists of his day. Osler, in turn, stimulated others in the field through his many articles and editorials on neurologic topics.

E. Steven Roach
DALLAS, TEXAS

Stephen Ashwal
LOMA LINDA, CALIFORNIA

REFERENCES

Abbott, M. E. 1939. *Classified and Annotated Bibliography of Sir William Osler's Publications*. 2d ed. Montreal: The Medical Museum, McGill University.

Cushing, H. 1925. *The Life of Sir William Osler*. Oxford: Clarendon Press.

Donaldson, H. H., and M. M. Canavan. 1928. A Study of the Brains of Three Scholars: Granville Stanley Hall, Sir William Osler, Edward Sylvester Morse. *J Comp Neur* 46:1–95.

Ebers, G. C. 1985. Osler and Neurology. *Can J Neur Sci* 12:236–42.

Golden, R., and C. Roland. 1987. *Sir William Osler: An Annotated Bibliography with Illustrations*. San Francisco: Norman Publishing.

McHenry, L. C. *William Osler, a Philadelphia Neurologist*. Unpublished (and unfinished) manuscript in author's possession, dated March 26, 1984.

Middleton, W. S. 1976. William Osler and the Blockley Dead House. *Okla State Med Assoc J* 69:387–89.

Mills, C. K. 1927. Dr. William Osler in Philadelphia. In *Sir William Osler Memorial Volume*. Philadelphia: International Association of Medical Museums.

Osler, W. 1880. On the Systolic Brain Murmur of Children. *Bost Med Surg J* 103:29–30.

______. 1881–82. Cases of Tubercular Meningitis. *Can Med Surg J* 10:603.

______. 1885a. The Primary Muscular Atrophies. *Med News* (NY) 47:681.

______. 1885b. A Contribution to Jacksonian Epilepsy and the Situation of the Leg Centre. *Am J Med Sci* 89:31–37.

______. 1886. Thomsen's Disease. *Med News* (NY) 49:292.

______. 1887a. The Cardiac Relations of Chorea. *Am J Med Sci* 94:371–86.

______. 1887b. On the General Etiology and Symptoms of Chorea — Based on the Records of 410 Cases at the Infirmary for Nervous Diseases, Philadelphia. Part 1. *Med News* 51:437–41, 465–70.

______. 1888a. Note on a Case of Friedreich's Ataxia, with Exhibition of Patient. *Trans Coll Phys Phila* 10:277–81.

______. 1888b. The Cerebral Palsies of Children (Clinical Lectures Delivered at the Infirmary for Nervous Diseases). *Med News Phila* 1:29–35; 2:57–66; 3:85–90; 4:113–16; 5:141–45.

______. 1889a. On a Case of Simple Idiopathic Muscular Atrophy, Involving the Face and the Scapulo-Humeral Muscles. *Am J Med Sci* 98:261–65.

______. 1889b. *The Cerebral Palsies of Children: A Clinical Study from the Infirmary for Nervous Diseases*. Philadelphia: Blakiston.

______. 1890. On the Form of Convulsive Tic Associated with Coprolalia, etc. *Med News* 57:645–47.

______. 1892. *The Principles and Practice of Medicine: Designed for the Use of Practitioners and Students of Medicine.* New York: Appleton & Co.

______. 1893. Remarks on the Varieties of Chronic Chorea, and a Report upon Two Families of the Hereditary Form, with One Autopsy. *J Nerv Ment Dis* 18:97–111.

______. 1894. *On Chorea and Choreiform Affectations.* Philadelphia: Blakiston.

______. 1897a. On the Classification of the Tics or Habit Movements. *Arch Ped* 14:1–5.

______. 1897b. Sporadic Cretinism in America. *Am J Med Sci* 114:377.

______. 1899. Cerebrospinal Fever. *Maryland Med J* (Baltimore) 41:291.

______. 1901a. On a Family Form of Recurring Epistaxis, Associated with Multiple Telangiectases of the Skin and Mucous Membranes. *Johns Hopkins Hosp Bull* 12:333–37.

______. 1901b. Sporadic Cretinism (Infantile and Juvenile Myxedema). In *Cyclopedia of the Diseases of Children*. Vol. 5, 359. Ed. J. M. Keating and W. A. Edwards. 2d ed. Philadelphia: Lippincott.

______. 1901c. Cerebrospinal Fever. In *Cyclopedia of the Diseases of Children*. Vol. 5, 1333. Ed. J. M. Keating and W. A. Edwards. 2d ed. Philadelphia: Lippincott.

Robbins, B. H. and A. Cristie. 1963. Sir William Osler the Pediatrician. *Am J Dis Child* 106:124–29.

Rogers, F. B. 1959. Neurology in Philadelphia: Personalities and Events. *Phila Med* 55:84–90.

______. 1970. Osler and Philadelphia. *Trans Coll Phys Phila* 38:118–23.

Spiller, W. G. 1935. The First Fifty Years of the Philadelphia Neurological Society. *Arch Neur Psych* 34:899–926.

HEINRICH QUINCKE

ON AUGUST 26, 1842, Heinrich Ireneaus Quincke (figure 1) was born in Frankfurt an-der-Oder, Germany, where his father, Hermann Quincke, was a doctor. The elder Quincke moved the family to Berlin and established a successful medical practice. After a classical education at Friedrichswerdersche Gymnasium in Berlin, Heinrich Quincke enrolled at the Friedrich-Wilhelm University in Berlin when he was only sixteen (Bethe, 1968) and later studied at the universities of Heidelberg and Würzburg. He received his medical degree in 1863 at the University of Berlin (Hochhaus, 1912). At age twenty-four he was appointed an assistant at the venerable Charité hospital in Berlin. His selection for this position marked the beginning of an atypical ascent in the German academic arena, which was known for interminable periods between promotions; Quincke's ascent can only be described as meteoric. By age twenty-eight he was a lecturer at the University of Berlin and at the age of thirty was appointed Professor of Internal Medicine at the University of Bern. After five intensely productive years at Bern, Quincke succeeded Karl Bartel as Ordinarius Professor at the University of Kiel where the next thirty years of his life resulted in an abundance of medical innovations and discoveries (Naunyn, 1922).

In Berlin Quincke studied under Johannes Müller, Albrecht von Gräfe, Ludwig Traube, and Rudolf Virchow, and at Heidelberg with Robert Bunsen and Hermann Helmholtz. In 1866 Quincke took an assistantship with Robert Wilms and the following year became assistant to Friedrich von Frerich. Under Frerich's influence Quincke became interested in liver diseases, which ultimately lead to his landmark publication at age twenty-three on the pathogenesis of neonatal jaundice (Quincke, 1885). A clinician of immense observational powers, Quincke was also acclaimed by his peers as a premier experimental pathologist. Although in later years he was revered by his contemporaries for his prolific work in hepatic disorders, Quincke authored four hundred publications on a dazzling variety of topics, some of which were of an abstruse nature. Over the course of his career, Quincke left virtually no aspect of medicine untouched. His research encompassed blood disorders, diabetic coma (Quincke, 1880), and syphilis. He also displayed a vivid interest in skin diseases. He was the first to describe the capillary pulse as a sign of aortic insufficiency or anemia, and the first to understand the nature of angioneurotic edema. He also wrote extensively on pernicious anemia.

It was his interest in the nervous system, however, that justifies Quincke's inclusion in this biographical collection. He described the function of the choroid plexus and performed pioneering studies of cerebrospinal fluid physiology (Quincke, 1872), investigations which led directly to his seminal work on hydrocephalus (Quincke, 1891) and meningitis (Quincke, 1893a).

What is now called pseudotumor cerebri was referred to as "Quincke's meningitis" in his day. In addition to hydrocephalus and meningitis, Quincke also investigated other neurologic disorders affecting children. Acute infantile hemiplegia (Quincke, 1893b) and cerebral palsy (Quincke, 1893c) were additional areas of child neurology that particularly interested him. The description of the late sequelae of acute infantile hemiplegia illustrates Quincke's meticulous nature. In this report, his case descriptions of infantile hemiplegia document in centimeters the asymmetric measurements of all limbs, including upper and lower extremities of each child!

Impressive as these contributions to child neurology and internal medicine were, it was the development of the lumbar puncture that his contemporaries considered to be Quincke's crowning clinical achievement. Although James Corning has been given credit for the first spinal puncture in a human, critical evaluation of this claim suggests that Corning did not actually enter the subarachnoid space and that priority should be given to either Walter Essex Wynter, who aspirated the lumbar subarachnoid space of children with tuberculous meningitis, or Quincke, who reported the lumbar puncture procedure the same year (Quincke, 1891; Gorelick and Zych, 1987). Quincke had laid the foundation for the spinal tap in humans with his animal experiments in Berlin twenty years earlier when he studied the flow of cerebrospinal fluid in dogs by injecting cinnabar into the lumbar thecal space. When Quincke went to Kiel, he expanded these experiments to include cadavers. In 1891 he performed lumbar punctures using a needle and stylet on two children with hydrocephalus for the purpose of relieving intracranial pressure, a therapeutic measure that survives to the present in selected cases of infantile hydrocephalus. Quincke did his first human spinal tap when he was fifty years old. The lumbar area was selected because he remembered that, in his experiments in Berlin, paraplegia could occur in animals when the puncture was done in the thoracic region. Quincke thus showed that when done by this technique, the spinal tap could provide a means by which meningitis, neurosyphilis, and other central nervous system disorders could be investigated with reasonable safety. Quincke's innovation directly led to the development of spinal anesthesia, pneumoencephalography, and provided the basis for Georges Guillain and Jean Alexandre Barré's studies on polyneuritis (Bethe, 1968, 96–97).

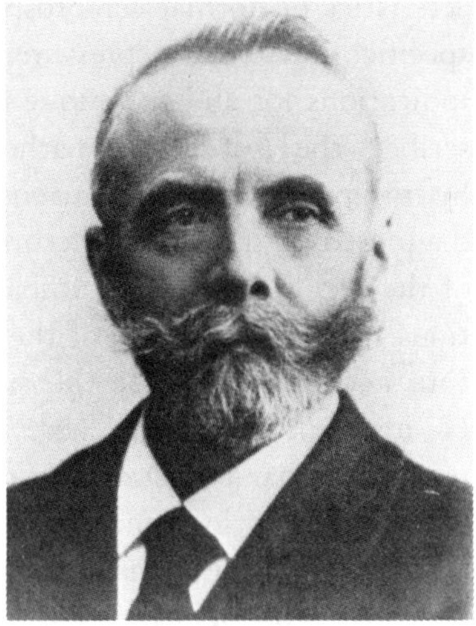

Figure 1: Heinrich Quincke (1842–1922).

A few years after his initial reports, Quincke described the characteristics of normal cerebrospinal fluid, including its appearance, specific gravity, and pressure, in a comprehensive review of the indications for and technique of the lumbar puncture. He also described the features of pathologic cerebrospinal fluid found in hydrocephalus and the various types of meningitis that could be diagnosed by lumbar puncture (Quincke, 1905). His descriptions of the technique of the lumbar puncture included precise instructions regarding the size of the canula used and depth of the puncture necessary to enter the subarachnoid space (Quincke, 1902). He also understood the necessity to perform the puncture in the midline. Characteristic of Quincke's generous nature, he gave credit to the instrument maker who was responsible for the fabrication of the spinal needle and stylets that he used. Quincke was also probably the first to record the ventricular pressure of infants by means of puncture of the open fontanelle.

Still in excellent health, Quincke seems to have heeded Osler's advice to professors of medicine and resigned the professorship at Kiel at age sixty-five and moved to Frankfurt-am-Main where he lived the remaining fifteen years of his life. He continued to serve as an editor of *Archiv für experimentelle Pathologie und Pharmakologie*, a journal that he helped found, and remained a regular participant at medical congresses. His research activities also continued well into his retirement years. In 1910 he published his results of one of the first investigations of medical disorders caused by hyperbaric conditions (Quincke, 1910). During World War I, Quincke resumed an active role in teaching students in the medical school at Frankfurt and later directed the installation of battlefield medical stations. After the war Quincke continued to publish until his death.

Quincke was nominated for the Nobel Prize several times for his work on the physiology of cerebrospinal fluid and for the development of the lumbar puncture. The archives of the Nobel committee reveal that Quincke's contributions to medicine and physiology were considered praiseworthy but the committee felt the stipulations of Alfred Nobel's will specifically excluded Quincke because his achievements in these areas were not of recent origin (Bethe, 1968, 91).

Tall and meticulous in appearance, Quincke gave the impression of being reserved and dry to those who did not know him well, but he was admired for his openness and integrity by those close to him. He was universally regarded as a person with genuine interest in the welfare of his fellow doctors and as one who possessed an old-fashioned chivalrous quality. On his seventieth birthday, a commemoration was held in Kiel at which his colleagues and former students lauded not only his formidable clinical and research accomplishments, but also his humanistic qualities.

Quincke was not a spellbinding speaker. His lectures have even been described as monotonous, but his ability to simplify complex issues at the bedside or in the clinic made Quincke highly regarded as a teacher by advanced students and resident doctors. Typical of medical academicians of the era, Quincke was broadly educated in a variety of subjects, including classical Greek. In a lecture at Kiel, Quincke sums up his own philosophy of life with a quote from Sophocles: "Nothing is more wonderful than the human being" (Bergman, 1923, 17).

Three months shy of his eightieth birthday, on the evening of May 19, 1922, Heinrich Quincke was at home working in his study when he wrote, "Lately I haven't been feeling well. I would prefer to have a sudden embolus than to slowly atrophy" (Kulbs, 1922). Having written this, he died peacefully in his sleep one hour later. Quincke's death seems to have marked the end of an era in which one individual could have such an extraordinary impact on astonishingly diverse areas of medicine.

Glenn W. Fowler
IRVINE, CALIFORNIA

REFERENCES

Bergman, G. von. 1923. Heinrich Quincke. Gedenkrede bei einer Trauerfeier der medizinischen Fakultat und des Arztlichen Vereins zu Frankfurt am Main. *Zeit klin Med Berl* 96:1–21.

Bethe, H. 1968. *Heinrich Quincke. Sein Leben und Werk.* Neumunster: Karl Wachholtz Verlag.

Gorelick, P. B., and D. Zych. 1987. James Leonard Corning and the Early History of Spinal Puncture. *Neur* 37:672–74.

Hochhaus, H. 1912. Heinrich Quincke zum 70. Geburstag. *Dtsch med Wschr* 38:1605–7.

Kulbs, F. 1922. Heinrich Quincke. *Dtsch Arch klin Med Leipz* 140:i–iv.

Naunyn, B. 1922. H. Quincke. *Arch exper Path Pharm* 93:i–iii.

Quincke, H. 1872. Zur Physiologie der Cerebrospinalflussigkeit. *Arch Anat Physiol Leipz*, 153–77.

______. 1880. Über Coma diabeticum. *Berl klin Wschr* 17:1–5.

______. 1885. Über die Entstehung der Gelbsucht bei Neugeborenen. *Arch exper Path Pharm* 19:34–38.

______. 1891. Die Lumbalpunktion des Hydrocephalus. *Berl klin Wschr* 28:929–65.

______. 1893a. Über Meningitis serosa. *Samml klin Vortrage* n.F. Nr. f67, 655–94.

______. 1893b. Über puerperale Hemiplegien. *Dtsch Zeit Nervenheilk* 4:291–98.

______. 1893c. Über cerebrale Muskelatrophie. *Dtsch Zeit Nervenheilk* 4:299–311.

______. 1902. *Die Technik der Lumbalpunktion.* Berlin: Urban-Schwarzenberg.

______. 1905. Die diagnostische und therapeutische Bedeutung der Lumbalpunktion. *Dtsch med Wschr* 31:1825–29.

______. 1910. Experimentelles über Luftdruckerkrankungen. *Arch exper Path Therapie.* 62:464–93.

EDOUARD SÉGUIN

MENTAL RETARDATION, or what was historically called "idiocy," is one of the major expressions of neurological dysfunction with which the child neurologist deals. Until the nineteenth century the plight of the retarded was one of neglect, shame, and hopelessness. It was the common belief that the retarded individual was incapable of being trained or educated and that his level of developmental or intellectual function could not be ameliorated. One of the foremost early pioneers of rehabilitation and education for mentally retarded children was Edouard Onesimus Séguin (1812–1880) (figure 1). By the age of thirty-five he had developed an educational system for the retarded and established a training school that was to become one of the models for such schools throughout the world. Our present-day programs are largely based upon the methods that he developed. Most of his professional life was spent as an advocate for the mentally retarded.

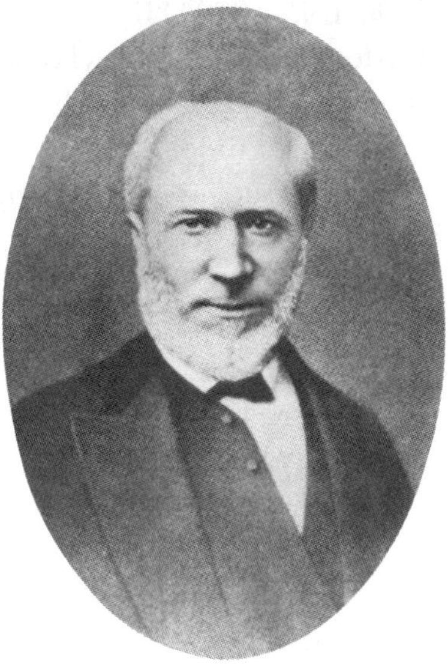

Figure 1. Edouard Onesimus Séguin (1812–1880).

Edouard Séguin was born January 20, 1812, in Clamacy, France. He came from a medical family and studied medicine in Paris under the tutelage of Jean Marie Itard and Jean Etienne Esquirol, both of whom were very interested in psychology, psychiatry, and the study of mental disorders. Inspired by Itard's attempts at educating a retarded boy known as the "Wild Boy of Aveyron," Séguin, at age twenty-five, formulated his own philosophy of educating the retarded. His basic premise was that "idiocy was largely a matter of arrested physical and mental development, which could be partly or wholly remedied by a scientific and thoroughly detailed education of all the senses" (Holman, 1914, 27). Under the direction of Esquirol, Séguin made his first attempts at educating a retarded child. His success with this child was declared by his mentor:

We the undersigned have pleasure in testifying that M. Edouard Séguin, born at Clamacy (Nièvre), has begun, with greatest success, the education of a child almost dumb and apparently an idiot — by reason of the small development of his intellectual and moral faculties. In eighteen months M. Séguin has taught his pupil to make use of his senses, to take care of himself, to speak, to write, to reckon, etc. The education has been done by M. Séguin, after the method of the late Dr. Itard, from whom he has received inspiration. From the character of his mind, and the extent of his knowledge, M. Edouard Séguin is capable of giving to this system of education all desirable extension. Signed: Esquirol and Guersant (Senior). Paris, the 18th of August, 1839.

After this initial success, Séguin opened a school for retarded children in 1839. His school flourished and was visited by French and foreign educators who were impressed with his method and who then incorporated his ideas into schools for the retarded throughout Europe.

Séguin's success was recognized by the minister of the interior of France who requested him to open the first public school for poor retarded children at the Hospital for Incurables (1841), which was later transferred to the Bicêtre. Two separate investigations of his school reported remarkable success, and Séguin was commissioned to expand his school to include more children. This expanded school was to be housed at the Hospital for the Aged. During this time period, he published two accounts of his work, *Théorie et pratique de l'éducation des idiots* (Séguin, 1841) and *Hygiène et éducation des idiots* (Séguin, 1843).

The latter work won recognition and endorsement by the Royal Academy of Sciences. Encouraged by the acceptance of his work, Séguin wrote his first book in 1846, the *Traitement moral, hygiène, et éducation des idiots et des autres enfants arrières.* The book quickly became the authoritative text on the education of the mentally retarded and was crowned by the Royal Academy of Sciences. Based on the humanistic philosophy of Saint-Simon and what Séguin considered physiologic principles, the latter felt that the child, especially the retarded child, had to develop control and proper use of his muscles and senses before the mind could be enlightened and trained. Instruction had to be individualized to the deficiencies and needs of each child. The first level of his educational plan was to train the motor system. Ambulation and then fine motor prehensile skills were systematically taught through imitation and repetition until the child mastered the skills and could incorporate them into spontaneous volitional activity. Once motor skills were mastered, attention was then centered on development of the senses, as "it is primarily through the senses that knowledge comes" (Séguin, 1846). Touch was considered the sensory modality to develop first after which focus was directed toward hearing and vision. Based upon the concepts developed by Jacob Rodrigues Pereire (whom he greatly admired and whose biography he wrote in 1847 [Séguin, 1847]) of using touch to teach deaf-mutes to speak, Séguin believed that the senses could be trained to compensate for each other if one was defective. Emphasis was placed on each sense until that sensory organ was used to its fullest potential. Séguin's papers on the training of the idiotic eye and hand illustrate the importance he placed on this concept (Séguin, 1879; Séguin, 1880).

Once the retarded child had developed motor and sensory skills, he was then taught to apply these skills in the performance of useful vocational activities. Séguin recognized the need of social interaction and the positive effect of meaningful work. "The most urgent need of the idiot, however, is the cultivation of these powers of body and mind which will enable him to do some useful work in the world" (Séguin, 1846).

Undergirding Séguin's physiological method was the belief that the child must always be treated with love and kindness and the dignity of the child must never be violated. He believed that women often made the best teachers of the retarded because of their natural inclination to gentle, loving ways (Kraft, 1961).

Although Séguin had gained notable success and recognition for his work with the mentally retarded, he received no money for his services. He supported his school and his pupils by practicing medicine, writing as an art critic, and penning commentary on political and economic topics of the day. In the 1840's he became part of

> *a group of the most brilliant literary men in Paris. Among these were included Ledru-Rollin, Pierre Leroux, Louis Blanc, Michel Chevalier, Jean Reynaud, and Victor Hugo. Of this circle of brothers, all of whom, some years later, achieved positions of distinction, Edouard Séguin was the youngest, but not, despite his modesty, the least brilliant.* (Holman, 1914, 35)

Because of his political activities, Séguin felt compelled to leave France after Louis Napoléon rose to power in 1848. In 1850, with his wife and young son (Edward Constant, who was born in 1843), he emigrated to America and settled in Cleveland, Ohio, where he practiced general medicine. Although living predominantly in Ohio for the next ten years, Séguin was very active in helping to establish institutions for the mentally retarded throughout the United States. In 1854 he spent the winter assisting Dr. H. B. Wilbur in Syracuse, New York, at the first public institution for the mentally retarded in the United States. He helped establish training schools in Connecticut, Ohio, and Pennsylvania, and was briefly the director of the Pennsylvania School for Idiots in 1857. In 1860 the Séguins moved to New York where Edouard started a general practice in Mount Vernon. In 1861 he received an M.D. degree at the University Medical College of New York, and in 1863 he moved to New York City where he established a private practice and helped organize the School for Defectives at Randall's Island.

In 1866, with the help of his son Edward, who was later to become a neurologist of note and the first department chairman of neurology at Columbia College of Physicians and Surgeons, Séguin wrote his second book on education: *Idiocy: Its Diagnosis and Treatment by the Physiological Method* (Séguin, 1866). The intent of this book was not only to further define his philosophy of education for the retarded but to also demonstrate that the physiological method was applicable to the education of all children regardless of their level of intelligence. In the late nineteenth and early twentieth century, Maria Montessori developed her method of early childhood education based largely upon Séguin's concepts (Boyd, 1914).

In the 1870's Séguin added to his medical activities an interest in medical thermometry (Séguin, 1871). He was active in promoting its use in medical practice as well as standardizing the medical charting of vital signs and use of the metric system in medicine. Also during this time he continued his work for the retarded. As a representative of the American Medical Association, he traveled to Europe several times to review their institutions for the retarded. In 1873 he was appointed one of the U.S. Commissioners of the International Exhibition at Vienna and reported on the educational section of the exhibition (Séguin, 1875).

In 1880, after being a widower for several years, he married one of his pupils' teachers, Elsie Mead, who was involved in helping to develop some of his new teaching methods (Dana, 1924). On October 28, 1880, a few months after his second marriage and following a two-week illness of dysentery he died at the age of sixty-eight. The last enterprise of his life was an attempt to establish a Physiological School for Weak-Minded and Weak-Bodied Children in New York City. In the prospectus of the school he wrote, "The application of physiology to education was the work of my youth and has been the main object of my thoughts for forty-two years. I give it my last years" (Boyd, 1914). Within two weeks of writing these words he had died. At his passing, a close friend and colleague, L. P. Brockett, provided the following insight into the driving force of his life:

His philanthropy was genuine and pervaded his whole nature. He loved his fellow-men intensely, because he saw through all their misfortunes, their weakness, deformities, and disabilities, the capacity for a higher and better life than they were then leading, and he desired to help them to attain to it. There was nothing morbid, nothing sour, nothing selfish, in his philanthropy, as there is in so much of what passes under that name. (Holman, 1914, 44)

Edouard Séguin was one of the key figures of the nineteenth century in revolutionizing the care given the mentally retarded. He provided a philosophy and a practical methodology of rehabilitation and education for these children who had been ignored and neglected by society. His contributions to the education of the mentally retarded can certainly be recognized in the physical therapy, occupational therapy, and educational programs found in our present day training schools for the retarded. His legacy is one of moral and humane treatment and care for the weaker and more vulnerable of the human family, an attitude and activity that he felt should and ought to make us a more compassionate race.

Paul Larson
TEMPLE, TEXAS

REFERENCES

Boyd, W. 1914. *From Locke to Montessori.* London: G. G. Harrax.

Dana, C. L. 1924. The Séguins of New York. *Ann Med Hist* 6:475–79. (Contains a complete bibliography.)

Holman, H. 1914. *Séguin and His Physiological Method of Education.* London: Pitman.

Kelly, H. A., and W. L. Burrage. 1920. *American Medical Biographies*, 1030–31. Baltimore: Norman, Remington Co.

Kraft, I. 1961. Edouard Séguin and 19th Century Moral Treatment of Idiots. *Bull Hist Med* 35:393–418.

Séguin, E. 1841. *Théorie et pratique de l'éducation des idiots.* Paris: Baillière.

______. 1843. *Hygiène et éducation des idiots.* Paris: Baillière.

______. 1846. *Traitement moral, hygiène et éducation des idiots et des autres enfants arrières*. Paris: J. B. Baillière.

______. 1847. *Jacob Rodrigues Pereire, premier instituteur des sourds et muets en France, analyse raisonnée de la méthode*. Paris: J. B. Baillière.

______. 1866. *Idiocy: Its Diagnosis and Treatment by the Physiological Method.* New York: W. Wood and Co.

______. 1871. *Medical Thermometry and Human Temperature.* New York: William Ward and Co.

______. 1875. *Report on Education. Vienna International Exhibition, 1873.* Washington, D.C.: Government Printing Office.

______. 1879. Psycho-Physiological Training of an Idiotic Hand. *Arch Med NY* 2:149–56.

______. 1880. Psycho-Physiological Training of an Idiotic Eye. *Arch Med NY* 4:217–33.

OTTO SOLTMANN

HERMANN JULIUS OTTO SOLTMANN (1844–1912) (figure 1) was born in Berlin, the son of Albert and Berta Wilhelmine Soltmann (née Herbig). His father, a pharmacist, was also proprietor of the well-known Dr. Struwe and Soltmann firm in the mineral water business. Nothing is known about his ancestry. On his mother's side, we find a "Royal Chamber Musician" and two painters, one in portraits and historical subjects, the other a landscapist. Otto Soltmann's father met an early death in 1856 when the boy was only twelve, a circumstance that explains his close relationship to his mother (Brüning, 1912; Rohleder, 1969).

Soltmann attended the Friedrich Wilhelm Gymnasium in Berlin. He was a good student, played the piano without ever having been instructed, and was an avid theater-goer. He excelled in calisthenics, having been awarded a gold medal for his school at an international competition in Leipzig. Even during his days in secondary school he was determined to become a physician. Thus, after having successfully passed his final exams in 1865, he began his medical studies at the University of Berlin. He spent some semesters in Würzburg, Zürich, Prague, and Vienna. It was under the guidance of Hermann Widerhofer in Vienna that he first became interested in pediatrics. In 1869 Soltmann graduated from the Friedrich Wilhelm University in Berlin, writing his thesis on lepra nervosa (Soltmann, 1869). In the same year, he passed his State exam.

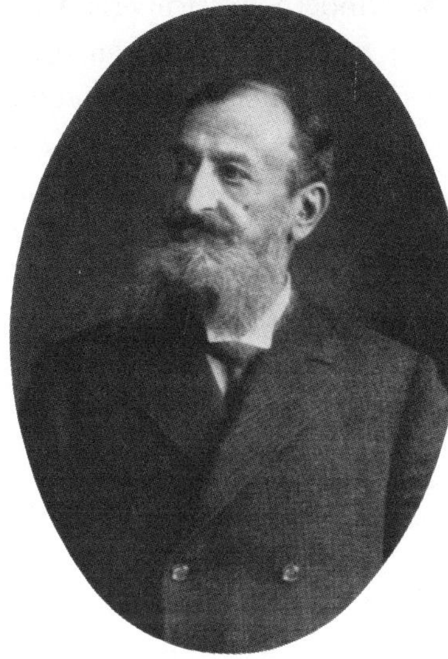

Figure 1. Otto Soltmann (1844–1912).

On March 14, 1870, Soltmann finished his training, became a full-fledged physician, and joined the army as a member of the Regiment Garde du Corps, serving as a doctor in the war against France. Returning to Berlin after the war, he soon opened a pediatric practice in Breslau. For a brief period, he went to Vienna, where he worked at the Institute of Anatomy, which was directed by Karl Langer (Soltmann, 1874).

Inspired by the discoveries of Eduard Hitzig (Fritsch and Hitzig, 1870), he became interested in neurophysiological studies of the central nervous system of neonatal and young mammals — all the while continuing his practice. He initially conducted his experiments in his apartment, but soon moved to the Institute of Physiology in Breslau, headed by Rudolf Heidenhain. The results of this research first appeared in 1875 (Soltmann, 1875a), and were primarily printed in the *Jahrbuch für Kinderheilkunde* (*Yearbook for Pediatrics*), of which Soltmann became coeditor in 1876.

That same year, Soltmann became director of the Wilhelm-Augusta Hospital, located in the outskirts of Breslau. This was a poorly equipped private children's institution with twenty beds. The following year he became docent for internal medicine and pediatrics at the University of Breslau, based on his work *Über einige physiologische Eigenthümlichkeiten der Muskeln und Nerven des Neugeborenen* (*On the Physiological Characteristics of Muscles and Nerves in Neonates*) (Soltmann, 1877b).

Soltmann was subsequently appointed director of the Kaiserliche Kinderheim (Imperial Children's Home) in Breslau/Grabschen, a care facility founded on his suggestion (1882). This was an institution for infants and women, mainly unmarried women, and was the first of its kind in Germany. He insisted on the natural feeding of infants by demanding that wet nurses or nursing mothers be present. He was in charge of this institution for twelve years and was able to reduce infant mortality to a relatively low level.

In 1883 he was appointed titular professor and five years later obtained a lectureship in pediatrics, accompanied by a nomination for associate professor. During this period he was not admitted to the university hospital and delivered his lectures in the Wilhelm-Augusta Hospital. In 1894 Soltmann was finally given the chair of pediatrics at the University of Leipzig. His inaugural lecture was entitled *Über die Beziehungen der physiologischen Eigentülichkeiten des kindlichen Organismus zur Pathologie und Therapie (The Physiological Characteristics of the Young Organism as Related to Pathology and Treatment)* (Soltmann, 1895). Based on his manifold experience and impressive pedagogical skills, he developed an almost exclusively clinically oriented teaching system designed to convey the most important elements of pediatrics to general practitioners. Having finally been appointed director of the Pediatric University Hospital and the Polyclinic, as well as the newly opened children's hospital, he was fully committed to the improvement and growth of these institutions.

In his attempts to lower the high infant mortality from nosocomial infections, Soltmann insisted on strictly separating patients with infectious diseases by constructing new buildings for these wards. As before, he also engaged wet nurses, and by implementing all these measures was able to reduce the infant mortality rate considerably. In addition to his clinical and research activities, Soltmann endeavored to improve the professional image of pediatrics. As early as 1875, at a meeting of German natural scientists and medical doctors in Graz, Austria, he criticized the Congress for suppressing the pediatric sections. He advocated the separation of pediatrics and internal medicine and was one of the founders of the Pediatric Society, established on September 18, 1883, in Freiburg/Breisgau. He served as a member of the board and subsequently served as its chairman several times (Hohlfeld, 1912; Risel, 1913).

Soltmann's private life was spent with his family. An excellent host, he enjoyed company and was also a popular "sometime poet." Even on the day of his death, September 10, 1912, he had guests for lunch, as was his custom. Later they played some music, and, in the afternoon, he died of a myocardial infarction at the age of sixty-eight.

Otto Soltmann gave numerous lectures and wrote many papers on various topics of pediatrics, particularly in regard to infantile gastrointestinal disorders, infectious diseases, and infant mortality (Soltmann, 1881a, 1896, 1904, 1907).

His significance for child neurology is primarily based on his early experimental studies in neurophysiology, which he carried out at the Breslau Institute with the physiologist Rudolf Heidenhain. As early as 1875, an article on his experiments was published in the *Centralblatt für die medizinischen Wissenschaften* (*Central Gazette for Medical Science*) under the title "Zur elektrischen Reizbarkeit der Großhirnrinde" ("On the Electrical Excitability of the Cerebral Cortex") (1875a). Referring to the studies on motor centers of the cerebral cortex published by Gustav Fritsch and Eduard Hitzig, he pointed out that the findings in newborn dogs were substantially different from those in adults. In the same year, he gave a talk on this topic at the forty-eighth meeting of the Society of German Scientists and Physicians in Graz (Soltmann, 1875b). In 1876 his first extensive neurophysiological study was published under the title "Experimentelle Studien über die Function des Großhirns der Neugeborenen" ("Experimental Studies on the Function of the Cerebrum in the Newborn"). After describing in detail the experiments in 132 dogs, he drew the following conclusions:

In the newborn the cerebral cortex does not trigger any muscle movements with electrical stimulation. They can be observed in the puppy as of day 10; first the movement for the opposite front paw, then for the rear paw and facial muscles (eyes). The cortical field that triggers the movement is first more extended than later. With the number of individual fields the isolation of each field increases; they correspond then to the locations indicated by Hitzig. In newborns and puppies up to 10 days old, extirpation of the cortex of the anterior lobe does not result in any motor impairment, neither immediately nor later. The corresponding anterior lobe of the opposite hemisphere seems to take the place of the lost one. In older animals extirpation of the cortex of the anterior lobe causes paralysis of the muscle sense, which increases with the age of the animal. In the newborn, extirpation of the cortex of both anterior lobes does not cause motor impairment, neither immediately nor, it seems, later. In the adult dog, extirpation of the cortex of both anterior lobes causes double-sided ataxia, which is not completely reversible. In newborn dogs the striate body is not voluntary. By means of electric stimulation of the fibre fascicles of the internal capsule, twitching of the opposite front paw may be triggered in newborn dogs. The point from where this is possible varies with age and the individual. Sometimes it is located closer to the surface, sometimes deeper. Stimulation of the fibre fascicles of the internal capsule, located between the thalamus and the striate body, never achieves twitching of the opposite rear paw nor movements of other body muscles in newborn dogs. (Soltmann, 1876, 122–23)

Soltmann was not able to provide an adequate explanation for these results, but he did believe he had proven in his experiments that movements of the newborn could only be involuntary. Continuing his neurophysiological studies, he published another experimental paper "Über das Hemmungsnervensystem der Neugeborenen" ("On the Inhibitory Nervous System of the Newborn") in 1877, in which he was able to show that the inhibitory centers of mammals identified by L. M. Simonoff in the cerebrum could be detected in newborns only fourteen to twenty-one days after birth. He considered this proof of the "increased reflex disposition" of the newborn, already discussed in the study on the cerebrum, and believed that he had found an explanation of the frequent spasms in newborns, that is, "spasmophilia" (Soltmann, 1877a). In this study he also dealt with the cardioinhibitory nervous system of the newborn and described how, in the first days of life, cardiac arrest could not be achieved by vagus stimulation or, if at all, only with much higher intensities of electric current than in adults.

He then turned to experimental studies on the peripheral nervous system in newborns. After he held a lecture on the topic at the fiftieth meeting of the German Scientists and Physicians in Munich in 1877, he received tenure the same year with his Habilitationsschrift "Über einige physiologische Eigenthümlichkeiten der Muskeln und Nerven des Neugeborenen" ("On Some Physiological Particularities of Muscles and Nerves in Newborns") (1877b). In this paper he presented the following findings:

The excitability of motor nerves in the newborn is less susceptible to electrical stimulation than in adults. . . . Excitability steadily increases from birth to the sixth week of life, when it reaches or even exceeds excitability in adults. . . . The myogram of newborns is similar to that of fatigued animals (muscles). It is characterised by a lower overall maximum, a flattening of the peak and increasing extension above all in its descending line. Muscles remain longer in their maximum contraction, and re-extension occurs gradually. 16 circuit interruptions per second are sufficient to produce complete tetanus in the newborn rabbit while more than 70 are needed in the adult. . . . Also tetanus in newborn animals is similar to that of fatigued animals. Direct and indirect muscle stimulation provide the same results. (Soltmann, 1877b, 17–18).

Continuing his work on the peripheral nervous system, Soltmann published the experimental study "Über die Erregbarkeit der sensibeln Nerven der Neugeborenen" ("On the Excitability of Sensory Nerves of Newborns") in 1879, in which he determined that stimulus conduction was slowed as compared to adults and steadily increased in the course of regular development (Soltmann, 1879). As a result of these findings, he revised his theory of newborn spasms. He now believed that the explanation was to be found in the physiologically caused disproportion between quick development of sensory and motor nerves and the slower maturation of inhibitory centers. Because of his studies on the physiology and development of the nervous system, Soltmann was qualified to write the section "Die funktionellen Nervenkrankheiten" ("Functional Nervous Disorders") in the first major standard reference book on pediatrics, the *Handbuch der Kinderkrankheiten*, edited by Carl Gerhard (Soltmann, 1880). In the introduction to his contribution in the fifth volume of this reference work, he wrote:

If we want to bridge the gulf that exists between matter and activity and gain an insight into the nature of the so-called functional nervous disorders, we must recognize beside pathological anatomy (and chemistry) clinical observation and experimental physiology . . . as the main pillars of our studies, testing ground of our knowledge and regulators of our actions. We shall, therefore, attempt in the following chapter to do justice in each disease to all three factors, and to proceed genetically by taking into consideration the functional particularities of the nervous system in the first few years of childhood in addition to anatomical development and the gradual formation of psychic and physical manifestations. (Soltmann, 1880, 3–4)

Soltmann's systematic presentation, consisting of more than three hundred pages, discussed the individual disorders in detail and was the major work in this field for many years. Among his later, almost exclusively clinical studies, are the following: "Über das Mienen und Geberdenspiel kranken Kinder" ("On Facial Expressions and Gestures of Sick Children") which deals especially with cerebral disorders (Soltmann, 1887); "Schrift und Spiegelschrift bei gesunden und kranker Kindern" ("Writing and Mirror-Writing in Healthy and Sick Children"), in which Soltmann demonstrated connections between handwriting and cerebral changes (Soltmann, 1890); contributions to the *Real Encyclopädie der gesamten Heilkunde* (edited by A. Eulenberg) on "Night Terrors," "Spasmus nutans," and "Eclampsia infantum" (Soltmann, 1881b, c, d); and to the French standard reference book of pediatrics, *Traité des maladies de l'enfance* (edited by J. Grancher and J. Comby), "Myélite transverse généralisée aiguë" and "Maladie de Landry" (Soltmann, 1905a, b).

Soltmann was able to supply experimental findings of fundamental significance for neurophysiology, especially in the newborn period, and gained recognition for his work in this field. His explanation of newborn and infant spasms, however, was controversial and proved to be incorrect. From today's viewpoint, the aspect of developmental neurology in his work, although it has received little recognition, deserves to be stressed.

Helmut Groger
VIENNA, AUSTRIA

REFERENCES

Brüning, H. 1912. Otto Soltmann. *Dtsch med Wschr* 46:2182.

Fritsch, G., and E. Hitzig. 1870. Über die elektrische Erregbarkeit des Groß-hirns. *Arch Anat Physiol* 545–64.

Hohlfeld, M. 1912. Otto Soltmann. *Jahrb Kinderheilk* 3.F. 26:505–6.

Risel, H. 1913. Otto Soltmann. *Mschr Kinderheilk* 11:233–35.

Rohleder, W. 1969. *Otto Soltmann (1844–1912). Pädiater in Breslau und Leipzig.* Thesis, Berlin: Freie Universität.

Soltmann, O. 1869. Lepra nervosa (anaesthetica). Thesis, Berlin: G. Lange.

______. 1874. Die Ausbreitingsbezirke der Congestions-Abscesse bei der Spondyloarthrocace der Kinder. *Jahrb Kinderheilk* n.F. 7:267–95.

______. 1875a. Zur elektrischen Reizbarkeit der Großhirnrinde. *Centralbl med Wiss* 13:209–10.

______. 1875b. Über die Functionen des Großhirns der Neugeborenen. *Tagebl 48 Vrs dtsch Naturf Ärzte Graz* 48:92.

______. 1876. Experimentelle Studien über die Function des Großhirns der Neugeborenen. *Jahrb Kinderheilk* n.F. 9:122–23.

______. 1877a. Über das Hemmungsnervensystem der Neugeborenen. *Jahrb Kinderheilk* n.F. 11:101–14.

______. 1877b. *Über einige physiologische Eigenthümlichkeiten der Muskeln und Nerven des Neugeborenen.* Leipzig: B. G. Teubner.

______. 1879. Über die Erregbarkeit der sensibeln Nerven der Neugeborenen. *Jahrb Kinderheilk* n.F. 14:308–15.

______. 1880. Die funktionellen Nervenkrankheiten. In *Handbuch der Kinderkrankheiten*, 5:3–332. Ed. C. Gerhardt. Tübingen: H. Laupp.

______. 1881a. *Über die Behandlung der wichtigsten Magen-Darmkrankheiten des Säuglings*. Tübingen: H. Laupp.

______. 1881b. Eklampsia infantum, 343–54. In *Real-Encyclopädie der gesamten Heilkunde*, 343–54. Ed. A. Eulenberg. Wien u. Leipzig: Urban & Schwarzenberg.

______. 1881c. Spasmus nutans. In *Real-Encyclopädie der gesamten Heilkunde*, 595–97. Ed. A. Eulenberg. Wien u. Leipzig: Urban & Schwarzenberg..

______. 1881d. Night Terrors. In *Real-Encyclopädie der gesamten Heilkunde*, 659–62. Ed. A. Eulenberg. Wien u. Leipzig: Urban & Schwarzenberg..

______. 1887. Über das Mienen- und Geberdenspiel kranken Kinder. *Jahrb Kinderheilk* n.F. 26:206–21.

______. 1890. Schrift und Spiegelschrift bei gesunden und kranker Kindern. In *Pädiatrische Arbeiten, Festschrift E. Henoch*, 432–60. Ed. A. Baginsky. Berlin: August Hirschwald.

______. 1895. *Über die Beziehungen der physiologischen Eigentülichkeiten des kindlichen Organismus zur Pathologie und Therapie*. Leipzig: Veit.

______. 1896. *Über die Erfolge mit Diphterieheilserum*. Leipzig: Veit & Co.

______. 1904. *Masern, Keuchhusten, Scharlach, Diphterie*. Leipzig: G. Thieme.

______. 1905a. Maladie de Landry. In *Traité des maladies de l'enfance*, 4:505–12. Ed. J. Grancher and J. Comby. 2d ed. Paris: Masson.

______. 1905b. Myélite tranverse géneralisée aiguë, 496–505. . In Grancher, J., and J. Comby (eds.) *Traité des maladies de l'enfance*. Ed. J. Grancher and J. Comby. 2d ed. Paris: Masson.

______. 1907. Die Säuglingssterblichkeit im Krankhenhaus. *Münch med Wschr* 54:5–8, 80–83.

______. 1922. Otto Soltmann. In *Das Leipziger medizinische Viertel*, 116–17. Ed. M. Weiser. Leipzig: Verlag von Alfred Lorentz.

WILLIAM ALLEN STURGE

BORN IN BRISTOL, England, William Allen Sturge (1850–1919) (figure 1) was the eldest son of William Sturge and his wife, Charlotte. His father was a wealthy land surveyor, and the family were members of the Religious Society of Friends (Quakers).

Sturge attended local schools until 1865, when he was sent to a Quaker school in London. There he injured his knees while playing soccer, and stayed with his uncle while he was recuperating. His uncle was a physician whose own sons were studying medicine, and it was during this time that Sturge developed an interest in medicine. This was contrary to the wishes of his father, who wanted him to continue the family business, but fortunately his father relented and permitted Sturge to pursue medical study.

He entered Bristol Medical School in 1868 to study for the Preliminary Scientific Examination for the London Bachelor of Medicine degree. During this time he did practical work at Bristol General Hospital. He was a very industrious young man who did not allow himself much time for meals and leisure. Perhaps partly as a result of overwork, he fell ill with diphtheria in June 1869. After recovering, he went on vacation in August to Switzerland with his family. There he developed rheumatic fever, an illness that lasted for several weeks. He subsequently was able to resume his studies, and in 1870 passed the Primary Examination of the College of Surgeons. Sturge then went to London in 1871 to continue his studies at University College, London, but he had a second attack of rheumatic fever the following year that forced him to discontinue work on his degree. His father sent him on a prolonged tour of the East in 1873. The following winter he accompanied a wealthy young man named Lucas to Egypt as medical attendant and, upon returning to London, resumed and completed his medical studies in 1875. After holding the post of physician's assistant, he became a resident medical officer and subsequently registrar of the National Hospital for Paralysis and Epilepsy. It was here that he laid the foundation for a wide and thoughtful survey of neurological diseases. He spent the years

1876 and 1877 in Paris doing further postgraduate studies. This was the era when Jean Martin Charcot was attracting neurologists from all over Europe to his clinic at the Salpêtrière. Sturge did not limit his studies to neurology. He worked in general pathology and medicine, as well as closely following Alfred Fournier's practice at the Hôpital St. Louis. Both Charcot and Fournier were highly impressed by Sturge's intelligence and originality. It was in Paris that he met his first wife, Emily Bovell, who was also a physician. They married in September 1877 and returned to London to set up a practice together. Sturge was appointed physician and pathologist to the Royal Free Hospital and was one of the lecturers at the Women's Medical School. Emily Bovell, after much difficulty, became one of the first six women who gained admission to the Medical School of Edinburgh University, only to be physically ejected by the male students and faculty. All of these women eventually completed their medical training elsewhere, and all achieved distinction in their own particular field. Bovell, who was older than Sturge, developed tuberculosis, a circumstance that prompted the couple to move to Nice in order to live in a milder and more salubrious climate. There they practiced together, treating mainly English and American visitors, most of whom were affluent and well known; among his patients were Queen Victoria and her family. It was in recognition of this service that he received from the Queen a special order and decoration for individuals who rendered service of a personal nature to the Royal family. Sturge stayed at Nice for twenty-seven years. His wife died in 1885, and the following year Sturge married Julia Sherriff, his nurse at Nice and daughter of a wealthy ironmaster in the north of England.

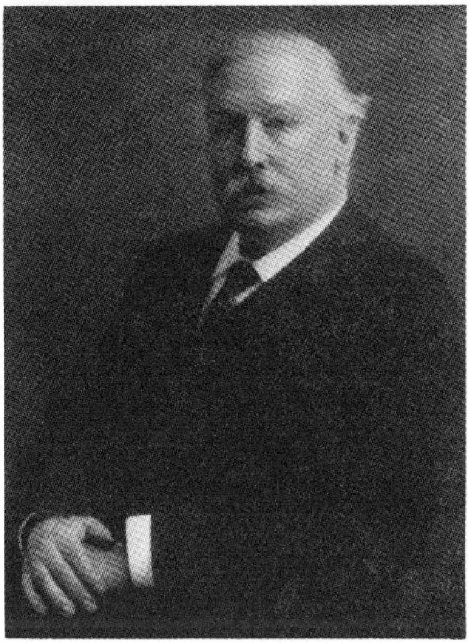

Figure 1. William Allen Sturge (1850–1919).

During his travels Sturge became greatly interested in archaeology and began collecting Greek vases and paleolithic and neolithic

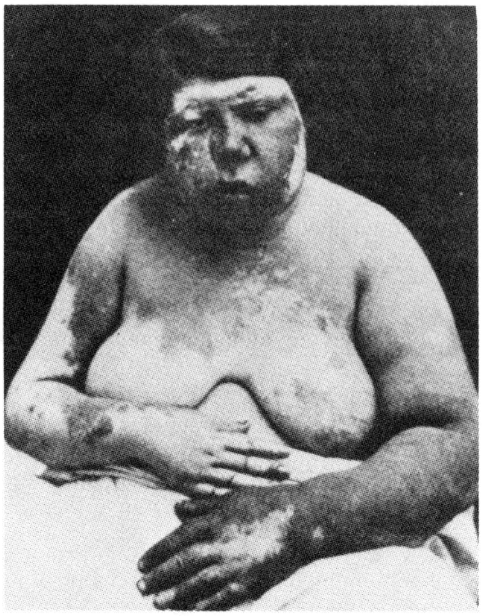

Figure 2. The first published photograph of Sturge-Weber syndrome (Weber, 1922). The patient is a 22-year-old female with a nevus involving both the face and body.

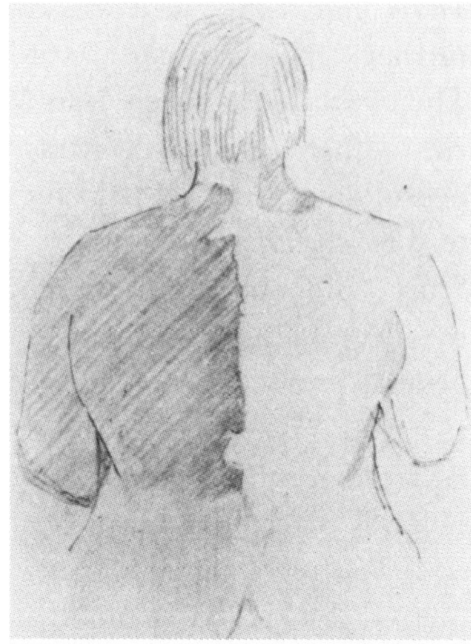

Figure 3. Drawing of the back of this patient showing that the nevus was limited to the midline.

flint implements. After his retirement in 1907, he returned to England, settling at Icklingham Hall, Suffolk, an area containing many neolithic flints, which provided material to satisfy his passion for archeology. In the winter of 1918 he suffered from influenza and nephritis and died in March 1919. He left no children to bear his name.

Sturge's name is associated with the well-known eponym Sturge-Weber syndrome, based on his description in 1879 of a patient he had originally seen when she was six and one-half years old. This child had enjoyed good health until she was six months old, when she began to have left-side twitching of her body. The attacks became stronger, but the child did not lose consciousness until some time later, when the twitching spread to her other side and she lost consciousness. The child appeared to benefit from potassium bromide. Of particular interest was that she had what was described as a "mother's mark" on the right side of the head and face. The skin lesion was pretty accurately demarcated in the midline and involved the upper lip, nose, forehead, scalp, and back of the neck, extending a little beyond the midline on the chin and the upper part of the sternum. It extended as low as the third or fourth dorsal vertebra behind and the second costal cartilage in front. The lips, gums, tongue, roof and floor of mouth, uvula, and pharynx were all similarly affected on the right side. The right eye was larger (buphthalmos; congenital glaucoma) and the sclera, choroid, and retina were all affected by a vascular malformation. There was in addition a patch about the size of the palm of the hand over the left eye and frontal and temporal regions. The mark was of a deep purple color, the color partially disappearing on firm pressure. The affected parts were distinctly larger than the corresponding parts on the other side. Sturge described this mark as "port-wine" colored. He postulated that the patient's neurological deficit was explained by a lesion that existed on the surface of the same side of the brain, though he could offer no proof for this hypothesis, for which he was greatly criticized by his peers when he presented his case to the Clinical Society in London on April 18, 1879. He did not suspect that the lesion could have arisen from the brain parenchyma itself because, in his view, had there been a parenchymal lesion the patient would have started with generalized seizures from the beginning since the immature brain has great "instability of gray matter" and thus allows for widespread dissemination of the "nerve-discharge." It is a great tribute to Sturge that he had such an incisive intellect to correctly postulate the underlying basis of the patient's disease. It was not until 1901 that Kalischer provided pathological proof of such an association. F. Parkes Weber of England described a 22-year-old patient with this syndrome (figures 2 and 3) and also published the first radiographs of this disorder in 1922 and again in 1928. It should be noted that Sturge also contributed toward the understanding of muscular diseases, in recognition of which he was awarded a silver medal by the Royal Society of Medicine for his dissertation on spinal muscular atrophy (Sturge, 1881).

Mohammad Sarwar
CHICAGO, ILLINOIS

ACKNOWLEDGMENTS

It was after an arduous effort that I was able to locate Dr. Sturge's two cousins, Ms. Margaret Goodbody and Dr. Sheila

Eades, who live in England. They provided immensely useful information. Ms. Goodbody identified a book entitled *Reminiscences* written by Sturge's sister, Elizabeth Sturge. This book was mainly designed for private use. I am greatly obliged to both Ms. Goodbody and Dr. Eades for their kind help. In addition, I greatly appreciate the efforts of my secretary, Claribel Olichwier, in the research and preparation of this manuscript.

REFERENCES

Kalischer, S. 1901. Ein Fall teleangiectasie (angiom) des Gesechts und der weichen Hirnhaut. *Arch Psych Nervenkrankh* 34:171–80.

Sturge, W. A. 1879. A Case of Partial Epilepsy Apparently Due to a Lesion of one of the Vasomotor Centers of the Brain. *Trans Clin Soc* 12:162–67.

______. 1881. On the Study of Muscular Atrophy as an Aid to the Physiological Investigation of the Spinal Cord. *Proc Med Soc London* 5:357–72.

Weber, F. P. 1922. Right-Sided Hemi-Hypotrophy Resulting from Right-Sided Congenital Spastic Hemiplegia, with a Morbid Condition of the Left Side of the Brain, Revealed by Radiograms. *J Neur Psychopathol* 3:134–39.

______. 1928. A Note on the Association of Extensive Hemangiomatous Nevus of the Skin with Cerebral (Meningeal) Hemangioma, Especially Cases of Facial Nevus with Contralateral Hemiplegia. *Proc Roy Soc Med* 22:431.

OCTAVIUS STURGES

THE TERM *chorea* used to describe the writhing movements seen in a variety of neurological disorders is based on a Greek word whose root means "to dance," and to most neurologists the word evokes the names of Sir Thomas Sydenham and George Huntington. In the field of child neurology, another and more recent name, should also be recognized, that of Octavius Sturges, who in the late nineteenth century published his own observation of choreiform disorders of childhood.

Octavius Sturges (1833–1894) (figure 1) was the eighth son and twelfth child of John and Elizabeth Sturges and was born in Connaught Square, London. His father was a merchant who spent much of his leisure time in learned and scientific pursuits, especially medicine. John Sturges not only studied surgical books but also frequently witnessed operations in several of the local hospital operating theaters. After attending King's College School, Octavius Sturges was nominated to the East India Company's Military College at Addiscombe, which he entered at the age of seventeen. In 1852 he finished his course, placing fifth in his term and received a commission in the Bombay Artillery. Although he had not yet considered a medical career, surgery had the same attraction for him that it had for his father. Sturges obtained permission to view surgeries at King's College Hospital, and when on leave from Addiscombe he would often stop on his way through London to view operations at the local hospitals (Donkin, 1895).

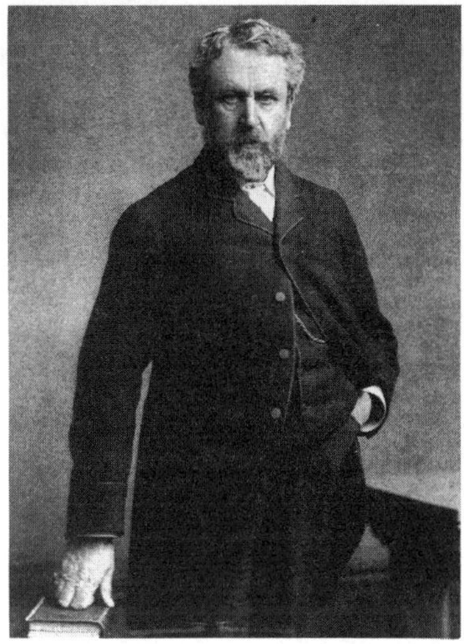

Figure 1. Octavius Sturges (1833–1894).

After two years in India, Sturges became ill and was misdiagnosed as having an aortic aneurysm. This diagnosis ended his military career and had a profound emotional effect on him, as he was given only several months to live. Eventually returning to London, he was diagnosed as having dilatation of the heart, presumably caused by the Indian climate. Rather than remaining idle, he entered Emmanuel College, Cambridge, in July 1858, at the age of twenty-five. Following his early inclinations and the advice of his nephew, W. Howship Dickinson, Sturges began his medical career and entered St. George's Hospital. He received his B.A. in 1861, his M.B. in 1862, and was appointed medical registrar to St George's and became a member of the College of Physicians in 1863. He received his M.D. from Cambridge in 1867 and in 1868 was appointed assistant physician to Westminster Hospital and lecturer on forensic medicine in the Medical School. From 1871 to 1874 he lectured on materia medica at Westminster and in 1874 was appointed chair of medicine at this institution, where he continued to lecture until 1893. Prior to this, because of his interest in children, he sought a position at the Hospital for Sick Children in Great Ormond Street. In 1873 he became assistant physician and was appointed full physician in 1884. Sturges also served as an examiner or censor at the College of Physicians and in 1894 was appointed senior censor, a position he held until he died. He frequently examined at Cambridge and also served for a time as dean of the School of Medicine at Westminster Hospital. At the time of his death he was the school's treasurer.

Sturges was highly regarded by his contemporaries. He was described as a man of great modesty, yet in defense of what he thought was right he was never reluctant to argue his position in any important debate. He was perceived to be religious in habit and mind, untainted by prejudice, always charitable in his judgment of others and among other things a "whole hearted liberal" to a degree that even in those days was considered advanced. Yet even his opponents could never accuse him of unreasoning hostility or blind adherence to a point of view. Sturges was also considered, in the true sense of the term, a skeptical physician. He had a reputation for being a nonbeliever in drugs, recognizing that in many instances particular remedies were useless or harmful. He was an excellent clinician, uniformly kind and considerate with his patients and well respected by the hospital staff. He apparently endeared himself especially to children, and had a singular influence over them, which greatly contributed to his successful treatment of many patients (Donkin, 1895). Sturges was held in high regard by the medical students. In 1870 he gave the introductory address for that session of school and was also a frequent lecturer (Sturges, 1870). He was one of the founding members of the Guthrie Society and was chosen as its president for the first two years of its existence.

In addition to his lectures on materia medica and forensic medicine, Sturges had a substantial interest in the diseases of children and made important observations in three areas, one of which, chorea, forms the basis of his contribution to child neurology. In 1876 Sturges wrote an exemplary book on pneumonia, *The*

Natural History and Relation of Pneumonia: A Clinical Study. The book was full of historical and clinically relevant information. In its second edition it embodied some of the recent teachings in regard to the specific bacteriological abnormalities occurring in these groups of disorders. Sturges prepared and delivered the Lumleian Lectures on heart diseases in children at the College of Physicians in 1894. This work was published posthumously with the assistance of W. H. Dickinson and was entitled *Heart Inflammation in Children* (Sturges, 1895).

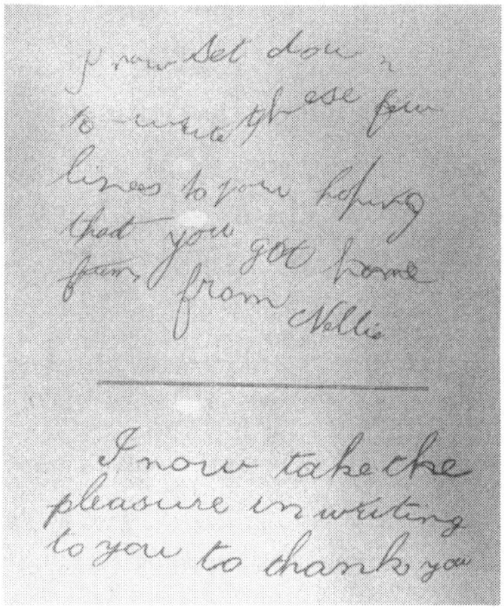

Figure 2. From the second, revised edition of Sturges's *On Chorea or St. Vitus's Dance in Children* (1893). The two samples of handwriting were taken several days apart during the acute episode of chorea.

Sturges's contribution to child neurology is based on his clinical studies of chorea, which were conducted primarily at the Hospital for Sick Children in Great Ormond Street. This was first published in 1881 in a volume entitled *On Chorea and Other Allied Movement Disorders of Early Life*. Sturges continued to collect patients and ideas, and a second edition entitled *On Chorea or St. Vitus's Dance in Children* was published twelve years later. This monograph of 188 pages was divided into eleven chapters and an appendix abstracting data on 132 consecutive cases in children and 45 cases in older subjects. Included is only one illustration, that of handwriting samples of a twelve-year-old girl with chorea (figure 2). The chapters in this work deal with a general description of chorea, its relation to rheumatic symptoms, cardiac involvement, pathology, chorea at school, functional involvement, treatment, and a series of illustrative cases.

The first epidemics of chorea occurred in the middle ages. Chorea was then believed to be due to either infectious disease, hysteria, or demoniacal possession. With the description of chorea minor or St. Vitus's Dance by Thomas Sydenham (1686), it was realized that chorea was a physical illness with certain characteristics. Descriptions of chorea also appeared in the eighteenth century, including the works of Richard Mead (1751) and William Cullen (1778–84). The first separate treatise on chorea was that of Etienne Michel Bouteille in 1810. German See, in a comprehensive treatise (See, 1850) reviewed 154 cases and distinguished the acute from chronic forms of this disorder. The studies of W. S. Kirkes provided some of the first case material implying a relation between cardiac disease and chorea minor; he suggested, however, that cardiac emboli might precipitate chorea. It was around this time that George Huntington described the adult-onset hereditary chorea (1872) that now bears his name. Charcot also described senile chorea, yet his *Tuesday Lessons* clearly showed that he was aware of the differences between hereditary and rheumatic chorea.

Sturges's work on childhood chorea thus appeared at a propitious moment. The following are some of his considerations on the disease from the 1893 edition of his work:

Various kinds of pain, rheumatic and other, headache, articular and other pains, are apt to precede and accompany chorea whether as cause or not. Again, the convalescence of scarlatina, and less obviously of measles, may be disturbed by its appearance. . . . It is beyond dispute that between chorea and endocarditis, whether rheumatic or not, there is during childhood a distinct connection. (1893, 30)

The duration of chorea is thus too variable to admit of any general statement, and it is not proportionate to its initial severity. . . . It is seldom recovered from under six weeks, and, as has already been mentioned, in the case of very young children, it may linger for months. (1893, 32)

I would insist, too, upon the cardiac symptoms of chorea as being special and unique, a part of the disease itself, coming and going with it, and exhibiting in many instances not only murmur, but marked unevenness of rhythm and even irregularity of action. (1893, 35)

It thus appears that 284 children with chorea include only 11 under six years old. One of these must be neglected owing to defective information. There remains 5 out of 10 who certainly and 6 out of 10 who probably, have had acute rheumatism. With such testimony, the conclusion is inevitable that the rheumatic element of chorea is conspicuous as regards the younger children. (1893, 48)

We thus establish the fact, making large allowance for error (which from the nature of the material cannot be wholly excluded), that the mortality of children directly from chorea is exceedingly small. . . . (1893, 53)

The best index of muscular infirmity tending to St. Vitus's Dance is the hand. Face mobility may be mere nervousness; the tongue may be tremulous by nature; the hand test is infallible. It is thus applied: bid the child hold up both hands open with extended arms and the palms towards you. If that be done steadily, both hands upright and both alike, no finger or thumb quivering, no falling back or hanging forward of either hand, then the child may be acquitted of chorea. (1893, 82)

Sturges's chapter on the pathology of chorea is both interesting and fascinating. He deftly balanced a wide variety of inconclusive material spanning almost one hundred years of investigation and came to the following conclusion:

In reviewing the several observations and conclusions which have now been enumerated, it is easy to see that the theories in reference to chorea which have successively gained acceptance represent so many attempts to accommodate this particular affection with the pathological doctrines of their day. (1893, 98)

Sturges died under somewhat unusual circumstances. Eight days prior to his death he was knocked down by a hansom cab in Cavendish Square, but suffered no significant external bruising (Cantab, 1894). He subsequently developed intestinal distension and respiratory distress, and then succumbed. The postmortem examination revealed no traumatic lesion, and his death was attributed to nervous shock and the failure of a feeble and dilated heart.

Stephen Ashwal
LOMA LINDA, CALIFORNIA

REFERENCES

Bouteille, E. M. 1810. *Traité de la chorée, ou danse de St. Guy*. Paris: Vancard.

Cantab, M. D. 1894. Obituary on Octavius Sturges. *Lancet*, Nov. 10, 2:1127.

Donkin, H. B. 1895. In Memoriam: Octavius Sturges. *Westminister Hosp Rep* 9:1–8.

McHenry, L. C. 1969. *Garrison's History of Neurology*. Springfield, IL: Charles C Thomas.

See, G. 1850. De la chorée. *Mém Acad Nat Méd* (Paris). 15:373.

Sturges, O. 1870. *Westminster Hospital Medical School: The Introductory Address for the Session. 1870–1871*. London: Strangeways.

______. 1876. *The Natural History and Relations of Pneumonia: A Clinical Study*. London: Smith, Elder & Co.

______. 1877. *Chorea and Whooping Cough: Five Lectures*. London: Smith, Elder & Co.

______. 1881. *On Chorea and Other Allied Movement Disorders of Early Life*. London: Smith, Elder & Co.

______. 1893. *On Chorea or St. Vitus's Dance in Children*. London: John Bale & Sons.

______. 1895. *Heart Inflammation in Children*. London: John Bale & Sons.

JULIUS THOMSEN

AMONG THE GENETIC muscle diseases affecting children, three common groups are well recognized: the muscular dystrophies; the myotonic dystrophies; and, more recently, the congenital myopathies. The clinical descriptions of the muscular dystrophies were carefully elucidated by Amand Duchenne, William Gowers, Wilhelm Erb, Louis Landouzy, Jules Dejerine, and many others. Myotonic dystrophy, a syndrome associated with muscle weakness and atrophy, wasting, cataracts, frontal baldness, and testicular atrophy, was described by Hans Steinert in 1909. Although myotonia had been noted by Thomas Willis, it was not until Steinert's work that myotonic dystrophy was clearly separated from muscular dystrophy. Prior to Steinert's work, two other myotonic disorders were recognized. Albert Eulenberg, in two papers in 1886 and 1916, characterized paramyotonia congenita, a disorder in which exposure to cold either induced or worsened myotonia (Dubowitz, 1980). Prior to this, myotonia congenita, a relatively benign but lifelong form of myotonia that begins in childhood, was described by Julius Thomsen in 1876.

Asmus Julius Thomas Thomsen (1815–1896) was born in

South Schleswig, Denmark, now part of West Germany. As a boy, he suffered physically and emotionally from myotonia congenita (Thomsen disease), a condition he later described; this description was his major contribution to child neurology (Thomsen, 1876).

From [those] who had no insight or understanding for this condition, I often received bad-mouthing and even physical punishment. . . . Since I was ambitious, these unjustified offenses affected my psyche severely and caused a great irritability, as also the attempts at concealing my condition since childhood had a negative influence on my overall character. . . .
(Thomsen, 1876, 709)

Thomsen attended the universities of Kiel, Copenhagen, and Berlin (Hirsch, 1887). He received his doctorate in medicine at Kiel in 1839 after successfully defending his doctoral thesis, "De Dipsomania." He then set up practice in Gelting, a small town in northeast Schleswig, but moved to Sieseby the following year. In 1853 he was appointed city physician and public health officer for the city of Kappellen. In this capacity, Thomsen published a number of articles on various poisons, narcotics, and abortives, as well as on health conditions in Iceland and the Faroe Islands (Hirsch, 1887).

Thomsen's most important medical work, "Tonische Krämpfe in willkürlich beweglichen Muskeln in Folge von erebter psychischer Disposition. (Ataxia muscularis?)" ("Tonic Cramps in Voluntary Muscles as a Consequence of a Hereditary Psychic Disposition [Ataxia muscularis?]") was published in 1876 as an indignant response to the accusation that his youngest son, who was afflicted with myotonia, was malingering to avoid military service (Thomsen, 1876). The manuscript had actually been ready for several years but remained unpublished because of the sensitivity with which Thomsen viewed this material.

From his own experience, Thomsen provided a clear, succinct description of myotonia, encompassing all of the clinical manifestations recognized today:

The first signs of this condition became manifest as far as my memory reaches back. Already as a boy it was often impossible for me to get out of a chair when I was called upon unexpectedly; if I got off the seat fast, a tonic cramp of my legs resulted which prevented any attempt at propulsion. If I then gathered all my willpower trying to force my legs to move, I would fall unavoidably and lay for awhile as stiff as a stick, unless I was able to grab support with my hands. Had I time to await the resolution of the cramp then my will would gradually and almost noticeably find its way along the paths of the nerves to the corresponding muscles. When everything was functioning properly again, I was just as swift as boys my age and had better running endurance than others. (Thomsen, 1876, 708)

Elsewhere in his report he identified the nonprogressive nature of the disorder, exacerbation with cold, muscular hypertrophy, and genetic transmission.

Since the functional disturbance involved all of the voluntary muscles and because several of the affected family members suffered from psychosis, Thomsen incorrectly concluded that the condition resulted from a disturbance of the central nervous system. In 1892 he reasserted this view, even though several reports in the interim suggested that the disorder was primarily of muscular origin (Thomsen, 1892). In addition, subsequent authors have argued that the psychiatric symptoms in Thomsen's family were probably unrelated to the muscle disorder and are presently not acknowledged as part of the syndrome, although they can be seen in the related disorder myotonic dystrophy (Nissen, 1934; Johnson, 1968). Nissen studied two additional generations of Thomsen's family and found that 64 out of 315 members were affected. Thomsen had also maintained that the disease was milder in his contemporaries than in earlier generations. However, neither Nissen nor even Eivind Thomasen in his later studies of Julius Thomsen's family (1948) found this to be true. It is now recognized that the symptoms of myotonia congenita are due to intrinsic muscular abnormalities rather than central nervous system dysfunction.

Thomsen traced the disease through five generations in his own family to his maternal great-grandmother, Frederikke Christiane Ludovica (von Grambow) von Barner, who was born in 1742 and is the first person known to have had myotonia (figure 1). Her son, Tugendreich Julius von Barner, was affected only mildly with myotonia. His second child was Thomsen's mother, Henriette, an intelligent and energetic woman who also had mild myotonic symptoms. Thomsen was the oldest of her thirteen children, of whom seven

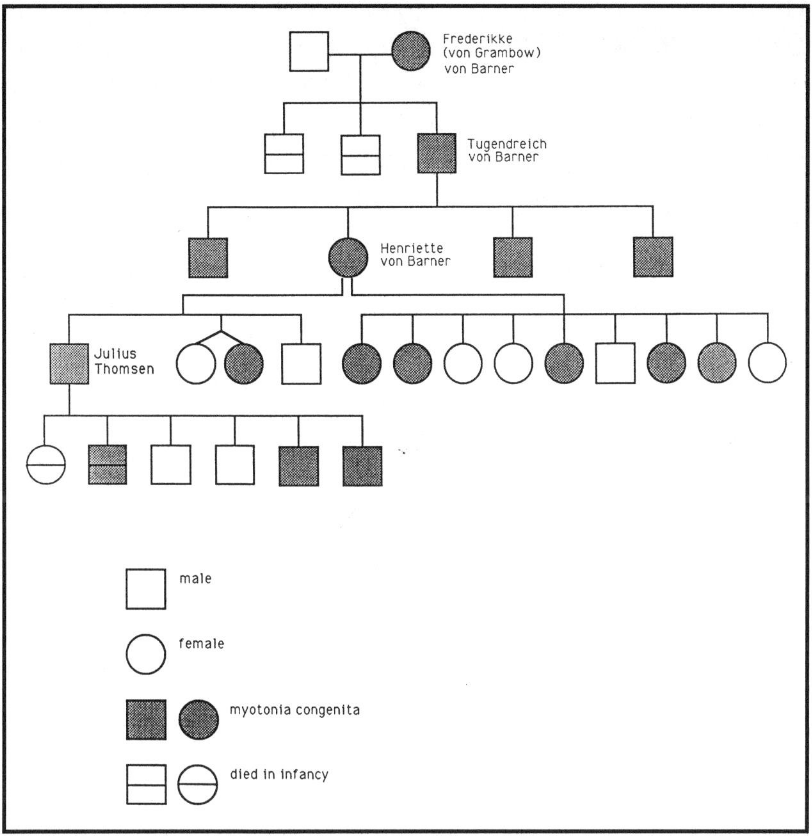

Figure 1. Pedigree of myotonia congenita in Thomsen's family, extracted from Thomsen, 1876, and Nissen, 1923.

were afflicted with myotonia. Thomsen himself had five sons and a daughter. One son died in infancy, having already exhibited symptoms of myotonia. Three of the other boys were also affected, the younger two severely so. The Thomsen pedigree was subsequently expanded by Nissen (1923, 1934) and Thomasen (1948).

Thomsen's original designation for his disorder, "ataxia muscularis," was not widely accepted, since it suggested a disturbance of coordination that is not present. Later, the condition was called myotonia congenita by Adolf Strümpell, and Thomsen's disease by Carl Westphal (Thomsen, 1892). In 1886 Wilhelm Erb published an exhaustive clinical description of this disorder in his classic monograph *Die Thomsen'sche Krankheit (Myotonia Congenita)*, which was written in celebration of the five-hundred-year jubilee of

Heidelberg University. Both Steinert (1909) in Germany and Frederick Batten and H. P. Gibb (1909) in England helped further delineate this disorder (Dubowitz, 1980). However, no greater work appeared on this disease until that of Nissen (1923), a grandnephew of Thomsen, who wrote on the genetics of this disorder and clarified the observations that many patients with Thomsen disease did not have behavior or cognitive impairments, as Thomsen originally suggested. Thomsen disease is among the few conditions in which the eponym applies to the person who both described the disease and suffered from it.

In addition to his medical contributions, Thomsen was a gifted poet. He published a number of original poems, several of which were set to music by Marschner (Johnson, 1968). Some of these contain disguised references to his muscular affliction, an "evil" that plagued him until his death in 1896 at the age of eighty-one.

Mary Jo Lanska

Douglas J. Lanska

Bernd Remler

CLEVELAND, OHIO

REFERENCES

Dubowitz, V. 1980. History of Muscle Disease. In *Historical Aspects of the Neurosciences. A Festschrift for Macdonald Critchley*, 213–22. Ed. F. C. Rose and W. F. Bynum. New York: Raven Press.

Erb, W. 1886. *Die Thomsen'sche Krankheit (Myotonia Congenita)*. Leipzig: F. C. W. Vogel.

Eulenberg, A. 1886. Über eine familiäre, durch 6 Generationem verfolghare Form congenitaler Paramyotonie. *Neur Centralbl* 5:265.

Hirsch, A. 1887. *Biographisches Lexikon der hervorragenden Aerzte aller Zeiten und Voelker*. Wien and Leipzig: Urban and Schwarzenberg.

Johnson, J. 1968. Thomsen and Myotonia Congenita. *Med Hist* 12:190–94.

Nissen, K. 1923. Beiträge zur Kenntnis der Thomsen'schen Krankheit (Myotonia congenita) mit besonderer Berücksichtigung des hereditären Momentes und seinen Beziehungen zu den Mendelschen Vererbungsregeln. *Zeit klin Med* 97:58–93.

______. 1934. Über der Erbgang der Myotonia congenita. *Verh dtsch Ges Med* 46:108–12.

Steinert, H. 1909. Myopathologischge Beiträge: I. Über das klinische und anatomische Bild des Muskelschwunds der Myotoniker. *Dtsch Zeit Nervenheilk* 37:58.

Thomasen, E. 1948. *Myotonia: Thomsen's Disease (Myotonia congenita), Paramyotonia, and Dystrophia Myotonica: A Clinical and Heredobiologic Investigation.* Copenhagen: Ejnar Munksgaard.

Thomsen, A. J. T. 1876. Tonische Krämpfe in willkürlich beweglichen Muskeln in Folge von erebter psychischer Disposition. (Ataxia muscularis?). Arch Psych Nervenkrankh 6:702–18.

______. 1892. Nachtraegliche Bemerkungen über Myotonia congenita (Strümpell), Thomsen'sche Krankheit (Westphal). *Arch Psych Nervenkrankh* 24:918–23.

HEINRICH UNVERRICHT

HEINRICH UNVERRICHT (1853–1912) (figure 1) was born in Breslau, Germany, where he remained for his undergraduate and graduate education. As a medical student, he wrote an award-winning thesis in 1877, "Studies on Pneumonia" (Schreiber, 1912). On April 23, 1883, he received his doctorate after publishing "Experimental and Clinical Studies on Epilepsy." In this fundamental paper, he concluded that all epileptic activity originated from the cortex and thus challenged the then prevalent view of Adolf Kussmaul and Hermann Nothangel that the seat of origin of epilepsy was in the medulla and pons (Unverricht, 1897). Unverricht demonstrated, through his experiments on dogs, that motor cortex was necessary for the origin and propagation of epileptic activity and that a seizure could be provoked by cortical stimulation. He also recognized that morphine had no effect on seizures, that chloral hydrate was the treatment of choice, and that the effects of chloroform and ether were temporary but effective. His doctoral thesis drew considerable attention and led to his appointment in 1886 as professor extraordinary and director of the Medical

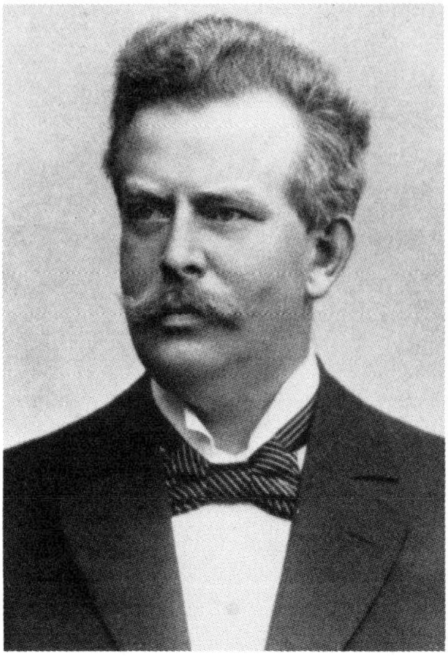

Figure 1. Heinrich Unverricht (1853–1912).

Polyclinic at the University of Jena (Obituary, 1912). In 1889 Unverricht became professor of internal medicine at the University of Dorpat, now in Estonia, where he remained for three years. It was there that his career as a teacher and researcher reached its pinnacle. He was perceived as a captivating and intriguing speaker and attracted as many as two hundred students to his lectures.

Unverricht continued his experimental work in epilepsy, but his most widely recognized contribution to child neurology was his description of progressive myoclonic epilepsy as a distinct clinical entity. He reported a detailed study of a familial degenerative disease characterized by myoclonic jerks and tonic-clonic seizures (Unverricht, 1891). In a family of eleven children born to healthy parents, four girls and a boy were afflicted by this malady. There was no family history of mental illness, epilepsy, or consanguinity. In all five children the disease evolved in a similar fashion, beginning between the ages of six and thirteen. Nocturnal generalized epileptic seizures were the first symptom. During the first year, the seizures occurred once a month. Over the following three years, there was a gradual increase in seizure frequency and, in the fourth year, the disease entered a new phase. The children developed myoclonia, which Unverricht described as lightning-like, arrhythmic, and asynchronous, with asymmetric muscle contractions involving the face, trunk, and extremities. Myoclonus occurred mainly during the day but occasionally was observed while the child was asleep. It was markedly enhanced by emotional excitement and intentional movement, and affected all aspects of voluntary activity, interfering with speech, swallowing, climbing stairs, writing, drawing, and playing the piano. For the girls, sewing was particularly difficult. Despite the progression of the disease, the intellect was spared in all affected children. Unverricht remarked about the poor prognosis regarding recovery and treatment. Herman Lundborg (1868–1943) reviewed the literature, reported several other cases, confirmed that myoclonic epilepsy was a progressive disorder and that its mode of inheritance was autosomal recessive (Lundborg, 1903).

There is a tendency by some to put Unverricht's and Lundborg's patients in separate groups because of the erroneous impression that Lundborg's patients had a milder course, more pronounced dementia, and increased longevity. In fact, dementia was not as marked a feature as Lundborg initially perceived it to be in his original cases. Also, only five out of eighteen of Lundborg's patients survived beyond age fifty. While it is not known how long Unverricht's patients lived, subsequent experience has shown that progression of this disease and survival vary greatly, even within the same family. Lundborg himself correctly considered his and Unverricht's patients as suffering from the same disease, which he called Unverricht's myoclonie. Furthermore, geographic distribution of the disease suggests that the cases of Unverricht and Lundborg may have had common ancestral origin (Norio, 1979). Unverricht's two families were Estonians, whereas Lundborg's patients were from a small rural area in Sweden. Both Estonia and Sweden are neighboring countries of Finland, where this disease is most prevalent. It is claimed that original ancestors of the Finns came from Estonia some two thousand years ago. The Swedes, as neighbors, have had contacts with both the Finns and Estonians. Thus, the gene for Unverricht-Lundborg myoclonic epilepsy in these three countries could very well have the same origin. It is because of this geographic preponderance that the disease is also referred to as Baltic/Nordic myoclonus.

Gonzalo Lafora described a seventeen-year-old boy who developed progressive dementia, epileptic seizures, and intense myoclonus (1911). Unique intracytoplasmic inclusions were found throughout the central nervous system at autopsy. The inclusions, known as Lafora bodies, consist largely of polyglucosans, are periodic acid-Schiff positive, and also are present in the liver, skeletal muscle, cardiac muscle, and skin. Compared to Unverricht-Lundborg myoclonic epilepsy, the onset of symptoms in Lafora disease is later, typically at eleven to eighteen years; behavioral and psychotic symptoms are more common; progressive dementia is universal; and prognosis is dismal, with death occurring two to ten years after disease onset.

Progressive myoclonic epilepsies are a heterogeneous group of disorders, resembling each other only superficially. A specific etiologic diagnosis is possible in many cases. In Unverricht-Lundborg disease, the biochemical cause is unknown and histology shows only nonspecific degenerative neuronal changes. Nevertheless, the concept of Unverricht-Lundborg myoclonic epilepsy as a distinct entity is now widely accepted.

Although from a very early stage in his career Unverricht took a special interest in epilepsy, he also wrote several original papers on more familiar topics, including the pathophysiology of pneumothorax, diseases of the pleura and diaphragm, and fever as it relates to polymyositis (Wenzel, 1912). He is also credited for coining the term dermatomyositis (McHenry, 1969).

In 1893 Unverricht left the University of Dorpat for political reasons to become director of a general hospital in Magdeburg-Sudenburg. Much to his regret, administrative demands left him little time to pursue his research. He served this institution until his retirement in 1911. During this time he founded the Magdeburg Medical Society and became its president. He also served as editor of the *Centralblatt für Innere Medizin* for eighteen years and edited the journal with great skill and diligence.

Unverricht was a keen observer, a good experimental researcher, and an excellent teacher. He died of hemiplegia complicating chronic nephritis on April 22, 1912, at the age of fifty-nine.

Svinder S. Toor
NORFOLK, VIRGINIA

REFERENCES

Lafora, G. R., and B. Glueck. 1911. Beitrag zur Histopathologie der myoklonischen Epilepsie (Unverricht's Myoclonie). *Zeit Neur Psych* 6:1–14.

Lundborg, H. 1903. *Die progressive Myoklonus-Epilepsie* (*Unverricht's Myklonie*). Uppsala: Almquist & Wiksell's Buchdruckerria.

McHenry, L. C., Jr., 1969. *Garrison's History of Neurology*. Springfield, IL: Charles C Thomas.

Norio, R., and M-L. Koskiniemi. 1979. Progressive Myoclonus Epilepsy: Genetic and Neurological Aspects with Special Reference to 107 Finnish Patients. *Clin Genet* 15:382–98.

Obituary. 1912. Heinrich Unverricht. *Boston Med Surg J* 166:910.

Schreiber. 1912. Heinrich Unverricht. *Dtsch med Wschr* 38:1294.

Unverricht, H. 1891. *Die Myoclonie*. Wien: F. Deuticke.

______. 1895. Über familiare Myoclonie. *Dtsch Zeit Nervenheilk* 7:32.

______. 1897. Über die epilepsie. *Samml klin Vortr inn Med* 196:1057–82.

Wenzel, G. 1912. In Memoriam: Heinrich Unverricht. *Centralbl inn Med* 33:445–46.

EUGEN VON HIPPEL

EUGEN VON HIPPEL (1867–1939) (figure 1) was born in Königsberg, Germany. He was the son of Arthur von Hippel, who had developed techniques for the first successful corneal transplant that restored vision, and who had extensively investigated the genetics of congenital color blindness (Pagel, 1901). Von Hippel received his primary education in Königsberg. His secondary education was obtained in the cities of Geissen and Heidelberg, where his father taught and practiced. At the encouragement of his father, Eugen studied medicine in Heidelberg, where his father had become professor of ophthalmology (Baurman, 1939). In 1890 he passed his state board examination and successfully defended his doctoral thesis, "Etiology of Keratitis," before the faculty of the Göttingen Medical School (Pagel, 1901, 740). He then joined Julius Arnold in the Heidelberg Pathological Institute in 1890, but was forced to resign one year later because of severe infection contracted from the cadavers (Baurman, 1939, 632).

In 1892 he joined the staff of the distinguished Professor Theodor Leber in Heidelberg. Leber recognized Von Hippel's assiduous and superior intelligence and promoted him to first assis-

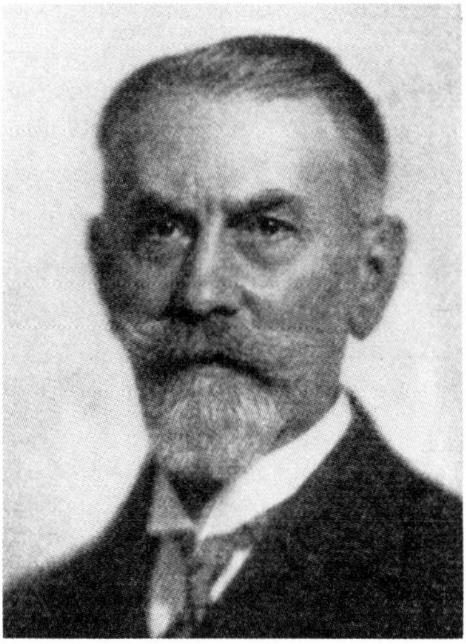

Figure 1. Eugen von Hippel (1867–1939) circa 1919.

tant after a remarkably short period of eighteen months. In 1893 Von Hippel was appointed privat docent, and he began exhaustive experimental research on siderosis of the eye. His research was recognized by the Von Graefe Prize in 1895, and he was subsequently promoted to associate professor in 1897 (Baurman, 1939).

From 1895 to 1904 Von Hippel was concerned with angiomatosis retinae. In 1895 he presented the case of a 23–year-old man to the Heidelberg Ophthalmological Congress (Von Hippel, 1904). The patient noticed dimming of his vision six weeks after falling downstairs on his back. The initial funduscopic examination of the right eye revealed dark red, enlarged, and convoluted veins and arteries, and white glistening flecks by the macula. The funduscopic examination of the left eye was normal. Progressive enlargement of the angioma caused retinal detachment. The macular flecks became confluent, resulting in amaurosis. The lens became opaque, ectopic, buckled, and finally came to rest in the periphery of the cornea. A second patient, aged twenty-eight, initially complained about poor vision in his left eye, and funduscopic examination also revealed a knot of distended veins and arteries (Von Hippel, 1904). The clinical course and funduscopic examination resembled that of the first patient, but this patient also had a conspicuous kyphoscoliosis. Because both patients had osseous disease, Von Hippel erroneously speculated that retinal angiomatosis may have been related to prior tuberculosis.

Perusal of "Über eine Seltene Erkrankung der Netzhaut" ("Concerning a Rare Retinal Disease") reveals Von Hippel's prodigious skills of observation and lucid writing. Unfortunately, he obtained a family history of only one generation. Von Hippel overlooked both the complaints of abdominal pain in a brother and the death due to an "internal disorder" in a sister of the first patient. Perhaps these were cases of pancreatic cysts or neoplasms associated with the Von Hippel-Lindau syndrome (Lindau, 1931).

Arvid Lindau (1892–1958) must be credited for describing the autosomal dominant inheritance of angiomatosis retinae, the presence of intracranial hemangiomatosis, and pancreatic and renal cysts (Lindau, 1926). Lindau recognized the association of angiomatosis retinae with adrenal neoplasms (pheochromocytomas), hypernephromas and cystic tumors of the cerebellum (Lindau, 1927). Lindau dismissed the association with Von Hippel and credited Treacher Collins with describing angiomatosis retinae in 1893 (Lindau, 1931).

In 1905 Von Hippel began experimental and clinical research significant to child neurology in the area of congenital ocular malformations. He described the pathological anatomy of keratopia and congenital corneal defects. Von Hippel induced lid colobomas, stars, lenticular opacities, and microophthalmia by irradiating the fetuses of gravid rabbits (Von Hippel, 1907). He concluded that radiation given at various times would produce different defects owing to its effect of inhibiting further development of the eye at different stages of embryogenesis. He suggested that no pregnant woman receive a roentgen examination, or if absolutely necessary, lead shielding be used. These recommendations are still followed today to prevent ocular malformations and cataracts.

In 1909 Von Hippel was appointed full professor at Halle, where his father had been professor and the successor to Albrecht von Graefe. At Halle, Von Hippel developed methods to treat glaucoma with trephining. He also published articles on the detailed anatomy of angiomatosis retinae. Von Hippel was later appointed professor at Göttingen in 1915, where he remained until his death. There he published articles on sympathetic ophthalmia, tuberculosis of the eye, and ocular malformations (Baurman, 1939).

Von Hippel's great success as an original investigator, exceptional physician, and able administrator reflected enormous energy and organizational skills, and an uncanny ability to perceive rapidly the essence of every problem. Somewhat reserved and given only to speaking when spoken to, he superficially appeared taciturn and even aloof. But all those who knew him beyond a casual acquaintance experienced his "deeply felt interest and concern" (Baurman,

1939). He had an extraordinary capacity to discover the interests of his house staff and colleagues and thus place them in the most challenging situations in the experimental laboratory or in the clinics. He was able to inculcate his students to adopt his rigorous approach to research and motivated them to assess their own work critically.

His clinics provided rich experiences for his house staff, enabling them to become adroit surgeons but also to investigate any clinical or experimental problem. Many of his graduates eventually became professors of ophthalmology.

Von Hippel inspired all of his colleagues and employees to provide the highest quality services to patients through his example of indefatigable concern for excellence in patient care and teaching. He kept instruction free of dogmatism by completely revising his lectures each year. Thus he always maintained "a spontaneous personal dialogue between a teacher who was willing to give and a student desiring to learn" (Baurman, 1939).

Von Hippel died July 5, 1939, at age seventy-one, shortly after he had retired from teaching and practice. Reflection upon Von Hippel's accomplishments, his clinical skills, ingenuity, and humanistic qualities affirmed the praise rendered in his obituary. His death was represented as "an irreplaceable loss," and those who knew him well reserved "eternal gratitude for him" (Baurman, 1939).

Edward J. Fine
BUFFALO, NEW YORK

REFERENCES

Baurman, A. 1939. Offene Korrespondenz. *Klin Mbl Augenh* 103:632–34.

Lindau, A. 1926. Studien über Kleinhirncysten: Bau, Pathogenesis, und Beziehungen zur Angiomatosis retinae. *Acta Path Microbiol Scand* 1(Suppl.):3–128.

______. 1927. Zur Frage der Anglomatosis retinae, und ihrer Hirnkomplicationen. *Acta Ophthal* 4:193–226.

______. 1931. Discussion on Vascular Tumors of the Brain and Spinal Cord. *Proc Roy Soc Med* 24:363–70.

Pagel, J. 1901. *Biographische Lexikon der Hervorragender Aerzte der Neunzehnten Jahrhunderts*, 739–40. Leipzig und Wien: Urban and Schwarzenberg.

Von Hippel, E. 1904. Über eine Seltene Erkrankung der Netzhaut: Klinische Beobachtungen. *Graefe Arkiv Ophthal* 59:83–10.

______. 1907. Über experimentelle Erzeugung von angeboren Star bei Kaninchen nebst Bemerkungen über gleichzeitig beobachteten Mikrophthalamus und lidcolobom. *Graefe Arkiv Ophthal* 65:326–60.

FRIEDRICH DANIEL VON RECKLINGHAUSEN

LITTLE IS KNOWN of the childhood of Friedrich von Recklinghausen (1833–1910) (figure 1), except that his family was of modest means and he grew up in Gütersloh, a community in an agricultural area of Westphalia, Prussia. The streams around Gütersloh may have provided his first exposure to fishing. Angling was a major avocation later in his life and may well have led to the story, probably apocryphal, that the first subject he dissected with multiple peripheral nerve tumors was a fish. Recklinghausen's mother died when he was an infant. His father was a teacher in a Protestant parochial school and, as was a tradition in the von Recklinghausen family, he was active in the political life of the community. The senior Recklinghausen was quite conservative and lost elections for mayor because of his social attitudes. His bitterness over having been rejected for the mayoral post remained with him until his death, when young Friedrich was but nineteen years old (Mortier, personal communication, 1988).

Much of Friedrich's higher education therefore took place after the death of both parents. After graduation from gymnasium in Bielefeld, Recklinghausen entered the Bonn medical school in 1852, matriculating for only one semester before transferring to Würzburg. After five semesters at Würzburg, he finished medical school in Berlin at the age of twenty-two. His thesis, "Theories of Pyaemia," was written in Latin. He continued at the Pathological Institute of Berlin as an assistant to the master pathologist, Rudolf

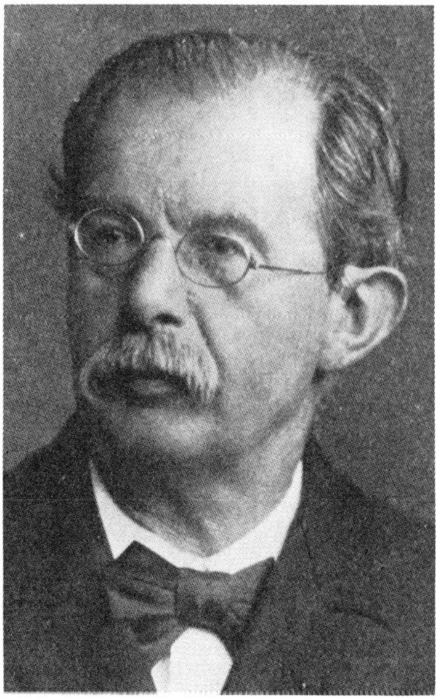

Figure 1. Friedrich Daniel von Recklinghausen (1833–1910).

Virchow. Except for brief sojourns in Vienna, Rome, and Paris, he remained under Virchow's tutelage for nine years.

Virchow took a special interest in Recklinghausen, not only because he recognized the young man's talent, but because he realized that Recklinghausen had almost no financial backing and might therefore be forced out of research (Remark, 1938). How important Virchow's influence was in Recklinghausen's meteoric rise from assistant to the professorial chair of pathology at the University of Königsberg in 1864 is not known. Recklinghausen's first major monograph, *Die Lymphgefasse und ihre beziehungen zum Bindegewebe* (*The Lymphatic Vessels and Their Significance in Connective Tissue*) (Recklinghausen, 1862), along with Virchow's influence, must have played an important role. Recklinghausen held the position in Königsberg only a few months before he was offered and accepted the chair at Würzburg, Bavaria. In 1872 he was appointed chairman of pathology at the newly founded University of Strasbourg in Alsace. He assembled a very productive and highly respected faculty at that institution and drew graduate students from all over Europe as well as the United States. He was named rector of the university in 1877 and remained in Strasbourg for the rest of his life.

Recklinghausen's scientific contributions were extensive, not only in pathology but also in biochemistry and physiology. In addition to his interest in the lymphatic system, he published papers on fat absorption, hemochromatosis (he coined the term), vascular disease, uterine myomas, and parasitic diseases. In the past his name has been associated eponymically with the bone disease associated with hyperparathyroidism (*Festschrift*, 1891), although only one of the sixteen patients he described in 1891 had hyperparathyroidism (Warkany, 1981).

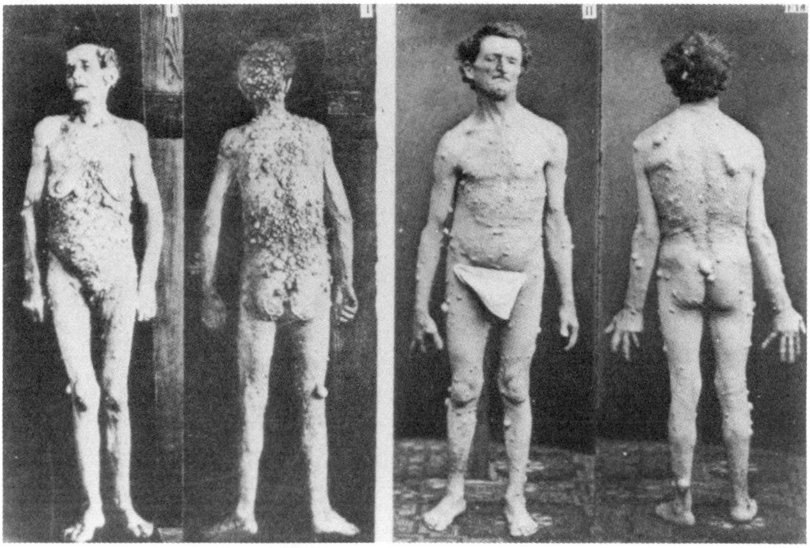

Figure 2. Two patients described by Recklinghausen in his monograph *Über die multiplen Fibrome der Haut und ihre Beziehung zu den multiplen Neuromen* (1882).

For child neurology, Recklinghausen's name is closely associated with neurofibromatosis. Recklinghausen's paper on multiple neuromas was presented as part of a festschrift honoring Virchow; his article described two patients (figure 2) (Recklinghausen, 1882). The first case was an autopsy on a 55-year-old woman, Frau Kientz, who had a "dirty brown color of her skin," as well as numerous brown spots and cutaneous tumors. Recklinghausen noted that the woman suffered from sexual excesses and was married twice. Although she bore eleven children, none were alive at the time she died. He was aware of the possibility of a familial disease, since he took the trouble to examine the brother of Frau Kientz, whom he described as having no spots but two possible fibromas. The second patient was a 47-year-old man who was alive at the time of the report and whose mother was similarly affected. Although similar patients had been reported as early as 1849, Recklinghausen reported the neural contribution to the tumors, which had not been previously described (Wilson, 1940).

In retrospect, Recklinghausen's most notable contribution to child neurology may have been his monograph on spina bifida (Recklinghausen, 1886). Recklinghausen is credited with defining the various types of spina bifida deformities and classifying them

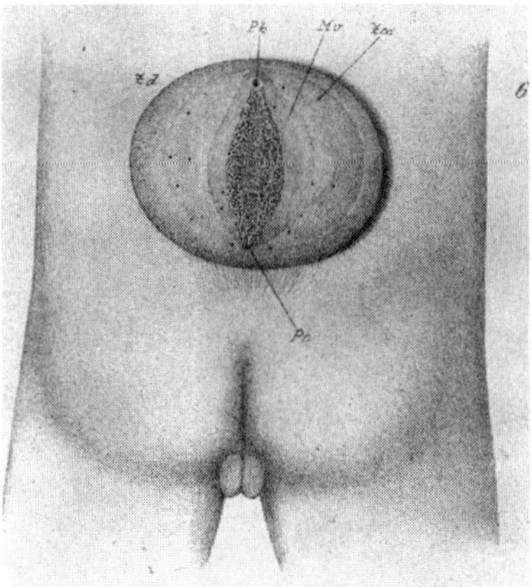

Figure 3a. Figure 6 from the *Untersuchungen über die Spina Bifida*, showing a young child with a meningomyelocele.

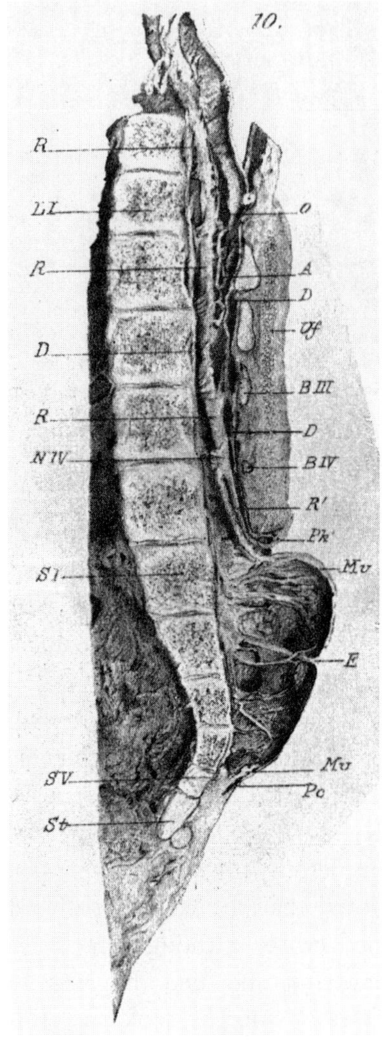

Figure 3b. Figure 10 from the same work, showing a sagittal view of a patient with a meningomyelocele.

according to the contents of the sac (figures 3a, b). Warkany et al. in 1958 defined the state of rachischisis by studying the morphogenesis of meningomyelocele in experimental animals. Warkany discovered, with considerable chagrin, that Recklinghausen, some seventy-two years previously, had come to almost identical conclusions after careful dissection of human material (Warkany, 1981). Such thoroughness in his researches is not surprising when one learns of Recklinghausen's scientific approach. He wrote, "I do not know how to spare myself. I have a duty and principle to research to the roots." He detested superficiality and dilettantism, as exemplified by his statement, "Whoever wants to be conversant with everything ends up being mediocre and a parrot-like repeater of conventional wisdom" (Remark, 1938).

Other insights into the personality of Recklinghausen written in English are limited to Warkany's somewhat whimsical biography (Warkany, 1981). Warkany drew a picture of an aloof and reluctant teacher. A biography of William "Popsy" Welch (Fleming, 1954), the noted Johns Hopkins pathologist who studied under Recklinghausen in Strasbourg, supplied evidence for this conclusion. Welch was initially rejected by Recklinghausen because he was not "advanced" enough. After finally securing the position, Welch was quoted as saying that Recklinghausen "practiced an almost total want of supervision." On those occasions when Recklinghausen did speak to Welch, the former would "convey some of the barely articulate wisdom that craftsmen of all kinds transmit by word of mouth or not at all." A possible explanation for this negative impression of Recklinghausen may be the effect of the liberal agitation for individual freedom going on within Germany at the time. Within scientific circles, the expression of this social movement resulted in the concept that scientific creativity was best served by the dictum "almost not to teach and never to force." A contrasting view of Recklinghausen's teaching was provided by Bernard Sachs, who also studied in Strasbourg and described the pathologist as "a vivacious and inspiring little man" (Haymaker, 1970).

Warkany also conveyed the impression that, to a certain extent, Recklinghausen's professional advance was aided by the fact that the pathologist distanced himself from the political and social turmoil rampant in Germany. Recklinghausen is compared unfavorably with his mentor Virchow. Virchow was a firebrand liberal who eventually ran for public office. Warkany points out with some relish that Virchow rejected the nobility's honorary title of "von". The implication is unjustified, since the "von" in von Recklinghausen's name indicates that the family came "from" the town of Recklinghausen and probably was acquired during the thirteenth century (Mortier, personal communication, 1988). But Recklinghausen was not immune from political struggles. During his early professional career, the political upheaval in part concerned the unification of Germany led by Protestant Prussia under Bismarck. Recklinghausen found himself a Prussian in Catholic Bavaria (between 1865 and 1872), where sentiment favored Austrian leadership in German unification. Recklinghausen thus experienced tension in his relationships with his Bavarian hosts (E. R., 1903). He met, in a nonconspiratorial fashion, and found solace with his

Prussian comrades in the local pub, which was nicknamed "Die Pickelhaube" — The Prussian Helmet. In 1866 Prussia went to war against Austria, and Bavaria sided with Austria. The Austrians were literally outgunned, pitting their old muzzle-loaded rifles against the newer Prussian breach-loaded variety. The war was mercifully short and became known as the Seven Weeks War. Bavaria eventually joined the German Empire in 1870.

In 1871, as a result of the war with France, Germany gained control of Alsace. Almost immediately, the German government established a new university at Strasbourg where Recklinghausen accepted the challenge by becoming the first chairman of pathology. In 1884 he was offered a prestigious chairmanship at the University of Leipzig, made vacant by the death of Cornheim. He turned the position down, in part, because he felt it was his patriotic duty to remain in Strasbourg (Remark, 1938). Recklinghausen may not have been a liberal, and he undoubtedly was not an activist, but he had a sincere commitment to the emerging German nation. He was also revered by most of his former students and colleagues, as evidenced by the flowery language, even by German standards, seen in German language journals celebrating his seventieth birthday (E. R., 1903). Recklinghausen died at the age of seventy-seven on August 25, 1910, after a brief illness associated with heart failure "ohne schweres Leiden" — without severe pain (Chiari, 1912).

Michael Blaw
DALLAS, TEXAS

ACKNOWLEDGMENTS

The author wishes to thank Ms. Kathy Rapport for help in translation, Mr. Mike Riedel for insights into the historical perspectives, and Professor Wilhelm and Dr. Roswitha Mortier of West Germany for providing literature not readily available.

REFERENCES

Chiari, H. 1912. Friedrich Daniel v. Recklinghausen. *Verh dtsch path Ges* 15:478–88.

E.R. 1903. Friedrich v. Recklinghausen. *Münch med Wschr* 50:2103–2105.

______. 1891. *Festschrift für Rudolf E. Virchow zu seinem 71. Geburststage gewidmet von den früheren und jetzigen Assistenten des Berliner Pathologischen Instituts.* Berlin: Reimer.

Fleming, D. 1954. *William H. Welch and the Rise of Modern Medicine.* Boston: Little Brown and Company.

Haymaker, W. 1970. Friedrich von Recklinghausen, 514. In *Founders of Neurology*. Ed. W. Haymaker and F. Schiller. 2d ed. Springfield, IL: Charles C Thomas.

Mortier, R. 1988. Personal Communication. Dr. Roswitha Mortier of Wuppertal, West Germany, provided information gained from Mr. Grimes, archivist of Gütersloh.

Recklinghausen, F. D. von. 1862. *Die Lymphgefasse und ihre beziehungen zum Bindegewebe.* Berlin: August Hirschwald.

______. 1882. *Über die multiplen Fibrome der Haut und ihre Beziehung zu den multiplen Neuromen*. Berlin: August Hirschwald.

______. 1886. *Untersuchungen über die Spina bifida*. Berlin: Druck und Verlag von Georg Reimer.

Remark, J. 1938. *Friedrich Daniel v. Recklinghausen und sein Werk, Dissertations.* Dusseldorf: Verlag G. H. Nolte.

Warkany, J., et al. 1958. Myeloschisis and Myelomeningocele Produced Experimentally in the Rat. *J Comp Neur* 109:35–64

Warkany J. 1981. Friedrich Daniel von Recklinhausen and His Times. In *Advances in Neurology*. Vol. 29, 251–57.

Wilson, S. A. K. 1940. *Textbook of Neurology.* Vol. 2, 1326. London: Williams and Wilkins.

GUIDO WERDNIG

GUIDO WERDNIG'S (1844–1919) (figure 1) name is connected with the disease first described by him in 1891, the infantile form of progressive spinal muscular atrophy, known today as Werdnig-Hoffmann disease. Werdnig himself was hardly known during his

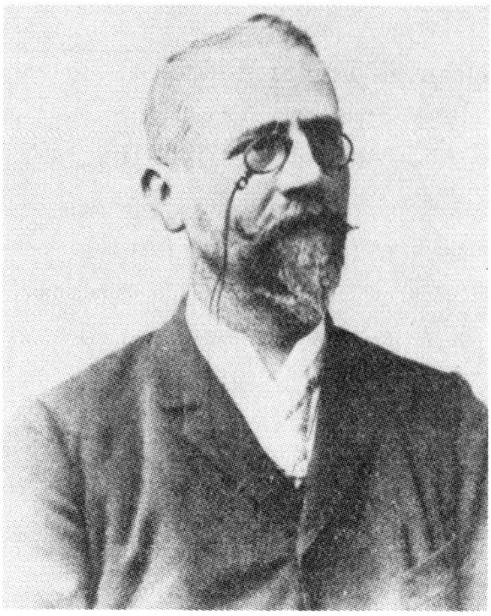

Figure 1. Guido Werdnig (1844–1919).

lifetime, and little information about him is available despite access to family documents (Beighton and Beighton, 1986; Pakesch, 1965). He was born the son of Anton Werdnig, a civil servant in the Austro-Hungarian Empire, on June 20, 1844, at Ratschach in the district of Krain (Slovenia), which is today part of Yugoslavia. He attended grammar school at Cilli (now Celje), from which he graduated with honors in 1862. He began his medical studies in 1863 at the Joseph Academy, an academy for the training of military physicians founded by Emperor Joseph II in 1785. Werdnig obtained his medical degree in 1868, and joined the army as a military physician, serving for over ten years, first in the rank of senior military physician and then as regiment physician. Military documents show that he was working as a physician with the military during the suppression of a revolt in South Dalmatia and during the occupation of Bosnia. He was first in charge of several military hospitals and then headed the medical training school of his regiment. There is evidence that he was interested in otology at that time. As early as 1870 he published an article, "Über die Mittel zum Transporte der Verwundeten des dalmatin Aufstandeson" ("Means of Transporting the Wounded During the Dalmatian Uprising"), in the *Allgemeine Militararztliche Zeitung*, a journal of military medicine published by Johann Schnitzler in Vienna (Werdnig, 1870). He worked extensively on the problems of improving the transport of wounded troops in mountainous terrain, and wrote two additional articles on this subject (Werdnig, 1874, 1875).

In 1877 Werdnig married Franziska Pummer, and their two children, Gisela and Otto, were born in 1880 and 1885, respectively. After his discharge from the army in 1879, with the rank of battalion physician, Werdnig settled in Vienna as a general practitioner, where he had lived since 1874.

In the course of his work as a physician, Werdnig became increasingly interested in neurology and worked in the laboratory of Heinrich Obersteiner, who founded the Institute of Anatomy and Physiology of the Central Nervous System at the University of Vienna. This center for neurological studies and training of future neurologists soon become recognized throughout the world. It was in that laboratory that Werdnig wrote his first articles on neurology, which were published in the *Medizinische Jahrbücher, Wien* in 1888; the two papers are histopathological studies on disorders of the central nervous system (Werdnig, 1888a, 1888b).

In 1888 Werdnig moved to Graz, where he worked in private practice and continued his scientific studies at the Institute of Pathological Anatomy of the University of Graz. He had contacts with Julius Wagner-Jauregg, who later won the Nobel Prize, and who headed the Department of Neurology and Psychiatry in Graz from 1889 to 1893. Most likely, Werdnig previously knew Wagner-Jauregg from his years in Vienna. Werdnig not only referred patients to the Department of Neurology and Psychiatry, but also examined them at the hospital and thus gained clinical experience in neurology.

On May 12, 1890, at the eighth monthly meeting of the Association of Physicians in Styria, he gave a lecture, "Über einen Fall von Dystrophia musculorum mit positivem Ruckenmarksbefunde" ("On a Case of Muscular Dytrophy with Positive Spinal Cord Findings"), in which he described the basic pattern of the disease that was to bear his name (Werdnig, 1890). The following year Werdnig published his contribution significant for child neurology, "Zwei frühinfantile hereditäre Fälle von progressiver Muskelatrophie unter dem Bilde der Dystrophie, aber auf neurotischer Grundlage" ("Two Early Infantile Hereditary Cases of Progressive Muscular Atrophy Appearing as Dystrophy, but on a Neurotic Basis") in the *Archiv für Psychiatrie und Nervenkrankheiten* published by Theodor Meynert, Vienna (Werdnig, 1891b). In 1894 he published another article on the subject, "Die frühinfantile progressive spinale Amyotrophie" ("On Early Infantile Progressive Spinal Amyotrophy").

Werdnig returned to Vienna in 1896, where he continued to work in private practice but published no further papers. In 1907 he suddenly developed spastic paraplegia of the lower extremities and was bedridden for the next twelve years. After the death of his wife, his daughter cared for him until 1918, when he was hospitalized at the public sanatorium at Steinhof. He died there on April 26, 1919 after many years of suffering, at the age of seventy-five.

In addition to his medical studies, Werdnig was an expert numismatist. In 1889 he published the monograph *Die Osellen oder Münz-Medaillen der Republik Venedig* (*The Coins of the Republic of Venice*), which is considered a classic on the topic (Werdnig, 1889). Werdnig was an accomplished linguist and, in addition to German and Slovene, he also spoke fluent Hungarian, French, and Italian. He loved music and played several instruments.

Werdnig's main contribution to medicine and child neurology was the detection of the infantile form of progressive spinal muscular atrophy. By careful observation and thorough investigation of all aspects, he managed to shed light on this rare disease, which, as he realized, did not fit into existing clinical classifications.

Werdnig began by documenting the case histories of two brothers of healthy parents. He examined one of the two brothers when the child was three years old. At the age of ten months the boy, who had been perfectly healthy until that time, developed progressive muscular weakness in both legs, became obese, and felt flabby. The muscles of the back began to weaken and sitting became increasingly more difficult. The ever-enlarging head could not be held up, and soon voluntary movements of the legs were no longer possible. The hands began to tremble, the boy developed difficulties in swallowing, and the eyes were not completely closed during sleep; patellar biceps and triceps reflexes were gone, but sensitivity was maintained. Some weeks after he had been admitted to the children's hospital, the boy died of pneumonia. Apart from hydrocephalus, pneumonia, and muscular atrophy in the spinal cord, the post-mortem findings showed nothing significant. Werdnig performed detailed histopathological investigations and detected a symmetrical involvement of the entire spinal cord afflicting the anterior gray columns with varying slight involvement of Gowers' tract and degeneration of the anterior roots and simple muscular atrophy. Werdnig managed to prove the hereditary nature of the disease by studying the younger brother, who developed almost identical symptoms at the same age. Two other siblings were not affected. The case history of the younger brother, compiled at the Department of Neurology and Psychiatry of the University Hospital in Graz in 1890, illustrates the problem of differential diagnosis. The original diagnosis of muscular pseudohypertrophy was replaced by one of progressive muscular atrophy, and the patient's history contained no reference to the spinal origin of the disease (figure 2).

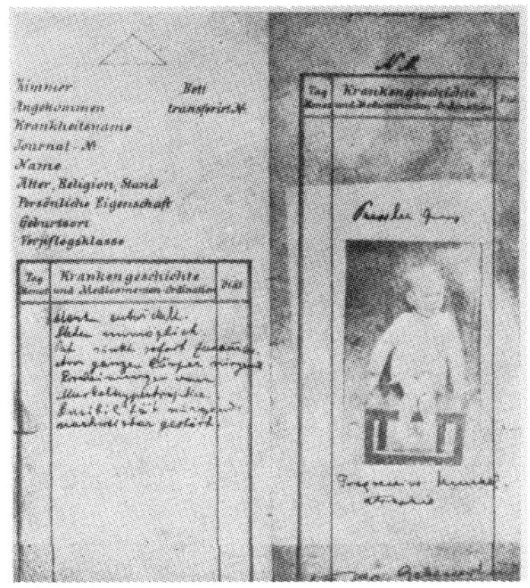

Figure 2. Case history and picture of the child from the University Hospital, Graz, 1890.

Werdnig, however, was familiar with the history of the older brother, and therefore assumed a spinal origin of the disease because of his clinical observations, and stated his belief in a lecture given in 1890 (Werdnig, 1890; 1891a). In his 1891 paper, Werdnig managed to prove this origin of the disease by submitting the detailed histories of the two brothers, an exact description of the histopathological findings of the spinal cord, and a comparison of the two cases regarding electrical excitability, which he had studied together with Wagner-Jauregg (1891b). The histopathological findings were confirmed in his 1894 article, published after the younger brother had died (Werdnig, 1894). In this publication, Werdnig also reported exact histological findings of various muscle groups and peripheral nerves and again confirmed the spinal origin and hereditary nature of the disease, taking into account the cases of the same clinical picture described by Johann Hoffmannn, a German neurologist from the University of Heidelberg (Hoffmann, 1893).

During his lifetime, Werdnig gained little recognition for the detection and description of a previously unknown syndrome. All that is left is a letter dated 1894 by Wagner-Jauregg (Pakesch, 1965), who by then held the chair of neurology and psychiatry at the University of Vienna, addressed to Werdnig, who had sent him his manuscript and the histological sections. Wagner-Jauregg wrote:

I have come to like the distinction of a new type of amyotrophy, which at first I did not quite appreciate, as you have been able to furnish good evidence and to correlate your new form with known types of dystrophy. After having ex-

amined the preparations, I quite agree with you regarding the presentation of the anatomical findings.

I should like to congratulate you on your solid work.

Helmut Groger
VIENNA, AUSTRIA

REFERENCES

Beighton, P. H., and G. J. Beighton. 1986. *The Man Behind the Syndrome*, 192–93. New York: Springer-Verlag.

Hoffmann, J. 1893. Über chronisch spinale Muskelatrophie im Kindesalter auf familiarer Basis. *Dtsch Zeit Nervenheilk* 3:427–70.

Pakesch, E. 1965. Dr. Guido Werdnig, 1894–1919. Ein Nervenarzt in Graz. *Wien klin Wschr* 77:445–47.

Werdnig, G. 1870. Über die Mittel zum Transporte der Verwundeten des dalmatin. Aufstandes. *Allg Militärärztl Zeit* 11:73–76, 81–85.

______. 1874. Über die Mittel zum Transporte im Gebirgskriege. *Allg Militärärztl Zeit* 15:249–51, 265–69, 276–79.

______. 1875. Über ein neuerfundenes Transportmittel für Verwundete im Gebirgskriege. *Allg Militärärztl Zeit* 16:69–73.

______. 1888a. Ein Fall von disseminirter Sclerose des Ruckenmarkes, verbunden mit sekundaren Degenerationen. *Med Jahrb Wien*, n.F. 3:335–50.

______. 1888b. Concrement in der rechten Substantia nigra Sommeringii mit auf-und absteigender Degeneration der Schleife und theilweiser Degeneration des Hirnschenkelfu Bes. *Med Jahrb Wien*, n.F. 3:447–77.

______. 1889. *Die Osellen oder Münz-Medaillen der Republik Venedig*. Wien: W. Frick.

______. 1890. Über einen Fall von Dystrophia musculorum mit positivem Ruckenmarksbefunde. *Wien med Wschr* 40:1796–98.

______. 1891a. Ein Fall von juveniler hereditärer Muskel-Atrophie mit Ruckenmarksbefund. *Mitt Ver Arzte in Steiermark Graz* 27:48–51.

______. 1891b. Zwei frühinfantile hereditäre Fälle von progressiver Muskelatrophie unter dem Bilde der Dystrophie, aber auf neurotischer Grundlage. *Arch Psych Nervenkrankh* 22:437–81.

______. 1894. Die frühinfantile progressive spinale Amyotrophie. *Arch Psych Nervenkrankh* 26:706–44.

The Merging of Pediatrics and Neurology into Child Neurology

THE EARLY TWENTIETH CENTURY

1900 – 1940

OVERVIEW

IN THE LATTER HALF of the nineteenth century the majority of physicians interested in pediatrics, except for a few of the major figures such as Abraham Jacobi, provided services on a part-time basis while still practicing general medicine, obstetrics, or surgery. This changed in the early twentieth century. This generation of pediatricians promoted pediatrics as a completely independent specialty and by the end of World War I "had institutionalized pediatrics as a consulting specialty and secured a favorable position within academic medicine" (Halpern, 1988, 57). Changing attitudes toward specialization contributed to the success of this independence. Opposition from within the medical community concerning specialization was beginning to decline in the early twentieth century. Another important trend was the shift in dominance from hospitals, which were critical for the support of specialists, to medical schools. Medical schools soon controlled the staffing, structure, and census of teaching hospitals. The rise of academic departments promoted research and helped create pediatrics as an independent specialty.

The focus of pediatrics that prompted its rapid growth during the early twentieth century related to both interest in the diseases of children, as well as to preventive medicine and the care of the well child. Although pediatrics was already regarded as a separate field in Europe and England, it was not until this period that it finally achieved recognition in the United States. The child welfare movements throughout France, Germany, England, and the United States prompted government assistance on many fronts and resulted in the establishment of many commissions, committees, organizations, and clinics to provide for the basic needs of children. Pediatricians became active and instrumental in advancing these causes and within time were leaders in advocating, organizing, and delivering this type of health care.

Pediatricians strived not only to be responsible for the care of children with diseases but also to monitor infant feeding and normal childhood growth and development.

Concern with infant mortality and children's diseases that dominated professional rhetoric in the early 1900s gave way to a focus on children's growth and development. . . . What separated the pediatrician from his medical colleagues was knowledge about children's physical growth and mental development. . . . The specialty's new domain included nothing short of the normative regulation of childhood. (Halpern, 1988, 96)

The social reform and public health movement of the late nineteenth and early twentieth century had established free infant care clinics and milk stations that parents were encouraged to use. These clinics, funded privately or by the government, were administered by pediatricians and nurses. Parents began consulting pediatricians in public clinics on a regular basis. While this is common today, during this period it was a dramatic innovation. As this practice became socially acceptable and eventually perceived as necessary, pediatricians began to see more and more patients in their private, more efficient offices. By the 1930s, about 30 to 40 percent of pediatric practice was devoted to well-baby care and full-time office-based pediatrics was emerging as a discrete career (Halpern, 1988, 92). By 1930 there were over fifteen hundred infant clinics in American cities. This is quite astounding when one considers that there were probably less than fifty pediatricians at the turn of the century.

A major factor in developing autonomy was the organization of the American Board of Pediatrics in 1933, which assumed responsibility for the establishment of training programs and certification. This was necessary because more physicians were now involved in direct primary pediatric care due to the rising demand for pediatric services, which were relegated mainly to the private-practice office setting. Parents began consulting child specialists in unprecedented numbers.

As outlined by Sydney Halpern, several major trends were implemented by pediatricians during this period. First, pediatricians systematized the techniques of well-child care and rendered child health supervision a recognizable component of the profession. Second, specialists brought this new service directly into the domain of pediatrics. Third, pediatricians transferred the practice of child health care from public clinics to both private medical offices and hospital-based practices. Fourth, pediatric leaders established formal certification and training programs that set certain standards to represent what they regarded as appropriate pediatric care. (Halpern, 1988, 94). With the proliferation of hospital-based residencies, young physicians no longer found dispensary appointments to be highly attractive. University-based clinics began to take over a lot of these infant-welfare clinics, and restrictions on the clientele visiting such facilities began to be implemented. It was at this time that pediatricians showed greater interest in the medical problems of the newborn, exemplified by the development of incubators, and slowly began to assume medical responsibility for their care from obstetricians.

PEDIATRICS

The numerous gains in pediatrics during the first half of the twentieth century are best reflected by the decline in the infant mortality rate from 165 per 1000 in 1900 to 26 per 1000 in 1955. Many of these clinical advances occurred in the field of infectious disease. The infectivity of poliomyelitis was demonstrated by serial passage of the virus in monkeys (1909). Clemens von Pirquet first demonstrated the delayed hypersensitivity reaction to intradermal tuberculin protein (1907) followed thirty years later by the more specific purified protein derivative (PPD) skin test. In the interim, the B.C.G. vaccine was introduced by Albert Calmette and Alphonse Guérin for the prevention of tuberculosis. Isolation of what is now called the Bordetella pertussis bacillus by Jules Bordet and Octave Gengou (1905) was soon was followed by the development of the pertussis vaccine by Louis Sauer (1926–33). Emil von Behring developed the diphtheria toxin-antitoxin immunization in 1912; this was later replaced by the safer toxoid vaccine. The investigations of Gaston Ramon from 1936 to 1947 led to the formulation of combined immunizations for diphtheria, polio, and tetanus. In the 1930s the relation between hemolytic streptococcal throat infection and acute rheumatic fever was established, and T. Duckett Jones introduced criteria for the diagnosis of rheumatic fever in 1944.

Perhaps the most important advance of this period was the introduction of antibiotics. Gerhard Domagk and his colleagues in Germany showed Prontosil's effectiveness against hemolytic streptococcal infections (1935). In France the active chemotherapeutic component of Prontosil was found to be sulfanilamide. Within a short period of time, Ernest Fourneau at the Pasteur Institute in Paris and Leonard Colebrook in England found these drugs to be effective against puerperal sepsis and meningococcal infections, and Coburn demonstrated their usefulness for rheumatic fever prophylaxis (1939). The discovery of penicillin by Alexander Fleming (1928) and its first clinical application in an Oxford policeman with staphylococcal septicemia on February 12, 1941, was the beginning of a momentous era in antibiotic research and therapeutics.

Gastrointestinal disease and infant nutrition also were intensively studied. These areas benefitted both from improvements in technology as well as the institutionalization of active clinical and basic science research programs, typified in the United States by the centers of L. Emmett Holt at Babies Hospital in New York and John Howland at Johns Hopkins. Some of the more important clinical investigations of this era were the studies of John Howland and William McKim Marriott, who proved that the major complications seen in infantile gastroenteritis were due to acidosis and dehydration (1920), and disproved other long-held theories of intestinal intoxication. These studies and those of James Gamble introduced a more rigorous and beneficial approach to fluid replacement therapy that has saved the lives of countless children. Soybean was introduced as a formula substitute by John Ruhräh. In 1912 Casimir Funk proposed the idea that diseases such as beriberi, scurvy, pellagra, and possibly rickets were due to a dietary deficiency of "vitamines." Over the next twenty-five years vitamins A, B, C, D, and E were identified, as were their biological properties and therapeutic benefits. It was also at this time that the relation between rickets and hypocalcemia was determined. The establishment of milk stations, certification and pasteurization of milk, and the opening of infant health care stations, gradually reduced the summer epidemics of diarrhea and the overall mortality from malnutrition. For the acutely ill child, rehydration was accomplished primarily by oral or intraperitoneal infusion; it was only much later that intravenous therapy was used.

Spurred by the development of the concept of hormones by William Bayliss and Ernest Starling (1902–1906), and by the discovery of insulin in 1921 by Frederick Banting and Charles Best, and its effectiveness in juvenile diabetes (1923), endocrinology developed as a subspecialty of pediatrics. Thyroxin was isolated and investigated by Edward Kendall (1913), and dessicated thyroid was used for the treatment of sporadic cretinism.

Interest in the medical problems of the preterm infant became more than just a curiosity. This interest was stimulated by the technological breakthroughs in environmental control and improved feeding methods that shifted care of the newborn from obstetrics to pediatrics. In France, Germany, and Austria, a great deal of investigation was already in progress. The incubator was developed by Stéphane Tarnier, a French obstetrician in 1889, and was improved upon by Thomas Morgan Rotch (1903); Julius Hess (1914); and Charles Chapple (1938), who added temperature and humidity controls and portholes for handling the infant. Vitamin K was introduced for the treatment of hemorrhagic disease of the newborn in 1939.

The area of environmental toxicology also evolved, as seen in the studies concerning acute and chronic lead poisoning in the first half of this century, followed by those on mercury poisoning and acrodynia (1948), and Minamata disease (1960). Preventive pediatrics and concerns about educational reforms also drew more widespread interest. The first public dental clinics were begun in Strasbourg and Darmstadt in 1902. The first International Congress on School Hygiene was held in Nuremburg in 1904 and the second in London in 1907. The Depression and World War II had a profound worldwide effect on the health of children. In spite of tremendous global socioeconomic and political turmoil, however, pediatric research continued and the care of children increasingly gained priority in subsequent decades.

The growth of pediatrics also was reflected in the continued growth of pediatric organizations, journals, and books in both general pediatrics and subspecialties. Thomas Cone in his *History of American Pediatrics* (1979) listed twenty new pediatric texts published from 1900 to 1925. In the United States, three new journals were established: the *American Journal of Diseases of Children* (1911), the *Journal of Pediatrics* (1932), and *Pediatrics* (1948). These continue to attract a wide variety of readers and topics that reflect all areas of pediatrics. The American Academy of Pediatrics was founded in 1930, followed in 1933 by the establishment of the American Board of Pediatrics. Similar developments occurred throughout Europe and England; the Société de Pédiatrie de Paris formed in 1899 and the British Paediatric Association was founded in 1928.

NEUROLOGY

Knowledge in all areas of the neurosciences continued to accelerate during the first half of the twentieth century. Anatomical investigations shifted towards cytoarchitectural studies, stimulated by Korbinian Brodmann (1908), Oscar Vogt (1903), and Walter Campbell (1905). Pio del Rio Hortega discovered microglia and oligodendroglia (1921). Neuropathology was illuminated by the works of Walter Spielmeyer, Max Bielschowsky, and J. Godwin Greenfield, among numerous others.

Neurophysiology benefitted from Charles Sherrington's investigations, particularly those on proprioceptive reflexes (1909). Nerve impulses were shown to be self-propagating (1914), and for the first time action potentials were recorded (1915). This was soon followed by Herbert Gasser and Joseph Erlanger's studies in which amplified nerve action potentials were demonstrated (1922), and proof that the velocity of nerve impulses was related to nerve diameter was provided (1928). Detlev Bronk's subsequent recordings of amplified single nerve fiber activity began a whole new era of investigative neurophysiology.

Animal brain electrical activity was first recorded in 1875 and the first electrical stimulation experiments of the sensory cortex in 1892. Human alpha and beta rhythms were recorded by Hans Berger via scalp recordings (1929) and were confirmed by Edgar Adrian and Brian Matthews, who developed the concept of EEG localization (1934). The first important studies on the mechanisms of epilepsy after the work of John Hughlings Jackson, David Ferrier, and Charles Sherrington, were those of Napolean Cybulski, who first showed paroxysmal EEG abnormalities from the cortical surface of dogs with electrically induced seizures (1914). Localization of cerebral tumors by EEG was first accomplished by W. Grey Walter at the Maida Vale Hospital in 1936.

The early twentieth century brought major changes in the field of neurology, a discipline previously devoid of meaningful therapy. Already mentioned was the introduction of antibiotics, which over the ensuing generations reduced the mortality of bacterial meningitis by more than 50 percent. Penicillin was also effective in treating syphilis, the most notorious of neurological diseases. Equally important was the introduction of anticonvulsants other than bromides, specifically phenobarbital by Alfred Hauptmann (1912) and diphenylhydantoin by H. Houston Merritt and Tracy J. Putnam (1938). Treatment of myasthenia gravis with prostigmine was reported by Mary Walker (1934), the first successful thymectomy for myasthenia by Ferdinand Sauerbruch in 1911, and the first successful removal of a thymic tumor by Alfred Blalock in 1939. Treatment of subacute combined degeneration with liver extract (1925), intrinsic gastric factor (1928), and later vitamin B_{12} (1948), essentially eradicated a previously common neurological disorder. In the 1930s, the relation between thiamin deficiency, chronic polyneuritis, and alchoholism was made. These are but two examples of several nutritional deficiency diseases that were recognized as having nervous system manifestations and that responded to vitamin treatment, as reviewed in John D. Spillane's *Nutritional Disorders of the Nervous System* (1947).

The second impetus to the dramatic changes that occurred in clinical neurology during this period were the technological advances in diagnostic testing, perhaps best exemplified in the field of neuroradiology. From the time of the first skull radiograph in 1896, to the introduction by Walter Dandy of pneumoencephalography (1918) and ventriculography (1919), followed soon thereafter by cerebral angiography by Antonio Egas Moniz in 1931, and then nuclear brain scanning by George Moore (1948), the neurological and neurosurgical evaluation of patients became increasingly more sophisticated.

Major advances were made in the clinical evaluation of epilepsy, pioneered by the work of William Lennox, Frederic and Erna Gibbs from the Harvard Medical School, and Wilder Penfield and Herbert Jasper at the Montreal Neurological Institute. Their accomplishments and the general advancements in the field during this era are described in detail in *Epilepsy and the Functional Anatomy of the Human Brain* (1954) and *Epilepsy and Related Disorders* (1960). The first classification (1938) and correlation of electroencephalographic recordings with clinical symptoms, the introduction of serial and long-term follow-up EEG recordings of patients, the establishment of multidisciplinary clinics for treatment of epileptic patients, and institution of formal training programs, are among the major contributions of Lennox and his collaborators over a forty-year period. The Montreal group received international acclaim for their surface and depth electrode studies of epileptic patients, their recognition of partial complex seizure activity originating from the temporal lobes (1941), and their refinement of the earlier attempts of surgical treatment of epilepsy, which originated with Otfrid Foerster after World War I. Additional historical landmarks related to the technical aspects of EEG recording and activation of seizures include the use of hyperventilation in the 1940s, photic stimulation by W. Grey Walter (1946), and sleep recordings by Frederic Gibbs (1947). The first application of the EEG for the study of behavioral disorders in children was that of Herbert Jasper, Philip Solomon, and Charles Bradley in 1938.

The influence of neurosurgery on neurology was quite pronounced during this period. Among the greatest contributions to the overall field shared by the two specialties was the classification of brain tumors proposed by Percival Bailey and Harvey Cushing in 1926. This underwent later modification by Bailey, and other classifications were later published by Wilder Penfield, James Kernohan and George Sayre, Klaus Zülch, Pio del Rio Hortega, and Dorothy Russell and Lucien Rubinstein.

To some degree, progress in the area of central nervous system infections paralleled the advances occurring in pediatrics. The field of neurovirology was still in its formative stages, with much interest still directed towards the study of poliomyelitis. Although the clinical manifestations associated with the epidemic of encephalitis lethargica were reported in 1917, the first isolation of viruses from the nervous system was not achieved until 1930 in an epidemic involving horses from the San Joaquin Valley in California. Between 1930 and 1939 the viral etiology of five different arthropod-borne encephalitides was determined. Another area in which major advances occurred was in the diagnosis of neurosyphilis, beginning with the discovery of *Treponema pallidum* in 1905, the Wassermann test in 1906, and isolation of the organism in 1913.

From the time that lumbar puncture was introduced by Heinrich Quincke (1891) to the monograph of William Mestrezat (1912), normal values for cerebrospinal fluid pressure, glucose and protein concentration, and cell and colloidal reactions were determined. In 1919 Lewis Weed and Paul McKibben made the important discovery that cerebrospinal fluid pressure could be markedly altered by the intravenous injection of saline solutions of various concentrations. The therapeutic implications of these studies, suggesting the use of osmotic agents to decrease intracranial pressure, are still employed today. The culmination of this research resulted in H. Houston Merritt and R. Fremont-Smith's classical text *The Cerebrospinal Fluid* (1937).

As interest in both clinical neurology and the neurosciences increased, a further desire for independence from internal medicine and psychiatry became evident, leading within a short time to strong clinical services within hospitals and the creation of major institutes. In England, the Institute for the Teaching and Study of Neurology was formed (1938). Later the National Hospital at Queen's Square joined the Maida Vale Hospital for Nervous Diseases (1948). In France, Charcot's death in 1893 resulted in the diminution of a once very strong neurological influence at the Salpêtrière. His students, such as Pierre Marie, Jules Dejerine, Fulgence Raymond, Edouard Brissaud, and Joseph Babinski, and even his major rival, Charles Bouchard, maintained the traditions of clinical neurology, although its emphasis and direction changed over the next twenty years. In Germany, several centers of neurological research and training were active. In Hamburg, Max Nonne, who was later succeeded by George Schaltenbrand, developed several strong clinical neurology services using the municipal hospital system. Neurological institutes were also founded at Breslau by Otfrid Foerster (1932), with support from the Rockefeller Foundation, and by Oskar and Cecile Vogt in Berlin (Zülch, 1987). In the United States, separate neurology wards and services were created in the larger medical centers, such as at the Philadelphia General Hospital (1877) and Bellevue Hospital Medical College in New York (1886). Other quite prominent neurological institutes were established during this era. The Psycho-Neurological Institute was organized in St. Petersburg by Vladimir Bechterev in 1908, and the Central Institute for Brain Research in Amsterdam was also established by Cornelius Ariëns Kappers (1908). The New York Neurological Institute, founded in 1909 by Joseph Collins, Joseph Fraenkel, Pearce Bailey, and Charles Elsberg, became formally affiliated with Columbia University in 1918. The Montreal Neurological Institute at McGill University was founded in 1930. In 1934 Ludo van Bogaert created the Institut Bunge in Antwerp, Belgium, and Percival Bailey formed the Illinois Neuropsychiatric Institute in 1941.

Existing professional organizations grew in the number of participants and new societies were formed. The number of journals devoted to neurology increased as did the number of books devoted to general clinical neurology or special areas of interest. The *Archives of Neurology*, the first official journal of the American Neurological Association, began publication in 1919. The famous *Handbook of Neurology* by Max Lewandowsky (1910–12) consisted of five volumes plus two supplemental volumes. This was later revised and expanded to seventeen volumes and edited by Oswald Bumke and Otfrid Foerster in 1936. The latest edition, edited by P. J. Vinken and G. W. Bruyn, began in 1969 and now contains over fifty volumes.

CHILD NEUROLOGY

Because of the decrease in childhood mortality, several trends occurred that prompted the development of pediatric subspecialty fields such as child neurology. In other fields of medicine and surgery, subspecialties concentrating on organ-specific diseases were appearing and it was now recognized that children likewise could have organ-related diseases, although quite different than those seen in adults. This became quite apparent in the fields of pediatric hematology and endocrinology. Children, to a limited extent, were thus able to receive medical treatment directed towards one particular organ, resulting in the saving of many lives but also in the emergence of a population with chronic diseases. The use of thyroid hormone, insulin, phenobarbital, vitamins, and other substances introduced during this period, predated the therapeutic advances that appeared after the 1940s. However, among the relatively few pediatricians or neurologists then practicing, some began to show interest in different subspecialties, including child neurology. Included in this first generation of child neurologists are such figures as Bernard Sachs, Frederick Batten, and Bronson Crothers.

A second achievement of this period was the continuation and significant improvement in the development of pediatric laboratory research. The development of simpler techniques for chemistry analysis of blood and cerebrospinal fluid, the ability to obtain blood specimens and infuse fluids intraperitoneally and later intravenously, as well as the development of radiography, further stimulated the growing interest in childhood diseases. With these advances, more specific diseases could be identified and studied, both in the laboratory and clinic. This progress led within a short time to the creation of a particular subspecialty. An excellent example of this were the remarkable studies of Walter Dandy and Kenneth Blackfan on hydrocephalus (1917), and the almost simultaneous introduction by Dandy of pneumoencephalography (1918) and ventriculography (1919); both of these procedures were instrumental in the development of pediatric neurosurgery and pediatric neurology. At the same time the neurosurgical and neuropathological achievements and contributions of Harvey Cushing and Percival Bailey also greatly stimulated the growth of these two subspecialty fields.

A third major factor was the development of pediatric organizations. Leaders in pediatrics realized the need to develop independent entities to promote both their own interests and the needs of children. Thus the growth of pediatric societies and organizations, independent departments of pediatrics within medical schools, residency programs, and, most importantly, strong hospital-based clinical services that provided improved care for children and patients. The progress of these patients was studied and used for teaching and clinical research. It was from these institutions, which typically served large urban populations, that child neurology developed. An example of this was the formation of the first cerebral palsy clinic at Johns Hopkins in the 1920s by Edwards Park, chief of pediatrics, and Adolf Meyer, chief of psychiatry and neurology.

Pediatricians were busy laying claims to the territory of caring for children and because of their general interest in social reform were also active in the care of handicapped children. Thus many state-run facilities for children were eventually headed by those who considered themselves pediatricians, or who were in allied health professions such as clinical psychology. The care needs of such children who were not hospitalized or in an institution also fell under the care of such pediatricians, who usually had a particular interest in neurology. Examples of such individuals include Alfred Tredgold, Clemens Benda, Henry Goddard, Edgar Doll, and Samuel Orton. In the quest to understand the etiologies of mental retardation, neuropathology also advanced the scientific basis for clinical pediatric neurology. The contributions of Paul Schilder, Walther Spielmeyer, Heinrich Vogt, Max Bielschowsky, Gonzalo Lafora, Jószef Baló, and Julius Hallervorden, among others, were instrumental in this regard. In conjunction with this new interest in the neuropathology of childhood nervous system disorders was the significant increase in clinical case reports of new neurological diseases, as described by Ludwig Merzbacher, Gertrud Hurler, Charles Hunter, Georges Marinesco, James Ramsay Hunt, and Knud Krabbe. Perhaps most important of all were the reports of Asbjörn Fölling that for the first time linked a specific inborn error of metabolism with mental retardation and seizures. The era of biochemical investigation was soon to unfold. The majority of these discoveries were usually presented at local meetings and later published in the many different journals of the day. There was yet no real forum for child neurology or any other pediatric subspecialty. However, childhood neurological disorders were covered very comprehensively in all of the standard pediatric texts, and separate works solely devoted to the field were written by Bernard

Sachs (1895), James Taylor (1905), Martin Thiemich and Julius Zappert (1910), Ludwig Bruns (1912), George Peritz (1912), Bronson Crothers (1926), and Frank Ford (1937). These works were of major importance for the future of child neurology. They were instrumental in developing a foundation for the organization and understanding of the many different nervous system diseases affecting children, they introduced specific forms of treatment directed towards children, they delineated the future scope of this emerging specialty, and perhaps most important of all, they helped towards the separation of child neurology from pediatrics, neurology, and psychiatry. (Please see the list at the end of the Introduction for references.)

PERCIVAL BAILEY

PERCIVAL BAILEY (1892–1973) (figure 1) remains one of the most composite scholars of the nervous system of the twentieth century. From a humble background in a portion of southern Illinois known as Little Egypt, the principal community of which is called Cairo, he emerged as one of the true luminaries of the neurosciences. Bailey defined his field of interest early on as the nervous system and throughout his life sought and attained skill in neuroanatomy, neurophysiology, neuropathology, neurology, neurosurgery, and psychiatry. He published more than 260 articles and was a member of twenty-five honorary societies (O. T. Bailey, 1986; Bucy, 1973).

His contribution to the field of pediatrics was no less than a major reclassification of the brain tumors of infancy and childhood, along with intricate and detailed descriptions of the associated clinical symptomatology (Bailey, Buchanan, and Bucy, 1939). This classification and the work engendered in its formation created the neuropathological foundation for the present school of thought on pediatric and adult brain tumors. Individually, and in

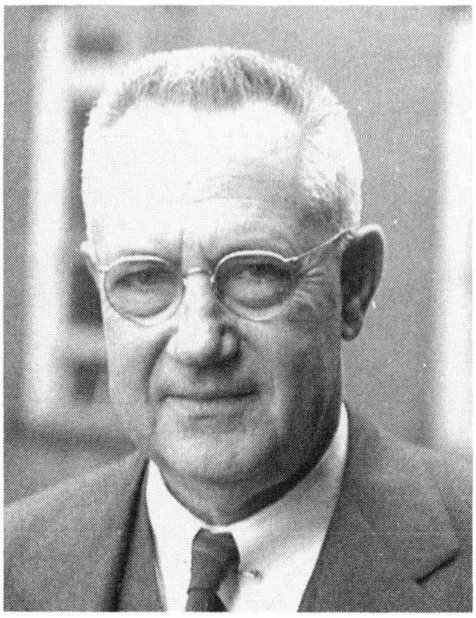

Figure 1. Percival Bailey (1892–1973).

collaboration with Harvey Cushing, he attempted to logically classify those central nervous system tumors arising from glia in a quantitative fashion so that clinicians would be able to predict patient length of survival, determine the efficacy of different types of operations, and evaluate the effects of supplemental radiation (Bailey and Cushing, 1926).

Bailey was born on May 9, 1892. His education began in a one-room country school (the Buckskin school); he then attended Southern Illinois Normal School at Carbondale for one year, going on to the University of Chicago to complete his undergraduate degree. His mother's death at this time turned his interests to science and medicine. Remaining at the University of Chicago under the tutelage of George W. Bartelmez, he developed an interest in neuroanatomy, specifically embryology, became an instructor in anatomy, and went on to earn a Ph.D. His thesis dealt with the development of the choroid plexus of the cerebral ventricles in man. He was later able to cauterize the choroid plexus of hydrocephalic infants with the cystoscope (Wortis, 1974).

At the time he was pursuing his doctoral studies at Chicago's Rush Medical College, he was also pursuing the study of medicine at Northwestern, having transferred there for the final year. The day after he received his M.D. degree from Northwestern he received his Ph.D. from the University of Chicago.

While at Northwestern, Bailey's intent was to study neurology, but he was frustrated by the latter field's inability to result in significant therapeutic cures. During his internship at Mercy Hospital, he studied neurology independently with Julius Grinker, one of the most eminent neurologists in Chicago, who had written the section on neurology in Tice's *Practice of Medicine*. However, Bailey did not wish to specialize solely in neurology, and at this stage a budding interest in psychiatry was nurtured through exposure to the Cook County Psychopathic Hospital where he noted the practice of both archaic and unfounded methods of treatment.

Bailey was also intrigued by neurosurgery, and in 1919 he wrote to Harvey Cushing at Harvard to offer his services. Simultaneously, he wrote to Adolph Meyer at Johns Hopkins to request an opportunity to train in psychiatry. Since Cushing responded to his inquiry first, he did not become a psychiatrist, and studied with Cushing intermittently for approximately nine years (Bucy, 1973; Bucy, 1974; Van Bogaert, 1975; Walker, 1974). In April 1919 Bailey became an assistant resident surgeon in neurosurgery at the Peter Bent Brigham Hospital and within a short period was considered Cushing's favorite resident. In his first scientific accomplishment in Boston, in collaboration with Frederick Bremer, he discovered that puncture of the infundibular hypothalamus provoked adiposo-genital dystrophy and diabetes insipidus, attributing the result to a disturbance of hypothalamic innervation of the pituitary (Wortis, 1974). However, since Bailey's results did not concur with those of Cushing, tension arose between the two men. During this early period Bailey found it extremely difficult to deal with Cushing's personality; such conflict became an ongoing theme between them. After less than a year with Cushing, he interrupted his training in neurosurgery to return to Chicago to pursue neuropathology under George Hassin at Cook County Hospital in 1920. Cushing procured a Field Service Fellowship that allowed Bailey a year's study in France (1921–22), where he studied neurology and psychiatry in Paris at the Salpêtrière with Pierre Marie. When Bailey returned to Boston in the summer of 1922, Cushing asked him to create a histological laboratory for the study of his collection of brain tumors (Bucy, 1974; Magoun and Clemente, 1976). Given Bailey's newly acquired expertise in neuropathology, this was quite important for Cushing, since he could not interest the senior neuropathologists at the "Brigham" in this project. Bailey was interested because a study of Cushing's material would fit his goal of investigating the nervous system from various approaches, combining neurosurgery with neuropathology and, as it turned out, neuroembryology.

Bailey's analysis of these tumors consisted of going through the cases in the order they came into the laboratory; then he arranged the cases in groups according to the length of clinical survival. He was thus able to isolate specific types of gliomas. The tumors separated in this manner did not fit into any schemes then in use for the classification of extracranial tumors. Moreover, they could not be arranged on an embryological basis. Bailey realized that very few gliomas were composed of purely one type of cell, and he decided to base his classification on the predominant element. He identified a glioma for each glial cell in its various stages of maturation, except for the microglia, a tumor, the derivation of which eluded him. In addition, he noted that several of Cushing's tumors were not primarily of glial origin, although presenting clinically and behaviorally like gliomas (Bailey, 1986).

Bailey's first representative study for publication involved a rapidly growing, midline glioma of childhood, which had a grave prognosis. He was unaware of the unpublished work of Joseph Globus and Israel Strauss and decided to call this glioma a spongioblastoma (Globus and Strauss, 1925; Bailey and Cushing, 1925). Both Globus and Strauss, as well as Bailey and Cushing, submitted papers for presentation at the 50th Annual Meeting of the American Neurological Association, June 4, 1924, with both papers being entitled "Spongioblastoma" (Bailey and Cushing, 1925). The four participants conferred behind closed doors, eventually agreeing that Globus and Strauss would identify their tumor as a spongioblastoma multiforme while Cushing and Bailey would call their tumor a medulloblastoma. Both papers were published consecutively in the *Archives of Neurology and Psychiatry*.

In 1924 Bailey secured one of the recently established Guggenheim fellowships and returned to France to study psychiatry with Pierre Janet. Prior to his departure, Bailey presented Cushing with a complete classification of the tumors of the glioma group. Cushing urged immediate publication, but Bailey felt that publication should take the form of a series of projects that would take several years.

When Bailey returned from Paris in 1926 after a year's stay at the Psychiatric Clinic at Sainte Anne, he was greeted with the news that Cushing had ignored his request, added a chapter on clinical correlation and sent it to the publisher as a monograph (Bailey and Cushing, 1926). Although Bailey's initial reaction was rage and horror, this soon turned to good humor — a hallmark characteristic of Percival Bailey. Although Cushing's monograph received international attention, its reception was mixed with less enthusiasm from neuropathologists due to the novel histopathological classification. This classification was also received with a grain of skepticism at the newly founded Boston Children's Hospital where a pediatric neurosurgical service had been established by Franc D. Ingraham, a Cushing trainee. When Bailey established his protocol of brain tumors, he considered other forms of childhood gliomas besides medulloblastomas, although this presented some problems with classification (Bailey, 1986; Bucy, 1974; van Bogaert, 1975).

Given Bailey's methodical approach, this work, which was published in 1926, assumed the format of a thesis. The dedication was to S. Ramon y Cajal, whose methodology Bailey employed throughout the study. The text spans 167 pages and had only 77 references. The key chapter, "A Classification of the Gliomata," gives a detailed histological description of the medulloblastoma, which is noted to have a pattern characterized by spongioblasts. Cushing's only contribution, the chapter entitled "Clinical Correlations," gives a detailed account of selected individual cases for which histology was correlated. The total series consisted of 414 cases.

Bailey remained in Boston for two more years after publication of this monograph. He expounded on the previous classification of gliomas, simplifying it by dropping the categories of medulloepithelioma, pineoblastoma, ependymoblastoma, and neuroblastoma, and the distinction between protoplasmic and fibrillary astrocytoma. He gave the spongioblastoma multiforme the new name *glioblastoma multiforme*, the term now most widely used.

In 1928 Bailey and Cushing published a second joint monograph dealing with tumors that arise from cerebral blood vessels — an outgrowth of some of the work of the 1926 monograph but characterized by a greater emphasis on detail than in their previous work (Cushing and Bailey, 1928). Unfortunately, this text remains somewhat overshadowed by the 1926 study and the future work on intracranial tumors in childhood. That same year Bailey left Boston to take a position at the University of Chicago, where he combined clinical neurosurgery and research on brain tumors. His most pressing interest was the oligodendroglioma, and by using metallic methods he was able to show that the tumors were made up of oligodendroglia. His classic paper on this subject of 1929 remains widely regarded (Bailey and Bucy, 1929).

Bailey accepted an associate professorship at Chicago with the idea of initiating a new division of neuroscience. During this period, the University of Chicago was considered progressive. It had not only the first full-time salaried faculty but also a mixed Flexnerian and Oslerian philosophy with regard to education and curriculum. Here Bailey developed a close association with many researchers of the nervous system: A. J. Carlson, Anro Lukhardt, Heinrich Kluver, Karl Lashley, Roy Grinker (Julius Grinker's son), and Stephen Polyak. Bailey's goal was to develop a clinical department of neurology and neurological surgery that would actually be a Department of the Neurosciences. Meanwhile, he was appointed head of the Division of Neurology and Neurosurgery. Bailey's vision of a Neurological Institute was encouraged by the Rockefeller Foundation. However, his grand scheme for an institute devoted to the neurosciences did not materialize because of the lack of insight and vision of those in authority at the University of Chicago. This frustration, which ended his dream for a Department of Neurosciences, should not be confused with an inactive period in his work. During the late 1930s he continued to elaborate on the pathology of brain tumors. Moreover, he trained and influenced a number of young men who later were to become distinguished in neurological surgery. Most notable were Clovis Vincent and his two associates, Pierre Puech and Marcel David. Vincent met Bailey in Boston, and the newly arrived Frenchman found that Bailey was the only member of Cushing's team who spoke fluent French. Vincent returned to the United States with his two associates to train with Bailey in the fall of 1930. Collectively, they were known as "The Three Musketeers." When Vincent became the first professor of neurosurgery in France in 1939 he dedicated his inaugural address to Bailey. During this same period, Bailey trained Chisato Arakai, Kenji Tanaka, and Kentaro Shimizu of Japan, who went on to become outstanding leaders in neurosurgery in their own country. He also worked with William Sweet (Boston), Ralph Cloward (Honolulu), and A. Earl Walker (Canada) (Walker, 1974).

While at Chicago, Bailey wrote his definitive text *Intracranial Tumors of Infancy and Childhood* with his collaborators Douglas N. Buchanan and Paul C. Bucy (1939). Buchanan, one of the outstanding Chicago neurosurgeons, was a major clinical collaborator for many years with Bailey when he was at the University of Chicago; he had a particular interest in head trauma and subarachnoid hemorrhage. Buchanan also was a collaborator with Bucy (Bucy and Buchanan, 1935), who was one of Cushing's first residents. Bucy not only had an exemplary career in neurosurgery, but was also Bailey's chief biographer. Typical of Bailey's "love-hate" relationship with his mentor, Harvey Cushing, is the dedication of this book to him. The text is extensive, spanning almost six hundred pages in fifteen chapters, and shows Bailey's ability to outgrow the thesis format and compile an integrated work. This remains his seminal work on the field of pediatric neurosurgery. It is interesting to note that he terminated childhood with the advent of one's sixteenth birthday, considering fifteen years as the upper limit of childhood. The majority of cases were obtained from the Children's Memorial Hospital of Chicago, as well as from the Milwaukee Children's Hospital and the Bobs Roberts Memorial Hospital in Chicago. The remaining cases came from local private practitioners. The theses of the authors in this work form the clinical basis for the study of pediatric neurooncology: 1. Tumors in infancy and in childhood are less frequent than in adult life, with the most common site being the cerebellum and neural axis. 2. Supratentorial lesions are less common than subtentorial lesions. Meningiomas, neurinomas, and pituitary adenomas are rare. The glioblastoma multiforme is rare in the hemispheric regions being more common in the pontine section. Pontine gliomas constitute 15 percent of childhood intracranial tumors below the age of 15 and are often misdiagnosed as encephalitis. 3. A brain tumor between the ages of 3 and 6 is likely to be a medulloblastoma of the vermis with a 3:1 male-female sex ratio. 4. The most important symptom in arousing suspicion of a brain tumor in children is rapid enlargement of the head associated with nausea and vomiting. 5. The medulloblastoma is the only intracranial tumor of childhood that is clinically responsive to radiotherapy.

After a decade of academic frustration, Bailey went to Belgium in 1938 as a visiting lecturer and to acquire more skill in neurophysiology. While Bailey was in Europe, Eric Oldberg offered him the professorship of neurology and neurosurgery at the University of Illinois, where a Neuropsychiatric Institute was under construction. Bailey accepted, and during the institute's construction, spent a period of time engaged in research at the physiology laboratory of Dusser de Barenne at Yale and, on the latter's death, transferred both the lab and its personnel to the institute in Illinois. He focused his efforts on determining the cytoarchitecture of the cerebral cortex of both man and the monkey and worked with the neuroanatomist Gerhard von Bonin. It was here that he developed temporal lobectomy as a treatment of psychomotor epilepsy and collaborated with his friend George Schaltenbrand of Würzburg, Germany, on a stereotactic atlas of the human brain that became a classic reference (Wortis, 1974).

Bailey remained at the new neuropsychiatric unit of the University of Illinois College of Medicine from 1940 until his retirement in 1959. He recognized two major needs in psychiatry, a scientific basis for diagnosis and treatment, and sound training for those who would be involved with patient care (Walker, 1974). In 1951 he became director of the Illinois State Psychiatric Training and Research Authority and fashioned a miniature model based on that of the National Mental Health Institute, which was supported by an eight million dollar grant from Adlai Stevenson, who was then the governor of Illinois.

In 1956 he delivered his sensational address "The Great Psychiatric Association" on the occasion of the Freud Centenary at the American Psychiatric Association; this was a sweeping public attack on psychoanalysis. Since 1894, when Silas Weir Mitchell gave his address on the state of psychiatry, no talk ever had more effect. He received resistance from the traditional psychoanalysts and responded with the text, *Sigmund, the Unserene* (Wortis, 1974). It was not that Bailey was anti-Freud, but rather he was wary of the vast influence that psychoanalysis was developing throughout the United States, overshadowing the biological aspects of psychiatry.

Bailey's greatness was recognized by many, for he was president of the Society of Neurological Surgeons in 1948, president of the American Neurological Association in 1954, and was awarded the Abraham Jacoby Prize. In 1949 he received the Doctor Honoris Causa from the University of Paris. His book on pediatric brain tumors was considered one of the best scholarly works of its kind, far surpassing the 1926 work on glioma classification in its complexity and depth. Being the perfectionist that he was, he went so far as to even pick the quality of the paper, avoiding glossy paper because the glare would impair readability.

In the 1960s Bailey's health began to deteriorate. He was plagued by recurring bouts of high fever during which he sometimes became delirious. No cause for these episodes was ever found. His vision deteriorated, and in 1967 he sustained a severe hip injury. Subsequently he developed pyelonephritis and was in the early stages of uremia. He never regained full mobility, and his health from that time was forever compromised. He remained confined to his home for the majority of his remaining life.

With the death of Percival Bailey on August 10, 1973, the world lost one of the great scholars of the nervous system. One of the testimonies of this is his comprehensive library collection on the neurosciences, which is now held at the University of Illinois (Cain, 1973). In addition to his other accomplishments, he ignited a growing interest in the study and classification of pediatric brain tumors.

Samuel J. Lassoff
NEW YORK, NEW YORK

REFERENCES

Bailey, O. T. 1986. Genesis of the Percival Bailey-Cushing Classification of Gliomas. *Ped Neurosci* 12:261–65.

Bailey, P., D. N. Buchanan, and P. C. Bucy. 1939. *Intracranial Tumors of Infancy and Childhood.* Chicago: University of Chicago Press.

Bailey, P., and P. C. Bucy. 1929. Oligodendrogliomas of the Brain. *J Path Bact* 32:735–51.

Bailey, P., and H. Cushing. 1925. Medulloblastoma Cerebelli: A Common Type of Midcerebellar Glioma of Childhood. *Arch Neur Psych* 14:192–224.

______. 1926. *A Classification of the Tumors of the Glioma Group on a Histogenetic Basis with a Correlated Study of Prognosis.* Philadelphia: J. B. Lippincott.

Bucy, P. C. 1973. In Memoriam: Percival Bailey. *Proc Inst Med Chicago* 29:373–74.

______. 1974. Percival Bailey, 1892–1973. *Trans Am Neur Assoc* 99:277–78.

______. 1974. In Memoriam: Percival Bailey. *Biol Psych* 8:343–45.

Bucy, P. C., and D. Buchanan. 1935. The Simulation of Intracranial Tumor by Lead Encephalopathy in Children. *JAMA* 105:244–50.

Cain, A. M. 1973. *A Catalog of the Percival Bailey Collection of Neurology and Psychiatry*. Chicago: University of Illinois.

Cushing, H., and P. Bailey. 1928. *Tumors Arising from the Blood Vessels of the Brain*. Springfield, IL: Charles C Thomas.

Globus, J. H., and I. Strauss. 1925. Spongioblastoma Multiforme. A Primary Malignant Form of Neoplasm: Its Clinical and Anatomic Features. *Arch Neur Psych* (Chicago) 14:139–91.

Magoun, H. W., and C. D. Clemente. 1976. Percival Bailey, 1892–1973. *Anat Rec* 186:235–37.

Van Bogaert, L. 1975. The Life and Work of Prof. Percival Bailey, Honorary Foreign Member (1892–1973). *Bull Mem Acad Roy Med Belgium* 130:263–71.

Walker, A. E. 1974. Obituary: Percival Bailey (1892–1973). *Surg Neur* 2:85–86.

Wortis, J. 1974. Percival Bailey. *Biol Psych* 8:263–64.

JÓZSEF MÁTYÁS BALÓ

JÓZSEF BALÓ (1895–1979) (figure 1) was born in Budapest, Hungary, on November 10, the son of minor Transylvanian nobility. He graduated in 1919 from the medical school of Pázmány Péter University, predecessor of the present Semmelweis Medical University. Although his medical studies were interrupted by World War I, Baló committed himself to pathology, where he felt able to deal with the entire diversity of medicine, unlike other specialities that were restricted to one organ system. As a medical student he had already participated in the ongoing work at the Institute of Pathology. After graduation, Baló joined this institute of the medical school in Budapest, with which he remained affiliated until his death. Here he worked under the guidance of Karoly Schaffer and Kalman Buday. In these early years his interest was focused on the pathology of the nervous system. His early publications dealt with the central nervous system involvement in pernicious anemia, periarteritis nodosa, and the pathological changes in herpes encephalitis and encephalitis epidemica of Von Economo.

As the recipient of a Rockefeller fellowship, he spent 1922–24 in Baltimore at the Johns Hopkins University and in Boston, where he began his work in virology. In 1926 he was appointed chairman of the Department of Pathology at the Szent István Korház (St. Stephen's Hospital), one of the major municipal hospitals in Budapest, where he stayed until 1928.

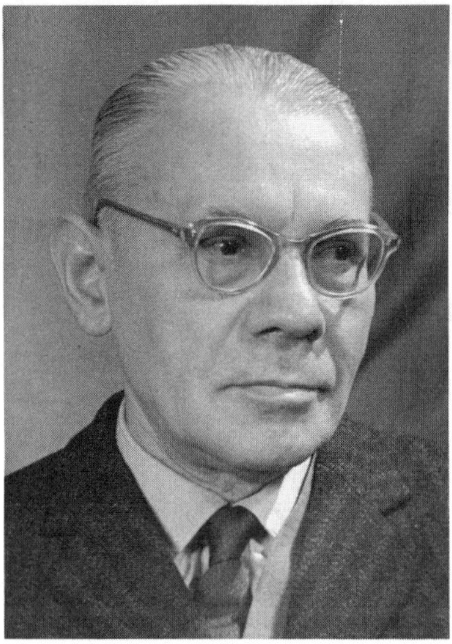

Figure 1. József Baló (1895–1979).

It was during this time that he encountered a 23–year-old patient who died after a rapidly progressing illness. His major complaints were expressive and receptive aphasia, right hemiparesis, nausea, headache, vomiting — findings suggestive of a left hemisphere space occupying lesion, for which he underwent exploratory craniotomy. The day following surgery the patient died. Baló did a detailed histological evaluation of the brain. His original description is as follows:

On cross-section, the corpus callosum was seen to be thickened and its right half was composed of stripes of alternating white and gray substance. Each stripe was from 2 to 3 mm in thickness. The white stripes were the same color as the white matter, while the gray stripes which were depressed, corresponded to the gray softening. The stripes extended from the gyrus cinguli in a winding manner perpendicular to the cross-section of the corpus callosum, becoming wider and forming curves up to the centrum semiovale. At about the middle of the corpus callosum three stripes presented somewhat concentric layers. On the same cut surface of the right centrum semiovale, an area 4 by 3 cm was found. The long axis of this area was situated in the transverse diameter of the brain. The area resembled the annual rings of trees, being composed of concentric lamellae. The center of the concentric focus was an elliptic area 3 x 1.5 mm. About this center, concentric rings composed of alternating gray and white lamellae were found. Near the center, the rings were about 1 mm thick, while the peripheral rings were wider. It was interesting to note that where the focus approached the cortex, the rings were interrupted. The cortical substance and a thin line of white matter adjoining it were not altered. The outside rings which were the largest, penetrated even to the inferior frontal gyrus and were situated in such a way that the stripes parallel to the cortical substance were formed. The orbital gyri seemed to be normal on this side. The white matter of the left hemisphere was spotted. Gray dots the size of millet seeds and lentils were scattered throughout this region, often fusing together. . . . (Baló, 1928, 245)

Baló's original report (1927) was translated into English and published the following year in the Archives of Neurology and Psychiatry, where it was received with great interest (Baló, 1928). In this report Baló described a new disease, "encephalitis periaxialis concentrica," which was later named after him, although a similar case had been reported earlier by Otto Marburg as "encephalomyelitis periaxialis scleroticans" (Marburg, 1906). Baló was the first to provide a detailed description of this disease. This new entity, which has since been confirmed by several authors, belongs to the loosely connected group of degenerative diseases whose common feature is primary demyelination (Poser and Van Bogaert, 1956). Because of the availability of more sophisticated technology, the recent descriptions of this disease are more detailed; however, its etiology remains obscure. Most authors consider it a form of multiple sclerosis (Castaigne et al, 1984; Moore et al, 1985). The fact that several cases have been reported in which Baló's concentric sclerosis could be found together with lesions typical of multiple sclerosis, certainly supports this hypothesis. A detailed review of the pathology of the cases published since Baló's original description is available (Courville, 1970).

In 1928 Baló was appointed chairman of the Pathological Institute at the University of Szeged in southeast Hungary. That same year he received the title Privatdozent (Private University Professor), which is roughly equivalent to the Ph.D. in English-speaking countries. Although the University of Szeged was newly organized, it was the legal successor to the University of Kolozsvár, which had fled its seat in the ancient Hungarian city of Kolozsvár, the capital of Erdély (Transylvania), at the end of World War I when Transylvania was transferred to Romania. The reestablished university bore the name of Franz Joseph, the penultimate ruler of the Austro-Hungarian Empire (it is currently known as the Medical School of Szeged). Along with József Baló, this university had among its chairmen F. Brúnó Straub, the former Hungarian head of state, and the recently deceased Albert Szent-Györgyi, who discovered vitamin C and was the only Nobel laureate to receive his prize (1937) for work done in Hungary. He served as dean of the Medical School in 1932–33 and in 1941–42, and as rector of the University in 1939–40.

As a professor of pathology, Baló returned to the United States to continue his research in virology. The results of these studies were published in 1935 in his pioneering work concerning the role of viruses in the pathogenesis of tumors, a rather revolutionary idea at that time (Baló, 1935; Baló and Korpássy, 1936). During his years in Szeged he continued his work on the pathology of the diseases of the central nervous system, and his monograph on the demyelinating diseases of the brain and spinal cord was published in 1940.

Baló's interests continued to be diverse. He did not limit himself to one field and subsequently becoming involved in research on the causes of atherosclerosis. He was especially intrigued by the role of the elastic fibers in this pathological process. World War II obviously hindered his work but, even during the endless hours spent in crowded bomb shelters, he continued to think about new experiments that he could carry out between attacks.

In 1940 he was elected correspondent to the Hungarian Academy of Sciences (a form of minor membership) and after the war was elected to full membership. In 1948 during the oppressive years of Stalinism, he was expelled from the Academy. He was at least in good company, as Szent-Györgyi was among the numerous scientists excluded at that time. His membership was not reestablished until 1956, when a thaw in the political situation gave him the opportunity to be readmitted to the privileges of the Academy as a correspondent member. His full membership was not restored until 1973, when he was seventy-eight.

After World War II Baló returned to Budapest to work at Hungary's major medical school, Pázmány Péter University. In 1945 he became chairman of the university's Institute of Forensic Pathology. The following year he became chairman of the Institute of Pathology, a post he continued to hold until his retirement in 1967. His first concern was to rebuild the institute, which suffered severe damage during the war, and within a short time he established a vibrant center for research. During his years at the Institute of Pathology, he founded the Cancer Research Institute at the university, which he directed until 1967. Even after his retirement, he participated actively in the work of this institution, maintaining a very busy schedule of research and lectures until his death on October 9, 1979 (Lapis, 1979).

Through his work in connective tissues, he met Ilona Banga, whom he married in 1945 at the age of fifty. She was an assistant of Szent-Györgyi's, and they continued to work together until his death. In 1948 they isolated the connective tissue enzyme, elastase, which Ilona Banga prepared in its crystallized form in 1952 (Banga and Baló, 1952). They had one son, Mátyás Jr., who is currently an academic dermatologist in Budapest.

During his long career Baló published more than 350 papers and was elected a member of several foreign scientific societies, among them the Deutsche Gesellshaft für Pathologie (1940), the Royal Society (1965), the Deutsche Akademie der Naturforscher-Leopoldina (1962) and the Pathology Society of the USSR (1962).

Baló's contribution to child neurology is a unique example of the role played by neuropathology in the development of our knowledge of several rare degenerative disorders. Although there has been little advancement in our understanding of the disorder he described in 1927, Baló's work demonstrated the need for careful and methodical study to distinguish among the different entities affecting the function and structure of myelin in the developing nervous system.

Laszlo J. Mate
LOMA LINDA, CALIFORNIA

REFERENCES

Baló, J. 1927. A Leukoenkephalitis Periaxialis Concentricaról. *Magy Orv Arch* 28:108–24.

______. 1928. Encephalitis Periaxialis Concentrica. *Arch Neur Psych* 19:242–62.

______. 1935. *Die unsichtbaren Krankheitserreger filterbare Vira*. Berlin: S. Karger.

______. 1940. *Die Erkrankungen der weissen Substanz des Gehirns und des Rückenmarkes.* Leipzig: J. A. Barth.

______. 1957. *Lungenkrebs und Lulngenadenom*. Budapest: Hungarian Academy of Sciences.

Baló, J., and B. Korpássy. 1936. *Warzen, Papillome und Krebs*. Acta litterarum scientiarum Reg. Universitatis Hung. Francisco-Josephinae, Sectio Med. 7. Leipzig: J. A. Barth.

Banga, I., and J. Baló. 1952. Elastin and Elastase. *Nature* 171:44.

Castaigne, P., et al. 1984. Sclérose concentrique de Baló. *Rev neur* (Paris) 140:479–87.

Courville, C. B. 1970. Concentric Sclerosis, 9: 437–51. In *Handbook of Clinical Neurology*, vol. 9, 437–51. Ed. P. J. Vinken and G. W. Bruyn. Amsterdam: North-Holland Publishing Company; New York: American Elsevier Publishing Co., Inc.

Lapis, K. 1979. Dr. József Baló. Obituary. *Orv Hetilap* 120:2902–4.

Marburg, O. 1906. Die sogenannte'akute multiple Sklerosis (Encephalomyelitis periaxilis scleroticans). *Jahrb Psych Neur* 27:211–312.

Moore, G. R., et al. 1985. Baló's Concentric Slerosis: New Observations on Lesion Development. *Ann Neur* 17:604–11.

Poser, C. M., and L. van Bogaert. 1956. Natural History and Evolution of the Concept of Schilder's Diffuse Sclerosis. *Acta Psych Neur Scand* 31:285–331.

FREDERICK BATTEN

FREDERICK EUSTACE BATTEN (1865–1918) (figure 1) must be considered among the first of the truly great modern pediatric neurologists. Along with Bernard Sachs and Désiré Bourneville, he showed a particular interest in children with neurological disorders. Yet his medical career was not confined to pediatric neurology or even to the general neurological sciences: many of his professional efforts delved into areas of more general medicine.

Batten was born in Plymouth, England, on September 29, 1865, the son of J. W. Batten. A younger brother, Rayner D. Batten, was also a physician. In fact, Rayner Batten published material on cerebroretinal degeneration (1897) that is often confused with his older brother's extensive contributions on the subject, especially his frequently cited report "Cerebral Degeneration with

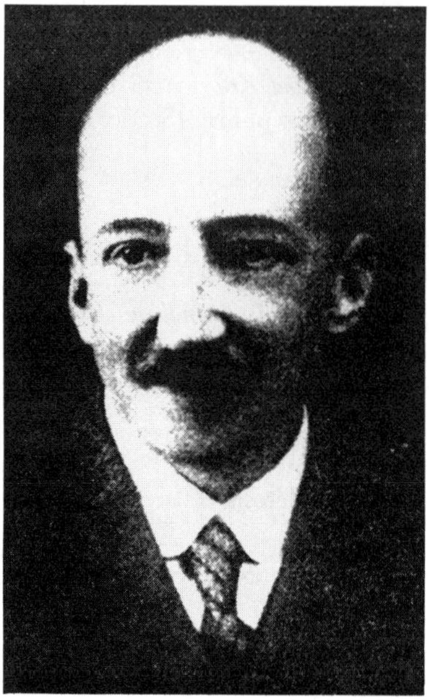

Figure 1. Frederick Batten (1865–1918).

Symmetrical Changes in the Maculae in Two Members of a Family" (Batten, 1903a). However, the cases reported by Rayner Batten had the onset of visual impairment at the age of fourteen years and were not associated with dementia or seizures.

Frederick Batten's early schooling was at the Westminister School. He later attended Trinity College at Cambridge and received a second-class honors degree in natural science in 1887. He then began study at St. Bartholomew's Hospital and there qualified for the M.B. in 1891. He became a member of the Royal College of Physicians in 1894 and an M.D. in 1895. Batten then became house physician to Sir William Church and later was appointed as a casualty physician. In the years after graduation, he studied in Berlin, where he is reported to have become fluent in German. In time, he returned to the Hospital for Sick Children and became medical registrar, assistant physician, and finally physician. In 1899 he was appointed pathologist at the National Hospital at Queen's Square and in 1900 was appointed to the honorary staff. He functioned as an outpatient physician for both the National Hospital and the King George Hospital.

Batten's publications were extensive: 106 items are listed in a commemorative article (Higgins, 1962). Some of his work published before 1900 concerned what some might consider to be non-neurological subjects. This work includes papers on empyema, tuberculosis, diphtheria, cholera and deformities. Yet even these studies showed his interest in child neurology, often commenting extensively on neurological implications. It is of interest, however, that Batten's first publications concerned his observations on three cases of progressive muscular atrophy; his initial publication was dated 1892, one year after the original description of muscular atrophy by Werdnig (1891) and one year before the more complete publication by Hoffmann (1893). Batten incorporated more detailed descriptions of progressive muscular atrophy into articles that appeared in *Brain* in 1897, 1903 (with H. M. Fletcher), and again in 1911. In one of his later papers on this subject, which he coauthored with Gordon Holmes (1912), Batten reported a fourteen-month-old child with this disorder. He included careful neuropathological examinations, including the spinal cord from normal children as well as a child who died with severe anterior horn cell degeneration. His rapidly maturing biological scientific skills were also reflected in several publications concerning the muscle spindle, early degenerative changes in the sensory end organs of muscles, and the effect of Marchi's fluids on the nervous system (Higgins, 1962). Batten also published works on disseminated sclerosis (Batten, 1908–1909).

As his age and education would suggest, Batten's most productive years were in the twentieth century. His publications covered a wide range of topics (Higgins, 1962), including studies on arrested neural development, cerebral diplegia, poliomyelitis, polioencephalitis, myopathies, cerebellar ataxias, cretinism, more on progressive spinal muscular atrophy (which he graciously called Werdnig-Hoffman's disease in 1903 and 1911), Mobius syndrome (1905a), partial epilepsy, Grave's disease, cerebroretinal degeneration, acute infective diarrhea, spinal cord tumors, diffuse neural sarcomatosis, myasthenia gravis, ophthalmoplegia, muscular dystrophy, meningitis, acute myelitis, functional astasia, celluloid splints in the rehabilitation of acute poliomyelitis, dystrophia adiposo-genitalis, brain tumors, atonic diplegia, Pelizaeus-Merzbacher's disease, Tay-Sachs disease, and post-traumatic encephalopathies. With Sir Archibald Edward Garrod and Hugh Thursfield, Batten was also coeditor of the first edition of *Diseases of Children* (1913). For this compendium Batten wrote two extensive chapters entitled "Organic Nervous Diseases" and "Diseases of Muscle," together consisting of 150 pages and 77 illustrations (Chaves-Carballo, 1978). Batten's last paper, "Epidemic Stupor," was written soon before his death in 1918, and was coauthored with George Frederic Still (Higgins, 1962).

Batten's most recognized and important accomplishments concerned his many years of work on progressive muscular atrophy

(1892, 1897, 1903, 1911), the cerebroretinal degenerations (1903a, 1903b; Batten and Mayou, 1915), the myopathies, the acute and chronic cerebellar syndromes, and poliomyelitis. The eponym Batten's disease has rightly been associated with both the juvenile and late infantile varieties of neuronal ceroid lipofuscinosis. He published several articles, including one on subacute combined degeneration of the spinal cord, (coauthored with J. S. Risien Russell and James Collier in 1900), myotonic dystrophy (coauthored with H. P. Gibb in 1909), infantile progressive muscular atrophy, congenital cerebellar ataxia or cerebellar diplegia and acute cerebellar ataxia (Batten, 1903b, 1905b,c). Batten is credited with distinguishing congenital from acquired forms of ataxia and with noting that congenital ataxia could be due to either damage to the cerebellum at birth or to developmental malformations of the brain. More careful study of several less-recognized works, such as the case he reported of ophthalmoplegia externa with blindness of acute onset in a child with fever (1903c), could in the future conceivably be considered as further examples of other "Batten's diseases."

Higgins eloquently described Batten as a "brisk lithe figure with the conspicuous domed head and lively eye." He possessed a "bubbling humor," was "able, enthusiastic, indefatigable," had an "unflinching honesty of purpose [and] no trace of arrogance or egotism." He was "practical and purposeful [and] children loved him" (Higgins, 1962). Batten was a perfectionist, and he insisted on accurate, up-to-date, typewritten notes, which meant late nights for the house physician. Yet he was held in high esteem by his students and colleagues, among whom he was known simply as Freddie. He consulted frequently and carried on spirited arguments with his Queen's Square colleagues Gordon Holmes and S. Kinnier Wilson. His adversaries in discussion "always found him a tough, though scrupulously fair and courteous antagonist" (Obituary, 1918). Observation of the kindly unassuming eyes of Frederick Batten as illustrated in figure 1 seems to support these descriptions. In 1918, at the age of fifty-three, he died from complications only two days after a prostatectomy.

Paul Richard Dyken
MOBILE, ALABAMA

REFERENCES

Batten, F. E. 1892. Notes on Three Cases of Progressive Muscular Atrophy Associated with Loss of Sensation to Heat and Cold. *St. Bart Hosp Rep* 28:211–20.

______. 1897. Hereditary Forms of Progressive Muscular Atrophy with Spinal Lesion in Young Children. *Brain* 20:536–42.

______. 1902. Three Cases of Family Progressive Spinal Muscular Atrophy (Werdnig-Hoffmann Type). *Trans Clin Soc Lond* 36:226.

______. 1903a. Cerebral Degeneration with Symmetrical Changes in the Maculae in Two Members of a Family. *Trans Ophthal Soc U.K.* 23:386–90.

______. 1903b. Congenital Cerebellar Ataxia (Cerebellar Diplegia). *Clin J* 22:81–88.

______. 1903c. A Case of Ophthalmoplegia Externa with Blindness of Acute Onset in a Child at 5 Years. *Trans Clin Soc Lond* 37:225.

______. 1905a. Congenital Affection of Sixth, Seventh and Twelfth Cranial Nuclei. *Brain* 28:359.

______. 1905b. Case of Acute Ataxia in a Boy. *Brain* 28:360.

______. 1905c. Ataxia in Childhood. *Brain* 28:484–505.

______. 1908–1909. Two Cases of Family Disease, the Symptoms of Which Closely Resemble Disseminated Sclerosis. *Proc Roy Soc Med* 2:35–37.

______. 1910. Progressive Spinal Muscular Atrophy of Infants (Werdnig-Hoffmann Type). *Proc Roy Soc Med* 4:115.

______. 1911. Progressive Spinal Muscular Atrophy of Infants and Young Children. *Brain* 33:433–63.

Batten, F. E., and H. M. Fletcher. 1903. Case of Progressive Muscular Atrophy of Spinal Origin in a Girl Aged 11 Years; With Autopsy. *Brain* 26:473–87.

Batten, F. E., and H. P. Gibb. 1908–1909. Two Cases of Myotonia Atrophica, Showing a Peculiar Distribution of Muscular Atrophy. *Proc Roy Soc Med* 2:32.

Batten, F. E., and G. Holmes. 1912. Progressive Spinal Muscular Atrophy of Infants (Werdnig-Hoffmann Type). *Brain* 35:38.

Batten, F. E., and M. S. Mayou. 1915. Family Cerebral Degeneration with Macular Changes. *Proc Roy Soc Med* 8:70–90.

Batten, R. D. 1897. Two Brothers with Symmetrical Disease of the Macula Commencing at Age of Fourteen. *Trans Ophthal Soc U.K.* 17:48.

Chaves-Carballo, E. 1978. Eponym: Frederick E. Batten: Father of Pediatric Neurology. *South Med J* 71:1428–29.

Garrod, A. E., F. E. Batten, and H. Thursfield. 1913. *Diseases of Children*. London: Edward Arnold.

Higgins, T. T. 1962. F. E. Batten. *Dev Med Child Neur* 4 (Suppl. 5):1–29.

Hoffmann, J. 1891, 1893. Über chronische spinale Muskelatrophie in Kindesalter, auf familiarer Basis. *Dtsch Zeit Nervenheilk* 1:95, 3:427.

Obituary. 1918. Frederick Batten. *Lancet* 2:157.

Russell, J. S. R., F. E. Batten, and J. Collier. 1900. Subacute Combined Degeneration of Spinal Cord. *Brain* 23:39–110.

Werdnig. G. 1891. Zwei frühinfantile hereditäre Fälle von progressiver Muskelatrophie unter dem Bilde der Dystrophie, aber auf neuratische Grundlage. *Arch Psych Nervenkrankh* 22:439.

CLEMENS BENDA

JOHN LANGDON DOWN'S classic paper, "Observations on the Ethnic Classification of Idiots," (1866) received scant attention until 1875, when John Fraser and Arthur Mitchell reported on a forty-year-old woman with "Kalmuc idiocy" (named after a Mongolian tribe) at a meeting of the Medico-Psychological Association held in the Royal College of Physicians in Edinburgh. William Ireland, who attended this meeting, rejected this term, observing that he did not think there were any Kalmucs in the east of Scotland. The chairman of the meeting, a physician named Jamieson, declared that there was "no reason for nicknaming an idiot by calling him a Kalmuc" (Kanner, 1964, 100). Mitchell described an additional sixty-two patients with the disorder in his presentation, emphasizing the short lifespan and brachycephaly. Two years later, Ireland included the disorder as a separate condition in his *Idiocy and Imbecility*. The majority of reports on Down syndrome at the turn of the century originated in England and the United States. It was not until 1899 that the first report of fifteen patients from continental Europe was published by Neumann in Germany. This was soon followed by case reports in France by Désiré Bourneville (1901), in Austria by Kassowitz (1902), in Norway by Holmboe (1905), and in Russia (1906) by Kowalewsky (Benda, 1946). After that time, clinical interest and research in patients with Down syndrome grew explosively. Many of these studies were carried out in institutions for the handicapped and developmentally delayed. Among the pioneers in the systematic studies of these patients was Clemens Benda.

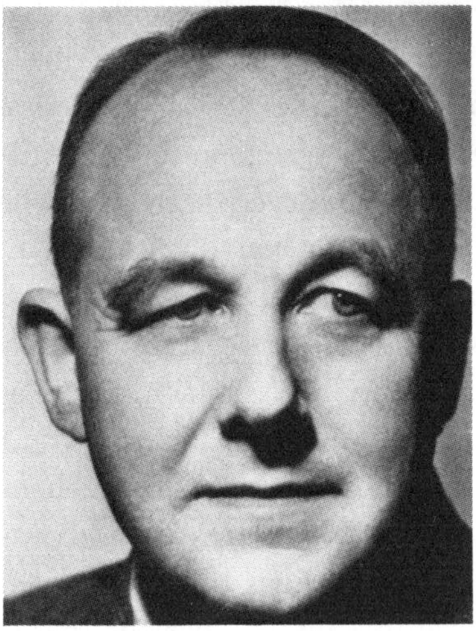

Figure 1. Clemens Ernst Benda (1898–1975).

Clemens Ernst Benda (1898–1975) (figure 1) was born in Berlin, Germany, on May 30. His father, Carl Benda, was a professor of pathology and his mother's family was noted for having produced several generations of scholarly theologians. He received his elementary and high school education in Berlin, attended the University of Heidelberg, and received his doctor of medicine from the University of Berlin in 1922. Benda was trained in the European tradition, leading to competence in neurology, psychiatry, and neuropathology. During his early training and professional career he was an assistant at the Psychiatric Clinic in Heidelberg, was associated with the State Hospital and Sanitarium in Switzerland, and trained in neurology at the Barmbek Hospital in Hamburg. He then became associate neurologist at the Red Cross Hospital in Berlin. In the early 1930s he became editor-in-chief of the journal *Die medizinische Welt* (*The Medical World*), which was noted for its socio-philosophical editorial content. The political climate in Germany at that time made it impossible for him to function there (Yakovlev, 1975). In 1935 he arrived in Boston, Massachusetts, with his wife, also a physician, and his two small sons. His arrival in Boston was fortuitous because his colleagues included, among others, such eminent physicians as Stanley Cobb, James Ayer, Houston Merritt, Raymond D. Adams, Charles Kubik, Derek Denny-Brown, and Paul I. Yakovlev. In 1935 Benda served as a research fellow in psychiatry and neuropathology with Stanley Cobb, head of the Department of Neurology at the Massachusetts General Hospital. Benda characterized Cobb's teaching as a "precision of thinking and awareness of facts and interpretations" (Benda, 1952a). James Ayer, his chief of neurology at Harvard Medical School, was instrumental in directing Benda toward research in mental retardation (Benda, 1970a). In 1936 a Research Center was completed at the Wrentham State School for Retarded

Children in Wrentham, Massachusetts. Ayer recommended that Benda be named director. In 1936 with his appointment as director of the Wallace Research Laboratory for the Study of Mental Deficiency, he became the first director of research in any institution for the retarded in the United States. Eleven years later, he became director of research and of clinical psychiatry at the W. E. Fernald School for Retarded Children in Waverly, Massachusetts. Disorders of mentation became the focus of his research and culminated in several books and over one hundred scientific publications (Benda, 1982).

Among Benda's more important contributions is a comprehensive study of Down syndrome that spanned thirty years and was based on over one thousand clinical observations and a detailed study of seventy-eight postmortem examinations on patients ranging in age from newborn to sixty-five years. Much of this work was accomplished more than two decades before Jerome LeJeune and his colleagues discovered the chromosomal abnormality in Down syndrome (LeJeune, Gautier, and Turpin, 1959). Benda's theories of the etiology of Down syndrome are, of course, no longer relevant; however, his detailed account of the clinical, anatomic, and pathologic features of Down syndrome represents the most comprehensive study of this disorder thus far published and remains a widely used reference. His first monograph on Down syndrome, *Mongolism and Cretinism*, was published in 1946. In this work he compared and contrasted these two congenital causes of mental retardation. The thrust of his research was aimed at determining why the child with Down syndrome grew and developed in a different way and to determine the cause for this deviation in fetal growth. He postulated that observed structural abnormalities in the endocrine glands (thyroid, adrenals, gonads, and pituitary) were the major factors interfering with normal growth and development. It was Benda's careful observations and analysis that categorized some of the common clinical physical findings, such as the simian crease, as well as other hand, foot, and ear abnormalities (figure 2). He felt that, from an anatomic point of view, Down syndrome represented a growth deficiency that was the opposite of acromegaly and suggested that acromicria was a more scientifically descriptive term (Benda, 1952b). A revised edition of his work, *The Child with Mongolism* (*Congenital Acromicria*), was published in 1960. In this volume he acknowledged the etiologic significance of the chromosomal abnormality but defended the scientific validity of his clinical, anatomical, and pathological observations (Benda, 1960). The third edition, entitled *Down's Syndrome: Mongolism and Its Management* (Benda, 1969) dealt with the long-term management of children with Down syndrome. He pointed out the tremendous impact of an abnormal child on the family and emphasized the need for counseling the parents. He discussed the question of institutionalization versus home care and cautioned that these decisions must take into account multiple factors. He stressed the need for individual educational evaluation since many of these children could function in society with appropriate training. He emphasized the need for an environment in which the children were treated with kindness and love, and was an early advocate of the establishment of sheltered villages for teenagers and adults with Down syndrome.

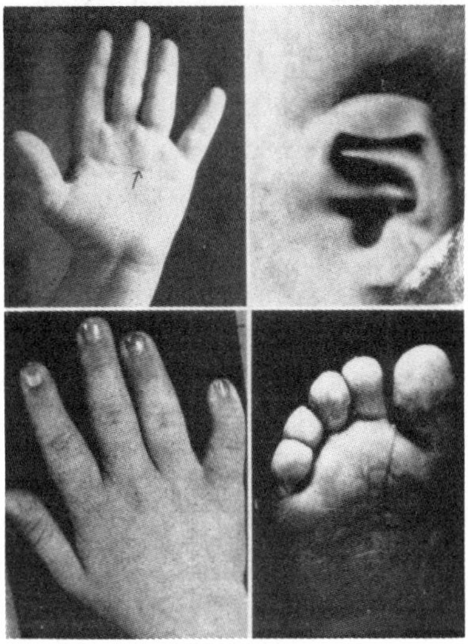

Figure 2. Benda's analysis of his case material was exceptionally detailed, helping to clearly differentiate mongolism from cretinism. He recognized physical features specific to Down syndrome. From Benda, C. E., *Mongolism and Cretinism* (New York: Grune and Stratton, 1946), figures 4–7, p. 21.

Another major contribution to our present day understanding of mental retardation is his textbook *Developmental Disorders of Mentation and Cerebral Palsies*, which was published in 1952 and today remains a widely used reference in the field of mental retardation (Benda, 1952a). He attempted to achieve a better understanding of the neuropsychiatric aspects of mental disorders in children by integrating clinical, neurological, physiological, and pathological findings. Clinical observations in congenital and acquired disorders of mentation were, for the first time, corroborated by postmortem and laboratory studies. Many of his observations have proven prophetic. "The prenatal health of the mother is an important factor for the well being of the fetus. Many irregularities may, therefore, be prevented if we learn to understand and control the factors that are involved" (Benda, 1952a, 32). As early as 1945 he attempted to differentiate those cases of mental retardation due to congenital malformations from those due to birth injury, a topic of major interest today (Benda, 1945). He analyzed one hundred autopsies on patients with mental retardation, first to determine the frequency of birth-related injury and second to document the permanent damage to the nervous system following such injuries. He concluded that a higher percentage of cases of "cerebral spastic infantile paralysis" is caused by congenital anomalies than by trauma at birth. "There is, however, no justification for neglecting the thirty to forty percent of post-traumatic cases because of the fact that fifty to fifty-five percent are congenital malformations" (Benda, 1945, 91). He further observed that seizures after birth or in early childhood are of major diagnostic value in the recognition of cerebral damage and that the diagnosis of cerebral damage can be made in the majority of cases immediately after birth: "Careful observation on the part of the pediatricians will reveal the seriousness of these cases in the first three months of life" (Benda, 1945, 93).

Benda retired in 1963 and entered the private practice of psychiatry. Under the influence of his early teachers, Karl Jaspers and Ludwig Binswanger, he became actively engaged in existential psychology and psychiatry. His later writings were concerned with the psychological and psychiatric aspects of conscience and guilt, which he applied to philosophy, religion, law, and politics. He presented the basis of his existentialist psychiatry in two books, *Der Mensch in Zeitalter der Liebloslichkeit* (*The Image of Love*) (Benda, 1961), and *Gewissen und Schuld* (*Conscience and Guilt*) (Benda, 1970). He died in Munich, Germany, on April 18, 1975, at the age of seventy-seven.

Benda was a member of the council of the Association of Existential Psychology and Psychiatry, a diplomate of the American Board of Psychiatry and Neurology, a fellow of the American Psychiatric Association, and a member of the American Association of Neuropathologists (president, 1952) and the American Academy of Mental Retardation (president, 1960). He was a member of the American Medical Association, American Association for Mental Health,

American Neurological Association and an associate member of the Royal Society of Medicine of Great Britain. In 1949 he received an award from the Association for the Help of Retarded Children for his outstanding contributions on behalf of the mentally retarded. In 1969 he was awarded the Heinrich Hoffmann Medal, which is given every fourth year in Germany to the psychiatrist who contributed the most to the science of child psychiatry. In the field of child neurology, he is recognized for his exhaustive clinical studies of Down syndrome and his pioneering efforts in separating the different causes of developmental retardation.

Gwendolyn R. Hogan
SHREVEPORT, LOUISIANA

REFERENCES

Benda, C. E. 1945. The Late Effects of Cerebral Birth Injuries. *Medicine* 24:71–110.

______. 1946. *Mongolism and Cretinism.* New York: Grune and Stratton.

______. 1952a. *Developmental Disorders of Mentation and Cerebral Palsies.* New York: Grune and Stratton.

______. 1952b. What is Mongolism (Congenital Acromicria)? *Internat Rec Med* 165:75

______. 1960. *The Child with Mongolism (Congenital Acromicria).* New York: Grune and Stratton.

______. 1961. *Der Mensch in Zeitalter der Liebloslichkeit.* Stuttgart: Schattauer.

______. 1969. *Down's Syndrome: Mongolism and Its Management.* New York: Grune and Stratton.

______. 1970a. Down's Syndrome: Beginning of the End. *Roche Report; Frontiers of Hospital Psychiatry* 7:1–11

______. 1970b. *Gewissen und Schuld.* Stuttgart: Schattauer.

Benda, C. 1982. Clemens Benda. In *National Cyclopedia of American Biography,* 53–54. Clifton, N.Y.: James T. White.

Down, J. L. H. 1866. Observations on an Ethnic Classification of Idiots. *Lond Hosp Clin Lect Rep* 3:259–62.

Fraser, J. 1876. Kalmuc Idiocy. *J Ment Sci* 98:169.

Ireland, W. W. 1887. *Idiocy and Imbecility.* London: Churchill.

Kanner, L. 1964. *A History of the Care and Study of the Mentally Retarded.* Springfield, IL: Charles C Thomas.

LeJeune, J., M. Gautier, and R. Turpin. 1959. Etudes des chromosomes somatiques de neuf enfants mongoliens. *Compt rend Acad Sci* 248:1721.

Mitchell, A. 1876. Notes on Kalmuc Idiocy. *J Ment Sci* 98:174.

Yakovlev, P. I. 1975. Clemens Ernst Benda. *J Neuropath Exp Neur* 34:549–50.

MAX BIELSCHOWSKY

ONE OF A GENERATION of distinguished German neuropathologists, Max Bielschowsky (1869–1940) (figure 1) was born in Breslau in what is now Poland. Goethe-Forscher Bielschowsky, coming from a family of merchants, encouraged his son to follow cousin Albert (a historian and biographer of Goethe) in the study of German, but young Bielschowsky preferred pursuing his childhood interest in the workings of the mind and began the study of medicine at the university in Breslau, as did his equally famous ophthalmologist cousin, Alfred. He later studied in Berlin and, in 1893, his degree was conferred *summa cum laude* in Munich (Lewy, 1941; Hallervorden, 1959; Weil, 1970).

Bielschowsky's contributions to neurology and pathology span many aspects of both fields. His most important discovery, and that which laid the groundwork for later investigations, was the development of the silver staining technique of myelin. Carl Weigert had already begun to develop crude myelin stains when Bielschowsky joined him after his medical school graduation at the Senckenberg Institute in Frankfurt-am-Main. Bielschowsky had moved on to head the lab of neurologist Kurt Mendel when his first publication of the staining technique appeared (Bielschowsky, 1902). At this same time, Santiago Ramón y Cajal in Spain and J. Fajersztajn in Hungary independently published their silver impregnation methods. Based on his silver stain technique, Bielschowsky and neurologist Paul Schuster wrote several papers characterizing the lesions of multiple sclerosis and a monograph dealing with myelitis and optic neuritis (Bielschowsky, 1901).

The year 1904 marked the beginning of what would be a long, productive, but stormy career for Bielschowsky with the Neurobiological Institute of the University of Berlin and its director Oskar Vogt. During the next thirty years, Bielschowsky worked with the finest medical minds in Germany. Together with Korbinian Brodmann and Maximilian Rose, he mapped the cytoarchitecture of the cerebral cortex and the corpus striatum (Bielschowsky, 1910, 1921a, 1935; Bielschowsky and Rose, 1929). In a foreshadowing of what was to become of Bielschowsky, Brodmann was forced to leave the institute and move to Tubingen in 1910 because of a soured relationship with Vogt (Ostertag, 1963). This did not decrease Bielschowsky's productivity. He contributed to the literature on topics from syringomyelia (Bielschowsky and Unger, 1920) and neurofibromatosis (Bielschowsky and Henneberg, 1922) to myotonia congenita (Weil, 1970). During World War I he studied trauma and surgery of the peripheral nerves with Unger and Valentin (Weil, 1970). He was one of the first to document hemiplegia and spasticity with lesions sparing the pyramidal tracts. He contributed directly to English medical literature with a chapter in Wilder Penfield's *Cytology and Cellular Pathology of the Nervous System* dealing with the histopathology of neurons and neuroblastic tumors of the sympathetic nervous system (Penfield, 1932).

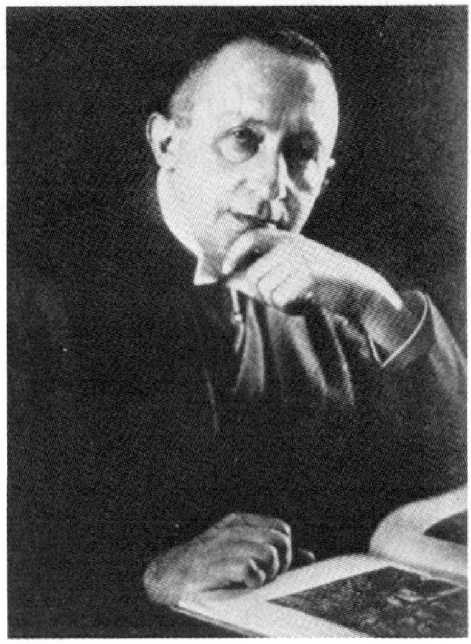

Figure 1. Max Bielschowsky (1869–1940). From Haymaker and Schiller, eds., *The Founders of Neurology*, 2d ed. (Springfield, IL: Charles C Thomas, 1970).

In 1914 Bielschowsky described three siblings with normal development, a mild speech disturbance, and the onset of severe generalized convulsions between the ages of three and four years (Bielschowsky, 1914). Dementia and blindness from retinal and optic nerve degeneration quickly progressed, with death ensuing in four years. The brains, in particular the cerebellum, showed marked atrophy. Microscopic examination revealed neurons swollen with lipopigments, an abnormality that had become known as the Schaffer-Spielmeyer cell process. At the end of the nineteenth century Bernard Sachs had seen similar changes in an infantile disease, which he had termed amaurotic family idiocy. Because of what seemed to be a unifying cellular pathology, Bielschowsky dubbed these new patients as having a late infantile form of the same disease. In 1921 Bielschowsky expanded on his original description, yet continued to mistakenly link his cases with Tay-Sachs disease (Bielschowsky, 1921b; Zeman, 1970; Volk, 1964).

The eponymic classification of what would become the neuronal ceroid lipofuscinoses (NCL) has had a long and muddled history. Jan Jansky, a Prague psychiatrist, described a family similar to that described by Bielschowsky in 1908, and the late infantile form of NCL has usually been referred to as Jansky-Bielschowsky disease. David Cogan, the prominent neuroophthalmologist, attempted to classify amaurotic familial idiocies by funduscopic changes as Bielschowsky-Stock-Spielmeyer disease (Cogan, 1958). Frederick Batten described cases of juvenile onset NCL, but some have mistakenly linked Batten and Bielschowsky to descriptions of the late infantile form. Despite this eponymic confusion, it is clear that Bielschowsky played a pivotal role in the early descriptions of the neuronal ceroid lipofuscinoses (Zeman, 1970).

In addition to being an outstanding researcher, Bielschowsky maintained his own weekly clinic and was considered by his colleagues to be an excellent diagnostician. Despite a tremendously productive career, which ultimately resulted in 187 publications, an honorary membership in the American Neurological Association, and becoming a fellow of the Kaiser Wilhelm Gesellschaft, his relationship with Oskar Vogt became increasingly difficult, forcing him to leave the Senckenberg Institute in 1933.

The final seven years of Bielschowsky's life were not happy. He became a nomad, first accepting a position in the laboratory of Wilhelmina Gusthuis in Amsterdam, only to move one year later to Utrecht to work in the laboratory of the university's psychiatric clinic with the support of a Rockefeller Foundation grant. In 1935 he moved to the Cajal Institute in Madrid but was forced back to Berlin under the threat of losing his old age pension. He then suffered a cerebellar infarct in June 1936, incapacitating him for three months. These final years saw his eldest son obtain a position as a physician and biochemist at the University of Madrid, only to become involved in that country's civil war. Another son joined the Royal Air Force as a pilot stationed in South Africa, while a third son accompanied his father to London before the outbreak of World War II. On August 14, 1940, Max Bielschowsky died of another stroke. His ashes were buried next to his friend Paul Schuster at Golders Green (Weil, 1970).

As Lewy stated in his obituary for the American Neurological Association:

With Bielschowsky passed away the last of a generation of scientists who had forged the tools for the development of neuropathology and have used them skillfully. . . . [H]is life was that of an unassuming German scientist and his end symbolizes the decline of a cultural period. (Lewy, 1941)

Henry J. Kaminski
CLEVELAND, OHIO

ACKNOWLEDGMENTS

I wish to thank Janina B. Kaminski for aid in translation of German manuscripts and Mary L. Hlavin for help with manuscript editing.

REFERENCES

Bielschowsky, M. 1901. *Myelitis und Schnerventzudung*. Berlin: Krager.

______. 1902. Die Silberimpragnation der Achsenzylinder. *Neur Centralbl* 21:579.

______. 1910. Allgemeine Histologie und Histopathologie des Nervensystems. In *Handbuche der Neurologie*. Ed. Max Lewandowski. Berlin: Springer.

______. 1914. Über spatinfantile familiäre amaurotische Idiotie mit Kleinhirnsymptomen. *Dtsch Zeit Nervenheilk* 50:7.

______. 1921a. Weitere Bemerkungen zur normalen und pathologischen Histologie des striaren System. *J Psych Neur* 23:233.

______. 1921b. Zur Histopathologie und Pathogenese der amaurotischen Idiotie mit besonderer Berucksichtigung der zerebellaren Veranderungen. *J Psych Neur* 26:123.

______. 1935. Allgemeine Histologie und Histopathologie des Nervensystems. In *Handbuche der Neurologie*. Ed. Max Lewandowski. Berlin: Springer.

Bielschowsky, M., and R. Henneberg. 1922. *Zur Histologie und Histogenese der zentralen Neurofibromatose*. Madrid: Del libro en honor de D. Santiago Ramon y Cajal.

Bielschowsky, M., and M. Rose. 1929. Über die Pathoarchitektonik der mikro—und pachygyren Rinde und ihre Beziehungen zur morphogenei normaler Rindengebiete. *J Psych Neur* 38:42.

Bielschowsky, M., and E. Unger. 1920. Syringomyelia und Teretoma und extramedullare Blastombildung. *J Psych Neur* 25:173.

Cogan, D. G. 1958. Amaurotic Family Idiocy, A Case for Eponyms. *NEJM* 258:1212.

Hallervorden, J. 1959. Zur Erinnerung an Max Bielschowsky 1869–1940. *Nervenärzt* 30:325–37.

Lewy, F. H. 1941. Max Bielschowsky. *Trans Am Neur Assoc* 67:243–44.

Ostertag, B. 1959. In Memoriam Max Bielschowsky. *Dtsch Med Wschr* 84:765–66.

______. 1963. Max Bielschowsky. In *Grosse Nervenärzte*. Vol. 3. Ed. Kille. Stutgart: Thieme.

Penfield, W. 1932. *Cytology and Cellular Pathology of the Nervous System*. New York: Hoeber.

Volk, B. W. 1964. *Tay-Sachs' Disease*. New York: Grune and Stratton.

Weil, A. 1970. Max Bielschowsky. In *The Founders of Neurology*, 319–22. Ed. W. Haymaker and F. Schiller. 2d ed. Springfield, IL: Charles C Thomas.

Zeman, W. 1970. Historical Development of the Nosological Concept of Amaurotic Familial Idiocy. In *Handbook of Clinical Neurology*. Ed. P. J. Vinken and G. W. Bruyn. New York: American Elsevier.

LUDWIG BRUNS

LUDWIG BRUNS (1858–1917) (figure 1) was born in Hannover, Germany, on June 25. His father was the director of the Hannover Land Insurance Company, and had planned a business career for him. However, by the age of twelve Ludwig was an orphan (Wollenberg, 1917). Financial reverses forced Bruns to attend trade school, but through the support of relatives, he was able to graduate from the gymnasium, attaining first class honors. He graduated with honors from the medical school in Göttigen and obtained his medical doctorate at Munich in 1882 (Wollenberg, 1917, 547).

Bruns spent his first two years of postgraduate training in ophthalmology but left that field for neuropsychiatry. He became an assistant to Eduard Hitzig at the Irrenanstalt Nietleban (Nietleban Insane Asylum) and continued when Hitzig moved his clinic to Halle. The appointment by Hitzig confirmed Bruns's competence, intelligence, and industry. However, Hitzig's bellicose nature had forced him to leave Zurich, where he displayed acerbic, hypercritical behavior (Edinger, 1917). Despite Hitzig's nature, Bruns acquired superlative skills from his tyrannical teacher, and did not assimilate Hitzig's fractious behavior or interest in experimental physiology (Gustav Fritsch and Hitzig had mapped out the cortical representation of movements in the dog by electrical stimulation [Fritsch and Hitzig, 1870]). For Bruns, the clinic would serve as his laboratory.

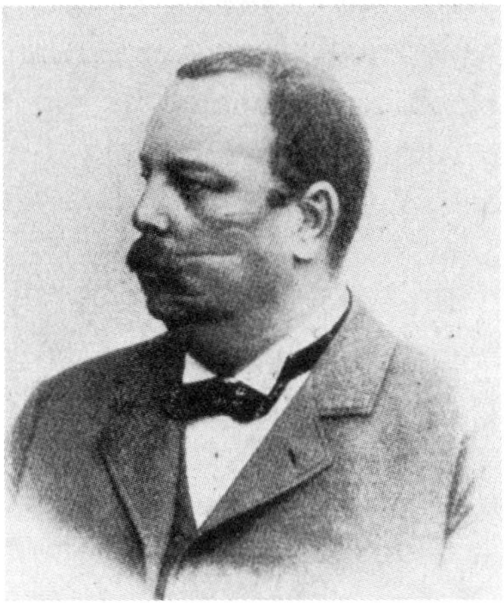

Figure 1. Ludwig Bruns (1858–1917). From Witte, J., "Zur Geschichte des aerztchen Vereins Hannover." *Dtsch Med Woch* 55(1929): 859-60.

After two years with Hitzig, Bruns joined Carl Westphal and Hermann Oppenheim at the Charité Hospital in Berlin. Bruns cultivated a life-long association of mutual respect with Oppenheim. Bruns also spent time in Paris with Jean Martin Charcot when his school at the Saltpêtrière was in full bloom. A short visit to England completed his training and forged links with the English school of neurology (Edinger, 1917). Bruns sustained this connection by translating English articles for publication in reviews that appeared in German journals.

Bruns returned to his native city of Hannover to practice adult and child neurology at the Polyclinic and the Clinic of the Child Health Institute. Bruns was often invited to consult in neighboring towns in Westphalia. As his reputation for intelligent leadership spread, he was elected to preside over regional medical societies (Witte, 1929). Bruns subsequently founded the German

Society of Neurologists and served as its first director. Later he represented this society at international meetings (Edinger, 1917). He was also honored by the Prussian government with promotion to professor of neurology in 1903 and received the Iron Cross, Second Class, in 1916 for organizing a consultation service for the army.

Bruns's influence on child neurology was significant and can be measured by the quality and volume of his publications. His writing was the quintessence of brevity and clarity. Bruns wrote several articles on dyslexia, myopathy, and congenital absence of muscle groups. He published a series of articles on the localization of brain tumors (Bruns, 1897), which were further augmented in *Die Geschwülste des Nervensystem* (*Tumors of the Nervous System*). This exhaustive handbook was one of the first to provide a numerical analysis of symptoms, record indications for surgery, and detail outcome (Bruns, 1908).

He prepared a succinct table, part of which is recorded below, to distinguish frontal from cerebellar ataxia (Bruns, 1897).

FRONTAL ATAXIA	CEREBELLAR ATAXIA
Monoparesis or hemiparesis, motor beginning sometimes with dysarthria and truncal weakness. . . . Jacksonian or more commonly generalized epileptic seizures. Often the eyes are deviated in tonic conjugate deviation to the side of the tumor. . . .	No monoparesis or hemiparesis. More commonly alternating paresis. Rare truncal weakness. Frequent dysarthria. No cortical seizures, but frequently . . . tonic cramps of truncal and neck muscles with appearance of *arc en circle*. Motor paralysis toward the side of the tumor. . . .

A report of an outbreak of poliomyelitis demonstrates his powers of observation and lucidity of description. The epidemic

affected equally children from good and poor circumstances. The most striking symptoms were severe pains with spontaneous twitching of muscles and Kernig's sign. In nearly all cases there was severe diaphoresis and a particular diarrhea

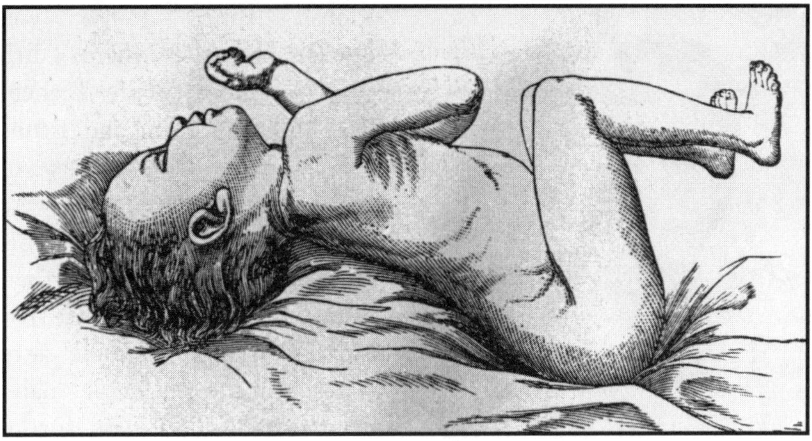

Figure 2. Child with opisthotonus due to tuberculous meningitis.

with intense abdominal cramps. Conspicuous was the predilection for the quadriceps. (Bruns, 1914)

In 1906 Bruns published *Die Hysteria im Kindesalter* (*Hysteria in Childhood*). In this work he observed that abnormal behavior often took a single form that expressed an internal conflict. Bruns remarked that parents of hysterical children were overbearing and harshly punished their children. Bruns advocated "benign neglect," restriction of corporal punishment, and reeducation of the parents.

His most significant publication was the nearly 900–page *Handbuch der Nervenkrankheiten im Kindesalter* (*Handbook of the Nervous Diseases in Childhood*), written in collaboration with August Cramer and Theodor Ziehen and published in 1912. The nosology, classification, and scope differs little from those of modern textbooks. Although Bruns wrote the chapters on peripheral nerve and brachial plexus disorders, and localization and pathology of tumors, his style permeated the book. Ziehen contributed chapters on infectious diseases (figure 2). The book is notable for including many X-ray and patient photographs, and other illustrations. Another example of this, derived from his interest on hysteria in children, is that of a young girl with epilepsy and persistence of abnormal posturing and weakness (figure 3).

Bruns presented a thorough review of the literature interwoven with his views of the topic. He published several papers on the congenital absence of muscles but included the observations of

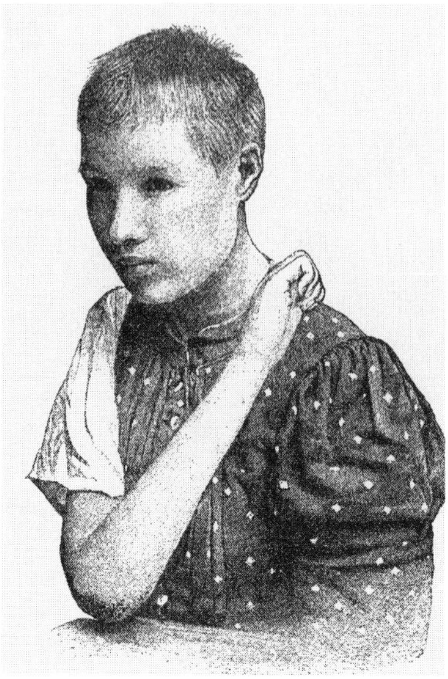

Figure 3. Hysterical posturing and possibly a hysterical seizure in a girl with known epilepsy.

Rudolph Bing, Hugo von Ziemssen, and Wilhelm Erb (Bruns, Cramer, and Ziehen, 1912, 449–53). Bing and Bruns observed that the defects of muscles of the chest wall were "mostly one sided, rarely bilateral, more on the right than on the left." Bruns believed that the excess number of male cases was due to the fact that males were examined for fitness during involuntary conscription or prior to taking up apprenticeships. He combined his cases with those from Bing's series to conclusively demonstrate that defects in the pectoralis major were accompanied most often by absence or defects in the pectoralis minor and sternocostal muscles. Often the muscular defects were combined with other severe developmental defects, the skin on the side of the absent muscle was "pigmentless, stretched, and lacked subcutaneous fat. The breast nipple was smaller and placed higher on the (defective) side." Polymastia was observed "with bony defects of the ribs and sternum." Bruns noted that, for the most part, adjacent muscles hypertrophied and "took on a vicarious function for the absent muscle," causing only a minimal functional defect (Bruns, Cramer, and Ziehen, 1912, 449–53).

Bruns's description of birth trauma to the brachial plexus is unsurpassed by modern authors:

Birth paralysis occurs above all after a long and difficult delivery, especially with a narrow pelvis . . . more often with a breech delivery than with a head first delivery and most frequently where the delivery is completed artificially.

He also included "pressure lesions caused by the finger of the obstetrician or instruments, crushing of the plexus between the clavicle and the first rib or . . . tugging or stretching the nerve fascicles or tearing them from the spinal cord" (Bruns, Cramer, and Ziehen, 1912, 486–90).

Rarely were birth injuries to the brachial plexus bilateral. Bruns and F. Jolly each observed a case of bilateral lower brachial plexus birth injury in which

all of the muscles of the hands and forearms were paralyzed, besides the triceps and the pectoralis major, and those muscles innervated by the cervical roots 5 and 6 were preserved. The preserved muscles were continuously contracted, causing abduction of the arm and bending of the forearm (figure 4).

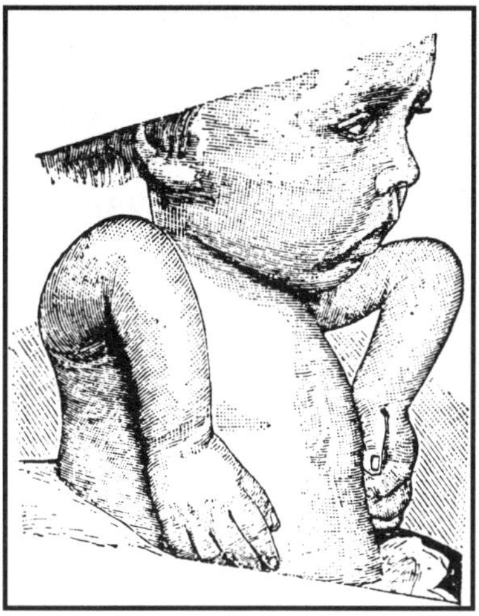

Figure 4. A young child with what is described as a bilateral brachial plexus injury; this illustration appeared as figure 98, p. 490, in the *Handbuch der Nervenkrankeiten im Kindesalter* and was credited to Jolly.

Bruns was of the opinion that the spinal cord was also involved in this case (Bruns, Cramer, and Ziehen, 1912, 490).

Bruns's last publication dealt with the diagnosis and treatment of war casualties. Always respecting his association with Hermann Oppenheim, Bruns credited his friend for suggesting treatments for peripheral nerve injuries. Bruns adeptly described the "pseudo-spastic paresis, irregular tremor and bizarre postures soldiers manifested feigning injury" (Bruns, 1915).

At age fifty-four, a widower, and suffering from diabetes mellitus, he volunteered for military service in the Tenth Army Corps. Although continuously plagued by complications of his diabetes, he was never absent from duty for any long period of time. On November 9, 1917, he died unexpectedly due to "cardiac arrest following a severe pulmonary infection," after being operated on for a "small right leg thrombosis" (Wollenberg, 1917). He left two young daughters and a second wife, having remarried in 1916.

Bruns was "heavy set, powerful, on the whole more solid than fleshy with a pale and intelligent face on which there was an inconspicuous sword cut" (Witte, 1929). He was "somewhat phlegmatic and reserved but had an excellent sense of humor. He always had the ear of the audience because he never spoke casually. He was most precise in speech and writing, often appearing crude when correcting errors made by others" (Wollenberg, 1917).

Bruns left behind a legacy of over eighty journal articles and three books. He was one of the major organizers and spokesman of German neurology. Although he "wrote nothing that was truly great or highly original, he represented all that was needed for the advancement of neurology" (Edinger, 1917). Indeed "he was a conscientious, well-educated, independent thinking man," superbly adept at recording what he had observed in an extensive clinical practice. Ludwig Bruns was "truly a splendid man" (Edinger, 1917), whose life was tragically truncated at the apex of achievement. His legacy to child neurology, aside from his numerous papers, is that of the voluminous and well-organized *Handbook of the Nervous Diseases of Childhood*, which he wrote in collaboration with Ziehen and Cramer.

Edward J. Fine
BUFFALO, NEW YORK

REFERENCES

Bruns, L. 1897. Ueber einige besonders Schwierige und praktisch wichtige differential-diagnostische Fragen in bezug auf die Localisationen der Hirntumoren. *Neur Centralbl* 16:922–23.

______. 1906. *Die Hysterie im Kindesalter*. Halle: Marhold.

______. 1908. *Die Geschwülste des Nervensystems*. Berlin: Karger Verlag.

______. 1914. Kurze Mittielungen ueber eine Epidemie spinaler Kinderlahmung in Hannover umgegend im Jahre 1913. *Neur Centralbl* 34:788–89.

______. 1915. Kriegsneurologische Beobachtungen und Betrachtungen. *Neur Centralbl* 34:12–15.

Bruns, L., A. Cramer, and T. H. Ziehen. 1912. *Handbuch der Nervenkrankheiten im Kindesalter*. Berlin: Karger Verlag.

Edinger, L. 1917. Ludwig Bruns. *Dtsch Zeit Nervenheilk* 56:1–8.

Fritsch, G. T., and E. Hitzig. 1870. Ueber die elektrische Erregheit des Grosshirns. *Arch Anat Phys Wiss Med* 37:300–32.

Witte, J. 1929. Zur Geschichte des aerztchen Vereins Hannover. *Dtsch Med Wschr* 55:859–60.

Wollenberg, R. 1917. Ludwig Bruns. *Arch Psych Nervenkrankh* 57:541–51.

MYRTELLE CANAVAN

THE STUDY OF pathology as we know it today is a well organized profession with many recognized subspecialties. However, in the late 1800s there were fewer than fifty pathologists in the United States (Ober, 1976). Prior to the mid-1800s, no university had a professorship devoted solely to pathology; most "pathologists" earned their living from clinical practice in addition to demonstrations of morbid anatomy. In 1847 J. B. S. Jackson, later curator of the Warren Anatomical Museum at Harvard, was appointed professor of pathology at Harvard Medical School, a chair devoted exclusively to the study of pathology. However, as William Ober outlined in his essay on American pathology in the nineteenth century, "the events which were to prove decisive for American pathology, indeed for all biological sciences, were taking place in Germany, France and England during the 1850s." Three important scientists were advancing new ideas: Rudolf Virchow, Louis Pasteur, and Charles Darwin. "Each of these investigators was making the same statement: living substance arises only from living substance. . . . It was in the reference of this *Zeitgeist* that pathology began to develop rapidly." Coupled with this new way of viewing biologic organisms were advances in microscope design, tissue-sectioning methods, and bacteriologic methods. Early American pathologists concentrated principally on morbid anatomy and, in the tradition of Pasteur, bacteriology.

The subspecialty of neuropathology in the United States did not formally develop until the early 1900s; however, interest in diseases of the nervous system had arisen much earlier (Bailey, 1988). Most of the responsibility for diagnosis of nervous system diseases fell to the general pathologist, while many neurosurgeons and neurologists also studied difficult cases and pursued research in nervous system disease.

Based on this historical perspective, it is easy to see that Myrtelle May Canavan (1879–1953) (figure 1) was one of a small group of practitioners: she was a woman, a trained pathologist, and an early neuropathologist. Her contemporaries were few but included Hugo Ribbert, Joseph Globus, and Hermann Strauss, as well as

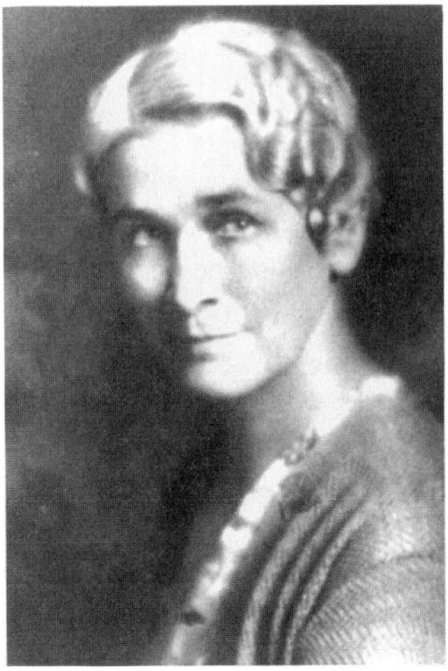

Figure 1. Myrtelle M. Canavan (1879–1953).

the excellent group studying tumors at the Peter Bent Brigham Hospital in Boston, including Harvey Cushing, Percival Bailey, and Louise Eisenhardt (Manuelides, 1979).

Myrtelle May Canavan was born June 24, 1879, in St. John's, Michigan, to Richard and Kate Moore. In 1898 she entered Michigan State College at the age of nineteen, continuing her studies the following year at the University of Michigan. Her academic pursuits took her to Philadelphia, where she obtained her M.D. in 1905 from the Women's Medical College of Pennsylvania, one of thirty-six women to graduate that year.

Upon graduation, she married another doctor, James Francis Canavan. In 1907 she became a laboratory assistant at the Danvers State Hospital in Hawthorne, Massachusetts. It was at Danvers that she had her first contact with Elmer Ernest Southard, Bullard Professor of Neuropathology at Harvard Medical School and director of the Boston Psychiatric Hospital. This association was to foster her interest in neuropathology, an interest that led to many meticulous descriptions of brain and spinal cord pathology in a variety of diseases. Canavan wrote of her association with Southard:

Elmer Ernest Southard had in his short life of 43 years a great inspirational effect on his students and friends. His remarkable memory for events and the literature, his sympathy and open mind, the mental shower bath effect his lectures and demonstrations had, made for him grateful, admiring friends and firm adherents. Many a logically trained mind felt new impetus because of the contact, however brief, and very few have left the field of neuro-psychiatry who were his pupils in it. (Canavan, 1939)

In 1909, while Canavan was at Danvers State Hospital, the first of her seventy-nine articles was published in the *Boston Medical and Surgical Journal*. Many of her early publications dealt with bacillary dysentery (Canavan, 1909). Her interest in bacteriology, part of the legacy to pathologists from Louis Pasteur, was evident throughout her medical career, which spanned thirty-eight years.

Canavan became resident pathologist at the Boston State Hospital in 1910, a post she held for four years. During this time, she continued her association with Southard and began to publish articles pertaining to neuropathology. Canavan's meticulous attention to detail and her tireless attempts at clinicopathologic correlation, in the tradition of Morgagni, were evident in these early publications. In 1910, together with Southard, she published "Bacterial Invasion of the Blood and the Cerebrospinal Fluid by Way of Mesenteric Lymph Nodes: A Study of Fifty Cases of Mental Disease" (Southard and Canavan, 1910).

Like many neuropathologists of her day, she was interested in the anatomical and clinicopathologic correlates of disease. Her tenure at Boston State Hospital and subsequently as pathologist to the Massachusetts Department of Mental Diseases (1914–24) allowed her to study the neuropathological substrate of mental disease. In one of several treatises on functional psychoses, Canavan stated:

Most studies of functional psychoses directly concern themselves with living concrete cases (if they do not merely content themselves with atmospheric or special theoretical statements). Accordingly we have turned the problem about and are seeking what can be learned of the history and various factors (including somatic lesions) in cases having normal brains. . . . We hope therefore to catch some true examples of the functional psychoses by scrutinizing the list of the normal-looking brain cases. By eventual careful microscopic examination of suitable cases we shall be able to approach closer and closer the desired aim. (Southard and Canavan, 1914, 776)

Over the next several years Canavan published numerous articles on pathology found in mentally defective patients. Her topics were limitless, carefully researched, and well illustrated. Her many papers included studies of optic nerve pathology, non-neural neoplasms, the spleen, and a study of a thousand autopsy cases in institutionalized patients (Canavan, 1916; Southard and Canavan, 1915; Canavan and Southard, 1918; Southard, Canavan, and Thom, 1919). She also wrote on a variety of neuropathological topics such as multiple sclerosis, sudden death, microscopic hemorrhage and glioma (Canavan and Maloney, 1941; Canavan, 1922; Canavan and Hemsath, 1931; Hemsath and Canavan, 1932).

In 1924 she became the curator of the Warren Anatomical Museum at Harvard University Medical School, a position she held until her retirement. She concurrently began her tenure as associate professor of neuropathology at the Boston University School of Medicine. Two years later she became an instructor in neuropathology at the University of Vermont School of Medicine. It was during this period that she published a paper in the *Archives of Neurology and Psychiatry* describing a disease that now bears her name (Canavan, 1931). The report, entitled "Schilder's Encephalitis Periaxialis Diffusa: Report of a Case in a Child Aged Sixteen and One-Half Months," begins with the following statement:

> *This report is made to emphasize the care needed to separate cases of macrocephalus due to diffuse degeneration of the brain from those due to hydrocephalus or tumor, with which they might become confused.* (Canavan, 1931)

The reported patient died at age sixteen months with a head circumference of 51.25 cm. At the time of death, the patient was severely developmentally delayed, could not sit, and had questionable vision.

Pathological examination revealed a large, soft brain weighing 1,890 grams after formalin fixation. Gross sections through the brain showed intact gray matter with soft, pink retractile white matter, the changes being more pronounced in the posterior portions of the brain. On microscopic examination there was a spongy degeneration of the white matter with "preservation of the glia but not in excess." The pattern was described by Canavan as a "lacy edema . . . with no perivascular changes and no evidence of any cellular reaction to the process in the subcortical regions" (Canavan, 1931). She concluded by stating "no hint of etiology can be given, except that in general one expects edema to be due to toxic action." As is well known, Ludo van Bogaert in collaboration with Ivan Bertrand published several additional cases after World War II and a classic monograph on this disorder entitled *Spongy Degeneration of the Brain in Infancy* in 1967. Despite extensive studies of spongy degeneration of the nervous system (Canavan's disease), it was only recently that a biochemical basis for this disorder has been suggested (Matalon et al, 1988).

Canavan continued to publish, teach, and be associated with the Warren Anatomical Museum until her retirement in 1945. In response to a questionnaire to alumnae of the Women's Medical College of Pennsylvania in November 1944, she stated that there was no longer a need for a separate medical school for women and that coeducation would be better. She also advocated more graduate work for physicians in accordance with the pupil's interest (Women's Medical College, 1944). In these statements, as in her meticulous, honest reporting of observations in neurologically and psychiatrically impaired patients, Canavan was innovative, saw trends in health care clearly, and set an example for all physicians to follow. She died August 26, 1953, in Boston of paralysis agitans.

Melinda L. Estes
CLEVELAND, OHIO

ACKNOWLEDGMENTS

The author wishes to thank Ms. Marion Dorner for her help in obtaining reference materials.

REFERENCES

Bailey, O. T. 1988. Neuropathology — Then and Now. *JAMA* 260:1891–93.

Canavan, M. M. 1909. The Blood Cell Picture in Bacillary Dysentery. *Boston Med Surg J* 161:694–702.

______. 1916. An Histological Study of the Optic Nerves in a Random Series of Insane Hospital Cases. *J Nerv Ment Dis* 43:217–30.

______. 1922. Sudden Deaths in the Feebleminded. A Report of Two Cases Due to Gland Disorder. *Proc Am Assoc Study Feebleminded* 46:186–99.

______. 1931. Schilder's Encephalitis Periaxialis Diffusa. Report of a Case in a Child Aged Sixteen and One-Half Months. *Arch Neur Psych* 25:299–308.

______. 1939. Lesions in Spinal Cord in Mental Disease and Defect Recognized by Myelin Sheath Stain. A Report of 600 Unselected Cases with an Appendix on Technique. *J Med Assoc Georgia* 28:324–31.

Canavan, M. M., and F. A. Hemsath. 1931. Glioma of the Fourth Ventricle of a Prematurely Born Infant. *Arch Neur Psych* 26:1234–36.

Canavan, M. M., and J. D. Maloney. 1941. Multiple Sclerosis in a Mental Defective. Report of a Case with Serial Sections of the Brain and Cord. *J Med Assoc Georgia* 30:14–18.

Canavan, M. M., and E. E. Southard. 1918. Microsplenia and Other Observations on the Spleen in Psychopathic Subjects. *Bull Mass Comm Ment Dis* 2:136–42.

Hemsath, F. A., and M. M. Canavan. 1932. Microscopic Cerebral Hemorrhage in Stillbirths and Newborn Deaths. *Am J Obstet Gyn* 23:471–78.

Manuelides, E. E. 1979. A Neuropathologist's Perspective on the Celebration of the 2000th Operation of Harvey Cushing. *J Neurosurg* 50:13–16.

Matalon, R., et al. 1988. Aspartoacylase Deficiency and N-Acetylaspartic Aciduria in Patients with Canavan Disease. *Am J Med Genet* 29(2):463–71.

Ober, W. B. 1976. American Pathology in the 19th Century: Notes for the Definition of a Specialty. *Bull NY Acad Med* 52:325–47.

Southard, E. E., and M. M. Canavan. 1910. Bacterial Invasion of the Blood and the Cerebrospinal Fluid by Way of Mesenteric Lymph Nodes: A Study of Fifty Cases of Mental Disease. *Boston Med Surg J* 163:202–9.

______. 1914. Normal Looking Brains in Psychopathic Subjects. Second Note (Westborough State Hospital Material). *J Nerv Ment Dis* 41:775–82.

______. 1915. Notes on the Relation of Somatic (Non-neural) Neoplasms to Mental Disease. *Interstate Med J* 22:738–51.

Southard, E. E., M. M. Canavan, and D. A. Thom. 1919. The First Thousand Autopsies of the Pathological Service of the Massachusetts Commission on Mental Diseases. 1914–1919. *Proc Am Medico-Psych Assoc* 26:459–66.

Van Bogaert, L., and I. Bertrand. 1967. *Spongy Degeneration of the Brain in Infancy.* Amsterdam: North-Holland.

Women's Medical College of Pennsylvania. 1944. Women's Medical College of Pennsylvania Alumnae Questionnaire. Sept. 15, 1944. Archives and Special Collections on Women in Medicine, The Medical College of Pennsylvania.

JAMES STANSFIELD COLLIER

JAMES STANSFIELD COLLIER (1870–1935) (figure 1) was born and reared in Cranford, near London (now a part of Heathrow Airport) (Critchley, 1964). His early education was completed at the City and Guilds Institute, London, and he then entered medical training at St. Mary's Hospital (Obituary, 1935). The M.B. with honors was presented to him in 1894 and the M.D. in 1896 by St.

Mary's Hospital. He became a clinical clerk to Thomas Buzzard in Queen's Square and later was house physician to Sir William Broadbent at St. Mary's Hospital. Collier then accepted an unusual position as companion and personal medical attendant to a wealthy patient of William Gowers. His interest in neurology developed early, and he was accepted for training at the National Hospital, Queen's Square (Critchley, 1964). Following this training, Collier was appointed pathologist to the National Hospital in 1901 and received an appointment to the visiting staff in 1902 (Denny-Brown, 1953). The following year he was elected assistant physician to St. George's Hospital and developed a neurology teaching unit that served as a model for many years. His weekly clinical demonstrations were well attended because of his excellent teaching style. Credit for the weekly clinical demonstration sessions at Queen's Square belongs solely to Collier, and he continued them for many years. They became a part of the London scene for medical visitors:

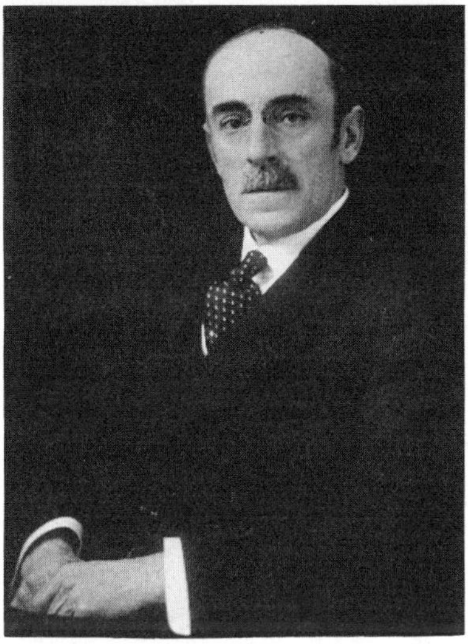

Figure 1. James Stansfield Collier (1870–1935).

In these demonstrations Collier would use every histrionic trick of display, eloquence, gesture and emphasis. Overemphasis too was not despised, for when Collier actually first began these demonstrations he told his resident medical officer not to attend. "Sometimes," he explained, "I am tempted to take liberties with the clinical history and I might be rather embarrassed if I realized that you were listening. . . ." Despite his dialectic tricks of exaggeration, he really did possess an uncanny clinical sense, and he stored up in his memory essential details of cases previously seen. (Critchley, 1964, 119–20)

Collier was the last of the English neurologists who taught at his clinic with great flair and drama in the tradition of earlier continental neurologists. Derek Denny-Brown credits Collier with the distinction of being the individual who did most to improve

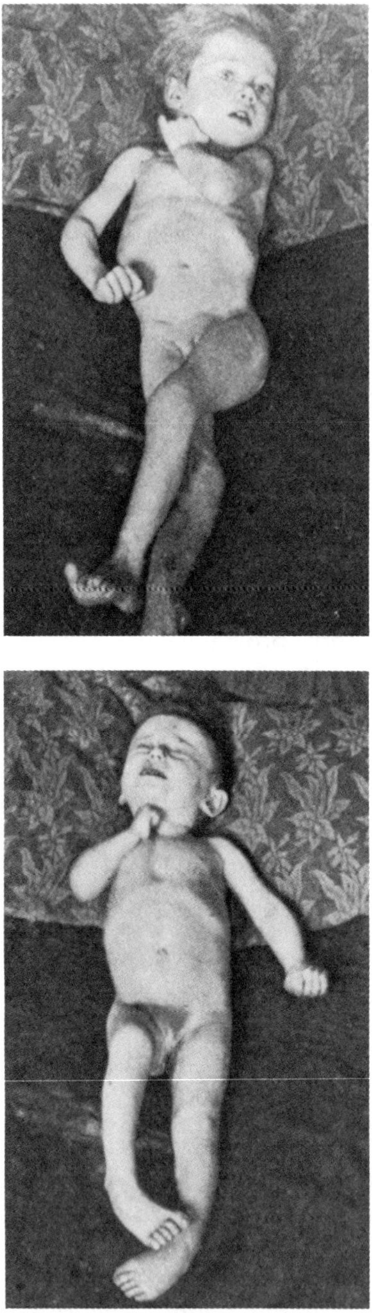

Figures 2a, b. Figures 1 and 2 from Collier's "Cerebral Diplegia," *Brain* (1899) 22:373-441.

the neurological ability of physicians of internal medicine (Denny-Brown, 1953).

Collier's significant contributions to the medical literature on nervous diseases of children began in 1899 when he published an article on cerebral diplegia in children (figures 2a, b). This work is an extensive summary of his clinical experience with the syndrome at National Hospital, Queen's Square, and includes three autopsy reports (Collier, 1899a). The most significant contribution in this particular article is his statement, "In diplegia the brain is usually affected during its development." Contrary to the general medical opinion that diplegia resulted from subdural and cerebral hemorrhage, Collier firmly believed that diplegia resulted from arrested development during formation and growth of the fetal brain. In that same year he wrote an article on Babinski's sign (Collier, 1899b). He, J. S. Risien Russell, and Frederick Batten published their classic article on subacute combined degeneration of the spinal cord in 1900, the work for which Collier is best remembered in the field of adult neurology (Collier, Russell, and Batten, 1900).

Collier's interest in nervous system diseases of infants and children continued, resulting in articles on hydrocephalus and seizures in 1904 and on tumors and seizures in 1905. He and S. Kinnier Wilson published an extensive article on amyotonia congenita in 1908 in which they credited Hermann Oppenheim with first drawing attention to this malady in 1901 (Collier and Wilson, 1908). They also suggested that Batten's "three cases of myopathy infantile type" were probably amyotonia congenita. They concluded the article with an abstract of twenty-one cases from the literature and a detailed account of four new cases. This article was followed in 1909 by another written jointly with Gordon Holmes, which unfortunately continued to add to the confusion in the literature between Werdnig-Hoffmann disease and amyotonia congenita. They presented the pathological report of two cases of amyotonia congenita and described

unmistakable pathological changes in the ventral horns at all levels of the spinal cord. The large cells of the motor type were much reduced in number, in places there appeared to be scarcely one-third of the normal number of these cells present, and those that were present were individually smaller and more angular and irregular in shape than are normal cells. (Collier and Holmes, 1909)

A revision of Charles Bastian's famous *A Treatise on Aphasia and Other Speech Defects* was completed by Collier with very little change from the original book that had been published in 1898 (Bastian, 1910). This work is useful because Bastian's book on aphasia is very difficult to locate, while Collier's revision is more readily available.

His article "Pathogenesis of Cerebral Diplegia" has been equally accepted and criticized (1924). Recent reports suggest that cerebral diplegia (cerebral palsy) is not related, in most instances, to complications during labor, delivery, or the newborn period:

These results suggest a relatively small role for factors of labor and delivery in accounting for cerebral palsy in this population. . . . This study indicates that a large proportion of cases of cerebral palsy remains unexplained. New contributions to [*the*] *explanation* [*of this disease*] *may come about as advances in the understanding of brain development and maldevelopment are translated from the basic to the clinical neurosciences.* (Nelson and Ellenburg, 1986, 86)

Recent developments in the pathogenesis of cerebral diplegia suggest that Collier's concept was correct even if some of the details in his article have not been generally accepted.

Macdonald Critchley was a resident house physician to Collier and has written an interesting commentary on his mannerisms:

Perhaps the most unforgettable characteristic of Collier was his tic-like spasms. Ordinarily quick, even jerky, in movement, he would frequently punctuate his conversation with a coordination of gestures which endeared him to all bystanders. He would abruptly hunch up one shoulder and then make a long and noisy sniff which contorted one side of his face and neck. This tic usually embellished some particularly outrageous statement on his part — like a challenge. (Critchley, 1964, 122)

Just before his sixty-fifth birthday, as he was preparing to retire from the active staff of the National Hospital, Queen's Square, Collier developed pneumonia and succumbed to heart failure. Thus, according to Macdonald Critchley, passed one of the true characters of English neurology.

Lucius Waites
DALLAS, TEXAS

REFERENCES

Bastian, C. 1910. *Aphasia and Other Speech Defects*. Revised by J. Collier. In *A System of Medicine*. Vol. 8, 385–446. Ed. C. Albutt and H. D. Rolleston. London: Macmillan Co.

Collier, J. S. 1899a. Cerebral Diplegia. *Brain* 22:373–441.

______. 1899b. Babinski's Sign. *Brain* 22:71–79.

______. 1904. The False Localizing Signs of Intracranial Tumour. *Brain* 27:490–508.

______. 1905. A Case of Acute Encephalitis Resulting in Partial Hemiplegia, and Complete Loss of Vision. *Brain* 28:589.

______. 1924. The Pathogenesis of Cerebral Diplegia: Presidential Address Delivered Before the Neurological Section of the Royal Society of Medicine, October, 1923. *Brain* 47(1):1–21.

Collier, J. S., and G. Holmes. 1909. The Pathological Examination of Two Cases of Amyotonia Congenita with the Clinical Description of a Fresh Case. Brain 32:269–84.

Collier, J. S., J. S. R. Russell, and F. E. Batten. 1900. Subacute Combined Degeneration of the Spinal Cord. Brain 23:39–110.

Collier, J. S., and S. K. Wilson. 1908. Amyotonia Congenita. Brain 31:1–14.

Critchley, M. 1964. *The Black Hole and Other Essays*, 115–23. London: Pitman.

Denny-Brown, D. 1953. James Stansfield Collier (1870–1935). In *Founders of Neurology*, 269–71. Ed. W. Haymaker. Springfield, IL: Charles C Thomas.

Nelson, K. B., and J. H. Ellenberg. 1986. Antecedents of Cerebral Palsy. *NEJM* 315:81–86.

Obituary. 1935. Collier, James Stansfield, M.D., F.R.C.P., London. Consulting Physician and Emeritus Lecturer in Neurology, St. George's Hospital. *Lancet* 1:403–4.

BRONSON CROTHERS

BRONSON CROTHERS (1884–1959) (figure 1) was one of the first doctors to spend his academic career exclusively in the field of child neurology. His early work on birth injury of the brain and spinal cord led to significant improvement in obstetric care. He pioneered the concept of mental hygiene for the handicapped child, especially those with cerebral palsy. Crothers came to feel that it was much more important to help children adjust to life rather than to concentrate on frequently futile attempts at specific treatment. For his many years' service as neurologist at the Children's Hospital in Boston and for his elucidation of many child neurology problems, he was selected posthumously to receive the American Pediatric Society's prestigious John Howland Award in 1960.

Crothers was born in Elmira, New York, during one of his father's shorter pastoral positions. Before Crothers's birth, his father was a minister in areas such as Carson City, Nevada, and Santa Barbara, California. During most of Crothers's young life, his family lived in St. Paul, Minnesota, later moving to Cambridge, Massachusetts, where his father was a minister in the Unitarian Church. Crothers attended Harvard College and finished Harvard Medical

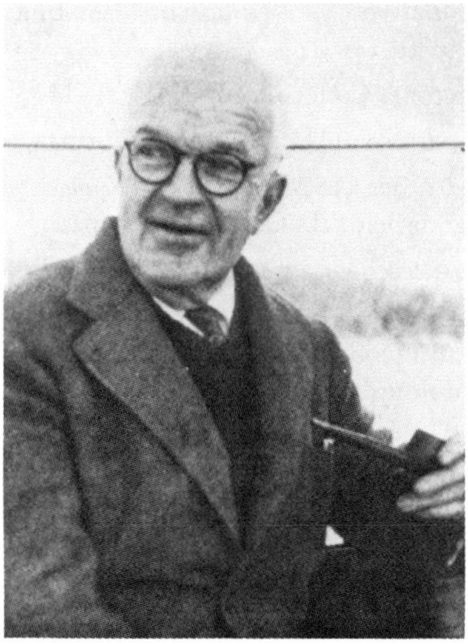

Figure 1. Bronson Crothers (1884–1959). From Byers, R. K., "Pediatric Profiles," *J Ped* 58(1961): 438–44.

School at age twenty-five. He did residency training at the Massachusetts General Hospital and the Children's Hospital in Boston. A brief period in private practice in St. Paul, Minnesota, did not seem exciting to him, but during this time he became reacquainted with his future bride, Alice Ames. In 1915 he joined the Massachusetts General Hospital unit of the British Army Medical Corps. He was cited during this period for "gallant and distinguished services in the field" by Secretary of State for War Winston S. Churchill. His association with British neurologists impressed him greatly, and his experience during World War I may have contributed to his later interest in birth injuries to the newborn nervous system.

When the United States entered the war, Crothers returned home to join the U.S. Army Medical Corps, but he took time to return to St. Paul and marry Alice Ames. After discharge, he studied at the New York Neurologic Institute and in 1920 was appointed neurologist of the Children's Hospital, as well as to the faculty of the Harvard Medical School. He kept this position until his retirement in 1952 and, even afterwards, continued to follow the patients with cerebral palsy whom he had seen over the years. With the help of Richmond Paine, Crothers published *The Natural History of Cerebral Palsy* in 1959 (Crothers and Paine, 1959).

Crothers was influenced among others by Frederick Shattuck, Stanley Cobb, George Riddock, and Sir Henry Head. Crothers was a contemporary of many medical giants in Boston, New York, and England, and his work was enhanced by his frequent contacts with them.

This influence is seen in Crothers's first book, *Disorders of the Nervous System in Childhood* (1926). Although overshadowed by the first American book on child neurology by Bernard Sachs (1895), by the later and more extensive publication of Frank Ford (1937), and actually by many of Crothers's own later and more popular works, it remains an important contribution. Consisting of 242 pages, 64 illustrations, and an admittedly brief bibliography, the book is organized into 18 chapters covering many of the major areas of child neurology, including congenital anomalies, hereditary and familial conditions, infections, hydrocephalus, tumors, convulsions, and the cerebral palsies. Philosophically, this volume covered two main areas. The first area, as alluded to, included work pertinent to specific childhood neurologic disorders. The second focused on Crothers's major concerns for the education and practical treatment of children with all types of neurological handicaps. Thus, there are chapters on psychological testing, speech evaluation, treatment and education of mentally defective or institutionalized children, and a cursory section on some of the functional disorders, such as tics and habit spasms. The book provided a general topical overview and was probably of great help to the pediatricians of the day. It conformed to the major trends of nosology and localization inherited from adult neurology but clearly had a pediatric feeling in its literature review and case descriptions. It contained many helpful illustrations, a good example being that related to the technique for performing lumbar punctures in children, as well as excellent examples of the diagnostic value of pneumoencephalography, which had just been introduced by Walter Dandy.

During his first six years at Children's Hospital, Crothers encountered 260 cases of cerebral palsy, 216 brachial plexus palsies, and 26 infants with spinal cord damage. He felt that all of these conditions could be attributed to birth trauma, especially with the use of traction. In fact, it was his paper in 1923 on spinal cord injury following breech extraction that drew attention to this very severe type of birth injury (Crothers, 1923a), although Parrott (1870) had published an excellent study of this problem. It was Crothers who advanced the theory that traction on the trunk during breech delivery may result in avulsion of the lower nerve roots from the cervical cord, as well as causing direct injury to the spinal cord. With Marian C. Putnam, he published this data in 1927; it initially appeared as an 85–page article in the journal *Medicine* (Crothers and Putnam, 1927a) but was published later

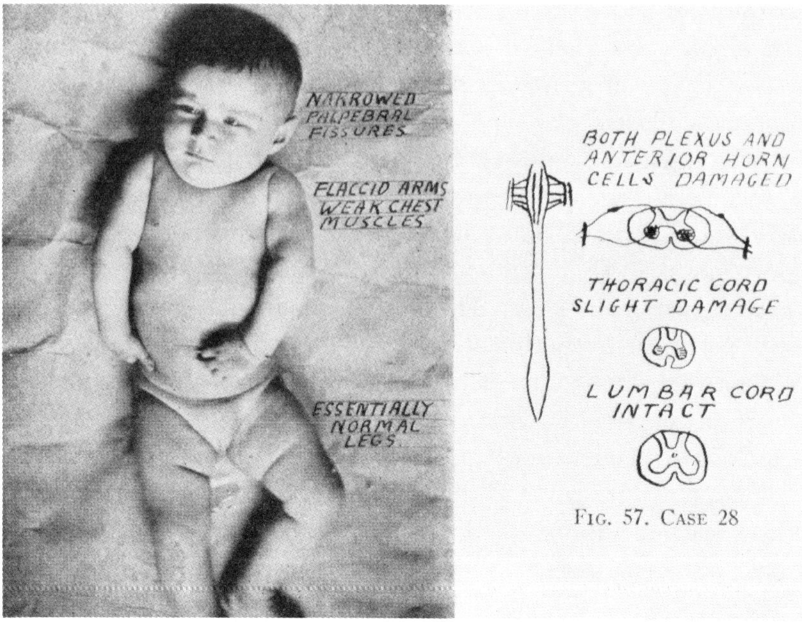

Figure 2. This two-month-old girl, seen in 1924, had bilateral flaccid paralysis of both arms. The photograph and drawing are one of many such helpful illustrations from "Cord Birth Injuries" (originally figures 56 and 57, p. 141) by Crothers and Putnam.

that year in *Birth Injuries of the Central Nervous System* (1927b). This volume was coauthored with Frank R. Ford, who contributed the first section, "Cerebral Birth Injuries." The section by Crothers and Putnam contained 28 case descriptions of almost every different type of spinal cord and brachial plexus injury. The 57 accompanying illustrations depicted the striking neurological findings on examination in a series of excellent photographs. Inserted onto these photos were notations demonstrating the pertinent findings (figure 2). With many of the clinical photographs Crothers and Putnam included a drawing illustrating either the dermatomal sensory loss, motor deficit, sphincter involvement, a cross section of the spinal cord pathology as it was found at autopsy, or the nature of the clinically suspected lesion. Crothers and Putnam also included a detailed review of the previous literature on this topic, referring, for example, to Ludwig Mauthner's 1844 monograph reporting two infants with breech presentation and flaccid paraplegia and the later and important case report of J. Parrot (1870), which was accompanied by autopsy findings showing spinal cord hemorrhage with complete separation of the cord in the cervical region. Crothers was appalled by the apparent lack of knowledge on the part of obstetricians that complications of birth were so prevalent. Although many of the cases of cerebral palsy may not have been due to birth injuries, as we suspect today, his work heightened awareness in the obstetrical community and led to significant improvement of the management of difficult deliveries. Among Crothers's other numerous observations was his finding that, during difficult deliveries, there was a tremendous increase in pressure on the tentorium, which was transmitted downward towards the spinal cord, and that infants who were frequently thought to be suffering from asphyxial injury actually had posterior fossa hemorrhage (Crothers, 1923b).

The advent of pneumoencephalography brought many improvements to child neurology, but Crothers pointed out one of the shortcomings in 1950 in a paper he wrote with H. V. Smith entitled "Subdural Fluid as a Consequence of Pneumoencephalography." He also appears to be one of the earliest investigators who realized that the size of the ventricular system was not necessarily related to the intelligence of the child. He is credited with publishing at least fifty-six papers and books, all dealing with the broad field of child neurology. Crothers also undoubtedly influenced many others to write papers in this field. He was president of the Boston Society for Neurology and Psychiatry in 1940 and of the Academy of Cerebral Palsy in 1951. His association with Elizabeth Lord and Edith Meyer-Taylor added much to current neuropsychological thinking in relation to children.

Crothers felt that the need for psychological support of children with neurological handicaps was great enough to warrant publishing a monograph entitled *A Pediatrician in Search of Mental Hygiene* (Crothers, 1937). Throughout his career he emphasized the importance of emotional well-being and adjustment to life in general. He found that treatments such as muscle training and speech therapy had limited results, and that overzealous efforts in these directions often led to disappointment and despair. Most of the suicides he encountered in palsied patients seemed to have this correlation.

The inability of the pediatrician to be omniscient was apparent to him, and he was one of the first to employ a team approach to his patients. He had a long association with psychologists, especially Elizabeth Lord, as well as with orthopedists and therapists (C. A. Smith, 1983). He made a great effort to point out that their relationship to the patient should not be considered subordinate to that of the medical doctor or even the neurologist. In this regard he was probably one of the first physicians to apply the team approach to treatment of the handicapped child. This is best exemplified by *The Natural History of Cerebral Palsy*, co-authored with Richmond Paine (1959) and based on his evaluations of more than 1300 children seen at the Boston Children's Hospital between 1930 and 1950. The early chapters contain sections reviewing the growth, development, and neurological examination of children. The main emphasis, however, is Crother's extensive experience and his comments on the etiologies of cerebral palsy, and more importantly, treatment programs, establishment of clinics and the psychological effects of this handicapping condition on children and their families.

A vivid insight into his personality is related to his work with Randolph Byers. Byers and Elizabeth Lord suggested that lead might be injurious to the development of the nervous system, then a rather new concept in medicine. Representatives of the lead industry visited them and seemed "bent on making trouble" about this suggestion. Crothers decided to take all parties to lunch. After he had hosted a very jovial meal, he calmed their anguish and obtained ten year's of financial support for the study of lead poisoning in children. This work resulted in the first systematic study of the psychological and developmental effects of lead poisoning in children (Byers and Lord, 1943).

As one frequently finds in a minister's child, Bronson Crothers was considered a "character." Early exploits have been implied but not recorded. Throughout his life he had a keen sense of humor. He could be caustic when discussing individuals whom he considered pompous or intellectually dishonest. For example, as moderator at a meeting on one occasion, he successfully admonished participants stating that "some of the discussers, whether through modesty or arrogance, are failing to give their names on arising." All participants thereafter quickly gave their names. He was usually soft-spoken, exceedingly polite, and was never self-aggrandizing. The citation he received from the British army was unknown even to his wife until she went through his effects after his death.

Neither did he mention his heroic actions when his airline flight crashed into Boston Harbor. Although he was then over sixty years of age, he is credited with saving several lives by helping them out of the plane and onto land. It was only through his secretary's comments that I learned about this deed. Crothers was typically modest when told of his selection to receive the Howland Award. Unfortunately, he died of spinal muscular atrophy before he actually received it.

Bronson Crothers was never significantly involved in a formal training program of other child neurologists. His influence was best seen in those who worked with him directly at the Children's Hospital in Boston, namely Randolph Byers, Richmond Paine, William Berenberg, and Kenneth Sands. The early child neurology trainees at this hospital had the opportunity of spending time with him and learning his philosophies firsthand. It is impossible to tell how many others were directly or indirectly influenced by his teaching. He had pupils from other parts of the world, such as Sir Peter Tizard from England and Thomas Ingram from Edinburgh.

There is no question that Bronson Crothers was one of the true giants of child neurology, and it is unfortunate that one has to search to learn about his achievements. He was a classic example of those who care less about who gets credit for a new idea than what it might possibly do for mankind. It is difficult to conceive of the breadth of his influence in this field, not only on his patients and their families, but equally on all physicians in whose training he had a part.

William T. McLean, Jr.
WINSTON-SALEM, NORTH CAROLINA

REFERENCES

Byers, R. K. 1961. Pediatric Profiles. *J Ped* 58:438–44.

Byers, R. K. and E. E. Lord. 1943. Late Effects of Lead Poisoning on Mental Development. *Am J Dis Child* 66:471.

Crothers, B. 1923a. Injury of the Spinal Cord in Breech Extraction as an Important Cause of Foetal Death and Paraplegia in Childhood. *Am J Med Sci* 165:94–110.

______. 1923b. Changes in Pressure Inside the Fetal Craniovertebral Cavity. *SGO* 37:790–801.

______. 1926. *Disorders of the Nervous System in Childhood.* New York: D. Appleton.

______. 1937. *A Pediatrician in Search of Mental Hygiene.* New York: The Commonwealth Fund.

Crothers, B., and R. S. Paine. 1959. *The Natural History of Cerebral Palsy.* Cambridge, MA: Harvard University Press.

Crothers, B., and M. C. Putnam. 1927a. Obstetrical Injuries of the Spinal Cord. *Medicine* 6:41–126.

______. 1927b. Cord Birth Injuries. Part 2 in *Birth Injuries of the Central Nervous System*, 79–164. Baltimore: Williams and Wilkins.

Ford, F. R. 1937. *Diseases of the Nervous System in Infancy, Childhood and Adolescence.* Springfield, IL: Charles C Thomas.

Sachs, B. 1895. *A Treatise on the Nervous Diseases of Children for Physicians and Students.* New York: William Wood and Company.

Smith, C. A. 1983. *The Children's Hospital of Boston: "Build Better Than They Knew."* Boston: Little, Brown.

Smith, H. V., and B. Crothers. 1950. Subdural Fluid as a Consequence of Pneumoencephalography. *Ped* 5:375–89.

OCTAVE CROUZON

OCTAVE CROUZON (1874–1938) (figure 1) was born of a French father and a Flemish mother in relatively humble surroundings outside the city of Paris. Indeed, he later recounted that had he not received a scholarship, he would not have been able to further his education. He attended high school at the Collège Rollin (1885–1892), where he came under the influence of Pierre Janet, an enthusiastic and ardent teacher who recently had presented his doctoral thesis on "psychological automatism." Janet served as an important model for Crouzon's own intellectual development and directed him towards medicine and the workings of the nervous system. Crouzon's scholarship was extended to allow university study. He diligently applied himself at the Paris Faculty of

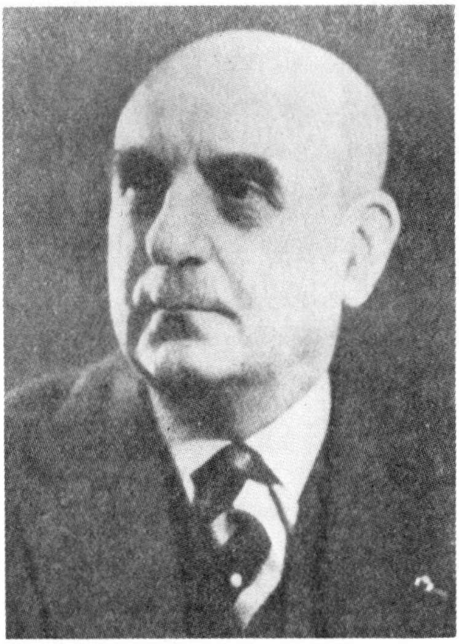

Figure 1. Octave Crouzon. (1874–1938).

Medicine, where he was captivated by the eloquence and mastery of Georges Dieulafoy, a professor of pathology whose primary area of interest was diseases of the central nervous system. Prior to receiving his Doctor of Medicine in 1904, Crouzon served an internship and then a residency at the Hôpital de Paris. In 1906 he was reunited with Dieulafoy at the Hôtel Dieu when he was appointed chef de clinique; six years later he was elevated to the position of Médicin des Hôpitaux. He served in this capacity until the outbreak of World War I.

In these formative years Crouzon trained under and associated with many of the great French neurologists including Désiré Bourneville and his proteges, Alfred Fournier and Joseph Babinski at La Pitié. Crouzon's most significant tutelage, however, came from Pierre Marie at the Salpêtrière. There Crouzon wrote his inaugural thesis on combined sclerosis, an impressive clinical and anatomical study based on work he performed in Pierre Marie's clinic at the Bicêtre (Crouzon, 1904). It was also at the Salpêtrière and in its stimulating environment that Crouzon became interested in the systematic study of neurological disorders and hereditary and familial dystrophies.

With the outbreak of World War I, Crouzon's administrative skills were recognized by the undersecretary of the state for military health services, who gave him the responsibility of originating a special neurology service for the armed forces. For his work in this area Crouzon received not only the War Cross Medal but also the Légion d'Honneur. The remainder of Crouzon's clinical career was spent almost entirely at the Salpêtrière, where in 1919 he became a member of the staff and subsequently a professor of medicine. He worked quite vigorously in the School for Nurses, where he maintained an active neurology service directed both toward diagnostic evaluation and education of those in training. Crouzon occupied numerous positions of prominence within the medical community. He succeeded Henri Meige as the general secretary of the Paris Neurology Society and at the *Revue neurologique*. For the ten years prior to his death he was a dominating force in French neurology. In 1935 Crouzon received what he considered to be his highest award when he was named a member of the French Academy of Medicine.

Crouzon had a longstanding interest in social medicine and public health issues. He recognized the importance of looking beyond a theory of medicine directed at treating only the individual and strove to make both medical students and fellow physicians understand the necessity for public health policy (Bezançon, 1938). Crouzon's ideas on these health care problems, which had been exacerbated by the war, were formally presented in a book entitled *Les assurances sociales, guide à l'usage du corps medical* (*Manual of Public Welfare*, Crouzon, 1930). In 1920 Crouzon was appointed a member of the Supervisory Council on Public Welfare and was a major participant in the work of renovating the French hospital system. Near the end of his career, Crouzon's dedication to social medicine was fittingly recognized by the City Council of Paris and the General Council of the Seine when he was named the first recipient of the Medical-Social-Welfare Chair at the Paris Faculty of Medicine.

Throughout his career, Crouzon made many valuable contributions in the field of child neurology, including his investigations on muscular dystrophies (Crouzon and Bouttier, 1919); congenital ophthalmoplegia (Crouzon and Behague, 1920); the familial cerebellar ataxias (Crouzon, Bouttier, and Bertrand, 1923); infantile encephalopathy and paralysis (Crouzon, 1925); and developmental anomalies of the spine, including spina bifida (Crouzon and Behague, 1921), and the Klippel-Feil syndrome (Crouzon and Liege, 1928). In later years Crouzon became very interested in epilepsy, especially myoclonic seizures, and he experimented with potassium bromide in the treatment of convulsions (Crouzon, 1928). Crouzon is best recognized, however, for his critical studies of hereditary craniofacial deformities, especially the syndrome that bears his name. He had observed a mother and her young son with identical craniofacial malformations when he was working at the Salpêtrière under the supervision of Pierre Marie (figures 2a,b). He later presented these

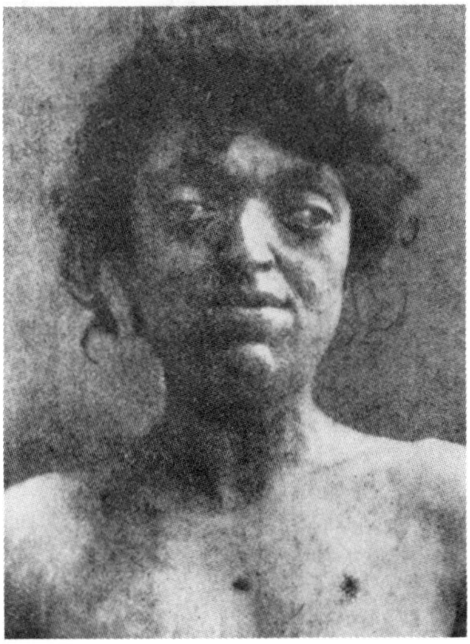

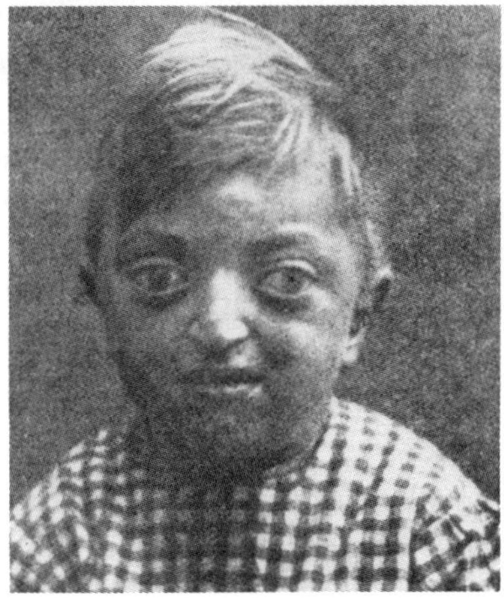

Figures 2a, b. Madame W. and son Roger W., the first patients that Crouzon described with "la dysostose cranio-faciale héréditaire." From Crouzon, *Etudes sur les maladies familiales nerveuses et dystrophiques*. Paris: Masson, 1929, 279–80.

two cases at a meeting of the Société Médicale des Hôpitaux de Paris as a specific familial syndrome (Crouzon, 1912). Crouzon remained deeply interested in the condition; he collected many other cases and subsequent publications contained clinical descriptions that even today are difficult to improve upon. From this work, a whole series of observations and research related to familial skeletal disorders arose, allowing Crouzon to postulate a classification explaining the hereditary and familial dystrophies affecting the skeletal system (Crouzon, 1932). Also at the Salpêtrière Crouzon initiated a series of clinical and pathological studies that systematically examined both typical and atypical familial nervous system disorders. These studies brought to this clinically complex and, at that time, pathologically obscure grouping of disorders, a precision that greatly served subsequent research in this area (Crouzon, 1929). It has been noted that in all of Crouzon's investigations the observations were solid, the presentations clear, and the methods and documentation firmly based.

In all his work Crouzon constantly sought to apply the principles of heredity formulated by Gregor Mendel to the pathogenesis of various neurological disorders. Initially, Mendel's ideas either were criticized or overlooked by most physicians. However, based on sound clinical and pathological observations by individuals like Crouzon, the importance of hereditary disorders slowly entered medical thinking. In all, Crouzon published over forty articles and books in which he elucidated familial patterns of neurological diseases, in some instances tracing the illness back through four generations. He was thus a seminal contributor to our recognition and understanding of genetic influences on disorders of the nervous system.

Outside formal medicine, Crouzon's interests were extremely varied and included anthropology and medicolegal issues. In the latter regard he graciously gave his time to the Law Court of the Seine, where his expert opinion was often instrumental in settling medicolegal disputes. He was described by colleagues as a man of firm intellectual qualities and enormous industry, and as possessing a clear sense of direction. He was valued by many as a highly appreciative listener and a man with great generosity (Jelliffe, 1939). Perhaps his most fitting tribute was provided by his colleague Gustave Roussy, who proclaimed, "Octave Crouzon was a friend, encompassing all that that word contains of vibrancy, of life, of sincerity, and of depth" (Roussy, 1938).

Michael J. Noetzel
ST. LOUIS, MISSOURI

ACKNOWLEDGMENTS

The author gratefully wishes to acknowledge the assistance of Joann M. Boczenowski for translating the original French references.

REFERENCES

Bezançon, O. 1938. Nécrologie: Décès de M. Crouzon. *Bull Acad Méd Paris* 120:165–67.

Crouzon, O. 1904. Anatomie pathologique des scléroses combinées tabétiques. *Nouv Icon Salpêtrière* 17:52–66.

______. 1912. Dysostose cranio-faciale héréditaire. *Bull Soc Méd Hôp Paris* 33:454–555.

______. 1925. Les encéphalopathies infantiles familiales. *Ann méd psych* 83:108–11.

______. 1928. *Le syndrome épilepsie*. Paris: Doin.

______. 1929. *Etudes sur les maladies familiales nerveuses et dystrophiques*. Paris: Masson.

______. 1930. *Les assurances sociales, guide à l'usage du corps medical*. Paris: Masson.

______. 1932. Sur le dysostose cranio-faciale et ses rapports avec l'acrocéphalo-syndactylie. *Bull Soc Méd Hôp Paris* 48:1568–74.

Crouzon, O., and P. Behague. 1920. Contribution à l'histoire d'une famille atteinte d'ophthalmoplégie congénitale dans trois générations. *Bull Soc Méd Hôp Paris* 44:372–77.

______. 1921. Fréquence à la bifidité des apophyses épineuses des vertèbres dorso-lumbaires. *Bull Soc Méd Hôp Paris* 45:403–5.

Crouzon, O., and H. Bouttier. Sur une variété singulière d'amyotrophie familiale. *Bull Soc Méd Hôp Paris* 43:1097–112.

Crouzon, O., H. Bouttier, and I. Betrand. 1923. A-propos d'une maladie familale du système nerveux proche de l'hérédo-ataxia cérébelleuse; étude anatomo-clinique. *Rev neur Paris* 30:314–27.

Crouzon, O., and R. Liege. 1928. Les anomalies du développement de la colonne cervicale côté cervicale. Syndrome de Klippel-Feil. *Monde méd* 38:737–47.

Jelliffe, S. E. 1939. Obituary. O. Crouzon. *J Nerv Ment Dis* 89:264–65.

Roussy, M. D. 1938. Notice nécrologique sur M. Octave Crouzon (1874–1938). *Bull Acad Méd Paris* 120:217–21.

HARVEY CUSHING

PROBABLY THE CHIEF architect and builder of the specialty of neurosurgery was Harvey Williams Cushing (1869–1939) (figure 1). Among Cushing's major accomplishments were his contributions to the neurosurgery of children and adolescents (Fulton, 1946; Thomson, 1950). To quote John Farquhar Fulton: "Harvey Cushing was widely known in three distinct capacities — as a great physician, as the founder of a school of neurosurgery, and as a humanist of unusual literary attainment" (Fulton, 1939, 477).

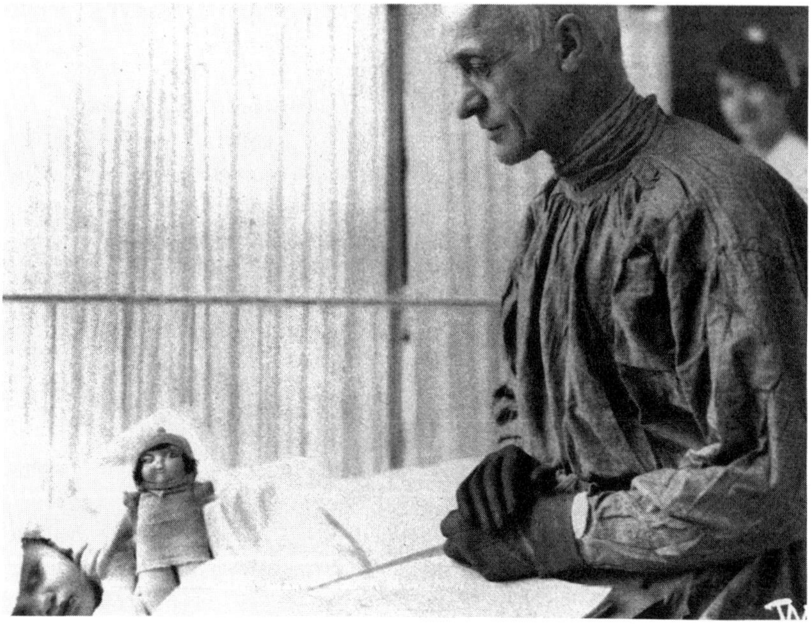

Figure 1. Harvey Cushing (1869–1939) examining a young patient a few days after removal of a cerebellar tumor.

Perhaps Cushing's greatest neurosurgical contribution was in the field of intracranial tumors, which became the main focus of his professional life. His meticulous surgical technique learned from the "Professor," William S. Halsted, was especially important in his development of this special field of neurosurgery. In addition, he developed technical aids that greatly enhanced the ability to remove tumors. These included the silver clip for occlusion of blood vessels (Cushing, 1911, 1927a) and the use of the electrosurgical instrument for tumor removal, which he introduced with William T. Bovie (Cushing, 1928a).

It is also important to emphasize Cushing's role as an investigator (Horrax, 1939). This is perhaps best shown in his investigations of the pituitary gland, beginning with the publication of his first monograph, *The Pituitary Body and Its Disorders* in 1912. His interest in pituitary pathology continued throughout most of his career, culminating in his 1932 paper on pituitary basophil adenomas (Cushing, 1932). This disorder became known as Cushing's disease. His other important monographs on tumors were those on acoustic tumors (1917) and the meningiomas

(1927a). The latter work, published with Louise Eisenhardt, was considered his greatest clinical treatise (Cushing and Eisenhardt, 1938). These monographs are noted because of their importance, despite the fact that tumors of the pituitary gland and acoustic nerve, as well as meningiomas, are uncommon in the pediatric population.

Cushing's first paper relating to pediatric neurosurgery, "Concerning Surgical Intervention for the Intracranial Hemorrhages of the New-Born," was published in 1905 (Cushing, 1905a). He reported four infants who, following either prolonged labor and spontaneous delivery or a difficult delivery, were depressed and developed seizures and other neurological signs. Cushing operated a few days after birth, finding massive subdural hematomas. Two of these newborns survived, one with apparently minimal sequelae. He thus demonstrated that surgery on such newborns could be successful.

Cushing's "Surgery of the Head," published in 1908 in William W. Keen's *Surgery, Its Principles and Practice*, was the first definitive American work on neurosurgery (Horrax, 1939). In this work, Cushing further discussed treatment of neonatal injuries to the skull and nervous system. He described the recognition and treatment of hydrocephalus, including congenital hydrocephalus in the newborn associated with spina bifida (meningomyelocele).

Among those patients in whom the ventricles communicated with the lumbar subarachnoid space, he reported twelve cases in which he operated using a new technique. He trephined the L5 vertebra through a laparotomy and transperitoneal approach, combining this with a laminectomy, and placed a silver cannula that connected and drained the subarachnoid space into the peritoneal cavity. Although he reported a "considerable measure of success" in twelve cases, long-term follow-up was wanting. Later, however, he noted that none of the surgical procedures gave uniform results (Cushing, 1910). A lumbar-subarachnoid-peritoneal shunt had not previously been reported. This principle of treating hydrocephalus, long abandoned, would eventually be rediscovered, improved upon, and adapted to the modern treatment of hydrocephalic infants.

In the Hunterian Laboratory of Surgical Research at the Johns Hopkins Medical School, Cushing initiated various studies on the cerebrospinal fluid (CSF) that profoundly influenced other investigators such as Walter E. Dandy, Lewis H. Weed, and Kenneth

D. Blackfan (German, 1969). Cushing's first paper on this topic was published in 1914.

Cushing's interest in CSF studies and hydrocephalus was unfortunately associated with one of the regrettable schisms in American neurosurgery. Cushing selected Walter Dandy to be his assistant resident and appointee in the Hunterian Laboratory for the year 1911–12. During that year, as Fulton noted, a conflict of personalities arose relating to Dandy's investigations. Dandy and Blackfan had begun their classic studies on experimental hydrocephalus in 1911. As Cushing was leaving Baltimore to take up his new appointment at Harvard and the Brigham Hospital, he placed Dandy's papers in a box of materials from the Hunterian Laboratory he was taking with him to Boston. As Fox later recounted, Dandy removed his records, announcing that it was his work, and that it would remain in Baltimore. For Cushing this apparently was the final straw, and shortly afterwards he informed Dandy that he would not be taking him to Boston (Fox, 1975). What part, if any, Cushing had in initiating these experiments other than allowing them to be performed in his laboratory is unknown. Cushing certainly had a strong interest in hydrocephalus in children (Cushing, 1910). The landmark experimental work by Dandy and Blackfan proved for the first time that CSF was secreted by the choriod plexus and absorbed diffusely by the pia-arachnoid veins (Dandy and Blackfan, 1913, 1914). These classic experiments formed the basis of our understanding of the nature and treatment of obstructive and communicating hydrocephalus.

Because of his rigid temperament and his precipitous decision concerning this affair, Cushing's Laboratory of Surgical Research at Harvard lost credit that it would otherwise have surely gained for this outstanding work. A great opportunity to find a solution to the problem of hydrocephalus was lost (German, 1969). It is a pity that Cushing did not recall that he had been in exactly the same situation as Dandy when he was working under Kocher's direction in Berne just a few years earlier (Fulton, 1946, 184).

Lewis Weed, who also had begun experimental studies on CSF and the pituitary gland in the Hunterian Laboratory, was invited by Cushing to go to Boston. Weed continued his important studies on CSF as a fellow in charge of the Laboratory of Surgical Research in 1912 (Weed, 1914; Thomson, 1950). Weed added to Dandy's work by demonstrating that CSF is principally absorbed in microscopic arachnoid villi found in the major cerebral veins, resembling Pacchionian granulations. This in itself was an important contribution to the understanding of hydrocephalus, a condition relatively more frequent in infants and children, and for which satisfactory surgical treatment lay in the future (Weed, 1914, 1917)

Cushing's most important contributions to pediatric neurology and neurosurgery were made over a period of five years, from 1926 to 1931 (German, 1969). This work had its genesis in the summer of 1922, when Cushing asked Percival Bailey, his assistant resident, and Arthur Tracy Cabot, a fellow in the surgical research laboratory, to create a histologic laboratory for the study of his collection of brain tumors. Bailey began first to classify the gliomas, working on this project intermittently for the next three years. Virtually all the work was done by Bailey, who later held some natural resentment toward Cushing for the latter's failure to acknowledge his contributions properly. Nevertheless, Bailey later generously expressed his affection for Cushing (Bailey, 1985).

The results of the glioma studies were first reported by Cushing in the Cameron Prize Lectures given at the University of Edinburgh in October 1925. The completed monograph by Bailey and Cushing, *A Classification of Tumors of the Glioma Group on a Histiogenetic Basis with a Correlated Study of Prognosis*, appeared in 1926. Here for the first time was an orderly classification of gliomas with their natural history and clinical course. This study included a total of 414 cases of glioma in Cushing's series; Bailey had done histologic tissue studies on 254. Based on the predominant cellular configuration, Bailey classified these tumors into thirteen categories. This histologic categorization was the first of its kind, and formed the basis for all subsequent classifications. From this study, it was determined that approximately 40 percent of gliomas had a relatively favorable prognosis if correctly diagnosed and operated (Bailey and Cushing, 1926; Horrax, 1944). The study also showed that certain of these tumors — for example, the ependymoblastomas, the unipolar spongioblastomas, and the medulloblastomas — were predominantly tumors of the pediatric age group.

Studying these cases further and adding another 159, Bailey reduced and simplified the glioma classification to ten groups. Cushing carefully reviewed the survival figures. The new classification of 1927 correlated the tumor types with survival (Bailey, 1927b). Bailey also published a valuable histologic atlas of these gliomas (Bailey, 1927b).

In 1923 Paul Martin and Cushing reported seven cases of optic nerve glioma. Four of the seven cases occurred in children. The authors emphasized the frequent finding of optic atrophy, a common finding of erosion of the anterior clinoid process on X ray, and the association of the tumor with von Recklinghausen's neurofibromatosis (Martin and Cushing, 1923).

Cushing's first report of his series of pediatric brain tumors in 1927 was "The Intracranial Tumors of Preadolescence." Of 1,108 verified tumors, 154 had occurred in patients under 15 years old (Cushing, 1927b). In this paper, Cushing noted that 40 percent of adult tumors — that is, meningiomas, acoustic tumors, and pituitary tumors — were "practically excluded from the children's list." The gliomas were found to make up 75 percent of childhood brain tumors, with cerebellar or infratentorial tumors being twice as common as those occurring above the tentorium. The other tumors included a small group of congenital tumors, such as craniopharyngiomas, tuberculomas and blood vessel tumors.

Cushing stressed the diagnostic vicissitudes that confront the physician who examines the child with a brain tumor, and urged careful and repeated examination of the optic fundi, as most children with posterior fossa tumors developed increased intracranial pressure with papilledema. In this report, Cushing cited a recent letter from a distinguished neurologist in another city whose experiences with operations on brain tumors in children had either been fatal or produced poor results. In contrast, the results in Cushing's clinic were hopeful in that cerebellar astrocytomas were twice as common as the more malignant medulloblastoma, and had an average postoperative survival of over six years. Moreover, the operative mortality had steadily dropped in the years preceding these reports.

Within the next two years, two additional seminal papers appeared on brain tumors in children. The first of these described Cushing's experiences with cerebellar medulloblastomas (Cushing, 1930) and the next, his experiences with cerebellar astrocytomas (Cushing, 1931).

The essay on medulloblastomas (the term was coined by Percival

Bailey (Bailey and Cushing, 1925)) was a classic that can hardly be improved upon today. The series of sixty-one cases includes six early cases operated at the Johns Hopkins Hospital in which the true nature and behavior of the tumors were not recognized. Also, these six surgeries were performed before the introduction of the suction apparatus and electrosurgical instrument (Cushing, 1928a).

Cushing described a "composite" of symptoms so typical of these tumors as follows:

A preadolescent child previously in good health begins to complain of headaches or of suboccipital discomfort and to have occasional attacks of vomiting without preliminary nausea, usually on first arising in the morning. Attendance at school meanwhile may continue but the teacher soon notices that the child is listless or inattentive and the character of its work noticeably falls off. Ere long it is apparent that there is some unwonted clumsiness of movement and awkwardness in gait. The mother may find that the child quickly outgrows its caps and she thinks the head enlarges unduly fast. In course of time it is noticed, at home or at school, that the child's sight is impaired; or a beginning squint of one eye may be detected, even in the absence of any complaint of double vision. The family doctor, who has previously suspected some gastro-intestinal disorder, may then have the eyegrounds examined and to the surprise of everyone a choked disk is found. Three or four months on the average have elapsed, and at about this stage of the malady many cases first come under hospital care.

Should the condition not be recognized so soon, the symptoms relentlessly progress. The clumsiness increases until the gait gradually becomes so ataxic walking without support is difficult; vomiting grows more frequent, the child begins to lose weight; the muscles become wasted and atonic; there may be a slight facial palsy; the internal squint may become bilateral and finally "fainting spells" occur, characterized by extensor rigidities that may be precipitated by slight changes in position. Ere this the child will have become bedridden. The whole story if uninterrupted by operation may cover a period averaging from eight to nine months. (Cushing, 1930, 43–44)

Diagnosis of such tumors at this time was largely clinical because today's sophisticated neuroimaging tests were unknown. Despite improvement in surgical techniques, survival was still measured in months. However, the problem of spinal seeding and the beneficial effect of radiation therapy were noted.

Further studies of Cushing's cases led to the conclusion that it was advisable to radiate the entire cerebrospinal axis following an operation for medulloblastoma, since a fatal outcome was inevitable once the patient developed symptoms from seeding (Bailey, 1930).

The 1931 article "Experiences with Cerebellar Astrocytomas" summarized Cushing's experience with these more favorable tumors. Here he acknowledged Bailey's "highly important contributory role." Again, though differing in some aspects from the medulloblastomas, a composite clinical progression was given:

A child apparently normal in all respects begins toward the end of the first decade, possibly after a fall or an attack of whooping cough, to have early morning headaches with vomiting. Nothing much is made of this by the family doctor, should he be called in, for the child subsequently feels perfectly well, has had breakfast and wants to go out and play. This daily performance may continue for a considerable time, the child even going to school meanwhile. There may then be a remission of weeks or perhaps months° and the episode [may] be forgotten. On their recurrence, the symptoms are likely to be more pronounced and are apt to be ascribed to some gastro-intestinal disturbance. This appears the more probable since the child finds that straining at stool brings on a headache and there is a tendency to become constipated. What is more, a mild daily laxative usually serves completely to mask the symptoms.

This sort of thing continues off and on until it becomes evident that the child is a little clumsy at play and gets knocked over easily. Very possibly, ere this, the periodic headache and vomiting will have ceased completely or at least have occurred at much longer intervals; and if parents are observant they may notice that the child's head in the interim has increased in size more rapidly than it should. This, however, is usually discounted for the child meanwhile has become free from complaints and in all respects appears alert and well.

Matters may run on in this way for an indefinite time, possibly with some increase in clumsiness of movement or in some instances with no noticeable change whatever until it suddenly becomes apparent, perhaps at school, that the child's sight is poor. To counteract this glasses are usually prescribed; but even should an opthalmoscope be resorted to, a child's retina is less easily examined than that of an adult and because of the decompressive effects of the enlarging head, the optic papillae often show no measurable swelling and the fact of their being pale and with margins blurred may easily pass unrecognized.

Due to the insidious nature of the symptomatic onset, it is in this pre-amaurotic stage of the process that even today the victims of these mid-cerebellar astrocytomas, unfortunately continue to be admitted to hospital. (Cushing, 1931, 147–48)

This series was based on seventy-six cerebellar astrocytomas. The children tended to become asymptomatic at an older age, have a longer duration of symptoms and greater loss of vision than the cases of medulloblastomas. Of perhaps greater importance was Cushing's discovery that removing the mural nodule in the cystic cerebellar astrocytomas would commonly lead to a long remission or cure. The importance of this surgical characterisic of the cystic cerebellar astrocytomas had not previously been recognized or reported.

These papers on brain tumors in children, illustrating the classic clinical picture and detailing the surgical aspects of the cases, including the beautiful illustrations drawn by Mildred Codding from Cushing's operative sketches, give some idea of the principles that made Cushing a great neurosurgeon (Matson, 1969). Cushing firmly believed that a surgeon should be familiar with all aspects of his cases; hence he did his own careful examination in each case and did not rely on a neurologist or someone else (Cushing, 1905b). He carefully recorded his cases, a habit he probably learned from William Osler. As Cushing pointed out in the cerebellar astrocytoma article:

What has been chiefly contributory in recent years to the success of operations for intracranial tumors has been the tendency of those interested in the subject to concentrate upon the behavior and traits of special tumors in special situations. (Cushing, 1931, 129)

This point is best illustrated by a case mortality of only 4 percent in the last twenty-five consecutive operations on these cerebellar tumors, a remarkable accomplishment in view of the prolonged and radical nature of the operations (Cushing, 1931).

This was Cushing's last major paper on brain tumors before his retirement in 1933. He undoubtedly had the largest operative experience in brain tumors in children, despite operating in the Brigham Hospital, which was not a children's hospital. Nevertheless, Cushing's reputation and skill brought him a wide referral of such patients.

In his 1925 Cameron Prize Lectures at the University of Edinburgh, Cushing included an assessment of the contributions from his students and fellow surgical investigators:

I do not know that I personally am to be credited with anything more than the introduction of a few trifling technical procedures which in time are almost certain to be superseded. However . . . a teacher's influence . . . should be centrifugal, his own ideas being far less important than the ideas which radiate from his pupils and theirs in turn. One of the greatest satisfactions of my professional life . . . has been my privilege to appoint annually some younger man who has been put in independent charge of a laboratory of experimental surgery. . . . (Cushing, 1926, xii)

Some events of Cushing's life are relevant to this presentation. He was born April 8, 1869, in Cleveland, Ohio. The sixth son and tenth child of Henry Kirke and Betsey Maria Williams Cushing, Harvey Cushing was raised in a comfortable upper middle-class home. Following graduation from Yale University and Harvard Medical School (*cum laude*, 1895) he spent a year (1895–96) as a surgical house officer at the Massachusetts General Hospital. In 1896 he joined William Stewart Halsted as an assistant resident at the Johns Hopkins Hospital. Stimulated by William Henry Welch, William Osler, Howard Atwood Kelly, and Halsted, Cushing developed a strong interest in the history of medicine bibliophilia, and dedicated his talents to the development of neurological surgery.

He spent a year (1900–1901) with Emil Theodor Kocher and Karl Hugo Kronecker in Berne, Switzerland, studing the physiology of intracranial pressure, and a month with Charles Scott Sherrington in Liverpool studying the motor cortex in apes (Fulton, 1946, 161ff).

In 1902 he married Katharine Stone Crowell (1870–1949), with whom he had five children. In 1912 Cushing left Baltimore for Boston as Moseley Professor of Surgery and departmental chairman at Harvard Medical School. He served as surgeon-in-chief at the Peter Bent Brigham Hospital until he retired. During World War I Cushing organized the Harvard ambulance service in France. Later he was made director of the Fifth Base Hospital and was senior neurosurgical consultant to the American Expeditionary Forces. Forced to retire at Harvard, in 1933 he became Sterling

Professor of Neurology at Yale University, serving until his death on October 7, 1939.

He bequeathed his library of eight thousand volumes and other items to Yale University, which, with the libraries of his two friends John Farquhar Fulton and Arnold Carl Klebs, became the nucleus of one of the world's fine collections in the history of medicine. Cushing published over three hundred scientific papers and reports, twenty-four books, and many other contributions. An additional three hundred papers were published by associates, fellows, students, and others from his clinics and laboratories (Harvey Cushing Society, 1939; Cushing, 1943). He was a dedicated pedagogue with considerable artistic abilities, which he displayed when lecturing, enjoying drawing on a blackboard with both hands.

His nonsurgical contributions included the Pulitzer Prize-winning *Life of Sir William Osler* (1925), his World War I experience *From a Surgeon's Journal 1915–1918* (1936), *Consecratio Medici and Other Papers* (1928b), and *The Medical Career and Other Papers* (1940).

Harvey Cushing made fundamental contributions to child neurology through his work in the field of neurosurgery. As noted by several biographers (Fulton, 1946; Thomson, 1950) he set an example in the application of scientific method to clinical problems, especially that of tumors of the brain. He trained and influenced most of the neurosurgeons of his era in America and many from abroad. His landmark papers secured his place as the pioneer surgeon dealing with brain tumors in children. Cushing's singular dedication to his major life's work can be understood in the following statement:

The surgery of brain tumors may be likened without being trivial to a form of major sport which is played against an invisible but utterly relentless antagonist quick to take advantage of every misplay and faulty move. And when the time comes to make public one's score, it is done somewhat apologetically, but with the expectation that others may profit by it and with the assurance they will come to improve upon it. (Cushing, 1931, 130)

Dee James Canale
MEMPHIS, TENNESSEE

Lawrence D. Longo
LOMA LINDA, CALIFORNIA

ACKNOWLEDGMENTS

The authors express thanks and appreciation to Ms. Florence M. Bruce and Mrs. Brenda J. Kreutzer for their editoral assistance and word-processing skills.

REFERENCES

Bailey, P. 1927a. Further Remarks Concerning Tumors of the Glioma Group. *Bull Johns Hopkins Hosp* 40:354–89.

______. 1927b. Histologic Atlas of Gliomas. *Arch Path Lab Med* 4:871–921.

______. 1930. Further Notes on the Cerebellar Medulloblastomas: The Effects of Roentgen Radiation. *Am J Path* 6:125–35.

______. 1985. Pepperpot. 73–89. In *Neurosurgical Giants: Feet of Clay and Iron*, 73–89. Ed. P. C. Bucy. New York: Elsevier.

Bailey, P., and H. Cushing. 1925. Medulloblastoma Cerebelli; A Common Type of Midcerebellar Glioma of Childhood. *Arch Neur Psych* 14:192–224.

______. 1926. *A Classification of the Tumors of the Glioma Group on a Histogenetic Basis with a Correlated Study of Prognosis*. Philadelphia: J. B. Lippincott.

Cushing, H. 1905a. Concerning Surgical Intervention for the Intracranial Hemorrhages of the New-Born. *Am J Med Sci* 130:563–81.

______. 1905b. The Special Field of Neurological Surgery. *Bull Johns Hopkins Hosp* 16:77–87.

______. 1908. Surgery of the Head. In *Surgery, Its Principles and Practice*, 17–276. Ed. W. W. Keen. Philadelphia: W. B. Saunders.

______. 1910. Hydrocephalus. In *Modern Medicine*. Vol. 7, 459–66. Ed. William Osler. Philadelphia: Lea & Febiger.

______. 1911. The Control of Bleeding in Operations for Brain Tumors. With the Description of Silver "Clips" for the Occlusion of Vessels Inaccessible to the Ligature. *Ann Surg* 54:119.

______. 1912. *The Pituitary Body and Its Disorders. Clinical States Produced by Disorder of the Hypophysis Cerebri. An Amplification of the Harvey Lecture for December*. Philadelphia: J. B. Lippincott.

______. 1914. Studies on the Cerebro-Spinal Fluid and Its Pathway. *J Med Res* 26:1–19.

______. 1917. *Tumors of the Nervous Acousticus and the Syndrome of the Cerebellopontine Angle*. Philadelphia: W. B. Saunders.

______. 1925. *The Life of Sir William Osler*. Oxford: The Clarendon Press.

______. 1926. *Studies in Intracranial Physiology and Surgery. The Third Circulation. The Hypophysis. The Gliomas*. London: Oxford University Press.

______. 1927a. *MacEwen Memorial Lecture: The Meningiomas Arising From the Ol-*

factory Groove and Their Removal by the Aid of Electro-Surgery. Glasgow: Jackson, Wylie & Co..

______. 1927b. The Intracranial Tumors of Preadolescence. *Am J Dis Child* 33:551–84.

______. 1928a. Electro-Surgery as an Aid to the Removal of Intracranial Tumors. With a Preliminary Note on a New Surgical-Current Generator by W. T. Bovie, Ph.D. *SGO* 47:751–84.

______. 1928b. *Consecratio Medici and Other Papers*. Boston: Little, Brown, and Co.

______. 1930. Experiences with the Cerebellar Medulloblastomas. A Critical Review. *Acta Path Microb Scand* 7:1–86.

______. 1931. Experiences with the Cerebellar Astrocytomas. A Critical Review of Seventy-Six Cases. *SGO* 52:129–204.

______. 1932. The Basophil Adenomas of the Pituitary Body and Their Clinical Manifestations (Pituitary Basophilism). *Bull Johns Hopkins Hosp* 50:137–95.

______. 1936. *From a Surgeon's Journal 1915–1918, with Illustrations and Maps*. Boston: Little, Brown, and Co..

______. 1940. *The Medical Career and Other Papers*. Boston: Little, Brown, and Co.

______. 1943. *The Harvey Cushing Collection of Books and Manuscripts*. New York: Schuman's.

Cushing, H., and L. Eisenhardt. 1938. *Meningiomas. Their Classification, Regional Behavior, Life History, and Surgical End Results*. Springfield, IL: Charles C Thomas.

Dandy, W. E., and K. D. Blackfan. 1913. An Experimental and Clinical Study of Internal Hydrocephalus. *JAMA* 61:2216–17.

______. 1914. Internal Hydrocephalus: An Experimental, Clinical and Pathological Study. *Am J Dis Child* 8:406–82.

Fox, W. L. 1975. The Cushing-Dandy Controversy. *Surg Neur* 3:661–66.

Fulton, J. F. 1939. Harvey Cushing: An Appreciation. *Sci Month* 49:477–79.

______. 1946. *Harvey Cushing: A Biography*. Springfield, IL: Charles C Thomas.

German, W. J. 1969. Cerebral Spinal Fluid. In *Harvey Cushing, Selected Papers on Neurosurgery*, 274. Ed. D. D. Matson and W. J. German. New Haven: Yale University Press.

______. Harvey Cushing Society. 1939. *A Bibliography of the Writings of Harvey Cushing*. Springfield, IL: Charles C Thomas.

Horrax, G. 1939. Harvey Cushing, 1869–1939. *SGO* 69:828–34.

______. 1944. Some of Harvey Cushing's Contributions to Neurological Surgery. *J Neurosurg* 1:3–22.

Martin, P., and H. Cushing. 1923. Primary Gliomas of the Chiasm and Optic Nerves in Their Intracranial Portion. *Arch Ophthal* 52:209–41.

Matson, D. D. 1969. Neoplasms. In *Harvey Cushing, Selected Papers on Neurosurgery*, 104–5. Ed. D. D. Matson and W. J. German. New Haven: Yale University Press.

Thomson, E. H. 1950. *Harvey Cushing: Surgeon, Author, Artist*. New York: H. Schuman.

Weed, L. H. 1914. Studies on Cerebro-Spinal Fluid. *J Med Res* 31:21–117.

______. 1917. The Development of the Cerebro-Spinal Space in Pig and Man. *Contrib Embryol Carneg Inst* 5:1–116.

WALTER DANDY

MOST OF US DOCTORS, shortly after our retirement or death, will be forgotten by all but a few patients and ex-residents. It is, therefore, a measure of Walter Dandy's (1886–1946) (figure 1) greatness that some forty years after his death, his biography is being featured, not in a neurosurgical volume but in a volume on the founders of child neurology. This is entirely justified as, throughout Dandy's career, he was particularly interested in childhood tumors but, more important, early in his career, he made outstanding contributions to the understanding of hydrocephalus that laid the foundation for management of this previously lethal condition (Fox, 1984).

Dandy was born in 1886 in Sedalia, Missouri, of English parents who had emigrated to America two years previously from Barrow-in-Furness in Lancashire. His father was a train driver, socialist, and member of the Plymouth Brethren. Had he stayed in Britain, the chances of his son receiving a university education, let alone becoming a doctor with that class background in the nineteenth century, would have been remote. Fortunately, he was able to attend the University of Missouri, where he was both an accomplished athlete and a first-class student, eventually being offered a Rhodes Scholarship. He was unable to study medicine at Oxford, however, so he elected to go to Johns Hopkins Medical School in Baltimore, qualifying for his degree in 1910.

From the beginning of his medical career he was attracted to surgery and was particularly influenced, like many others at that time, by William Halsted. After graduating, he was taken under

Halsted's wing and set to work in the Hunterian Laboratory under the supervision of Harvey Cushing. This period saw the beginning of a long feud between these two different personalities, who were ultimately to be the foremost neurosurgeons of their time (Rizzoli, 1987). Dandy's first research project was on blood flow to the pituitary gland, which he undertook with Cushing. Also during this time, he began his celebrated collaboration with the pediatrician Kenneth Blackfan on the study of cerebrospinal fluid (CSF) dynamics and its relation to hydrocephalus. Although hydrocephalus had been well described since the time of Hippocrates, little was understood about the formation and circulation of cerebrospinal fluid, and no effective treatment was available. One reason for this was that no effective animal model of hydrocephalus had been developed, and this contribution was the first major success for Dandy and Blackfan. They produced hydrocephalus by obstructing the Aqueduct of Sylvius, using a gelatine cap inserted in the aqueduct from the fourth ventricle causing obstructive hydrocephalus (Dandy and Blackfan, 1913, 1914). They then went on to study CSF absorption in the laboratory and in patients, using phenolsulfonphthalein injected into the subarachnoid space, which was then secreted by the kidneys. Thus, by comparing patients with no hydrocephalus, communicating hydrocephalus, and obstructive hydrocephalus, they delineated different absorption rates in the different patients (Dandy and Blackfan, 1917). With an understanding of production, circulation, and absorption of CSF, Dandy was able to devise a number of procedures for logically treating hydrocephalus. Communicating hydrocephalus he treated by cauterization or removal of the choroid plexus (Dandy, 1918, 1938a). Aqueductal stenosis was treated initially by cauterization of the aqueduct and, after 1922, by anterior third ventriculostomy, the latter operation (figure 2)

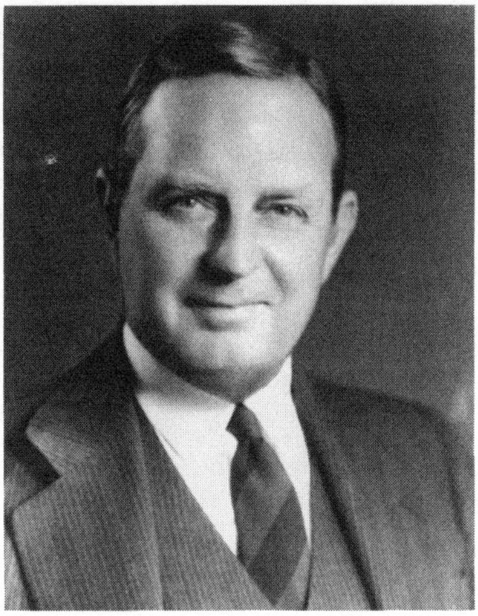

Figure 1. Walter E. Dandy (1886–1946).

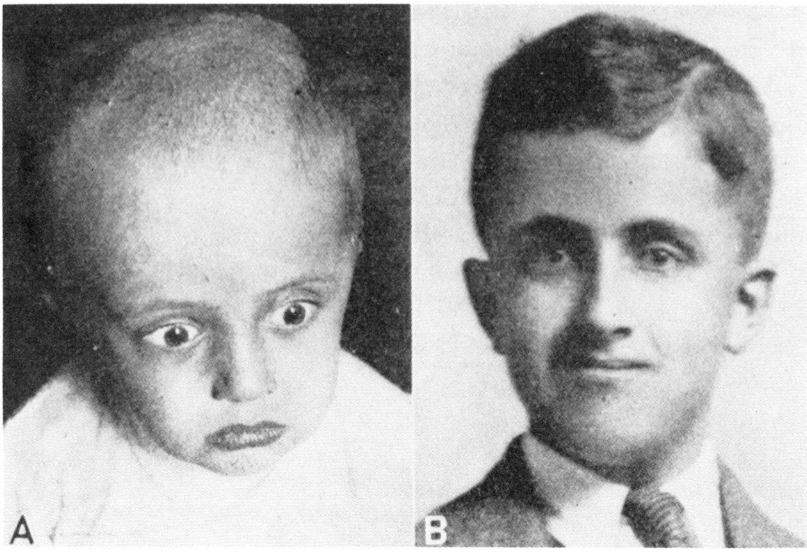

Figure 2. At age two years with a head circumference of 62.5 cm, this child had a third ventriculostomy performed by Dandy on January 17, 1930 (originally figure 9 from Dandy's article). At follow-up for treatment of aqueductal stenosis in 1944, the patient was doing well. From Dandy, "Diagnosis and Treatment of Stricture of the Aqueduct of Sylvius," *Arch Surg* 51(1945): 9. Copyright 1945, American Medical Association.

also being used for treatment of hydrocephalus caused by the congenital fourth ventricular outlet syndrome (Dandy, 1945) or adhesions at the base of the brain. It was from the paper entitled "The Diagnosis and Treatment of Hydrocephalus Due to Occlusion of the Foramina of Magendie and Luschka" (Dandy, 1921a), as well as his and Blackfan's previous work (Dandy and Blackfan, 1914), for which Dandy is especially credited with describing the Dandy-Walker syndrome (figure 3). He thus became the first surgeon to logically treat hydrocephalus, and his methods remained standard practice until the introduction of shunts.

Dandy was eventually appointed to the staff of Johns Hopkins and rapidly gained a reputation as a skilled surgeon, developing an enormous practice, which he ran with precise efficiency. He would write brief, concise clinical notes and operative descriptions, which included all relevant details. He expected and maintained dedication and hard work in his residents. His surgical skill was outstanding, particularly helped by above average eyesight that allowed him to see fine structures that others were unable to appreciate until the era of the operating microscope. He was particularly keen on posterior fossa surgery and developed the posterior fossa approach to the trigeminal nerve, cutting it as it enters the pons; he used this technique for the treatment of trigeminal neuralgia (Rizzoli, 1987). Dandy noted the presence, in these cases, of an artery compressing the nerve at this point, and although he did not act on this observation, it has now been appreciated that pressure of these arteries on the nerve is the likely cause of trigeminal neuralgia and a procedure to move the artery away from contact with the nerve is the definitive modern treatment for this condition. Dandy was also the first surgeon to directly clip an intracranial aneurysm (Dandy, 1938b). He also performed an extensive series of operations on arteriovenous malformations and advocated the complete removal of acoustic neuromas. Much of his work concerned childhood tumors, and he devised a transcallosal approach to pineal tumors (Dandy, 1921b) and was also the first to suggest a transcranial approach to orbital tumors (Rizzoli, 1987).

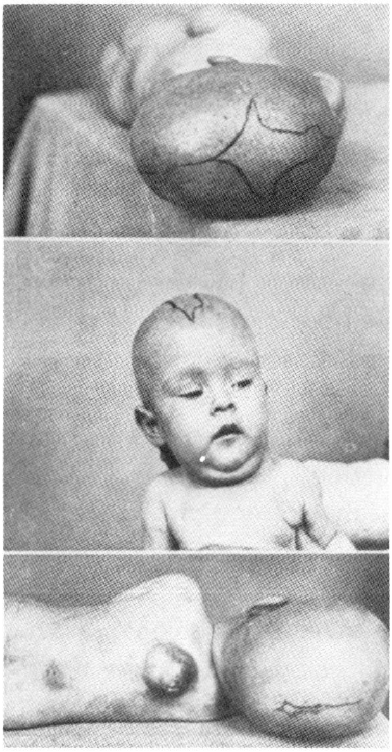

Figure 3. This three-month-old infant was found by Dandy at surgery to have an inflammatory process occluding the foramen of Magendie with a large fourth ventricle (originally figure 1 from Dandy's article). The black lines outlined the fontanelles. From Dandy, "The Diagnosis and Treatment of Hydrocephalus Due to Occlusions of the Foramina of Magendie and Luschka," *SGO* 32(1921): 115.

As well as being a skilled and busy operator, he was a prolific writer, producing numerous papers on trigeminal and glossopharyngeal neuralgia, Meniere's Disease and hydrocephalus. He wrote the neurological section of Lewis's Practice of Surgery, which for many years was the standard guide to the aspiring neurosurgeon.

As if these achievements were not enough, Dandy will be remembered for an outstanding contribution to the development of neurosurgery as a specialty, in that he described the first radiological method of localization of intracranial masses, namely pneumoencephalography (Dandy, 1918). He developed this method following the observation of air collecting under the diaphragm following intraabdominal visceral rupture, and realized that air in the subarachnoid space, introduced either spinally or into the ventricles, could be used to delineate the ventricular system and its displacement by intracranial masses (Dandy, 1919). In terms of intracranial localization, this was the only method of reliably visualizing the position of tumors until Egas Moniz introduced angiography in the early 1930s, and it was used routinely by most neurosurgeons until the mid 1970s when it was superseded by computed tomographic scanning. There are still occasional indications for performing ventriculography, although with improved technology, the technique is no longer taught and ultimately will no longer be used. However, it can be confidently said that, without pneumoencephalography, neurosurgery would not have developed at the rate it did, and many surgeons and patients worldwide owe a debt of gratitude to Dandy for applying this simple technique to the specialty.

While there is little doubt that Dandy was an extremely successful surgeon, an innovator, and brilliant researcher, there was one aspect of his career that was, unfortunately, not so successful, and that was his relationship with his peers. He had a reputation for being a very difficult man with whom to work, both demanding the highest standards from his juniors and having a tendency to be outspokenly critical of other neurosurgeons. When the Association of American Neurosurgeons, now known as the Cushing Society, was first established, virtually all American neurosurgeons joined—with the exception of Dandy, who, it is said, refused to join because of Cushing's involvement. The feud between Cushing and Dandy is legendary, and although the reasons for it are obscure, it is thought to have originated when they worked together in Halstead's Laboratory. Whatever the reason, although they were initially friends, they spent most of their working lives refusing to talk to each other. It is sad that the two giants of this fledgling specialty never collaborated. One wonders what they could have achieved.

The neurosurgeons of my generation no doubt have a relatively easy time. We have computed tomographic and magnetic resonance imaging scans to allow us accurate visualization of lesions before we operate, and then, thanks to good anesthesia, corticosteroids, mannitol, microscopes, lasers, and ultrasonic aspirators, we are able to operate unhurriedly on our patients under good conditions, safe in the knowledge that our patients are likely to do well. Despite this, disasters still occur and most people consider neurosurgery to be a high-stress specialty requiring a special form of dedication to its practice. Contrast this with Dandy's time, when many operations were performed based on clinical judgment alone, without good radiology, with patients under local or light anesthesia, and without the luxuries of blood transfusions and antibiotics. One realizes the stresses and strains under which these surgeons performed. To have worked in that field in those days must have taken a very special kind of person, and to work more or less in isolation, not only in clinical practice, but at the same time researching and innovating, must have required superhuman qualities. The fact that one may have difficulty getting on with one's colleagues pales into insignificance compared to the rest of the qualities required to work in such circumstances. One can only look back at the achievements of Dandy with awe and wonder. From the point of view of pediatricians and child neurologists, his work on hydrocephalus alone was the stimulus that changed this condition from an untreatable to an easily treatable condition. On a broader front, however, his thinking and innovation helped to advance neurosurgery from its infancy to its highly advanced modern state. He will be remembered as a giant among neurosurgeons, to whom many doctors and their patients owe a debt of gratitude.

Peter Richards
LONDON, ENGLAND

REFERENCES

Dandy, W. E. 1918. Extirpation of the Choroid Plexus of the Lateral Ventricles in Communicating Hydrocephalus. *Ann Surg* 68:560–79.

______. 1918. Ventriculography Following the Injection of Air into the Cerebral Ventricles. *Ann Surg* 68:5–11.

______. 1919. Roentgenography of the Brain After Injection of Air into the Spinal Canal. *Ann Surg* 70:397–403.

______. 1921a. The Diagnosis and Treatment of Hydrocephalus Due to Occlusion of the Foramina of Magendie and Luschka. *SGO* 32:112–24.

______. 1921b. An Operation for the Removal of Pineal Tumors. *SGO* 33:113–19.

______. 1938a. The Operative Treatment of Communicating Hydrocephalus. *Ann Surg* 108, 194–202.

______. 1938b. Intracranial Aneurysm of the Internal Carotid Artery Cured by Operation. *Ann Surg* 107:654–59.

______. 1945. Diagnosis and Treatment of Stricture of the Aqueduct of Sylvius. *Arch Surg* 5:1–14.

Dandy, W. E., and K. D. Blackfan. 1913. An Experimental and Clinical Study of Internal Hydrocephalus. *JAMA* 61:2216–17.

______. 1914. Internal Hydrocephalus: An Experimental, Clinical, and Pathological Study. *Am J Dis Child* 8:406–82.

______. 1917. Internal Hydrocephalus. *Am J Dis Child* 14:424–42.

Fox, W. L. 1984. *Dandy of Johns Hopkins.* Baltimore: Williams & Wilkins.

Rizzoli, H. 1987. Dandy's Contribution to the Foundation of Neurological Surgery. *Ped Neurosci* 13:316–22.

EDGAR DOLL

EDGAR ARNOLD DOLL (1889–1968) (figure 1) was born in Cleveland, Ohio. After earning an A.B. in education at Cornell University in 1912, he became an instructor and Fellow in Psychology at the University of Wisconsin for one year. From 1912 through 1917 he trained under Henry Goddard at the Training School in Vineland, New Jersey, as a research and clinical psychologist. He simultaneously continued his education and was awarded a Pd.M. in education from New York University in 1916 (E. E. Doll, 1969).

Doll volunteered for the U.S. Army in 1917 and entered the Sanitary Corps, where he was assigned to the Psychological Examining Board. During his army service he was invited by Edward Ransom Johnstone, superintendent of Vineland who was also serving as vice-president of the Board of Managers of the state prison, to examine prisoners under consideration for parole (Doll, 1988). Doll began this work while still a doctoral student at Princeton. He was awarded his Ph.D. in 1920.

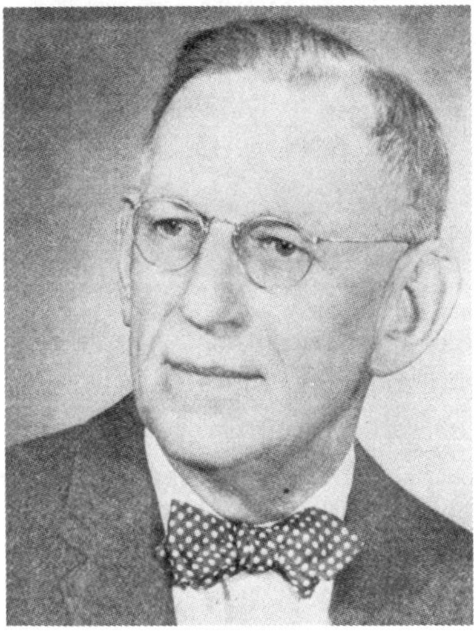

Figure 1. Edgar A. Doll (1889–1968). From the *American Journal of Mental Deficiency* 73(1968):680.

In 1919 Doll became director of the Division of Education of the Department of Institutions and Agencies of the State of New Jersey. He held this position until 1923, when Goddard invited him to teach at Ohio State University as an assistant professor.

In 1925 he was appointed director of research at the Vineland Training School and kept this position until 1949. Following his retirement from Vineland he served as coordinator of research at the Devereux School and as consulting psychologist to the public schools of Bellingham, Washington.

Doll married Agnes Martz, Johnstone's niece through marriage, in 1914. They had two sons. His first wife died in 1937, and he subsequently married Geraldine Longwell; this second marriage produced a son and daughter. Edgar A. Doll died in 1968 at the age of seventy-nine (Doll, 1969).

Early in his career Doll became convinced that the Binet Test of Intelligence was not accurate for children more than ten years of age (Doll, 1913). He stated that in designing a test it was important to have knowledge of the psychological abilities and behavior of children of various age groups, that one must carefully select those mental functions that best contribute to intelligence, and that item selection must be objective. He used these concepts in his work throughout his career.

In 1924 he presented a major analysis of the state of art in mental testing (Doll, 1924). Among his major criticisms was that the discipline was uncertain about the age at which intellectual development ceases and what the average mental age of an unselected adult population was. He believed that the role of nationality and color was not clear, that there was no agreement on methods of calculating IQs, and that statistical methods used in standardizing and interpreting tests were often wrong or misused. His major theme, however, was that it was important to determine the types of ability shown by patients, as well as the overall level of intelligence. He further pointed out that special talents might offset general disabilities, and that these special talents could determine how an individual functioned in society.

The work in this area eventually led to the publication of the Vineland Social Maturity Scale. The purpose of this scale was to separate socially competent and socially incompetent individuals with mental retardation. Doll argued that for an individual with mild mental retardation social competence was the critical factor in overall adjustment. This scale was also designed to provide a characterization of individual differences and deficits, because the test allowed calculation of a social age and a social quotient. Although the original prototype was published in 1936 (Doll, 1936a), the final scale was not published until 1953 (Doll, 1953).

In his 1936 presidential address to the American Association on Mental Deficiency, Doll stated, "Intellectual subnormality alone cannot safely be used as a criterion for mental deficiency, for to intellectual subnormality we must add at least social inadequacy and arrested development" (Doll, 1936b). He criticized the Binet for not taking into account social competence and felt that the various levels of mental retardation could be more accurately divided by using social age or a social quotient.

Doll's longstanding interest in social competence was demonstrated by his formulation of a six-part definition of mental retardation (Doll, 1941). The essential criteria were social incompetence due to mental subnormality that was developmentally arrested, present at maturity, of constitutional origin, and essentially incurable. The first four of these criteria formed the basis of the definition of mental retardation used by the American Association on Mental Retardation. The questions of constitutional origin and incurability became controversial. Other researchers had pointed out that under certain circumstances an individual can show an increase in IQ, and they also begin to define a subcultural type of mental retardation. Doll responded that if there were no physical abnormalities and if the individual was from certain subcultural groups the diagnosis of mental retardation should not be used (Doll, 1947a) and that if the IQ improved the problem was one of mistaken terminology and uncertain diagnosis (Doll, 1947b).

Another professional interest of Doll's was the origin of mental retardation (Doll, Phelps, and Melcher, 1932). He began studying this area with Johnstone's first grandson, who had cerebral palsy. An analysis of twelve cases led him to the conclusion that 5 to 10 percent of institutionalized individuals with mental retardation had this condition because of birth injuries. At that time, a hereditary etiology for all mental retardation was widely accepted, and Doll's work helped focus research on possible environmental causes. He later stated that when cases with known pathology and etiology were examined, approximately one-third had hereditary diseases, one-third were clearly not hereditary, and the remaining third were best classified as unknown (1936b).

At the time of Doll's 1936 presidential address there was a shift away from the concepts of the eugenics movement and the use of compulsory sterilization. Doll acknowledged these changing ideas and pointed out that a problem with sterilization was the frequent lack of an adequate diagnosis and inadequate knowledge about the hereditary nature of the condition in a given case. He did note that one remaining argument for sterilization was the inadequacy of the mentally retarded individual as a parent, whether or not the child was also mentally retarded.

Doll was also ahead of his time in his view of segregation of individuals with mental retardation in institutions. He pointed out that an institution might be appropriate for some individuals but that 90 percent of persons with mental retardation lived at home. He felt that the institution should provide training, assistance, and supervision for this group.

Although Doll made many contributions that have had an impact on pediatric neurology, the most significant were his conceptualization of an operational definition of mental retardation that is still in use and his demonstration that not all mental retardation has a hereditary basis. He also helped formulate a policy for care of individuals with mental retardation in the community which, unfortunately, some fifty years later is still not fully implemented.

Gerald S. Golden
MEMPHIS, TENNESSEE

REFERENCES

Doll, E. A. 1913. Suggestions on the Extension of the Binet-Simon Measuring Scale. *Transactions* 5:665–69.

______. 1924. Capabilities of Low-Grade Feeble-Minded. *Training School Bull* 21:65–77.

______. 1936a. *The Vineland Social Maturity Scale: Revised Condensed Manual of Directions*. Training School at Vineland, New Jersey, Department of Research: Series 1936, number 3.

______. 1936b. President's Address: Current Thoughts on Mental Deficiency. *J Psycho-Asthenics* 35:40–41.

______. 1941. The Essentials of an Inclusive Concept of Mental Deficiency. *Am J Ment Defic* 46:214–19.

______. 1947a. Feeble-Mindedness Versus Intellectual Retardation. *Am J Ment Defic* 51:456–59.

______. 1947b. Is Mental Deficiency Curable? *Am J Ment Defic* 51:420–28.

______. 1953. *The Measurement of Social Competence: A Manual for the Vineland Social Maturity Scale*. Minneapolis: Educational Testing Bureau.

Doll, E. A., W. M. Phelps, and R. T. Melcher. 1932. *Mental Deficiency Due to Birth Injuries*. New York: Macmillan Co.

Doll, E. E. 1969. Edgar Arnold Doll, 1889–1968. *Am J Ment Defic* 73:681–82.

______. 1988. Before the Big Time: Early History of the Training School at Vineland, 1888 to 1949. *Am J Ment Retard* 93:1–15.

HUGO EHRENFEST

DURING THE NINETEENTH century a number of writers described various injuries and neurological sequelae in newborn infants and children, many of which were secondary to trauma at birth. For instance, in 1827 Jean Baptiste Cazauvielh first described congenital paralysis in children (Cazauvielh, 1827), and the following year Charles Michel Billard published his work based on several hundred autopsies in children in which he correlated the pathologic findings with their clinical and neurologic symptoms, including those associated with birth trauma (Billard, 1828). In 1843 Frederic Rilliet and Antoine Charles Ernest Barthez described neuromuscular problems following childbirth (Rilliet and Barthez, 1843).

In 1843 William John Little first described cerebral palsy, asserting that it followed lack of development of the cerebrum or meningitis (Little, 1843). He recorded only in passing that this condition may follow prolonged and difficult labor and delivery, often by forceps, and that in such instances, it may have been due to intracranial hemorrhage. It was only in his later work that he came to ascribe three-quarters of the cases of cerebral spastic paralysis to brain damage from birth injury (Little, 1862). About this time Guillaume Duchenne de Boulogne described upper extremity palsy in a newborn in whom the brachial plexus had been injured at birth. A decade later Duchenne described several mechanisms of injury to the brachial plexus at birth (Duchenne, 1872). Shortly thereafter, Wilhelm Heinrich Erb published his monograph on traumatic brachial paralysis, noting that the fifth and sixth cervical nerves were commonly involved (Erb, 1873–77). This was followed by William Richard Gowers's *Clinical Lecture on Birth Palsies* (Gowers, 1888), which differentiated between "cerebral" and "peripheral" paralysis; Gowers was one of the first to use the term *cerebral palsy*, noting that not all such disorders followed traumatic childbirth (Gowers, 1886–88, 1888). Other writers of this era on cerebral palsies following childbirth included William Osler (1889), Sigmund Freud (1897), and Bernard Sachs (1891).

The work of John William Ballantyne of Edinburgh drew attention

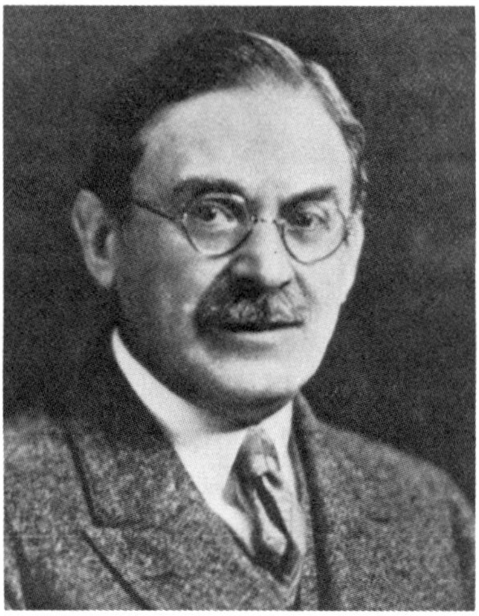

Figure 1. Hugo Ehrenfest (1870–1942), about 1930. From *Album of the Fellows of the American Gynecological Society, 1876–1930* (1930), 196–97.

to the importance of prenatal care and pathology of the fetus and newborn infant (Ballantyne, 1902–1904). John Whitridge Williams, professor of obstetrics at the Johns Hopkins Medical School and a leader in American obstetrics, also promulgated the idea of prenatal care and played a key role in founding the American Society for the Study and Prevention of Infant Mortality (Longo, 1981). In the first edition of his textbook (Williams, 1903), Williams mentioned skull fractures (p. 388), paralysis of the arm and other injuries secondary to birth trauma (p. 806), but gave little attention to birth injuries per se. Joseph Bolivar DeLee, obstetrician at the Chicago Lying-in Hospital, devoted a chapter of his textbook, *The Principles and Practice of Obstetrics*, to "accidents to the child," in which he considered asphyxia neonatorum and injuries at birth, presented criteria to distinguish caput succedaneum from cephalhematoma, and discussed fractures of the spine and paralysis of the extremities (DeLee, 1913). Other writers, particularly of the French and German schools, described injuries to the head, brain, face, extremities, and trunk. This was not unexpected, because during the late nineteenth and early twentieth centuries aggressive management of labor with operative delivery became relatively common. For instance, pituitrin was used to induce or augment labor; premature induction of labor was used in cases of pelvic contraction; "twilight sleep" with large doses of morphine and scopolamine was popularized; "mid" to "high" forceps deliveries were used to shorten the second stage of labor; and version and extraction, difficult breech extractions, and rather rough resuscitative measures for the newborn infant were widely used, often by individuals with little or no formal specialty training (Longo, 1989).

In his 1922 monograph *Birth Injuries of the Child*, Hugo Ehrenfest

(1870–1942) (figure 1) of St. Louis presented the first comprehensive survey of the various injuries associated with childbirth. In 17 chapters covering 221 pages with just over 300 references, he reviewed the literature on almost every conceivable injury and neurological sequelae from laceration of the scalp and fractured cranial bones to trauma to the neck, vertebral column, trunk, and extremities. Although drawn chiefly from German and American publications that he had studied in the original, and contributing relatively few original observations of his own, Ehrenfest explored in considerable detail the spectrum of disorders reported. He justified his failure to include many personal observations, as no practitioner "could ever be expected to accumulate sufficient personal experience to write authoritatively on every form of injury. . ." (Ehrenfest, 1922, xi).

The basic outline of each chapter was as follows: introduction, pathology, classification, etiology, frequency, symptomotology, diagnosis, differential diagnosis, prognosis, prophylaxis, and treatment, followed by a list of references.

In the preface Ehrenfest pointed out a paradox: while "intracranial traumatic lesions of some sort are discovered" in at least 40 percent of all autopsies properly performed on stillborn infants and those dying within the first few days of birth, "official and unofficial tabulations of the causes of death in earliest infancy or of stillbirth, 'injury in birth' is assigned a most inconspicuous place" (Ehrenfest, 1922, vii). He also noted the relatively high incidence of injuries to the vertebral column and abdominal viscera, particularly the liver, pancreas, and adrenal glands. He acknowledged that there was no uniform agreement as to what constituted a birth injury, and stated that he would not consider toxicologic and drug-related disturbances. Even so, he could claim, correctly, that such an exhaustive review of the subject had not heretofore been made.

Ehrenfest admitted that

> *the attending physician excusably hesitates to pronounce the infant's death the result of a parturitional injury, because, unfortunately and unjustly, it has remained the prevalent conception, both among the profession and laity, that fatal injuries are the result of, and thus signify, a lack of proper skill on the part of the accoucheur.* (Ehrenfest, 1922, viii)

Nevertheless, he noted that

practically without any exceptions every known type of parturitional traumatization has also been observed subsequent to spontaneous labors. . . . [Thus] no physician should feel any reluctance in pronouncing and reporting the infant's death as the result of birth injury if, in his opinion, this is the case. (Ehrenfest, 1922, viii-ix)

He warned:

[M]ost clearly it has become the duty of those who advocate the artificial termination of labor under general anesthesia in order to overcome the unquestionably slower and more painful process of spontaneous delivery, to prove that such methods do not imply a greater immediate and later risk to the life and health of the infant. . . . Mere mortality figures will not suffice to settle this complex problem. (Ehrenfest, 1922, ix, x)

The volume's first four chapters, on caput succedaneum, cephalhematoma, injuries to the scalp, and those of the cranial bones, respectively, present careful descriptions of the pathologic details. In the last of these chapters Ehrenfest distinguished fissures that parallel the radii of ossification from traumatic fractures. In addition, he presented a lengthy and insightful discussion of the problem of infanticide and the need to clarify and avoid wrongly charging the mother or birth attendant of a child's death.

The centerpiece of the volume, occupying a third of the monograph, is the chapter on intracranial injuries. With seventy-seven references, plus several dozen other authors quoted or referred to in the text without a citation, Ehrenfest compiled what was undoubtedly the finest survey of this problem to date. He first described the proper post-mortem technique, as described by Beneke, which avoided inadvertant tearing of the tentorium so as to diagnose lesions and their extent with certainty, and noted the significance of tentorial tears. Then he presented a useful classification of intracranial hemorrhages and related lesions.

After recording that intraventricular hemorrhages "do not occur often," he devoted a dozen pages to the etiology of intracranial birth injuries. Confessing that the "immediate" causes of such lesions were "undeniably . . . mechanical," he questioned why such factors "at play in all labors, only at times should become responsible for serious intracephalic injury." During the period of this publication and thereafter, Ehrenfest opposed the indiscriminate and injudicious use of "twilight sleep," pituitrin in labor, high forceps to shorten the second stage of labor, Dührssen's incisions, and cesarean section, procedures that were in widespread use and that were associated with alarmingly high maternal and perinatal morbidity and mortality (Longo, 1989). He also emphasized trauma to the aftercoming head in breech delivery, other mechanical factors, and the role of the accoucheur upon whom the onus of responsibility lay as the primary causes of injuries.

Ehrenfest held that predisposing causes of brain damage included syphilis, prematurity, asphyxiation, and quick release of the molded head. He also included the contributing factors hemorrhagic diathesis and inappropriate newborn resuscitative manipulations, such as the Schultze swinging method, in the etiology of these lesions.

Ehrenfest warned that the frequency of intracranial lesions was much greater than suspected and stressed the need to define carefully the clinical picture and recognize the symptoms. Suggested evidence for proper diagnosis included the newborn "crying almost incessantly or . . . strikingly quiet," increased heart rate, retinal hemorrhages, edematous blurring of optic discs, and convulsions. He also included prolonged bleeding and coagulation times, and lumbar puncture, which he believed also could be therapeutic, as useful diagnostic tests. Later in the chapter he asserted that the former tests were not always to be relied upon. He therefore encouraged as diagnostic tools routine funduscopic examination and lumbar puncture when intracranial bleeding was suspected.

He associated birth trauma with the later development of internal hydrocephalus. In addition, he presented criteria for linking abnormal childhood development with birth trauma, for example, by directly associating a developmental anomaly with evidence of an intracranial lesion recorded at birth, and by careful follow-up of the life histories of a large number of individuals whose birth histories were known in great detail.

Ehrenfest reviewed the divergent viewpoints of neurologists and obstetricians, the former attempting to link neurological deficiencies in childhood and later life with an abnormal labor and delivery, and the latter noting the association of such neurological problems with "normal" as well as abnormal parturition. He observed that such injuries could be discovered at autopsy in at least one-half of stillborn infants or in those dying within the first few days of life, that autopsies later in infancy frequently showed residue of hemorrhage at birth, and that many apparently normal individuals experienced intracranial injuries at birth. Nonetheless, he stressed ". . . without fear of contradiction . . . [that] in a large number of cases today definite symptoms of intracranial parturitional injuries are overlooked. The obstetrician . . . still fails to appreciate his responsibility in this matter" (Ehrenfest, 1922, 87–88). He advocated avoidance of sudden or excessive head compression digitally or with forceps and careful examination of the newborn with continual observation for several days. "Better results . . . can be hoped for only when the obstetrician will have come to a full realization of his responsibility for a most careful observation of the newborn infant immediately after birth and during the first few days of life" (Ehrenfest, 1922, 98).

In the chapter on injuries to the vertebral column and spinal cord, Ehrenfest stressed that such injuries were observed only following operative deliveries, particularly version and extraction, difficult forceps delivery, and breech delivery of the aftercoming head, particularly if it was hyperextended. On the topic of facial paralysis he distinguished between "central" and "peripheral" lesions, noting that while such injuries were most commonly seen following a difficult forceps extraction, they could also occur in association with a normal spontaneous delivery. Subsequent chapters considered injuries to the face, eye, neck, sternocleidomastoid muscle, clavicle, brachial nerves, upper extremities, thorax, abdomen, and lower extremities.

Overall, Ehrenfest stressed that many conditions previously regarded as congenital, simply because they existed from birth, were, in fact, traumatic injuries. He maintained that the obstetrician had a two-fold obligation in regard to such injuries. The first of these was prevention. He observed that the incidence of serious injuries decreased in proportion to the expertise of the attending obstetrician and the avoidance of "heroic" obstetrical intervention. Second, he maintained that should such injuries occur it was the obstetrician's duty to diagnose them, which often required a careful autopsy.

Despite the volume's notable contributions, it contains a modest number of errors, such as referring to Little, an orthopedic surgeon, as a neurologist, and giving incorrect dates. A major problem is that Ehrenfest cited numerous authors and works without proper reference. In addition, Ehrenfest's main observations are anecdotal rather than being a formal series of cases; however, this was a common practice at that time.

Prior to the appearance of *Birth Injuries*, Ehrenfest had published about two dozen papers, chiefly on preeclampsia, eclampsia, and related topics (Ehrenfest, 1902, 1905, 1906, 1907, 1908). His first report on birth trauma was read before the Section on Obstetrics, Gynecology, and Abdominal Surgery at the 1921 meeting of the American Medical Association (Ehrenfest, 1921). In this paper he briefly reviewed the salient aspects of intracranial injury (which later appeared in his monograph), stressing the need for proper diagnosis, the etiologic role of mechanical factors, asphyxia, prematurity, and hemorrhagic diathesis. In a paper read before the St. Louis Gynecological Society the year *Birth Injuries* appeared, Ehrenfest stated that

even expert obstetricians appear to be slow in appreciating their own obligations towards the problem of parturitional traumatization of the infant, and in recognizing the relation of this problem to that "better" obstetrical care which must be furnished to the women as well as to the newborn babies of this country. (Ehrenfest, 1922b, 61)

He also noted that

the very traumatization of the child in birth will produce a clinical picture closely resembling that of deep asphyxiation, which, if not properly interpreted, necessarily leads to additional traumatization by the efforts of resuscitation. (Ehrenfest, 1922b, 62)

He again observed that obstetricians had been too willing to accept the judgment of neurologists to avoid difficult labors by means of interference. In closing his essay, Ehrenfest called for a keener appreciation of the obligation to better obstetrics, and recognition that birth injuries provided a "wide and virgin field for many interesting and valuable observations and investigations" regarding their etiology, diagnosis, and prognosis (Ehrenfest, 1922b, 66).

For the following two decades Ehrenfest continued to champion diligent and considerate obstetrical care, writing on various aspects of birth injury (Ehrenfest, 1929). To an Illinois county medical society he observed that such injuries may result from a ". . . lack of diagnostic ability, a lack of judgment, or mere awkwardness of technique, not rarely super-induced by bewilderment or by undue haste" (Ehrenfest, 1923a, 26–27). The same year he cautioned obstetricians not to accept the opinion of many pediatricians that most such pathology resulted from a "hemorrhagic diathesis" (Ehrenfest, 1923b). To the Section of Obstetrics, Gynecology, and Abdominal Surgery of the American Medical Association he posed the question "Can intracranial birth injuries be prevented?" (Ehrenfest, 1929), answering in the affirmative.

In the mid 1920s several other researchers wrote on this topic. For instance, in 1926 Bronson Crothers published *Disorders of the Nervous System in Childhood.* The following year Frank R. Ford and Bronson Crothers with Marian C. Putnam published a 164–page work, *Birth Injuries of the Central Nervous System: Part 1, Cerebral Birth Injuries* , and *Part 2, Cord Birth Injuries* without referring to Ehrenfest's contributions to the field other than his 1923 paper (Ford, Crothers, and Putnam, 1927). In the same year, both Philip Schwartz and Albert Dollinger contributed major reviews in *Ergebnisse der inner Medizin und Kinderheilkunde* (Schwartz, 1927; Dollinger, 1927).

In 1925 and 1928 Ehrenfest circulated supplements to his original volume, and in 1931 published the second edition of *Birth Injuries* (Ehrenfest, 1931a). In the preface he noted that several chapters had been greatly expanded and many new references included, citing the major works of Crothers, Crothers and Putnam, Dollinger, Ford, and Schwartz. The chapter on intracranial injuries was almost doubled in size, to 138 pages, and included much new material. A new Chapter 10 was devoted to injuries of the ear, especially as related to deafness and deaf-mutism. Nonetheless, the basic format of the volume was similar to the original monograph, with detailed accounts of the pathology, etiology, and diagnosis of birth trauma.

At the 1931 White House Conference "Child Health and Protection," sponsored by President Herbert Hoover, Ehrenfest chaired the Subcommittee on Factors and Causes of Fetal, Early Infant, and Maternal Morbidity and Mortality of the Committee on Prenatal and Maternal Care. In reviewing medical complications of pregnancy that accounted for perinatal morbidity and mortality, he stated that it was unfortunate that the term *birth injury* had become synonymous with *intracranial injury*, since so many systems other than the brain were involved (*White House*, 1932; Ehrenfest, 1933). To counteract the rise in the numbers of babies so injured, his committee recommended improved prenatal care, eschewing interference in pregnancy and labor except when definitely indicated, increased awareness among women and their physicians that shorter and more comfortable labors increase the risk for infant and mother, and increased precision of data recorded on birth and death certificates. Ehrenfest also considered the relation of birth trauma to neonatal morbidity and infant mortality, emphasizing many of the principles of conservative obstetrics that he had previously stressed (Ehrenfest, 1931b, 1932). In a 1934 paper to the Nebraska State Medical Society (his last publication on the subject) he presented a series of thirty lantern slides, which graphically illustrated the unfortunate sequelae of birth injuries (Ehrenfest, 1934).

Some details of Hugo Ehrenfest's life are relevant to this review. Born in Vienna on March 31, 1870, he received his medical degree from the Imperial University of Vienna (Medizinisce Fakultät der Universität, Wien) in 1894. He then served as intern and assistant surgeon in the Austrian Military Hospital in Laibach (1894–95), and as assistant surgeon at Franz Joseph Hospital in Vienna (1896–97). For a short period he also worked at the Jewish Hospital, Berlin, and in the laboratories of the Koch Institute, Berlin. From 1897 to 1899 he was an assistant in Professor Schauta's obstetrical clinic (Universitäts Frauenklinik, Allgemeine Krankenhaus) in Vienna.

Ehrenfest emigrated to America in 1900, settling in St. Louis at the suggestion of George Gellhorn, a German friend from Vienna. He rapidly became a leader in obstetrics and gynecology in the Midwest and America (Kosmak, 1942). Practicing at the Jewish Hospital, from 1904 to 1920 he served on the faculty of St. Louis University. He was gynecologist and chief of staff at the Jewish Hospital Dispensary (1903). In 1904 he became physician-in-chief at St. Louis Obstetric Dispensary and was appointed instructor of obstetrics and gynecology at St. Louis University. That same year he married Sophie Schwab, a member of an established St. Louis family; the Ehrenfests had two sons and a daughter. He served as obstetrician at the Jewish Hospital, St. Louis (1906). In 1907 the American Gynecological Society elected him to fellowship (he was vice-president of the society in 1921), and the following year he was promoted to assistant professor of obstetrics and gynecology at St. Louis University. At that time he became director of the division of obstetrics and gynecology at Jewish Hospital, a post he held until 1936. He served as coeditor of of the *Interstate Medical Journal* from 1909 to 1919. In 1910 he was appointed visiting gynecologist at St. Louis City Hospital, and the following year was promoted to professor of obstetrics and gynecology at St. Louis University. In 1920 he was appointed associate editor of the *American Journal of Obstetrics and Gynecology,* becoming coeditor in 1935, in which capacity he served until his death. In 1920, he resigned his position at St. Louis University.

The year 1922 saw the publication of his *Birth Injuries of the Child* and his appointment as associate professor of obstetrics and gynecology at Washington University in St. Louis. He translated and edited Robert Koehler's *Therapy of Puerperal Fever* (1925), was appointed professor of clinical obstetrics and gynecology, Washington University, in 1926, and in 1929 was elected to membership in the Central Association of Obstetricians and Gynecologists. In 1936 Washington University elevated him to professor emeritus. During his active professional life Ehrenfest championed sane, conservative obstetrics. He scrupulously avoided fads and opposed the indiscriminate use of "twilight sleep," Dührssen's incisions, and "meddlesome midwifery" of any sort.

As a pedagogue he was a role model and inspiration to those whose lives he touched. He is said to have been an effective teacher because of his large fund of knowledge and experience, his lucid analysis of problems, and his droll wit. Axel N. Arneson recalled of his former teacher:

During labor, he exorted patients to, "B-r-r-e-e-z-z-e deeply." This was repeated frequently, often loudly, and always with a strong trace of Austrian accent. Could he have been trying to increase oxygen delivery to the fetus? During my year of residency in OB/GYN Pathology, I recall performing several autopsies upon stillborn infants. . . . There was a sort of "code" that sought the necessary permits. I suspect this may have been an effort by Dr. Ehrenfest to obtain more data explaining the loss. (Arneson, 1989)

Willard M. Allen recalled that Ehrenfest often lectured on birth trauma to both medical and lay audiences. He had an extensive collection of fetal skulls and skeletons with various traumatic injuries and would illustrate his points with specimens from this collection. To conclude the lecture Ehrenfest would often show a fetal head with a tentorial tear--and then state that it had occurred during a relatively uncomplicated spontaneous vaginal delivery (Allen, 1989).

Ehrenfest is said to have exuded Viennese charm. He was a man of many accomplishments and had a genial personality, He was unassuming, with a keen sense of humor, and spirit of kindness toward all. He was a serious pianist and developed ties with leading musicians of the St. Louis Symphony Orchestra (Taussig, 1942). On July 24, 1942, at age seventy-two, following a busy morning at the Jewish Hospital and in his office, he died peacefully during an afternoon nap.

Hugo Ehrenfest's *Birth Injuries of the Child* played a key role in focusing the attention of physicians on the many complications of childbirth. For obstetricians, the work forced them to face the reality of the sequelae of "radical" obstetrics and "meddlesome midwifery." For pediatricians and neurologists it emphasized the etiology of many neurological deficits in childhood and later life, and stressed that "child neurology" begins at the time of birth, if not before. For public health workers the volume highlighted an important area of preventive medicine. For all health professionals the work summarized a wealth of literature from various specialties and different countries, synthesizing it into a coherent, reasonably complete whole that was a seminal contribution to obstetrics and gynecology and pediatric neurology, a masterpiece of its time.

Lawrence D. Longo
LOMA LINDA, CALIFORNIA

REFERENCES

Allen, W. M. 1989. Personal communication.

Arneson, A. N. 1989. Personal communication.

Ballantyne, J. W. 1902–1904. *Manual of Antenatal Pathology and Hygiene.* Vol.1: *The Foetus*; Vol. 2: *The Embryo.* Edinburgh: W. Green & Sons.

Billard, C. M. 1828. *Traité des maladies des enfans nouveau-nés et à la mamelle.* Paris: J. B. Baillière.

Cazauvielh, J. B. 1827. Recherches sur l'agénésie cérébrale et la paralysie congénitale. *Arch gén méd* 14:5–33, 347–66.

Crothers, B. 1926. *Disorders of the Nervous System in Childhood.* New York: D. Appleton.

Crothers, B., and M. C. Putnam. 1927. Cord Birth Injuries. In *Birth Injuries of the Central Nervous System.* Vol. 11, Part 2. Ed. F. R. Ford, B. Crothers, and M. C. Putnam. Baltimore: Williams & Wilkins.

DeLee, J. B. 1913. *The Principles and Practice of Obstetrics.* Philadelphia: W. B. Saunders.

Dollinger, A. 1927. Geburtstrauma und Zentralnervensystem. *Ergeb inn Med Kinderheilk* 31:373–455.

Duchenne de Boulogne, G. B. A. 1872. *De l'électrisation localisée et de son application à la pathologie et à la thérapeutique.* 3me. éd. Paris: J. B. Baillière.

Ehrenfest, H. 1902. The Impropriety of Cesarean Section in Placenta Praevia, with Remarks on a Rational Method of Treatment. *Am Med* 3:64–68.

______. 1905. The Etiology of Eclampsia. *St. Louis Cour Med* 33:200–7.

______. 1906. The Present Status of Pelvimetry. *Am J Obstet* 53:465–78.

______. 1907. The Influence of the Central Nervous System in the Causation of Uterine Hemorrhages. *Trans Am Gyn Soc* 32:522–58.

______. 1908. Brachial Birth Palsy in the Newborn. A Review of Recent Literature. *Interstate Med J* 15:747–53.

______. 1921. Intracranial Birth Trauma of the New-Born from the Standpoint of the Obstetrician. *JAMA* 77:103–7.

______. 1922a. *Birth Injuries of the Child.* New York: D. Appleton.

______. 1922b. A Better Obstetrics and the Problem of the Birth Injuries of the Newborn Infant. *Am J Obstet Gyn* 4:61–66, 99–101.

______. 1923a. The Prevention of Birth Injuries of the Child. *Illinois Med J* 44:20–27.

______. 1923b. The Causation of Intracranial Hemorrhages in the New-Born. *Am J Dis Child* 26:503–14.

______. 1929. Can Intracranial Birth Injuries be Prevented? *JAMA* 92:97–99.

______. 1931a. *Birth Injuries of the Child.* 2d ed. New York: D. Appleton.

______. 1931b. Factors and Causes of Fetal, Newly Born, and Maternal Morbidity and Mortality. *Am J Obstet Gyn* 21:867–80.

______. 1932. The Relation of Birth Trauma to Neonatal Mortality and Infant Morbidity. *Am J Dis Child* 43:426–30.

______. 1933. *Fetal, Newborn, and Maternal Morbidity and Mortality. Report of the Subcommittee on Factors and Causes of Fetal, Newborn, and Maternal Morbidity and Mortality*. New York: D. Appleton-Century.

______. 1934. Birth Injuries of the Child. *Nebraska State Med J* 19:313–16.

Erb, W. H. 1873–77. Über eine eigenthümliche Localisation von Lähmungen im Plexus brachialis. *Verh Nat-Med Vereins Heidelburg*, n.F. 1:130–36.

Ford, F. R. 1927. Cerebral Birth Injuries. In *Birth Injuries of the Central Nervous System.* Vol. 12, Part 1. Ed. F. R. Ford, B. Crothers, and M. C. Putnam, Baltimore: Williams & Wilkins.

Freud, S. 1897. *Die Infantile Cerebrallähmung*. Wien: A. Hölder.

Gowers, R. 1886–88. *A Manual of Diseases of the Nervous System.* London: J. & A Churchill.

______. 1888. Clinical Lecture on Birth Palsies. *Lancet* 1:709–11, 759–60.

Koehler, R., and H. Ehrenfest. 1925. *The Therapy of Puerperal Fever*. St. Louis: C. V. Mosby.

Kosmak, G. W. 1942. A Tribute. *Am J Obstet Gyn* 44:369.

Little, W. J. 1843–44. Course of Lectures on the Deformities of the Human Frame. Lecture IX. *Lancet* 1:350–54.

______. 1862. *On the Nature and Treatment of the Deformities of the Human Frame.* London: Longman.

Longo, L. D. 1981. John Whitridge Williams and Academic Obstetrics in America. *Trans Studies Coll Phys Phila* 5th ser., 3:221–54.

______. 1989. The Professionalization of Obstetrics: Invention of a Specialty. In *Women and Health*. Ed. R. D. Apple. New York: Garland.

1942. Obituary. Hugo Ehrenfest, M.D. *JAMA* 120:65.

Osler, W. 1889. *The Cerebral Palsies of Children: A Clinical Study from the Infirmary for Nervous Diseases*. Philadelphia: Blakiston.

Rilliet, F., and A. Barthez. 1843. *Traité clinique et pratique des maladies des enfants*. Paris: G. Baillière.

Sachs, B. 1891. Contributions to the Pathology of Infantile Cerebral Palsies. *NY Med J* 53:503–10.

Schwartz, P. 1927. Tramatischen Schädigungen Zentralnervensystems durch die Geburt. Anatomische Untersuchungen. *Ergeb inn Med Kinderheilk* 31:165–372.

Taussig, F. J. 1942. In Memoriam. Hugo Ehrenfest 1870–1942. *Am J Obstet Gyn* 44:367–69.

1932. *White House Conference on Child Health and Protection. Proceedings*. New York: Century.

Williams, J. W. 1903. *Obstetrics. A Text-Book for the Use of Students and Practitioners*. New York: D. Appleton.

ASBJÖRN FÖLLING

A CENTURY AGO the son of a struggling Norwegian farmer could hardly have been expected to achieve a university education, let alone develop into a world renowned scientist. Yet this scenario describes the career of Asbjörn Fölling (1888–1972) (figure 1), whose research led to the identification of phenylketonuria, the first inborn error of metabolism for which a prenatal diagnosis could be made through biochemical analysis. Folling's discovery laid the foundation for the study of those diseases of children resulting from the accumulation of neurotoxic substances secondary to genetically determined enzyme deficiencies. His later experiments, which excluded phenylalanine from the diet of phenylketonurics led to a new concept — that of dietary restriction — in the treatment of certain progressive diseases of childhood. These pioneering studies appropriately place Asbjörn Fölling at the forefront of the founders of child neurology.

Fölling was born on August 23, 1888, the youngest of six children in a farming family not far from Trondheim, Norway. He attended an every-other-day school where local children of all ages were taught together in a common room. Even though he loved books and reading and had both the ability and motivation, his education would no doubt have ended in that small schoolroom, had he not had an older married sister living in Trondheim. He was able to stay with her family to continue his education beyond high school, finally graduating from the local technical college in 1916 as a biochemist.

Fölling's desire to attend medical school at the University of Oslo was looked upon as strange by his parents, who considered that he had enough education. But Fölling was determined, supporting himself entirely through teaching and working in the physiology laboratory. During the summers he helped his family on the farm. He completed his medical studies in 1922 and for the next six years worked in the University of Oslo clinics. In 1928 he received a Rockefeller Foundation travel grant, which he used in the United States, studying metabolic diseases at the Mayo Clinic and at Harvard, Yale, and Johns Hopkins medical schools. He received a doctoral degree in 1929 at the University of Oslo, defending his thesis "The Mechanism of Ammonium Chloride Acidosis."

Fölling at this point had every intention of following a clinical career. When a patient was admitted in diabetic coma, however, the professor of medicine sent for Fölling to ask him "to make some insulin," and his laboratory studies began. Although he became professor of nutritional medicine at the University of Oslo in 1932, he did not like being removed from contact with students, so two years later he eagerly accepted a new position that allowed him both to continue with his laboratory investigation and to return to teaching. In 1934 Fölling was appointed professor of biochemistry and physiology in the newly opened Veterinary College in Oslo. That same year he made the discovery that would bring him international acclaim.

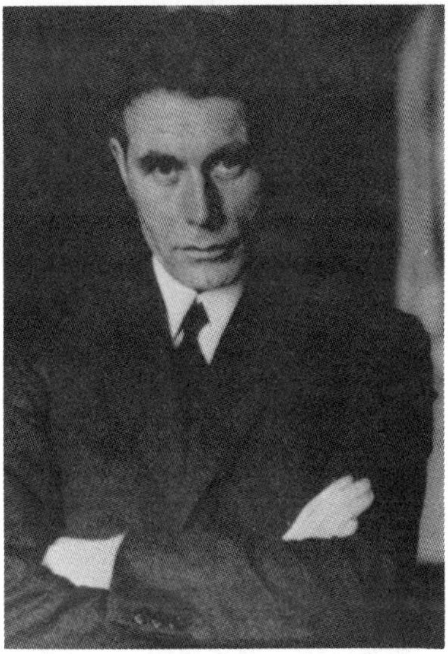

Figure 1. Asbjörn Fölling (1888–1972). This photo was taken in 1934 shortly after his first diagnosis of patients with phenylketonuria.

A dental colleague had suggested that the mother of two mentally retarded children consult Fölling in the hope that his biochemical expertise might help her. The children's father, an asthmatic dentist, felt that his attacks of asthma were accentuated by the peculiar odor that clung to the children, which was particularly strong in their urine. The problem was to discover the source of the odor. Physical examination of the two retarded patients revealed little beyond a fair skin, a slightly stooped posture, and, in one of the two, eczema (figure 2). The odorous urine exhibited no sign of infection; however, the test for ketones provided the first clue. Ferric chloride, which would have colored ketotic urine purple, instead tinged the fluid bluish-green. At Fölling's request, the mother then provided him with an additional twenty liters of her children's urine. Working in a nitrogen atmosphere to prevent the inevitable oxidation that occurred in the presence of oxygen,

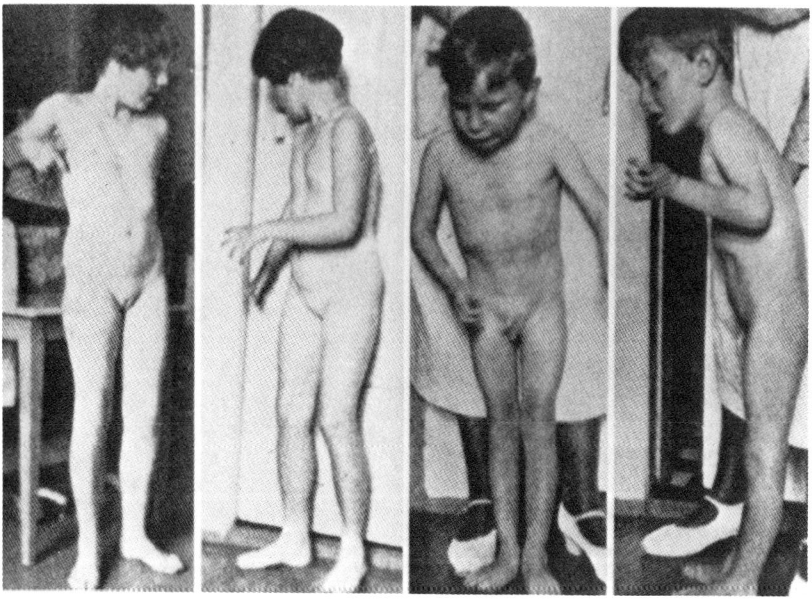

Figure 2. The first children to be diagnosed with phenylketonuria by Fölling in 1934.

Fölling was able to obtain a pure compound within a month and to identify that compound as phenylpyruvic acid in another six weeks.

Once the odorous compound was identified, Fölling tested urine specimens from several hundred patients in psychiatric clinics and in homes for the mentally retarded. In addition to his first two patients, he found nine others to be retarded and to excrete phenylpyruvic acid. He concluded that the condition was a disorder of phenylalanine metabolism, and, since four of the total of eleven patients were siblings, that the condition was hereditary as well.

Fölling then labeled the condition *imbecilitas phenylpyruvica*. After the original description appeared in the Norwegian literature, his countrymen adopted the designation of "Fölling's disease" (Fölling, 1934a). In the United States, it was referred to as phenylpyruvic oligophrenia. Since additional manifestations, such as seizures, gait and postural changes, and abnormal involuntary movements may accompany the retardation, that terminology was considered too restrictive. Fölling's disease is now recognized under the name of phenylketonuria.

In 1934 Fölling first published his initial identification of phenylpyruvic acid in Norwegian (1934a) and in German (1934b) and also published a paper in German on the elevation of phenylalanine in the brain and blood of involved patients in 1938 (Fölling and Closs, 1938).

World War II and the five years of German occupation interfered with many scientific studies in Norway and inhibited publication of those studies that were performed — for it was considered unpatriotic to publish during the German domination. Fölling's laboratory remained active, however, and made a unique contribution toward Norway's struggle to regain its freedom. It was at Fölling's benches that Ole Jacob Malm worked to perfect the invisible ink that the Norwegian Resistance used for its critical communications, undetected throughout the occupation (Malm, 1987).

Fölling continued his work on phenylketonuria. After developing an assay for serum phenylalanine, he demonstrated increased excretion of phenylacetic acid in the urine. Together with professor O. Louis Mohr and a medical student, Lars Rudd, he proved phenylketonuria to be an autosomal recessive disease (Fölling, Mohr, and Rudd, 1945), and then reported, together with Sverre Sydnes, delayed excretion of a phenylalanine load in carriers of that condition (Sydnes and Fölling, 1962).

In 1953, at the age of sixty-five, Fölling was recalled to the University of Oslo to reorganize the Clinical Laboratory for which he had laid the groundwork some twenty years earlier. Five years later, he "retired" and returned to the Veterinary College to continue his research.

Professor Fölling received many honors for his pioneering work in the discovery of phenylketonuria and his subsequent studies of that condition. In 1960 he received the Jahre Prize, known in Norway as the "little Nobel Prize" and, in 1962, the Kennedy Prize. He received the Order of St. Olav in Norway and the Danneborg Order in Denmark. He was elected to the Norwegian Academy of Sciences and Letters. He valued most, however, the Order of St. Blasius, the Patron Saint of the Veterinary Students, which he received in recognition of his teaching and his friendship for the students.

Asbjörn Fölling died at the age of eighty-four and, in accordance with his wishes, was buried in his local churchyard near the soil he had worked as a young man (Elgjo, 1985).

Maynard M. Cohen

Doris Vidaver

CHICAGO, ILLINOIS

REFERENCES

Elgjo, R. F. 1985. Asbjörn Fölling, His Life and Work. In *Medical Genetics, Past, Present, Future*, 79–81. Ed. K. Berg. New York: Liss.

Fölling, A. 1934a. Utskillelse av fenylpyrodruesyre i urinen som stoffskifte anomali i forbindelse med imbecillitet. *Nord Med Tidskr* 8:1054–59.

______. 1934b. Über Ausscheidung von Phenylbrenztraubensaure in den Harn als Stoffwechselanomalie in Verbindung mit Imbezillitat. *Hoppe-Seylers Zeit physiol Chem* 227:169–76.

Fölling, A., and K. Closs. 1938. Über das Vorkommen von l-Phenylalanin in Harn und Blut bei Imbecillitas phenylpyrouvica. *Hoppe-Seylers Zeit physiol Chem* 254:115–16.

Fölling, A., O. Lous Mohr, and L. Rudd. 1945. *Oligophrenia Phenylpyruvica. A Recessive Syndrome in Man*. Oslo: Det Norske Videnskap Akademi, Skrfter I. Math. Naturv. Klasse No 13:44.

Malm, O. J. 1987. Personal communication.

Sydnes, S., and A. Fölling. 1962. On Detection of Heterozygotes for Phenylpyruvic Oligophrenia. *Scand J Clin Invest* 14:44–46.

HENRY HERBERT GODDARD

THE DEVELOPMENT OF psychological testing and educational reform was a culmination of substantial religious, scientific, and political changes in attitudes toward the developmentally disabled that occurred from the seventeenth through twentieth centuries.

As observed by Edward Brett, pediatric neurologist at The Hospital for Sick Children in Great Ormond Street:

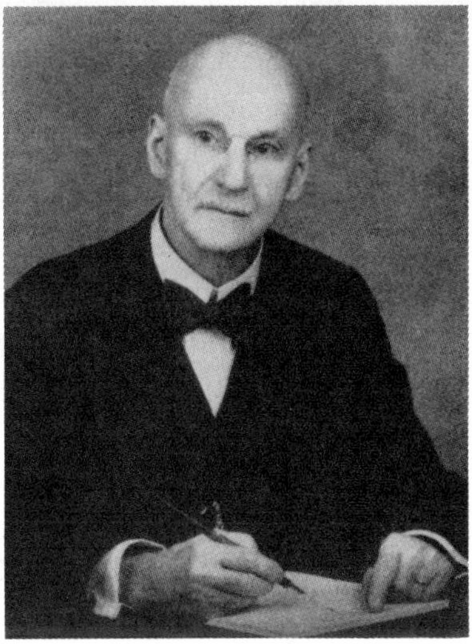

Figure 1. Henry Herbert Goddard (1866–1957). From *American Psychologist* 1 (1946): 381.

> *Abandoned and exposed in Ancient Greece and Rome; cared for in asylums and seen as 'les enfants du bon dieu' in mediaeval times; whipped and chained 'Children of Satan' in the 16th century, sold by Parish authorities to mill owners in the 18th century, the lunatics and the idiots were finally rescued by the great educational reformers of the 19th century.* (Brett, 1983, 349)

Serious interest in the evaluation and treatment of such individuals began in France with the works of Phillipe Pinel, Jean Etienne Esquirol, Jean Itard, and Edouard Séguin; in Switzerland with Johann Jacob Guggenbuhl; in England with William Twinning; in Germany with Carl Wilhelm Saegert; and in the United States with Samuel Gridley Howe (Kanner, 1964). Séguin's influence was substantial. In 1842 he convinced the French authorities of the need to educate the "idiots" and "imbeciles" at the Bicêtre and from this effort dates the origins of the first state schools for retarded children and recognition that the state had a responsibility to train and educate the handicapped (Brett, 1983, 350). Subsequently, the work of Sir Francis Galton in England and Wilhelm Wundt in Germany pioneered the development of the scientific approach to understanding intelligence and sensorimotor function. These investigations were continued by many others, including James Cattell, a student of Wundt; Alfred Binet in France; Stanley Hall in the United States; and one of Hall's students, Henry Herbert Goddard.

Henry Herbert Goddard (1866–1957) (figure 1) was born in Vassalboro, Maine. He received a master's degree from Harvard in 1889 and, after teaching at the University of Southern California for a year, served as a high school principal in Ohio and Maine for six years (Scheerenberger, 1983). Goddard then entered a doctoral program at Clark University and received his degree in 1889. His work was carried out under G. Stanley Hall, a major figure in psychology and one of the early workers in developmental psychology (Rosen, Clark, and Kivitz, 1976). At the time Goddard was pursuing his education, the individual with mental retardation was rarely differentiated from other "degenerates." This group also included the blind, deaf, epileptic, and insane, as well as delinquents and criminals (Wolfensberger, 1974). Much of Goddard's early work supported this general concept and was used by the eugenics movement, but in his later career he began to modify his views.

After receiving his degree, Goddard took a position teaching at Pennsylvania State Teacher's College; then, after a one-year interlude of study in Germany, he was appointed director of the research laboratory of the Vineland Training School in New Jersey in 1908. This was the first psychological laboratory devoted to the study of individuals with mental retardation, and it was here, until his resignation in 1918, that he did his best-known work, which formed the basis of his contribution to child neurology.

The laboratory at Vineland attempted expansion into three divisions: psychology, biochemistry, and neuropathology; however, for a number of reasons continuous research was sustained only in psychology (Doll, 1988). Goddard's work at the laboratory covered a number of areas, three of which are of importance to child neurology. These are: the measurement of intelligence and classification of mental retardation, the effect of education and training on intelligence, and the hereditary basis of mental retardation and antisocial behavior.

In 1906 Alfred Binet and Theodore Simon published a test for the assessment of intelligence in children designed to differentiate normal children from those designated as feeble-minded (Rosen, Clark, and Kivitz, 1976). They revised the test in 1908, introducing the concept of mental age. In 1909 Goddard translated the Binet-Simon Scale into English, standardized it on two thousand school children in the Vineland public schools, and applied it as a research tool for the study of individuals with mental retardation. The results of a study of four hundred such children was presented at the Thirty-Third Annual Meeting of the American Association for the Study of the Feebleminded, subsequently the American Association on Mental Deficiency and now the American Association on Mental Retardation (Sloan and Stevens, 1976). The importance of this study was the use of an objective criterion, mental age, in the classification process. Goddard continued to use the then accepted terms of idiot and imbecile, but substituted the term moron in place of feebleminded (Goddard, 1910). The terms idiot (severe mental retardation), imbecile (moderate mental retardation) and moron (mild mental retardation) are now archaic and are only used as they were used by Goddard. He also devised the category of moral imbeciles, those individuals who have only developed intellectually to the moron level and so have failed to develop adequate reasoning and control of their instincts.

Further work at the Vineland laboratory under Goddard's supervision attempted to extend the usefulness of the Binet scales. This research included a pilot program to detect mentally retarded individuals among immigrants to the United States and the development of the Army Alpha and Beta tests, used by the U.S. Army to classify recruits drafted for military service (Doll, 1988). The tests provided a wealth of data that was used in research for many years. One initial problem was Goddard's recommendation that a mental age of twelve years be the cutoff for feeblemindedness; 47.3 percent of draftees fell into this category.

Goddard provided an additional insight that has become an important component of the classification of mental retardation. In 1928, at the Fifty-Second Annual Meeting of the American Association for the Study of the Feebleminded, he presented a paper in which he suggested that mental age alone was insufficient to classify feeblemindedness, but that it was more important to determine if the individual could care for himself and his own needs and act with ordinary prudence (Sloan and Stevens, 1976). This definition was the forerunner of the current definition of mental retardation that depends on deficits in both intellectual and adaptive function.

Goddard took a strong position for many years that education was of little or no use in the management of individuals with mental retardation. He felt that intelligence scores were fixed, based on a study in which three annual administrations of the Binet scale were given to 346 children (Goddard, 1913). He in

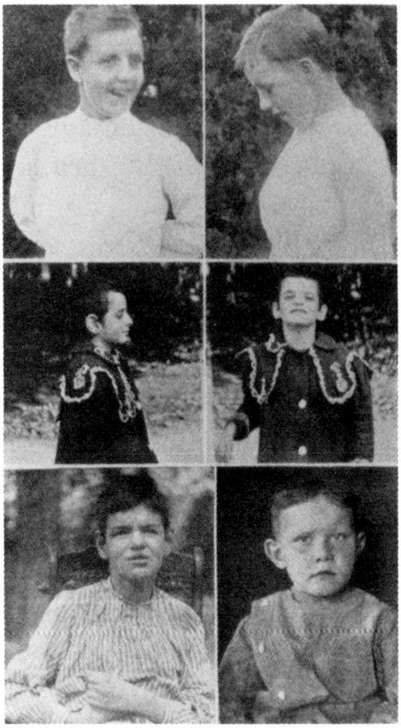

Figure 2. "Nellie E." (top) from *Feeble-Mindedness: Its Causes and Consequences*. The other children are from subsequent case histories. Goddard noted that Nellie's family was the second most affected family he evaluated, the most severely affected being the Kallikaks.

fact held this belief to such an extent that he argued that the only reasons for having feeble-minded children attend school were if they were too small to work or if they needed entertainment (Scheerenberger, 1983).

In 1928, however, Goddard publicly reversed his position (Goddard, 1928). He now blamed the educational system for the existence of morons, and felt that with a proper system of education these individuals could manage their own affairs. He also stated that the condition was not incurable and that most of the feebleminded did not require institutionalization.

The third area of interest, that of the inheritance of mental retardation, is best demonstrated by Goddard's study at Vineland (figure 2), which resulted in his renowned studies of the Kallikak family (Goddard, 1912) and the publication of *Feeblemindedness: Its Causes and Consequences* (1914). Deborah Kallikak (a fictitious name) was admitted to Vineland Training School when she was eight years old. A detailed genetic history revealed that her great-great-great grandfather had two groups of lineal descendents by two different women. Deborah's line, initiated by a liaison with a feebleminded woman, gave rise to 408 individuals, 143 of whom were mentally retarded; many others suffered from various forms of social pathology (Scheerenberger, 1983). The second line consisted of 496 people, none of whom were mentally retarded, and many of whom assumed prominent places in the community. Only one was insane and three were socially degenerate. In the conclusion of his paper, Goddard states that *it is inevitable that all this degeneracy has come as the result of the defective mentality and bad blood having been brought into the normal family of good blood. . . . The biologist could hardly plan and carry out a more rigid experiment or one from which the conclusions would follow more inevitably.* (Goddard, 1912, 69)

Despite the obvious methodological problems in the study, the data were among those used by a very active eugenics movement, resulting in restrictive immigration laws, sterilization of mentally retarded individuals, and a great increase in the number of people placed in institutions. Although the eugenecists drew upon Goddard's work, he became more liberal with time and in 1928 spoke out against sterilization (Goddard, 1928). Based on his recent acceptance of the idea that morons could be self-sufficient if given appropriate education, he affirmed that they should have the right to marry and have children, and that they could live happy and useful lives.

From 1918 to 1922 Goddard was director of the Ohio State Bureau for Juvenile Research and, from 1922 until his retirement in 1938, he was professor of clinical psychology at Ohio State University. In these two latter positions he published several works in the areas of mental retardation, juvenile delinquency, multiple personalities, and the education of gifted children (Scheerenberger, 1983). Goddard died in 1957 at the age of ninety-one.

Gerald S. Golden
MEMPHIS, TENNESSEE

REFERENCES

Brett, E. M. 1983. *Paediatric Neurology*. London: Churchill Livingstone.

Doll, E. E. 1988. Before the Big Time: Early History of the Training School at Vineland, 1988 to 1949. *Am J Ment Retard* 93:1–15.

Goddard, H. H. 1910. Four Hundred Feeble-Minded Children Classified by the Binet Method. *J Psycho-Asthenics* 15:17–30.

______. 1912. *The Kallikak Family: A Study in the Heredity of Feeblemindedness*. New York: Macmillan Co.

______. 1913. The Improvability of Feeble-Minded Children. *J Psycho-Asthenics* 17:121–31.

______. 1914. *Feeblemindedness: Its Causes and Consequences*. New York: Macmillan Co.

______. 1928. Feeblemindedness: A Question of Definition. *J Psycho-Asthenics* 33:219–17.

Kanner, L. 1964. *A History of the Care and Study of the Mentally Retarded*. Springfield, IL: Charles C Thomas.

Rosen, M., G. R. Clark, and M. S. Kivitz. 1976. *The History of Mental Retardation*. Baltimore: University Park Press.

Scheerenberger, R. C. 1983. *A History of Mental Retardation*. Baltimore: Brookes Publishing Co.

Sloan, W., and H. A. Stevens. 1976. *A Century of Concern: A History of the American Association on Mental Deficiency, 1876–1976*. Washington, D.C.: American Association on Mental Deficiency.

Wolfensberger, W. 1974. *The Origin and Nature of Our Institutional Models*. Syracuse: Syracuse University Division of Special Education and Rehabilitation, Center on Human Policy.

JULIUS HALLERVORDEN

THE NAME OF JULIUS Hallervorden (1882–1965) (figure 1) has become familiar to neurologists and to many pediatricians in connection with Hallervorden-Spatz disease, a rare cerebral disorder that manifests itself during childhood. Its recognition as a distinct disease is due to the clarity and completeness of the original description, which was the result of a close collaboration between Hallervorden and his long-time associate, Hugo Spatz. It is appropriate that both names appear together in the name of the syndrome, since both men participated equally in delineating it, but Hallervorden has been singled out for this biographical essay, partly because of seniority and partly because of his lifelong interest in pediatric neurological problems.

Hallervorden's contribution to the development of child neurology was in neuropathology — the detection and study of pathoanatomic changes in the tissues of the nervous system with the purpose of achieving a better understanding of the clinical phe-

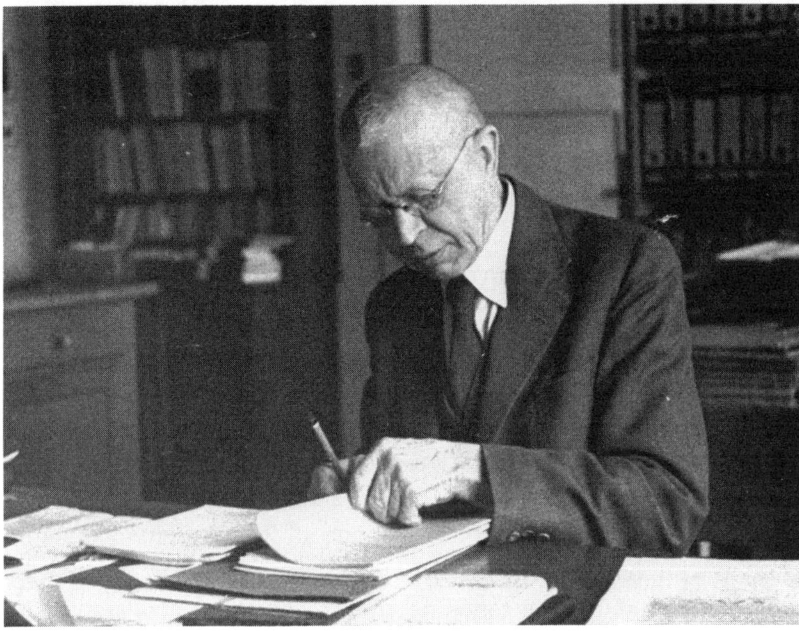

Figure 1. Julius Hallervorden (1882–1965) at his desk in Giessen, 1956.

nomena of nervous system diseases. In his long professional life he published original investigations and review articles on a wide range of topics from neonatal encephalopathies to aging in the brain.

In all probability, Hallervorden's earliest experiences determined the ultimate choice of his life's work. He was born in 1882 in Allenberg in East Prussia, which then belonged to Germany, where his father was a staff psychiatrist in an asylum for the mentally ill (Spatz, 1966; Krücke, 1966). Later the family moved to Königsberg (now Kaliningrad), where his father became director of a psychiatric hospital and Hallervorden studied medicine at the university, obtaining his doctoral degree in 1909. He spent the next four years acquiring additional experience in internal medicine and psychiatry in Berlin. Then, in 1913, he was appointed staff psychiatrist in the psychiatric hospital in Landsberg an der Warthe (now Gorzów Wielkopolski), where he remained until 1936. Soon after arriving in Landsberg, he became interested in studying the pathological anatomy of the brains of his deceased patients as a means of gaining further insight into the disease states that had afflicted them. Before long he established a small laboratory, where, largely self-taught, he started to undertake systematic postmortem neuropathologic studies, which he documented in meticulous detail with both clinical and anatomical observations. From time to time he presented these case studies at meetings of the Berlin Society for Psychiatry and Neurology, a forum known for its lively discussions. Apparently because of his contributions to the meetings, he attracted the attention of Walther Spielmeyer, who in 1912 was head of the newly established Neuropathological Laboratory at the University Hospital for Psychiatric and Neurologic Diseases. This institution later became the German Research Institute for Psychiatry in Munich. In 1921 Spielmeyer invited Hallervorden to his laboratory for a period of study. When he arrived in Munich, Hallervorden brought with him from Landsberg the brain of one of his patients, a young woman who had died with a familial disorder characterized by abnormalities of muscle tone and movement and a progressive dementia. At that time there was already a lively interest at the laboratory in diseases of what had come to be called the extrapyramidal motor system, and Hugo Spatz, who had been a pupil of Franz Nissl, was especially active in these investigations. Spatz had shown, in a study of the distribution of iron in the brain, that certain components of the extrapyramidal system, the globus pallidus, and the closely related pars reticulata of the substantia nigra contained a considerably greater quantity of iron than any other cerebral structures (Spatz, 1922). Together Hallervorden and Spatz undertook the examination of the brain of Hallervorden's patient. It was their report of this case that established Hallervorden-Spatz disease as a nosologic entity (Hallervorden and Spatz, 1922).

The patient, Martha S., died at twenty-three years of age with a gradually progressive incapacitating neurologic illness. She developed normally at first and started school uneventfully, but between the ages of seven and nine her legs became spastic, with inward rotation of her feet, so that walking was impaired. Meanwhile, it became evident that her mental abilities were deteriorating. At nineteen she became incontinent and unable to care for herself, and was admitted to the psychiatric institution in Landsberg. Ultimately flexion contractures and scoliosis developed, with total incapacitation. The exact cause of death was not determined; autopsy was confined to the brain and spinal cord.

Investigation of the family history, which was laborious because of the difficulty of obtaining records, indicated that of nine surviving children of a total of twelve (three had died in early infancy), five had been afflicted with an illness that appeared identical to that of Hallervorden's patient. An older sister, who died at twenty-two, had choreoathetotic movements in addition to spastic contractures of the limbs. A younger sister also died at twenty-two; the examination of her brain was reported later (Hallervorden, 1924). The other two children, who were twins, died at age sixteen.

On their examination of the brain of Martha S., Hallervorden and Spatz found, to their surprise, that instead of the atrophic changes in the basal ganglia they had expected, there was "an intense rust-brown discoloration," coupled with a greatly increased iron content, in the very structures that are normally especially rich in iron — the globus pallidus and the pars reticulata of the substantia nigra. Otherwise, the brain was of normal appearance and weight (1250 grams), and there was no evidence of gross atrophy. On microscopic examination, however, the cortex was seen to be thinner and the basal ganglia were smaller than normally expected. Sharply localized to the grossly discolored regions were massive accumulations of pigment granules that were easily visible as yellowish areas in unstained sections; these regions, when stained for iron, gave an abnormally intense positive reaction. The pigment granules, which were found within the cytoplasm of large glial cells and in perivascular aggregates, were of many kinds. In addition to those that were iron-positive, there were others that stained for lipids, and still others that took up hematoxylin strongly in the manner of calcium but were negative with the von Kossa stain for calcium. Astrocytes were increased in size and numbers. Scattered about in the background were numerous rounded structures that were often larger than the nerve cells of these regions. These structures were identified by silver staining (devised by Bielschowsky) as swollen axons (now generally referred to as spheroids). They were found to be present not only within the basal ganglia but at all levels of the central nervous system, including the spinal cord, and in both white and gray matter. In longitudinal sections of the spinal cord they were seen along the course of axons in long tracts, suggesting that they were not exclusively in axonal terminals. They were especially numerous in the subthalamic nucleus. In the cerebral cortex there was widespread loss of neurons, diffusely distributed but relatively greater in the third layer. There also was some loss of Purkinje cells in the cerebellum and of some of the motor neurons in the brainstem and spinal cord. The corticospinal tracts were intact.

The authors considered that the disorder they had described was without exact parallel in previous experience. They emphasized that an outstanding feature was the presence of an excessive content of iron in cerebral structures that normally contain relatively large amounts of this element, and also drew particular attention to the widely disseminated axonal swellings. They related the motor abnormalities to the lesions in the globus pallidus and substantia nigra and attributed the dementia to the neuronal loss in the cerebral cortex. Their conclusion was that this was an endogenous metabolic disorder of undetermined type, probably hereditary, as indicated by the family history.

Two years later Hallervorden reported the findings in the brain of the patient's sister, Alma S., who died with a clinically similar illness at the age of twenty-two (Hallervorden, 1924). In all essential respects, the neuropathological changes were identical to those described in the case of Martha S. In this report, Hallervorden pointed out that all of the affected members of the family were girls. He attempted to obtain more details of the family history but was unsuccessful.

Hallervorden went on to attain international fame as a neuropathologist. When, in 1938, Spatz became director of the recently established and well-financed Kaiser-Wilhelm Institute for Brain Research in Berlin, he invited his old friend Hallervorden to become head of the Neuropathological Department. Meanwhile, during the Nazi regime in Germany, and during the war, a systematic program of euthanasia was carried out on individuals officially not considered suitable for the kind of society the leaders were trying to create (Lifton, 1986). In addition, there were the now well-known horrors of the Holocaust. Hallervorden, as well as Spatz, was accused of having carried out examinations on anatomical materials deriving from victims of these massacres (Aly, 1989). Spatz's work focused largely on adult neuropathology and comparative neuroanatomy, and thus he did not contribute to child neurology in his later work as much as did Hallervorden, who had an active interest in the pathology of mental retardation, neonatal neurologic disorders including cerebral palsy, and hereditary neurologic diseases. Hallervorden published extensive reviews on these topics, but it is impossible to escape the suspicion that some of the observations included were made without appropriate consideration of the provenance of the material on which they were based.

Following the war, the part of the city in which the institute was located was incorporated into East Berlin. Together with their colleagues in other divisions of the institute, Hallervorden and Spatz were forced to move, but they were able to find new laboratories for their respective neuropathological and neuroanatomical departments in what is now the Federal Republic of Germany. After temporary stays in Dillenburg (Hessen) and in Giessen, their departments, by this time divisions of what had become the Max-Planck-Institute for Brain Research, ultimately found suitable quarters in Frankfurt. Here, both Hallervorden and Spatz continued scientific work to the end of their lives.

In 1955, when the institute was still in Giessen, I had the opportunity to spend nearly six months working with Hallervorden and became acquainted with him. He was of a quiet, reserved nature, wholly devoted to science and to neuropathology, and at the same time, warm, friendly, and an inspiring teacher. He was one of the last great figures of the classic period of German neuropathology. His description, with Spatz, of Hallervorden-Spatz disease still ranks as a major contribution to child neurology, even though the disorder remains nearly as mysterious as at the time of the original report.

Edward P. Richardson, Jr.
BOSTON, MASSACHUSETTS

REFERENCES

Aly, G. 1989. Je mehr, desto lieber. Über den Umgang mit Präparaten von Nazi-Opfern vor 1945 und danach. *Die Zeit* (10 February) 6: 21–22. Hamburg: Kommanditgesellschaft Zeitverlag Gerd Bucerius GmbH & Co.

Hallervorden, J. 1924. Über eine familiäre Erkrankung im extrapyramidalen System. *Dtsch Zeit Nervenheilk* 81:204–10.

Hallervorden, J., and H. Spatz. 1922. Eigenartige Erkrankung im extrapyramidalen System mit besonderer Beteiligung des Globus pallidus und der Substantia nigra. *Neur Psych* 79:254–302.

Krücke, W. 1966. Julius Hallervorden, 1882–1965. *Acta Neuropath* 6:114–16.

Lifton, R. J. 1986. *The Nazi Doctors. Medical Killing and the Psychology of Genocide.* New York: Basic Books.

Spatz, H. 1922. Über den Eisennachweis im Gehirn, besonders in Zentren des extrapyramidal-motorischen Systems. *Zeit Neur Psych* 77:261–390.

______. 1966. Erinnerungen an Julius Hallervorden (1882–1965). *Nervenarzt* 37:477–82.

JAMES RAMSAY HUNT

JAMES RAMSAY HUNT (1874–1937) (figure 1) is best known for his description of inflammation of the geniculate ganglion of the facial nerve (Ramsay Hunt syndrome, 1907, 1910). He also gave his name to a syndrome beginning in adolescence consisting of seizures, myoclonus, and cerebellar ataxia, which is also known as Ramsay Hunt syndrome. Other Ramsay Hunt syndromes include an ulnar nerve entrapment syndrome and static epilepsy (Jelliffe, 1938).

Hunt was born in Philadelphia on February 1, 1874, of Quaker parentage. He attended the Friends School in Philadelphia and then the University of Pennsylvania, receiving his medical degree in 1893. He remained there for his internship and developed lifelong friendships with Charles Karsner Mills and Charles Camac, both of whom influenced his career. He also began a long-term infatuation with music, later being a regular at Carnegie Hall (Cobb, 1938).

After two years of internship, Silas Weir Mitchell arranged for Hunt to care for a patient abroad. After visiting Japan, China, and India, Hunt studied pathology in Vienna with Albert Neisser and Ferenc Kovaacs, and neurology with Heinrich Obersteiner. In Berlin he studied with Hermann Oppenheim and Richard Cassirer, and in Paris he visited Pierre Marie, Joseph Babinski, and Jules Dejerine in their clinics (Jelliffe, 1938). On his return to the United States he spent a year in Philadelphia and was then appointed assistant instructor at Cornell University Medical School under Charles Loomis Dana, where he remained until 1910 (Wechsler, 1953).

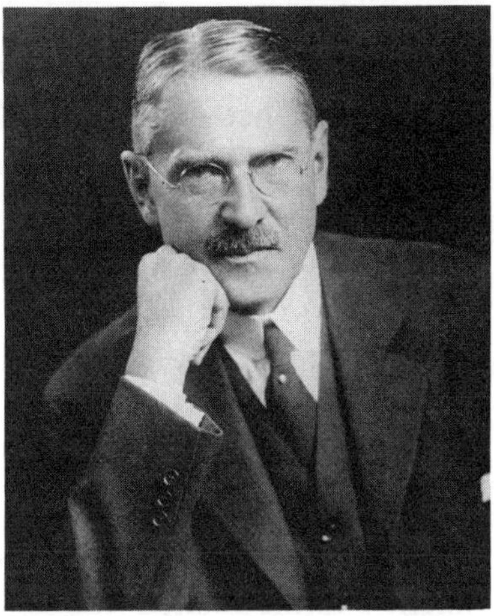

Figure 1. James Ramsay Hunt (1874–1937).

While at Cornell, he first reported on herpetic inflammation of the geniculate ganglion (Hunt, 1907). He later published a masterful review of inflammation of the geniculate, auditory, glossopharyngeal, and pneumogastric (vagal) ganglia with the meticulous diagrams that were to be the hallmark of his work (Hunt, 1910).

In 1910 Hunt joined what was later to become the Neurologic Institute as associate professor of neurology at Columbia University. There he began his lifelong work of investigating movement disorders. His descriptions of paralysis agitans (Parkinson's disease) are classic. He considered this a clinical syndrome, attributing symptoms to degeneration of the globus pallidus and corpus striatum (Hunt, 1916a, 1917). Hunt was the first to describe a juvenile form of Parkinson's disease with familial features pathologically characterized by atrophy of the caudate nucleus and sparing the substantia nigra. His patient had the onset of a pill-rolling tremor at age fifteen, with generalized rigidity and anarthria (Hunt, 1917). The clinical course was progressive, with death occurring at the age of forty. He described the clinical features of dystonia musculorum deformans and stressed that this was an organic disease, noting the preservation of intellectual functions despite torsion spasm (Hunt, 1916b). His pathologic and clinical descriptions were exhaustive, and his publications frequently exceeded fifty pages.

In his presidential address to the American Neurological Association in 1920, Hunt summarized current knowledge of the systems of movement and control, dividing movements into three types: reflex, automatic, and associated and isolated synergistic. He related these to the reflex systems of the neuraxis, "a paleoencephalon" and "neo-encephalon." He regarded the cerebellum as "the great correlating center for static functions of motility" and the corpus striatum and rolandic area "the essential correlating centers for the control of their respective forms of kinetic function." Regarding muscles, he said "the disc" was "the end organ of the kinetic system" and "the sarcoplasm was the end organ of the static system." He divided motor symptoms into the "paleo-kinetic" (corpus striatum) and "neo-kinetic" (cortical) systems, or extra pyramidal and pyramidal systems. He divided the cerebellum into "paleo-static" (vermis) and "neo-static" (dentate nucleus) systems. Hunt related various clinical disorders to these systems, such as epilepsy to cortical motility and Huntington chorea to striatal motility (Hunt, 1920).

The following year Hunt described "dyssynergia cerebellaris myoclonica," now known as the Ramsay Hunt syndrome (1921). Hunt described four patients who developed generalized major motor seizures during adolescence with myoclonus and appendicular cerebellar tremors. There were no cranial nerve, sensory, or reflex abnormalities on examination. There was no family history of similar neurologic disease. One patient also had akinetic seizures or drop attacks. He presented two additional patients with myoclonus, epilepsy, and Friedreich's ataxia with a positive family history and later development of myoclonus and seizures. Hunt termed these seizures "the astatic type of epilepsy," describing drop attacks or akinetic seizures. In his paper, he stressed the clinical features of intention tremors and their correlation with atrophy of the dentate nuclei, and stated that the cerebellum regulates "posture synergies of motility" (Hunt, 1921).

Hunt served as a consultant at Fort Myer, Virginia, during World War I, and later was a lieutenant colonel with the American Expeditionary Forces. In addition to the Neurologic Institute at Columbia, he was associated with the Charity Hospital on Wards Island, and the Lenox Hill, Babies, New York, Montefiore, and New York Lying-in hospitals, as well as the New York Eye and Ear Infirmary, the Psychiatric Institute, Letchworth Village, and the Craig Colony (Jelliffe, 1938). He had a summer home in Katonah, New

York, where he died of hypernephroma on July 22, 1937, at the age of fifty-three (Cobb, Draper, and Meyer, 1938).

Hunt was known for his exhaustive meticulous work. His obituarists regarded him as having "great natural dignity" and described him as "Olympian" (Jelliffe, 1938).

Fred Haruda
SALINAS, CALIFORNIA

REFERENCES

Cobb, S., G. Draper, and A. Meyer. 1938. Obituary. *Trans Assoc Am Phys* 53:12–13.

Hunt, J. R. 1907. Herpetic Inflammation of the Geniculate Ganglion. *J Nerv Ment Dis* 34:73–96.

______. 1910. The Symptom Complex of the Acute Posterior Poliomyelitis of the Geniculate, Auditory, Glossopharyngeal and Pneumogastric Ganglia. *Arch Int Med* 5:631–71.

______. 1916a. Progressive Atrophy of the Globus Pallidus. *Trans Am Neur Assoc* 42:104–65.

______. 1916b. The Progressive Torsion Spasm of Childhood (Dystonia Musculorum Deformans). *JAMA* 67:1430–37.

______. 1917. Progressive Atrophy of the Globus Pallidus. *Brain* 40:58–145.

______. 1920. The Static and Kinetic Systems of Motility. *Arch Neur Psych* 4:351–69.

______. 1921. Dyssynergia Cerebellaris Myclonica-Primary Atrophy of the Dentate System: Contribution to the Pathology and Symptomatology of the Cerebellum. *Brain* 44:490–538.

Jelliffe, S. E. 1938. James Ramsay Hunt, 1874–1937. *Trans Am Neur Assoc* 64:219–22.

Wechsler, I. S. 1953. James Ramsay Hunt (1874–1937), 302–5. In *The Founders of Neurology*, 302–5. Ed. W. Haymaker and F. Schiller. Springfield, IL: Charles C Thomas.

CHARLES HUNTER

SIR ARCHIBALD GARROD'S clinical and biochemical studies on alkaptonuria at the turn of the century introduced the concept of heritable disorders of metabolism, which he later named inborn errors of metabolism (Garrod, 1902, 1923). Although specific biochemical defects for most of these disorders would not be elucidated until much later, their clinical manifestations were distinct enough to permit clinical recognition and classification. Central nervous system involvement was a frequent feature of these unusual conditions and, therefore, developmental delay, mental retardation, seizures, visual impairment (amaurosis), and other symptoms brought these conditions to the attention of those interested in neurologic diseases of children. In 1917 Charles Hunter of Winnipeg and in 1919 Gertrud Hurler of Munich, independently described brothers with diffuse abnormalities of the skeletal system, coarse facial features, mental retardation,and hepatosplenomegaly. Thus, confusion engendered by the use of the eponyms Hunter disease, Hurler disease, Hunter-Hurler disease, as well as by the introduction of the unfortunate term "gargoylism," prevailed until biochemical studies clarified the specific defect in mucopolysaccharide or glycosaminoglycan metabolism for each disorder; iduronate sulfatase deficiency in Hunter disease and alpha-l-iduronidase in Hurler disease.

Charles Hunter (1873–1955) (figure 1) was born on February 7 in Auchterlass, Aberdeenshire, Scotland. He received from the University of Aberdeen his M.A. degree in 1894, his M.B. and Ch.B. degrees in 1899, and his M.D. degree in 1904. He did postgraduate work in internal medicine in London and Berlin from 1901 to 1904. In 1902 he became a member and in 1930 was elected Fellow of the Royal College of Physicians of London (Munk's Roll, 1968).

In 1904 Hunter went to Canada and established an extensive consulting practice in Winnipeg, where he was regarded as a profound scholar. He possessed remarkable diagnostic acumen, and his opinion on obscure and difficult cases was sought by practitioners from many parts of western Canada. He served on the

Faculty of Medicine at the University of Manitoba from 1910 through 1933 and was associate professor of medicine from 1919 to 1928 (Bell, 1964). Upon the retirement of E. W. Montgomery, Hunter was appointed professor and head of medicine on a half-time basis in December 1927. However, administrative work did not appeal to him, and he resigned eight months later, at which time he was reappointed associate professor so that he could continue his teaching duties (Beamish, 1988). Hunter continued to teach until his retirement in 1933, when he was named professor emeritus of medicine. He remained in active practice until 1952 (Obituary, 1955a). He was one of the early members of the Winnipeg Clinical Society, a forerunner of the Winnipeg Medical Society, and a charter member of the Royal College of Physicians and Surgeons of Canada (Obituary, 1955b).

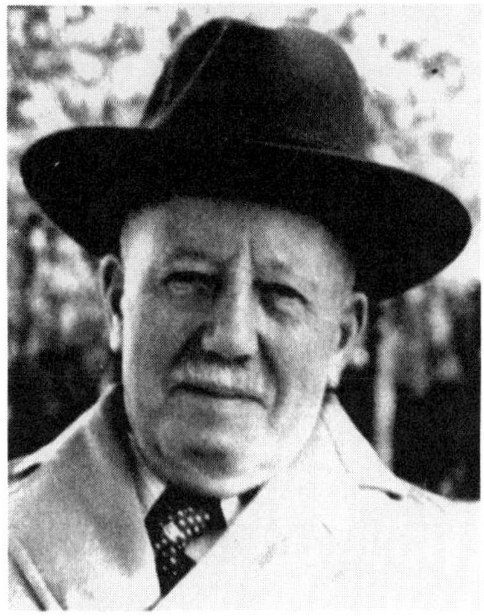

Figure 1. Charles Hunter (1873–1955).

Hunter served overseas during World War I with the Royal Canadian Corps from 1915 to 1919 and attained the rank of lieutenant colonel (Bell, 1964). In 1917, while serving in Europe, Hunter presented a paper entitled "A Rare Disease in Two Brothers" at a meeting of the Royal Society of Medicine in London. This paper later appeared in the *Proceedings of the Royal Society of Medicine* (Hunter, 1917). The article described two Canadian children, eight and ten years old and of British parentage, who were admitted to Winnipeg General Hospital in 1915 with shortness of stature, a large head, coarse facial features, a very large tongue, deafness, skeletal deformities, protruding abdomen, hepatosplenomegaly, and curtailed movement of the extremities (figure 2). Eight of the twelve patients in this article showed skeletal abnormalities now encompassed by the term dysostosis multiplex. Hunter did not use the unfortunate term gargoylism to describe this condition.

According to Victor McKusick (1966), the younger brother

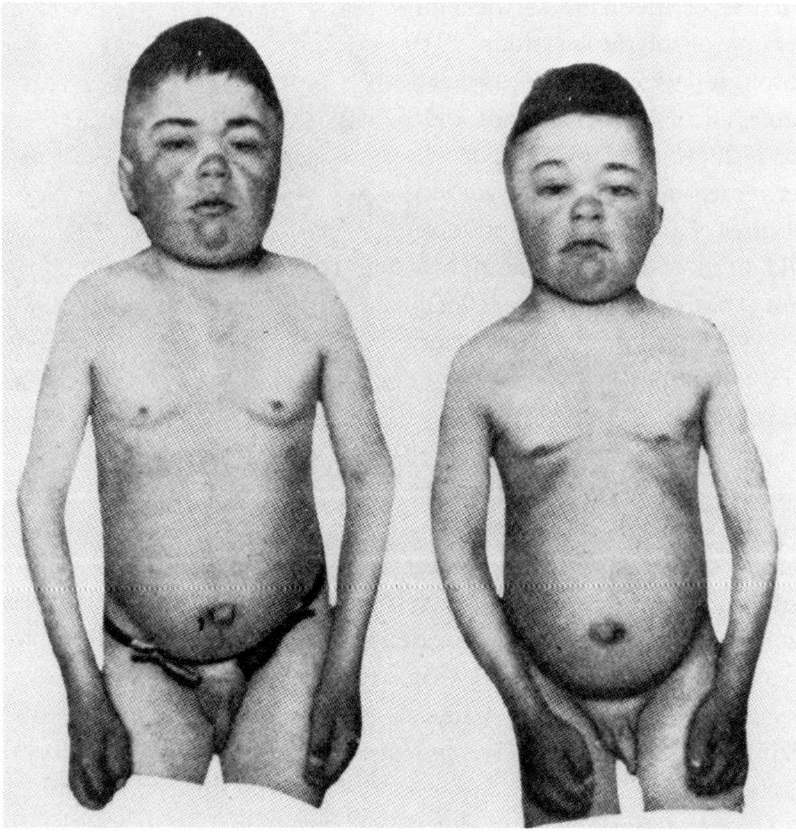

Figure 2. R. C. and G. C., brothers aged ten and eight years, described by Hunter as showing "an extraordinary appearance with very large heads and bulging of the squamous portion of the temporal bone and of the frontal bones, deep burnt-red complexion, puffy eyes, saddle nose with large thick nostrils, thick lips, short neck, broad chest, protruding abdomen, slightly forward inclination of the trunk, arms abducted and flexed so that hands rest on the front of the thighs instead of on the side, hands broad, short and thick, and fingers short and bent" (Hunter, 1917).

died of pneumonia in 1918 and the older one of dropsy in 1920 (McKusick, 1966). Hunter ended his detailed clinical and radiographic description of this rare disorder thus: "Owing to the limited library facilities of Winnipeg, I have been unable to find any reference to such a symptom complex." This was Hunter's first publication and the only one among his works about what is now known as mucopolysaccharidosis type II, or Hunter syndrome. The disorder is due to iduronate sulfatase enzyme deficiency with accumulation of dermatan and heparan sulfate and is inherited as an X-linked recessive disorder.

Charles Hunter was described as "a man of small stature, slim and compact. He moved with a restless energy that matched the quick incisive workings of his mind" (Bell, 1964). He entered discussions with an open mind, led them calmly, and never lost his temper. He was gifted with a sense of humor that enriched many of his tales, including those of his misfortunes (Moorhead, 1955). His personal life, however, was austere and regular. He was up at 5 a.m., worked in his garden for an hour and then spent some time reading the medical books and journals that regularly arrived from Germany. Outside of medical publications, his reading consisted mostly of history and biography; his familiarity with the speeches and writings of the great statesmen of the British Empire during the last two centuries was the fruit of those studies. Music gave him much happiness, and his liking for it seems to have developed during his medical studies in Germany. The hour from 7 to 8 a.m. was spent in walking the two or three miles from his house at the corner of Stafford Street and Yale Avenue (McLean, 1988) to the Winnipeg General Hospital, where he was a member of the honorary attending staff (Beighton and Beighton, 1986).

Following is an account of Hunter's ward rounds at Winnipeg General Hospital:

Just before 8 he appeared on the public ward to make his rounds. The interns and residents assigned to his service were expected to be on the ward with all their histories and progress notes completed and all routine laboratory work finished with the results duly recorded for his inspection. On Dr. Hunter's service there were no acceptable excuses for tardiness or for incomplete records and the intern who once had been subjected to his scorn and sarcasm would slave all night rather than to appear unprepared at early rounds. Each history was perused by the chief who checked each point with the patients and scrawled in the margins or crossed out whole passages with a red pencil. His physical examination was swift and exhaustive — sometimes almost acrobatic. Because of his short stature he would often kneel or half-lie on the bed to carry out auscultation. With this bedside routine would go a rapid fire commentary on the patient's symptoms and signs climaxing with a brilliant summary in which the relevant facts were assembled into a diagnosis. His basic teaching was somewhat didactic but always interspersed with provocative questions to his students, questions designed to make them think clearly in any given clinical situation. When Charles' ward rounds were over and he had bristled off the ward, he left the nurses, interns and residents quaking, sweating and drooping but always stimulated by the certain conviction that they had experienced the touch of a great clinician. Charles did not tolerate fools gladly, or condone any laxness of clinical discipline, but for the intern or resident or student who displayed an alert interest, he could be both genial and helpful. His acerbity was designed to keep everyone on their toes, he was not a martinet and his passion for accuracy, detail and method influenced everyone who worked under his guidance. (Bell, 1964)

Hunter died of hypertensive cerebrovascular disease on March 18, 1955, at age eighty-two.

Enrique Chaves-Carballo
NORFOLK, VIRGINIA

REFERENCES

Beamish, R. E. 1988. Personal communication.

Beighton, P. H., and G. J. Beighton. 1986. *The Man Behind the Syndrome*, 79. New York: Springer-Verlag.

Bell, L. G. 1964. Hunter, Charles. University of Manitoba Medical Library Files.

Garrod, A. E. 1902. The Incidence of Alkaptonuria: A Study in Chemical Individuality. *Lancet* 2:1616.

______. 1923. *Inborn Errors of Metabolism*. London: Oxford University Press.

Hunter, C. 1917. A Rare Disease in Two Brothers. *Proc Roy Soc Med* 10:104–15.

McKusick, V. 1966. *Heritable Disorders of Connective Tissue*, 326. 3d ed. St. Louis: C. V. Mosby.

McLean, J. 1988. Personal communication.

Moorhead, E. S. 1955. Coronach, 305. *Manitoba Med Rev* (July).

Munk's Roll. 1968. *Lives of the Fellows of the Royal College of Physicians of London*. Ed. R. R. Trail. 5:208.

1955a. Obituary. Dr. Charles Hunter. *Can Med Assoc J* 72:712.

1955b. Obituary. Dr. Charles Hunter, 1873–1955. *Winnipeg Clin Quart* (March 1955), 27.

GERTRUD HURLER

GERTRUD HURLER (1889–1965) (figure 1) was born in Taberwiese, Prussia, on September 1. She was educated in Königsberg and qualified in medicine at the University of Munich. Her father had been a general practitioner, and this tradition was passed on to several generations, as both her daughter and granddaughter became internists (Knorr, 1988). Hurler trained in pediatrics at Hauner Children's Hospital under Meinhard von Pfaundler. In 1919 she moved to Neuhauser where she practiced pediatrics for more than forty-five years. She was described as

an exceptional clinician and was greatly liked and respected by her patients. In addition to her clinical activities, she was associated with the local orphanage, served on many medical committees and was a pioneer in the establishment of a maternal postnatal service. (Beighton, 1986)

She remained in active practice until her death at age seventy-six in 1965.

While training with Pfaundler, Hurler reported in 1919, at his suggestion, two cases of "multiple abnormalities prevalent on the skeletal system" that had been presented earlier that year to the Munich Pediatric Society (Hurler, 1919). A follow-up report by Pfaundler on these cases was also published in 1920 (Pfaundler, 1920).

The cases described by Hurler were Paul O. and George O., brothers who first concerned their mother because of a "crookedness" of the spine and "strange-looking" heads. Delayed physical and mental development, as well as arrest of speech development, became apparent by age two. The head was enlarged and beaked at the vertex. The forehead and chin were prominent, while the orbits and nasal bones were small, resulting in a concave configuration to the face. Coarse facial features consisted of broad massive eyebrows, broad flattened nose, and full lips. Other dysmorphic features included a small, compact trunk, concave sternum, broad clavicles, kyphotic thoracic and lumbar spine forming a gibbus, broad and stocky hands with contractures, and a protruding ab-

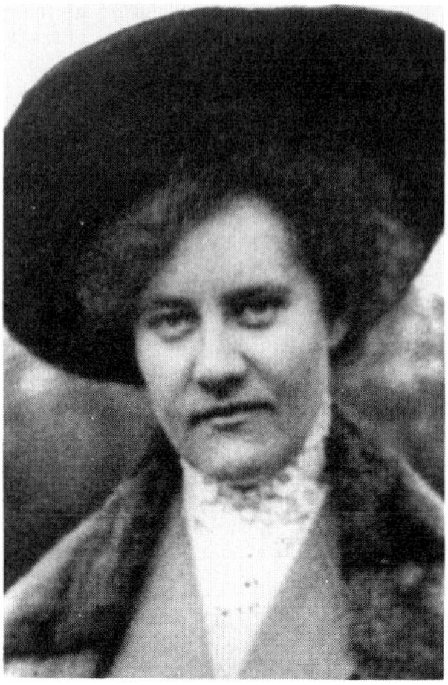

Figure 1. Gertrud Hurler (1889–1965).

domen. Hurler mentioned the presence of corneal haziness, which is an important distinguishing feature from Hunter's disease.

Because of World War I, it is unlikely that Hurler was aware of Hunter's similar cases (Hunter, 1917). Although the patients described independently by Hunter and Hurler shared many similarities, they differed in the severity of the clinical abnormalities, degree of central nervous system involvement, presence or absence of corneal clouding and, most important, in the mode of inheritance. The nosologic status of these disorders remained uncertain until subsequent biochemical studies identified this disorder as due to alpha-l-iduronidase deficiency and resultant accumulation of heparan and dermatan sulfate.

According to John Lewis Henderson, the disorder may have been recognized earlier by John Thompson of Edinburgh, who had encountered the first of three siblings affected by 1900 and the second in 1908 (Henderson, 1940). Realizing that he was dealing with a disease that had not been previously described in the literature, Thompson called it "Johnny McL— disease" after his first case. The cases were followed at the Royal Edinburgh Hospital for Sick Children and later were demonstrated by Thompson at a meeting of the Edinburgh-Glasgow Paediatric Club in 1924.

Gertrude Hurler's contribution to child neurology is representative of many similar types of early case reports and descriptions that are now recognized as being due to complex neurometabolic disorders. She was of a generation in which women were not generally accepted in many fields of medicine or surgery, aside from pediatrics. Like Madame Louis-Bar, Cornelia de Lange, Sarah McNutt, and Myrtelle Canavan, she made a unique contribution to child neurology.

Enrique Chaves-Carballo
NORFOLK, VIRGINIA

REFERENCES

Beighton, P. H., and G. J. Beighton. 1986. *The Man Behind the Syndrome*, 82–83. Berlin: Springer-Verlag.

Henderson, J. L. 1940. Gargoylism. A Review of the Principal Features with a Report of Five Cases. *Arch Dis Child* 15:201–14.

Hunter, C. 1917. A Rare Disease in Two Brothers. *Proc Roy Soc Med* 10:104–15.

Hurler, G. 1919. Über einen Typ multipler Abartungen, vorweigend am Skelettsystem. *Zeit Kinderheilk* 24:220–34.

Knorr, D. 1988. Personal communication.

Pfaundler, M. 1920. Demonstrationen über einen Typus kindlicher Dysostose. *Zeit Kinderheilk* 92:420.

KNUD KRABBE

KNUD HAROLDSEN KRABBE (1885–1961) (figure 1) was one of the great men in Danish neurology. He was not only an outstanding clinician but had a wide interest in the neurosciences, ranging from the embryology of the nervous system to comparative neuroanatomy and neuropathology. He helped establish neurology as a separate branch of medicine in Scandinavia in the first half of the twentieth century and had a particular interest in the neurological disorders of children.

Krabbe grew up in academic surroundings; his father who was the first member of a military family, had become a physician and had been appointed professor of anatomy at the Veterinary and

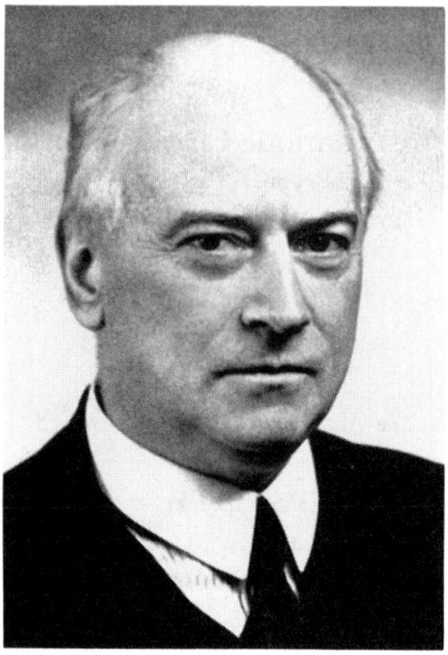

Figure 1. Knud H. Krabbe (1885–1961). From *Acta Psych Neur Scand* 36(1961): 4.

Agricultural Institute in Copenhagen. The elder Krabbe had a particular interest in helminthology and young Knud often visited his father's laboratory, where the boy's enthusiasm for biological science was kindled (Krabbe, 1956). Inspired by his father at the age of ten, he wrote his first paper, which was concerned with the preparation of tapeworms. In high school he was interested in cataloguing flowers as well as other scientific projects. Krabbe had many cultural interests, particularly in art and philosophy. He initially intended to be a zoologist, but at the last moment he changed his mind and entered medical school. Within medicine, he was first interested in psychiatry but subsequently became interested in neurology.

After his graduation from Copenhagen University in 1909, he married a law graduate, Thora Agnete Hindenburg. With a scholarship of three hundred dollars, they went to London, where they lived in a boarding house on Gower Street (near University College) for five months at a cost of twenty-four shillings per week, including board.

Krabbe visited the National Hospital for Nervous Diseases in Queen's Square and was deeply impressed by the physicians and surgeons and the great numbers of patients at that neurological center. He began to dream of establishing a similar hospital in Copenhagen with departments of neurology and neurosurgery. From London he went to Paris, where he met the great neurologists of the day.

While dissecting a human brain in his kitchen corner in his hotel room in Paris, he observed that the pineal gland was prominent and full of cavities and calcareous grains. He discussed this observation with Pierre Marie, who encouraged him to carry out research on this organ. Marie provided him with fifty human pineal glands, which he studied with some assistance from Gustave Roussy. From this work resulted his paper "Sur la glande pinéale chez l'homme" in the *Nouvelle Iconographie de la Salpêtrière* in 1911. After three months in Paris he returned to Copenhagen in June 1910, where he first held an internship at the Copenhagen mental hospital. He later became an assistant at the Municipal Hospital (Kommunehospitalet) from 1911 to 1914. While working on Ward 6, which was later devoted to neurology, he succeeded in procuring a supply of fetuses to study the development of the pineal. Upon completion of this research, he submitted his thesis on histological investigations of the pineal body. He successfully defended this thesis in 1915, wearing his military uniform, because World War I was in progress.

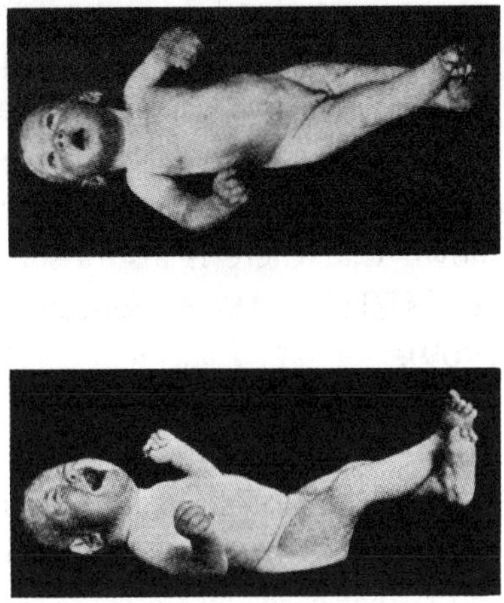

Figure 2. Photographs of Krabbe's Case 1 with diffuse brain sclerosis showing the infant's characteristic posture. Reproduced with permission from *Brain* 39(1916): 76.

Meanwhile, his wife had given birth to their two daughters in 1912 and 1913. In the latter year, Krabbe began some private neurological practice. He also became interested in diffuse brain sclerosis in children. In 1913 he first published the case of a one-year-old infant who had a similarly affected sibling and came to autopsy (Krabbe, 1913). At that time, there were only two known types of cerebral sclerosis in infants: a syphilitic form and Schilder's encephalitis periaxialis diffusa, the latter being a demyelinating disease of unknown cause. To these, Krabbe was able to add a third type, a familial infantile form. By 1916 he had collected five cases in three families and published them in his classic paper in *Brain* (Krabbe, 1916). He reported that the disease usually began somewhat acutely around the fifth month in a child who was previously healthy. It gradually progressed and culminated with death five to six months after onset. Characteristic symptoms were universal rigidity of the musculature (figure 2), violent tonic spasms that were liable to be brought on by touching or noise, and periodic fever without perceptible cause. As a rule, nystagmus was present and optic atrophy later supervened. Finally, extensive paresis and pronounced debility closed the scene. Krabbe also noticed that knee jerks could not be elicited in any of the affected infants and attributed this to rigidity. It was later shown that there is also a segmental demyelination of peripheral nerves (Lake, 1968; Sourander and Olsson, 1968; Dunn et al, 1969).

The main gross pathological anatomical finding was a marked hardness of the white matter of the brain without alteration of its shape. Microscopic examination of three cases showed relative intactness of cortex, basal ganglia, and central gray matter in brain and spinal cord, while there was destruction of myelin sheaths and axis cylinders throughout the white substance of the cerebrum apart from a two-millimeter layer immediately under the cortex. There was also complete destruction of the white matter of the cerebellum and degeneration of the spinal nerve tracts. The destroyed tissue was replaced by dense fibrillary gliosis, in which variously shaped glial cells were seen, including gigantic polynuclear cells. These were the characteristic cells that James Collier and J. Godwin Greenfield later named "globoid" (Collier and Greenfield, 1924). Krabbe commented on the absence of newly formed vessels and of any perivascular infiltration with plasma cells, lymphocytes, or leucocytes. He concluded that the affection should be regarded as purely degenerative, that it presented a certain relationship to Pelizaeus-Merzbacher disease and the Tay-Sachs form of familial amaurotic idiocy, but differed conspicuously from both these conditions.

Krabbe mentioned a few isolated reports of similar cases in the literature, but there is no doubt he deserved to have this disease named after him, inasmuch as he first summarized all the salient facts concerning this leukodystrophy, including its occurrence in siblings and its degenerative nature, which is now known to be due to a metabolic error inherited by an autosomal recessive gene (Suzuki and Suzuki, 1970).

In 1917 Krabbe's interest in the development of the pineal led him to establish contact with Professor Ivar Broman in Lund, Sweden, whose histological laboratory had a vast collection of fetuses. This led to fruitful cooperation during the next forty years.

Krabbe supplemented the material by procuring animal fetuses from the Zoological Garden and obtaining brains from the cattle market. After World War I he went to Amsterdam, where he worked at the Netherlands Central Institute for Brain Research, headed by Ariens Kappers. This cultured man had a wealth of knowledge concerning the comparative anatomy of the brain, and Krabbe found vast series of sections that he needed in his studies of the pineal. On that occasion, he discovered the subcommissural organ, which he described in a series of mammals. To his chagrin, he found that an Austrian woman, Marianne Bauer-Jokl, had previously described the organ. However, he contributed to the knowledge of its comparative anatomy (Krabbe, 1923).

While this research was in progress, Krabbe continued his clinical work. He was a prolific writer, publishing about two hundred articles and several books. In 1922, after having held temporary positions at the University Hospital (Rigshospitalet) and Public Hospital (Almindelig) in Copenhagen, he obtained a position at the Municipal Hospital as a staff member, under neurologist Viggo Christiansen. In 1924 he traveled to the United States, where he admired the organization of neurological and neurosurgical services and was particularly impressed by Harvey Cushing.

In January 1926, after consultation with Dutch, Swedish, and Norwegian colleagues, he founded the *Acta Psychiatrica et Neurologica Scandinavica*. He remained the sole editor until the beginning of the 1950s. Under his leadership, the journal attained an international reputation and published an increasing number of supplements. The subsequent division of the journal into a psychiatric and neurological section met with his full approval.

In 1927 Krabbe published a book in Danish for medical students and general practitioners entitled *Lectures on Nervous Diseases*. This was widely read in Scandinavia, going through seven editions, and was translated into Spanish and English (Krabbe, 1941, 1959a). In 1928 he travelled to Poland and Soviet Russia, where he found the health care system interesting but gained very little new neurological experience.

In the following year, psychiatry and neurology were first granted separate professorships at Copenhagen University. Krabbe did not apply for the professorship in neurology because he did not wish to compete with his senior colleague, Viggo Christiansen. The latter was duly appointed. Krabbe may have afterwards regretted this gentlemanly decision. He later moved to the position of senior neurologist at the Municipal Hospital and in 1933 established a Department of Neurology with 130 beds. During the day he was always busy with his clinical duties at the hospital, and only after 8 p.m. was he able to concentrate on his scientific work, which he continued far into the night.

His wide interest in the neurology of childhood is evident from many publications. He had already written a paper on fetal reflexes in the *Revue neurologique* (Krabbe, 1912). In 1916, apart from describing the disease named after him, he began to participate in the discussion on the distinction between amyotonia congenita, described by Oppenheim, and congenital familial progressive spinal muscular atrophy (the congenital type of Werdnig-Hoffmann disease). This culminated in a publication in *Brain* (Krabbe, 1920). He was also interested in endocrine problems in children, like the congenital or early acquired froms of pluriglandular insufficiency, precocious puberty, and the relation between the adrenal cortex and sexual development. He continued to have a particular interest in the pineal gland. In 1925 he wrote about varicella myelitis, first in a Scandinavian journal, and then in *Brain* (Krabbe, 1925), and later in *Acta Paediatrica* (Krabbe, 1927). He described the facial and meningeal angiomatosis associated with calcification of the cerebral cortex, to which the names of William A. Sturge and F. Parkes Weber have also become attached (Krabbe, 1934).

Krabbe presented a paper to the Danish Neurological Society in 1946 concerning a patient with congenital universal muscular hypoplasia (Krabbe, 1947). This interesting disorder was also observed by Frank Ford, who mentioned it in his textbook *Diseases of the Nervous System in Infancy, Childhood and Adolescence* (Ford, 1960). Both authors described a congenital, nonprogressive hypoplasia of muscle with associated weakness. The affected children were said to have normal stature, normal electrical reactions, and normal histological appearance of muscle, apart from some slightly slender fibers. The mother of Ford's patient displayed the same muscular deficiency but life was not shortened. Similar observations by other authors were quoted, and it is evident that these were the first descriptions of congenital, nonprogressive or slowly progressive myopathies, which have since been differentiated into special types by histochemical and electron microscopic studies.

Erna Christensen and Krabbe also described poliodystrophia cerebri progressiva (infantilis) (Christensen and Krabbe, 1949), which was previously reported by Alpers in 1931 as a diffuse progressive degeneration of the cerebral gray matter (Alpers, 1931). It is evident from this work that Krabbe was in the forefront of clinical neurology.

In 1937 the professorship in neurology at the University of Copenhagen again became vacant. Krabbe applied for the chair, but Mogens Fog, who was twenty years younger and highly qualified in neurophysiology, was appointed. Krabbe was undaunted. In 1939 he began publication of the first volume of his monumental studies on the morphogenesis of the vertebrate brain. The first volume was concerned with the brains of reptiles, while later volumes described the development of the brain in lower mammals, rodents, birds and other vertebrates (Krabbe, 1959b). The eighth volume was published in 1952, and he nearly completed the ninth volume before he died in 1961.

During his lifetime, Krabbe was awarded many honors. He was given two honorary doctorates in Sweden, at the University of Lund and the Karolinska Institute in Stockholm. He was made an honorary member of the American Academy of Neurology and the French, Spanish, and Dutch neurological societies. He was appointed a Chevalier de la Légion d'Honneur in France in 1949.

A special issue of the *Acta Psychiatrica et Neurologica Scandinavica* was dedicated to him in 1955 as a festschrift containing articles by friends, colleagues, and pupils. Professor Henning Pakkenberg, the editor of the *Acta Neurologica Scandinavica*, had worked with him during the previous five years when Krabbe was between sixty-five and seventy years old. He found Krabbe to be an active teacher with a comprehensive view of the clinical situation, who wished to help suffering patients (Pakkenberg, 1982).

Krabbe retired in 1955 as chief neurologist at the Municipal Hospital. In his retirement he continued to do scientific work in a small laboratory at the hospital but was increasingly afflicted by Parkinson disease. It is said that he never complained and worked with unique stoicism to the very last few months, dragging himself to his laboratory at the hospital, which was his second home. He died peacefully in his former ward.

Henry G. Dunn

Eva E. Thomas

VANCOUVER, BRITISH COLUMBIA

CANADA

ACKNOWLEDGMENTS

The authors wish to thank Professor Henning Pakkenberg for his assistance and for permission to publish the photograph of Krabbe; also Pierre Terrisse, Librarian at the University Library in Copenhagen, for his contribution, and Margaret R. Norman for her advice.

REFERENCES

Alpers, B. J. 1931. Diffuse Progressive Degeneration of the Gray Matter of the Cerebrum. *Arch Neur Psych* 25:469–505.

Christensen, E., and K. H. Krabbe. 1949. Poliodystrophia cerebri progressiva (infantilis). *Arch Neur Psych* 61:28–43.

Collier, J., and J. G. Greenfield. 1924. The Encephalitis Periaxialis of Schilder: A Clinical and Pathological Study, with an Account of Two Cases, One of Which was Diagnosed During Life. *Brain* 47:489–519.

Dunn, H. G., et al. 1969. The Neuropathy of Krabbe's Infantile Cerebral Sclerosis (Globoid Cell Leukodystrophy). *Brain* 92:329–44.

1955. *Opuscula Neurologica Knud H. Krabbe. Festschrift for Knud Krabbe. Acta Psych Neur Scand.* Vol. 30.

Ford, F. R. 1960. Congenital Universal Muscular Hypoplasia (Krabbe). In *Diseases of the Nervous System in Infancy, Childhood and Adolescence*, 1258–60. 4th ed. Springfield, IL: Charles C Thomas.

Krabbe, K. 1911. Sur la glande pinéale chez l'homme. *Nouv Icon Salpêtrière* 24:257–72.

______. 1912. Les réflexes chez le foetus. *Rev neur* 20:434–35.

______. 1913. Beitrag zur Kenntnis der Frühstadien der diffusen Hirnsklerose (die perivasculäre Marknekrose). *Zeit Neur Psych* 20:108–15.

______. 1916. A New Familial, Infantile Form of Diffuse Brain-Sclerosis. *Brain* 39:74–114.

______. 1920. Congenital Familial Spinal Muscular Atrophies and Their Relation to Amyotonia Congenita. *Brain* 43:166–91.

______. 1923. The Pineal Gland, Especially in Relation to the Problem on Its Supposed Significance in Sexual Development. *Endocrinology* 7:379–414.

______. 1925. Varicella Myelitis. *Brain* 43:535–39.

______. 1927. Myelitis varicelosa. *Acta Paed* 6:117–19.

______. 1934. Facial and Meningeal Angiomatosis Associated with Calcifications of Brain Cortex. *Arch Neur Psych* 32:737–55.

______. 1941. *Neurology Lectures for Medical Students and General Practitioners.* Copenhagen: Munksgaard.

______. 1947. Kongenit generaliseret muskelaplasi. *Nordisk Med* 35:1756.

______. 1956. *Livserindringer*, 1–244. Copenhagen: Munksgaard.

______. 1959a. *Latinsk mikrogrammatik for laeger og medioinske studerende.* Copenhagen: Munksgaard.

______. 1959b. *Studies on the Morphogenesis of the Brain in Some Amphibia.* Copenhagen: Munksgaard.

Lake, B. D. 1968. Segmental Demyelination of Peripheral Nerves in Krabbe's Disease. *Nature* 217:171–72.

Pakkenberg, H. 1982. Knud Krabbe and the Pineal Gland. *European Pineal Study Group Newsletter* (March) 7:20–23.

Sourander, P., and Y. Olsson. 1968. Peripheral Neuropathy in Globoid Cell Leucodystrophy (Morbus Krabbe). *Acta Neuropath* 11:69–81.

Suzuki, K., and Y. Suzuki. 1970. Globoid Cell Leukodystrophy (Krabbe's Disease): Deficiency of Galactocerebroside-Galactosidase. *Proc Natl Acad Sci* 66:302–9.

GONZALO RODRIGUEZ LAFORA

UNTIL THE WORK OF Ramon y Cajal, Spanish neurology had presented a bleak landscape. Cajal's seminal work triggered a lush growth of brilliant disciples; Nicolás Achucarro, Pio del Rio Hortega, Lorente de Nó, and many others. Among them, the young Gonzalo Rodriguez Lafora (1887–1971) (figure 1) became one of his most favored pupils, an influential figure in Spanish neurology, and an important figure in child neurology (Rodriguez-Arias, 1972).

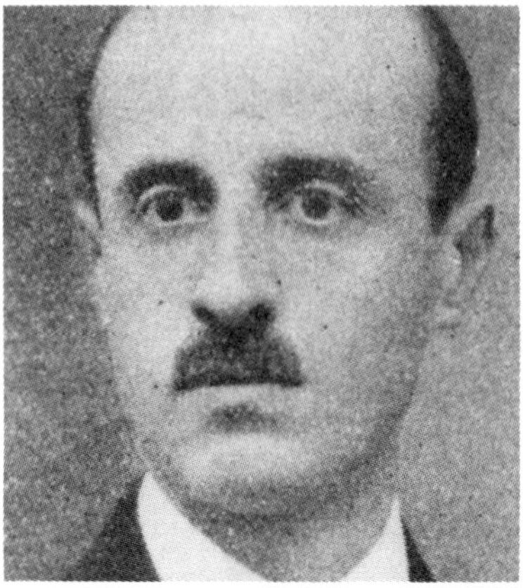

Figure 1. Gonzalo Rodriguez Lafora (1887–1971) at the age of forty-three.

Born and reared in Madrid, Lafora received his medical doctorate at the Complutense University of Madrid in 1908. In 1909 he was awarded a grant by the Council for Research Development, chaired by Cajal, to finish his education in Germany. In Berlin he had the opportunity to work under the direction of Theodore Ziehen, Oskar Vogt, and Korbinian Brodmann. A sojourn in Alois Alzheimer's laboratory in Munich broadened his neuropathological knowledge. His later interest in senile dementia may have its roots in his study during this period. His contributions to the neuropathology of Alzheimer's disease are extensive (Valenciano-Gaya, 1965).

Lafora achieved a solid reputation and as a result was appointed to the Government Hospital for the Insane, later known as St. Elizabeth Hospital, in Washington, D.C., where he went to take the place of Nicolás Achucarro, also a disciple of Cajal and another great figure in the Spanish school of neuropathology. There he directed the Laboratory of Cerebral Histopathology until his return to Madrid in 1913. During his stay in the United States he studied the brain of a seventeen-year-old boy and made the discovery that has since been attached to his name: the Lafora bodies (Lafora, 1911). The description of the large, round, intraganglionic deposits in the brain is Lafora's most important contribution to pediatric neurology (Lafora and Glueck, 1911). The boy suffering from this disease had been noted to have intellectual retardation in school and epileptic seizures since 1908. In 1909 he started having myoclonic jerks in his eye muscles and lips, later spreading to his extremities and trunk. A severe decrease in his visual acuity was also noted. He was admitted to the Government Hospital for the Insane in 1910, where he was found to have generalized hypotonia, constant diffuse myoclonic jerks, increased tendon reflexes, bilateral Babinski signs, and a pronounced Romberg sign. A severe dementia was present, characterized by irritability, poor attention, perseveration, and echolalia. He underwent a decompressive craniotomy, but a few weeks later his seizures worsened, he became emaciated, and died. The histopathologic study of the brain showed the presence of amylaceous bodies in the cerebral cortex and in the subcortical gray matter. They were particularly abundant in the second and third cortical layers, especially in the visual cortex, and were absent from the Betz motor cells. The amylaceous bodies, sometimes multiple, sometimes single, were located in the neuronal cytoplasm and at times displaced the nuclei towards the periphery. After examining multiple stains with different reagents, Lafora was certain about the amylaceous composition of the bodies.

Lafora made additional observations in a series of histochemical articles that were published in Spanish in *Trabajos del Laboratorio de Cajal* in 1913, insisting on the amylaceous nature of the bodies and differentiating them from the similar-looking bodies discovered by Lewy in Parkinson disease.

These carbohydrate deposits have only been found in patients suffering symptoms of the Unverricht-type of myoclonus and are of pathognomonic significance. Lafora disease is characterized by the onset of epileptic seizures between ages of ten and seventeen, soon followed by myoclonic jerks, blindness, and early and rapidly progressive dementia with death occurring after a period averaging six years. The disease is inherited as an autosomal recessive disorder. Harriman and Millar were the first to describe the extracerebral location of similar deposits in the heart and liver (Harriman and Millar, 1955).

Lafora's initial report of corpora amylacea was received with incredulity. Shortly after the publication of the case, Stürmer, one of Alzheimer's disciples, wrote that "Lafora's drawings lack any verisimilitude, even when considering them purely schematic" (Stürmer, 1913). The drawings from the original article actually have great clarity and an almost photographic likeness. Nevertheless, further publications on this topic by Max Bielschowski, Carl Westphal, and especially Walther Spielmeyer (Spielmeyer, 1922) soon afforded assurance to the soundness of Lafora's description of corpora amylacea. However, in Spielmeyer's review the chronological order of publications was inaccurate, casting doubt on Lafora's priority in the discovery. In this case, the inaccuracy was all the more blatant, because the original work was published in German and in the same journal that was later edited by Spielmeyer. In 1923 Lafora reviewed all the published cases of myoclonus with amylaceous bodies and justly claimed the priority of his discovery (Lafora, 1923). In the article he wrote this poignant remark:

It often happens that investigators from countries with scanty academic production have to endure the loss of credit for their discoveries. Authors of books and articles from affluent countries, in their historical reviews, tend to give improper credit for discoveries to their own countrymen, while ignoring the earlier works of scientists from poor countries.

Shortly after Lafora's return to Madrid he was invited by Cajal to join his institution, where he organized the Laboratory of Cerebral Experimental Physiology. A continuous outflow of experimental research originated from his laboratory. Lafora's experiments on cats and monkeys demonstrated the phenomena of contralateral apraxias after lesions of the corpus collosum. The broad scope of his work made him a pioneer in the study of multiple aspects of cerebral localization. He performed extensive experimental work on choreoathetosis, achieving the experimental verification of the Binderarm Chorea of Karl Bonhoeffer with lesions of the superior cerebellar peduncle. Lafora was also among the first to study the role of the hypothalamus and other regions around the third ventricle in the physiology of sleep (Rodriguez-Somoza, 1965).

In 1932 Lafora was made director of the psychiatric department of the Provincial Hospital in Madrid. As a clinician he considered himself a neuropsychiatrist and saw no contradiction in alternating the practice of psychoanalysis of neurosis with malarial treatments of neurosyphilis (Alberca-Lorente, 1965).

Lafora enjoyed much prestige and had a distinguished clientele among the aristocracy and upper classes of Madrid. His advanced liberal ideology often brought him into conflict with some of his more conservative patients. He would chuckle when telling the anecdote of a physician — most certainly himself — making a house call to a duke; the duchess sprinkled his footsteps with holy water while saying, "His science belongs to God but his ideas to the Devil" (Valenciano-Gaya, 1974).

Lafora was a prolific writer. He published approximately two hundred papers over a period of five decades. His many clinical and histopathological contributions about general paresis, senile dementia, and schizophrenia are noteworthy. His stimulating monograph on the subject of the mentally abnormal child attests to his continuing interest in child neurology and psychiatry (Lafora, 1917).

Versatile in many fields of neuropsychiatry, Lafora was also actively interested in philosophical, artistic, and historical issues. In the public forum, he was known as an impassioned champion of progressive ideology. His proud and polemic character and his quixotic devotion to truth brought him into various journalistic disputes. His cross-fire series of articles in which he debated with a vicar over the superstitious belief in miraculous cures became notorious throughout Spain. An influential physician of his time described Lafora as "someone that in the street of scientific polemics always takes his stand on the opposite sidewalk" (Llavero, 1965). His somewhat aloof sense of personal dignity did not prevent good rapport with his colleagues and a large following of disciples, for he was known as a man of uncompromising honesty who chastised ideas and not individuals.

The Spanish Civil War interrupted his work. His political ideas forced him to join the exodus of Spanish intellectuals known as the "Generation of the Diaspora" (Obrador, 1965). Banished from his native country, he lived in Mexico until 1947, when he was allowed to return to Spain to rejoin the Institute Cajal and the Provincial Hospital in Madrid until his retirement in 1957. He remained active in his areas of interest until his death in 1971 at the age of eighty-four.

Emilio Soria-Duran
BUFFALO, NEW YORK

REFERENCES

Alberca-Lorente, R. 1965. Lafora como psiquiatra. *Arch neurobiol* (Madrid) 28:365–76.

Harriman, D. G., and J. H. Millar. 1955. Progressive Familial Myoclonic Epilepsy in Three Families: Its Clinical Features and Pathological Basis. *Brain* 78:325–49.

Lafora, G. R. 1911. Über das Vorkommen amyloider Korperchen im Innern der Gangliezellen; zugleich ein Beitrag zum Studium der amyloiden Substanz im Nervensystem. *Virchows Arch Path Anat* 205:295–303.

______. 1913. Nuevas investigaciones sobre los cuerpos amilaceos del interior de las células nerviosas. *Trabajos del Laboratorio de Cajal.* T.XI, fasc. 1.

______. 1917. *Los niños mentalmente anormales.* Madrid: La Lectura.

______. 1923. Les myoclonies et les corps amylaces dans les cellules nerveuses. *Rev neur* 39:399–413.

Lafora, G. R., and B. Glueck. 1911. Beitrag zur Histopathologie der myoklonischen Epilepsie. *Zeit Neur Psych* 6:1–14.

Llavero, F. 1965. Lafora, maestro en el Hospital Provincial. *Arch neurobiol* (Madrid) 28:331–39.

Obrador, S. 1965. Lafora y la neurocirugia. *Arch Neurobiol* (Madrid) 28:354–57

Rodriguez-Arias, B. 1972. Influencia del Doctor Gonzalo R. Lafora en el auge de la neurologia patria. *Anales de medicina y cirugia* (Barcelona) 52:291–300.

Rodriguez-Somoza, R. 1965. Lafora y el Instituto Cajal. *Arch neurobiol* (Madrid) 28:341–352

Spielmeyer, W. 1922. *Histopathologie des Nervensystems.* Vol 1, 94. Berlin: Springer-Verlag.

Stürmer, R. 1913. Die "Corpora amylacea" des Zentralnervensystem. Histol. u. histopathol. Arbeiten de Nissl et Alzheimer.

Valenciano-Gaya, L. 1965. Lafora, el hombre. *Arch neurobiol* (Madrid) 28:322–29.

______. 1974. Las polemicas periodisticas del Doctor Lafora. *Arch neurobiol* (Madrid) 37:61–78.

GEORGES MARINESCO

GEORGES MARINESCO'S (1864–1938) (figure 1) life and work were closely associated with French and Romanian neurology. He was born in Bucharest, where he studied at the Theological Seminary and Medical School. Marinesco was a pupil of Victor Babes, who sent him to Paris to study under Charcot at the age of twenty-four. While there, he associated with Pierre Marie, Joseph Babinski, Georges Gilles de la Tourette, Alexander Souques, Emil Brissaud, Paul Blocq, and other well-known neurologists. From the famous

Salpêtrière Hospital, the cradle of modern neurology, he went to Frankfurt to study with the neuropathologist Carl Weigert, then to Berlin to work with the neurophysiologist Emil du Bois-Reymond. He returned in 1897 to his native country to receive a doctorate for his thesis "La main succulente de la syringomyelie" and was appointed to the Pantelimon Hospital in Bucharest. Soon after this, a chair of clinical neurology was created for him, which he occupied for the remainder of his life. Marinesco was the founder of the Romanian school of neurology, which supplied many important contributors to this field. Among these were his pupils Anghel Radovici, Ion Minea, State Draganesco, Arthur Kreindler, Oscar Sager, Constantin Parhon, Nicolae Ionescu-Sisesti, and Ion Nicolesco.

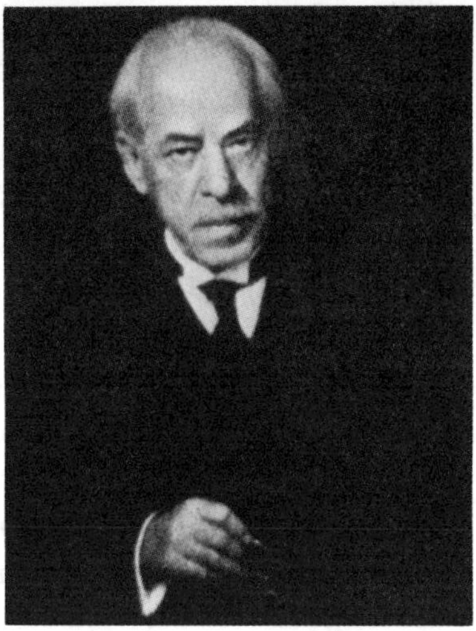

Figure 1. Georges Marinesco (1864–1938). From *La Presse médicale* 46 (1938): 1547.

Marinesco visited France on many occasions. In 1914, with the outbreak of World War I, he went to Paris to enter the service of the French army, which permitted him to devote his clinical skill to the wounded, as well as to promote his outstanding neuropathological studies. For his extensive participation in French neurology, he was greatly honored by the Société de Neurologie and the University of Paris. Shortly before his death, he was notified that he had been chosen to receive the degree of doctor honoris causa from the University of Paris. Marinesco was a member of seven academies (Paris, Bucharest, Madrid, Halle, Maryland, Buenos Aires, and Montevideo) and of twenty-three scientific societies.

Marinesco was a hard worker dedicated to his research and to his patients. His long hours of activity were legendary; he was the first to arrive in the Department of Neurology (usually before 7 a.m.) and the last to return home in the evening. He was married and had three children, two sons and one daughter, but was devastated by the accidental death of one of his sons and overcame his grief only after many years. His life was very modest, quiet, and private; he always wore the same dark suit and very rarely attended parties with his coworkers or his family. He read immensely, kept himself up-to-date with scientific progress in neurology, and immediately applied new research methods to histochemistry and electroencephalography and also to his work with tissue cultures and experimental nerve transplantations. He was active to the last day of his life, dying in his sleep of a massive myocardial infarction. Marinesco was an enthusiastic advocate of multidisciplinary research on the nervous system based on clinical, pathological, experimental, physiological, and biochemical studies. His publications illustrate well this concept and approach.

Marinesco contributed to a much-needed atlas of the gross pathological anatomy of the nervous system. He wrote it in collaboration with Babes between 1892 and 1906 (Babes, Blocq, and Marinesco, 1906). His clinicopathological description with Blocq of the lesions in the substantia nigra produced by a peduncular tumor (1893) was the basis of the theory of the nigral origin of Parkinsonism (Marinesco and Rascano, 1921). He also studied the effects of experimental removal of the pituitary gland in the cat. This physiological investigation clarified the pathogenesis of acromegaly that had previously been described pathologically by Pierre Marie and Marinesco (Marie and Marinesco, 1891).

Marinesco studied the regeneration of peripheral nerves at the level of the amputation neuroma, showing that hyperplasia of the connective tissue compressed the regenerating nervous endings and accounted for the excruciating pains (Marinesco, 1892). In 1909 Marinesco published *La cellule nerveuse*, his first book on normal and pathological neurons. This book, whose foreword was written by Ramon y Cajal, the Nobel laureate in histology, synthesized the development of new laboratory techniques. These included the study of living neurons using the ultramicroscope, incorporating new methods using vital stains, and the reactions of oxidases. Marinesco studied the oxidative activity of neurons histochemically during senescence and various neurological diseases and showed that autolysis of the tissues was related to the presence of excess acid phosphatases. Marinesco postulated that evolution and involution of neurons were dependent on the ratio of oxidative and hydrolytic enzyme activities. Prevalent activity of the first led to increased metabolic synthesis and neuronal regeneration, while dominant activity of the latter accounted for neuronal atrophy and accumulation of yellow pigment. He also suggested that normal neurons inhibited the proliferation of the glial cells, in contrast to involuted or atrophic neurons, which stimulated proliferation of glial cells. Neuronophagia, a term coined by Marinesco that indicated phagocytosis of the neurons, was thought to be implemented by macroglial cells (Marinesco, 1930). In 1958 the famous Canadian scientist Murray Barr emphasized the originality of Marinesco's ideas expressed in *La cellule nerveuse*: "All neurological scientists should not ignore this brilliant book written in Europe fifty years ago" (Voiculescu, 1970, 24).

Marinesco made an important contribution to our understanding of progressive bulbar palsy of childhood, or Fazio-Londe disease (1915), which had been described earlier by P. Londe (Londe, 1893–94). He described a twelve-year-old girl and her eight-year-old brother with this disorder. The major findings included speech impairment, mastication and swallowing difficulties, bilateral facial weakness, an absent gag reflex, and lack of pyramidal tract involvement.

Other infantile and juvenile neurological genetic conditions received Marinesco's particular attention. In Charcot-Marie-Tooth (CMT) neuropathy, he demonstrated spinal cord ventral horn involvement (Marinesco, 1894). He also expressed the opinion that CMT and Dejerine-Sottas neuropathy were variants of the same disease, a hypothesis that has been confirmed in recent years. His pathological studies of the spinal cord also revealed degeneration of the posterior and lateral columns, as well as the dorsal horns in patients with Friedreich ataxia (Marinesco and Tretiakoff, 1920), and he investigated brain neuronal lipid storage in amaurotic idiocy, or Tay-Sachs disease (Marinesco, 1921). In 1927 he wrote a chapter on muscle diseases for the medical textbook *Nouveau traité de médecine*, which included an excellent clinical and pathological description of Duchenne muscular dystrophy. The proliferation of the muscle nuclei was considered an early constant feature possibly leading to the formation of abnormal muscle fibers, some fibrotic and others with lipid degeneration (Marinesco, 1927).

With Radovici, Marinesco described the palmomental reflex in amyotrophic lateral sclerosis (1920). Subsequently, this reflex was found to be a good indicator of bilateral involvement of the upper

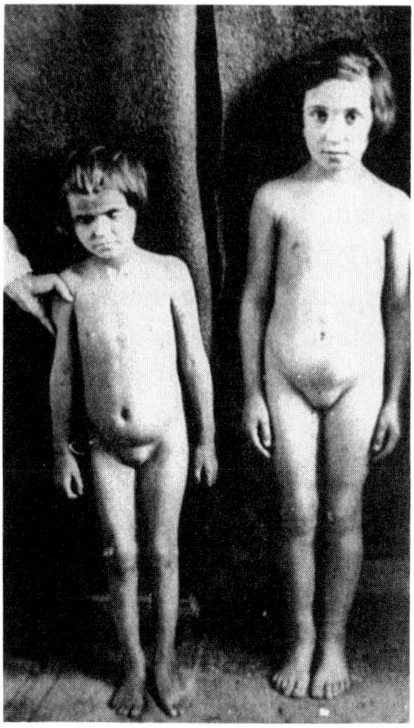

Figure 2. Marinesco-Sjögren Syndrome. This photograph is figure 4 from *Encéphale* 26(1931): 97–109. On the left, a nine-year-old female patient with congenital cataracts, mental retardation, and delayed growth. Next to her, on the right, a normal girl of the same age.

motor neuron at the cortical and subcortical level in many other neurological conditions.

In 1931 Marinesco, in collaboration with State Draganesco and Dumitru Vasiliu, described a new pediatric neurologic disease characterized by mental deficiency, ataxia, and bilateral congenital cataracts (figure 2). Four affected siblings in a Romanian sibship were affected. The condition is known by the eponym Marinesco-Sjögren syndrome (MSS). Sjögren (1950) emphasized that five out of six of his sibships were the product of first-cousin marriages. Pathologically, there was atrophy of the cerebral and cerebellar cortex, but this excluded the nodulus, flocculus, and the paraflocculus as shown by later studies. More recent studies have suggested that the genetic locus for this disorder might be linked with that for hypergonadotrophic hypogonadism or that MSS may be a lysosomal storage disorder (Walker, Blitzer, and Shapira, 1985). Electron microscopy studies in four patients revealed numerous enlarged lysosomes containing whorled lamellar or amorphous inclusion bodies.

Studies on infections of the nervous system, such as bacterial myelitis, syphilis, Von Economo encephalitis (1921), and zoster (1922) occupied an important role in both the early and later research of Marinesco. He demonstrated with Draganesco that the herpes virus inoculated on the rabbit's cornea reached the brain through the peripheral nerves (Marinesco and Draganesco, 1923).

Marinesco did not accept the purely psychological approach to hysteria because he believed that hysteria must be understood psychophysiologically (Marinesco, Sager, and Kreindler, 1930). In 1935, he published a work with Arthur Kreindler on the conditioned reflexes of Pavlov, the reflexes constituting for him a physical avenue by which he penetrated psychoneurotic manifestations and those of mental deterioration (Marinesco and Kreindler, 1935). Marinesco also collaborated with Sager and Kreindler, applying the new method of electroencephalography in experimental studies on sleep in newborn animals and in the investigation of epilepsy and brain tumors (Marinesco, Sager, and Kreindler, 1936).

An important book by Marinesco, Ionesco-Sisesti, Sager, and Kreindler, entitled *Le tonus des muscles striés* and which has a foreword by Sherrington, the outstanding English neurophysiologist, focused on additional experimental and clinical studies of muscular tone and was published in 1937, one year before his death (Marinesco et al, 1937).

The work of Marinesco, enlightened by a warm humanity, was nicely summarized in a speech given at the Romanian Academy in 1906. "If the goal of a scientist is to find the truth then his ideal is to contribute to the well-being of humanity" (Voiculescu, 1970, 90). Marinesco's enthusiasm and dedication to neurological research inspired his numerous pupils.

Victor Ionasescu
IOWA CITY, IOWA

REFERENCES

Babes, V., P. Blocq, and G. Marinesco. 1906. *Atlas der pathologischen Histologie des Nervensystems*. Berlin: Hirschwald.

Londe, P. 1893–94. Paralysie bulbaire progressive infantile et familiale. *Rev méd* 13:1020, 14:212–54.

Marie, P., and G. Marinesco. 1891. Sur l'anatomie pathologique de l'acromégalie. *Verhandlungen X International Congress, Berlin*, 4:129–32.

Marinesco, G. 1892. Über Veranderungen der Nerven und des Ruckenmarks nach Amputationen. *Neur Centralbl Leipzig* 11:569–76.

______. 1894. De l'amyotrophie Charcot-Marie. *Arch méd exp anat path* 6:921–26.

______. 1897. *La main succulente de la syringomyelie.* Thèse Faculté de Médecine, Bucharest.

______. 1909. *La cellule nerveuse.* Paris: Doin.

______. 1915. Sur deux cas de paralysie bulbaire infantile et familiale. *Compt rend Soc Biol* 78:481–83.

______. 1921. Contribution à l'étude de l'histologie pathologique et de la pathogénie dans l'idiotie amaurotique. *Compt rend Soc Biol* 34:1021–24.

______. 1922. Contribution à la pathogénie et à la physiologie du zona zoster. *Bull Acad Méd Paris* 37:487–500.

______. 1927. Les maladies musculaires. In *Nouveau traité de médecine,* 349–95. Ed. G. H. Roger, F. Widal, and P. J. Teissier. Paris: Doin.

______. 1930. Recherches sur la structure normale et pathologique de la microglie. *Ann path* 7:153–59.

Marinesco, G., and S. Draganesco. 1923. Recherches expérimentales sur la nevraxité herpétique du lapin. *Compt rend Soc Biol* 38:894–98.

Marinesco, G., S. Draganesco, and D. Vasiliu. 1931. Nouvelle maladie familiale caracterisée par une cataracte congénitale et un arrêt du développement somato-neuro-psychique. *Encéphale* 26:97–109.

Marinesco, G., et al. 1937. *Le tonus des muscles striés. Etude expérimentale et clinique.* Bucharest: Etat. Imprim. Nat.

Marinesco., G., and A. Kreindler. 1935. *Des Réflexes conditionnels: étude de physiologie normale et pathologique.* Paris: Edition Akan.

Marinesco., G., and A. Radovici. 1920. Sur un réflexe cutané nouveau: Réflexe palmomentonier. *Rev neur* 27:237–40.

Marinesco, G., and V. Rascano. 1921. Contribution à la physiologie pathologique du parkinsonisme. *Compt rend Soc Biol* 34:1017–20.

Marinesco, G., O. Sager, and A. Kreindler. 1930. Hystérie et réflexes conditionnels. *Rev neur* 1:721–31.

______. 1936. Etudes électroencéphalographiques. Les phénomènes de restitution et de compensation dans les lésions de l'encéphale. *Bull Acad Méd Paris* 116:383–85.

Marinesco, G., and C. Tretiakoff. 1920. Etude histopathologique des centres nerveux dans trois cas de maladie de Friedreich. *Rev neur* 27:113–31.

Sjögren, T. 1950. Hereditary Spinocerebellar Ataxia Accompanied by Congenital Cataract and Oligophrenia: A Genetic and Clinical Investigation. *Confin Neur* 10:293–308.

Voiculescu, V. 1970. *Georges Marinesco.* Bucharest: Edition Meridiane.

Walker, P. D., M. G. Blitzer, and E. Shapira. 1985. Marinesco-Sjögren Syndrome: Evidence for Lysosomal Storage Disorder. *Neur* 35:415–19.

LUDWIG MERZBACHER

THE EPONYM Pelizaeus-Merzbacher disease describes a rare inherited childhood neurological disorder that was recognized more than one hundred years ago. Originally described by Friedrich Pelizaeus in 1885, it was the subsequent clinical, and more important, pathological studies of Ludwig Merzbacher (1875–?) in 1910 that contributed to the classification of this clinical disorder as one form of cerebral "diffuse sclerosis."

Ludwig Merzbacher was born on February 9, 1875. Little is known of his early life except that he studied in Munich, Strasbourg, and Berlin, and received his medical degree from Strasbourg in 1900. He served as assistant at the Physiology Institute in Strasbourg from 1900 to 1902, and for the next eight years worked in the psychiatric clinics at Freiburg, Heidelberg, and Tübingen, where he also served as lecturer (Fischer, 1962). In 1910 he was appointed director of the laboratories at the Psychiatric Clinic in Buenos Aires, Argentina, and in 1924 he became director of the German Hospital in Buenos Aires. Surprisingly little else has been written about the rest of his life, and the date and cause of his death are unknown.

Merzbacher published several articles on experimental physiology, including "Winterschlaf, Regeneration und Degeneration der Nerven" ("Hibernation, Regeneration and Degeneration of Nerves") and "Abraumzeilen, reaktives Gliom" ("Cellular Debris and Reactive Gliomas"). Later in his career he wrote several articles in Spanish dealing with therapies for malaria and progressive paralysis (Fischer, 1962).

The term *diffuse sclerosis* was used for a variety of different disorders after Adolph Strümpell first employed the term in 1879. By 1910 patients with idiocy, lead intoxication, and senile or vascular degeneration had been reported as having diffuse sclerosis or "pseudosclerosis," in contrast to "multiple sclerosis" as described by Jean Martin Charcot (1868) and Edward Müller (1904).

The beginning of our understanding of these disorders in children is attributed to Paul Schilder, who in 1912 reported a patient with "encephalitis periaxialis diffusa," felt by later writers to be related to multiple sclerosis. The following year, Schilder reported another child whose disorder was familial and later considered to be the prototype for the genetically determined leukodystrophies. This was followed by the reports of Knud Krabbe (1916), Willibald Scholz (1925), and Armando Ferraro (1927), with additional isolated cases of diffuse sclerosis, and then by József Baló's description of "encephalitis periaxialis concentrica" (1928). That same year Max Bielschowsky and Richard Henneberg proposed the term leukodystrophy, dividing the entities with "diffuse sclerosis" into either an exogenous inflammatory type or an endogenous, familial, progressive type (Schumacher, 1975). The studies of Ludo van Bogaert and Ivan Bertrand (1933), L. Einarson and A. V. Neel (1938), Ronald Norman (1947), Joseph Greenfield (1952), and Charles Lumsden (1955) all contributed to the reclassification of these disorders proposed by Charles M. Poser and Van Bogaert in 1956. In this classification, the "diffuse scleroses" were divided into three groups: 1) Schilder's cerebral sclerosis; 2) leukodystrophies under which category Pelizaeus-Merzbacher's disease was included; and 3) subacute encephalitis. Five years later, Poser again reclassified these disorders into two major subgroups, the myelinoclastic and dysmyelinating disorders, with Pelizaeus-Merzbacher disease in the latter category (Schumacher, 1975). Based on the work of Hugo Moser and others, Schilder's disease, one of the myelinoclastic disorders, has been shown to be associated with a defect of peroxisomal long-chain fatty acid metabolism (Lazarow and Moser, 1986). The defect in Pelizaeus-Merzbacher disease is yet unknown.

In 1885 Pelizaeus described a neurologic disorder affecting fourteen members of a family, twelve of whom were male. The children developed an eye-movement disorder in the first decade of life, very slow progressive cerebellar and corticospinal tract signs, and mild dementia. Pelizaeus's paper was entitled "Über eine eigenthuemliche Form spastischer Laemung mit Cerebralerscheinungen auf hereditaer Grundlage" ("Concerning a Specific Form of Spastic Paralysis with Cerebral Manifestations on a Hereditary Basis") (Pelizaeus, 1885). Pelizaeus emphasized the spastic paralysis of his patients and the fact that this was a hereditary disorder. This is of interest, as Strümpell's classic paper on hereditary spastic paraplegia was not published until the following year. At this time in clinical neurology, the concepts of demyelinating diseases were just evolving because the field of neuropathology was still in its formative stages. In addition to the work of Alois Alzheimer and Franz Nissl, other researchers such as Carl Weigert were beginning to make definitive contributions; for example, the development of a specific myelin sheath stain in 1882, three years before Pelizaeus's paper was published (McHenry, 1969). Likewise, there had been numerous reports of primary lateral sclerosis, including the early works of Abercrombie (1828) and Turck (1857) and the more definitive studies of Charcot (1868). In none of these patients was a familial tendency observed. Thus both Pelizaeus's and Strümpell's papers for the first time clearly defined a group of patients for whom a genetic and potentially a neurometabolic rather than an infectious or inflammatory etiology could explain the clinical symptoms.

In 1908, twenty-three years after the original report of Pelizaeus, Merzbacher had the opportunity to describe other members from the same family that had been originally examined (Merzbacher, 1908). This report was a brief three-page case review that obviously provoked his interest in this disorder. Two years later, Merzbacher published a 138–page article in the *Zeitschrift für Neurologie und Psychiatrie* entitled "Eine eigenartige familiar hereditaire Erkrankungform (Aplasia Axialis Extra-Corticalis Congenita)" ("A Peculiar Familiar and Hereditary Form of Illness [Congenital Extracortical Axial Aplasia]") (Merzbacher, 1910). This paper was an exhaustive work and included a compilation of the literature, the clinical case histories of the patients examined by Merzbacher, a few photographs of the adult patients with this disorder, and several drawings of pathological material. What is interesting to note is that, although Merzbacher designated the lesions as "diffuse sclerosis" because of the demyelination and gliosis, he nevertheless termed the primary white matter lesion "extracortical axial aplasia" because he believed the disorder was due to a failure of myelin development.

Following Merzbacher's extensive clinical and pathological study of the same family that Pelizaeus had described, their names were conjointly used to describe this syndrome of familial chronic infantile diffuse sclerosis. Periodic reports on Pelizaeus-Merzbacher disease continued to appear over the next half-century. Walther Spielmeyer (1923) and later M. Liebers (1928) examined another brain from the same family. In 1933 K. Lowenberg and T. S. Hill described a very rare adult onset form of this disorder in an American family (Lowenberg and Hill, 1933). In 1954 the scope of this disorder was further expanded by Franz Seitelberger's description of the congenital form (Seitelberger, 1970), and Seitelberger later reclassified the different clinical forms. To date, the biochemical etiology of Pelizaeus-Merzbacher disease remains elusive, as does much information about the life of this unusual neurologist, whose intrigue with an isolated case report led to the recognition of a rare childhood hereditary degenerative disease of the nervous system.

Frederick B. Cochran
SAN FRANCISCO, CALIFORNIA

Stephen Ashwal
LOMA LINDA, CALIFORNIA

ACKNOWLEDGMENTS

The help of the following individuals is greatly appreciated: Mr. Lenger, Director of Information Services, Karl-Marx University, Leipzig; Gudrun Greck, Information Service, Niedersaechische Landesbibliothek, Hanover; Mr. Schwinger, North Rhine-Westfallen State Archives, Detmold.

REFERENCES

Charcot, J. M. 1868. Histologie de la sclérose en plaques. *Gaz hôp* (Paris) 41:554, 557, 566.

Fischer, I. 1962. *Biographisches Lexikon der hervorragenden Aerzte der letzten fuenfzig Jahre*, 1027–28. Zweiter Band. Muenchen: Verlag von Urban & Schwarzenberg.

Lazarow, P. B., and H. W. Moser. 1989. Disorders of Peroxisomal Biogenesis. In *The Metabolic Basis of Inherited Disease*. Ed. C. Scriver et al. New York: McGraw-Hill Information Services.

Liebers, M. 1928. Zuer Histopathologie des zweiten Falles von Pelizaeus-Merzbacherscher Krankheit. *Zeit Neur Psych* 115: 487–509.

Lowenberg, K., and T. S. Hill. 1933. Diffuse Sclerosis with Preserved Myelin Islands. *Arch Neur Psych* (Chicago) 29:1232.

McHenry, L. 1969. *Garrison's History of Neurology*. Springfield, IL: Charles C Thomas.

Merzbacher, L. 1908. Weitere Mitteilungen über eine eigenartige hereditaer-familiaere Erkrankung des Zentralnervensystem. *Med Klin* 4:1952–55.

______. 1910. Eine eigenartige familaere Erknankungsform (Aplasia extracorticalis congenita). *Zeit Neur Psych* 3:1–138.

Mueller, E. 1904. *Die multiple Sklerose des Gehirns und Rueckenmarks*. Stuttgart: Gustav Fischer Verlag

Pelizaeus, F. 1885. Über eine eigenthuemliche Form spastischer Laemung mit Cerebralerscheinungen auf hereditärer Grundlage (Multiple Sklerose). *Arch Psych Nervenkrankh* 16: 698–710.

Schilder, P. 1912. Zur Kenntnis der sogenannten diffusen Sklerose: Über Encephalitis periaxialis diffusa. *Zeit Neur Psych* 15:359.

Schumacher, G. A. 1975. The Demyelinating Diseases. In *Clinical Neurology*. Vol. 2, 1–92. Ed. A. B. Baker and L. H. Baker. New York: Harper and Row.

Seitelberger, F. 1970. Pelizaeus-Merzbacher Disease. In *Handbook of Clinical Neurology*. Vol. 10. Ed. P. J. Vinken and G. W. Bruyn. Amsterdam: Elsevier.

Spielmeyer, W. 1923. Der anatomische Befund bei einem zweiten Fall von Pelizaeus-Merzbacherscher Krankheit. *Zeit Neur Psych* 32: 202–3.

SAMUEL ORTON

THE UNDERSTANDING of developmental language disorders and their relation to learning problems was rudimentary during the first two decades of this century. Congenital word blindness had been described in the last decade of the nineteenth century in England, and the syndrome was slowly gaining acceptance in America as a clinical entity (Waites, 1980). The oral language disorders in children were described as congenital word deafness, idioglossia, or simply speech impediments. The concepts of developmental motor coordination and attention deficit disorders did not gain recognition and acceptance until the middle of this century. It is interesting that Samuel Orton included developmental alexia, developmental agraphia, developmental word deafness, developmental motor

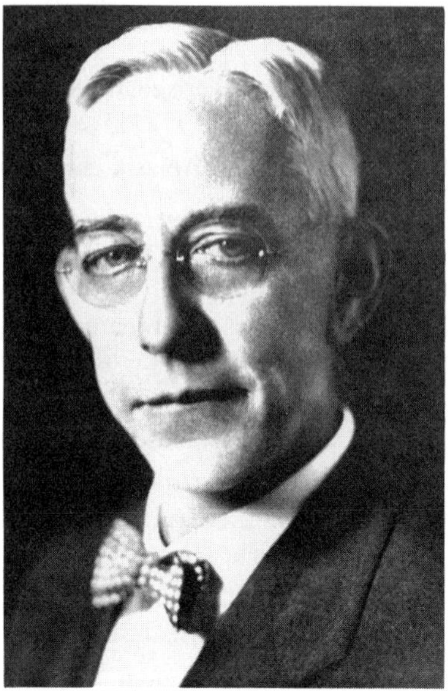

Figure 1. Samuel Torrey Orton (1879–1948).

aphasia, and developmental apraxia in his monograph, *Reading, Writing and Speech Problems in Children*, in 1937.

Samuel Torrey Orton (1879–1948) (figure 1) was born in Columbus, Ohio. He was the son of Edward Orton, a noted geologist and president of Ohio State University, and Anna Torrey, the aunt of President William Howard Taft. Orton attended elementary school in Columbus and completed high school at Taft School in Watertown, Connecticut. He received his B.S. degree from Ohio State University in 1901 and his medical degree from the University of Pennsylvania in 1905 (Orton, 1966).

Orton's interest in neuropathology led him to the laboratory of Frank B. Mallory at Boston City Hospital for further training. There he was influenced by Ernest Southard, who made it possible for Orton to complete further neuropathology training at the Danvers State Hospital, Massachusetts. He served as pathologist at the Worcester State Hospital from 1908 to 1912. In 1913 he trained in the laboratories of Alois Alzheimer in Breslau, Germany. Upon returning to the United States, Orton was appointed clinical director and pathologist of the Pennsylvania Hospital for Mental Diseases in Philadelphia, serving in this capacity from 1914 to 1919. In 1918 one of his first papers was on the technique and importance of cytoarchitectural studies of the brain (Orton, 1918). This was followed several years later by several excellent detailed neuropathologic studies of the hereditary disorders affecting both the peripheral and central nervous systems (Orton, 1925a).

From 1919 to 1927 Orton established and chaired the department of psychiatry at the State University of Iowa Medical School and was director of the State Psychopathic Hospital in Iowa City, Iowa, where he was also professor of neuropathology (Orton, 1966).

In the early 1920s, Orton was preoccupied with the problems

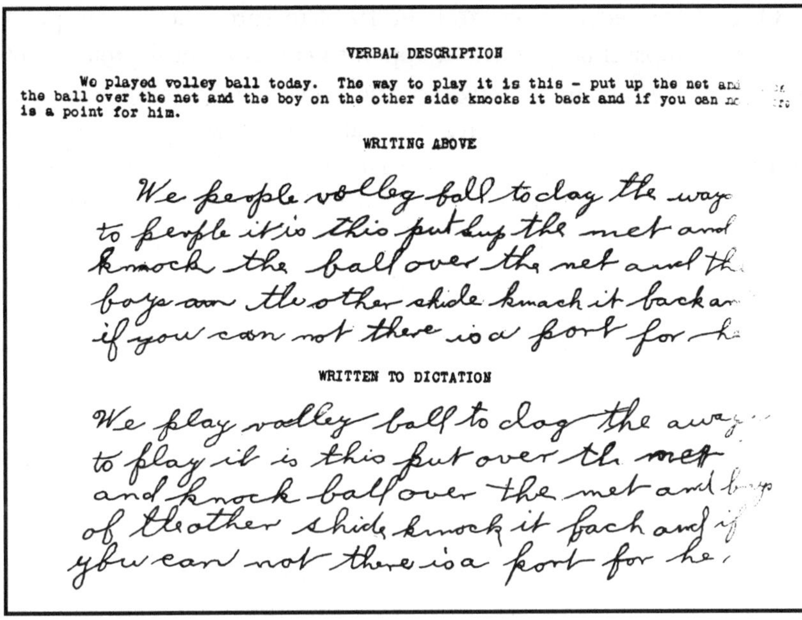

VERBAL DESCRIPTION

We played volley ball today. The way to play it is this - put up the net and
the ball over the net and the boy on the other side knocks it back and if you can n
is a point for him.

WRITING ABOVE

We people volley ball today the way
to perple it is this put bup the met and
knock the ball over the net and th
boys an the other shide knach it back an
if you can not there is a port for h

WRITTEN TO DICTATION

We play valley ball to dog the away
to play it is this put over th met
and knock ball over the met and boys
of the other shide knock it fach and if
you can not there is a port for he.

Figure 2. An example from Orton's "'Word Blindness' in School Children" originally figure 4. The sample is that of M. P., who was studied at age sixteen, and included his verbal description of his hospital day, a reproduction of his writing of the same material, and his production on writing to dictation. From *Arch Neur Psych* 14(1925): 588. Copyright 1925, American Medical Association.

some children had in learning to read. He was excited about the implications of the study of brain development and function: the possible relationship to dominance in the cerebral cortex, the frequency of reversals in reading and writing, the familial trends and evident importance of heredity, and the apparent specificity for all language functions — reading, writing, spelling, and speaking. Orton recognized that a patient, M. P., was suffering from the same condition that had been described in a monograph entitled *Congenital Word-Blindness* by the English ophthalmologist James Hinshelwood (1917). This experience resulted in an article entitled "'Word Blindness' in School Children" (Orton, 1925b). Orton provided some of the first examples of differences in auditory and visual processing of information in children (figure 2). He pointed out that letter reversals were not uncommon in school children and suggested the term strephosymbolia (twisted symbols) to describe the problem of reversals in dyslexia (Orton, 1928). However, this term never became popular.

Orton returned to New York in 1928 to enter the private practice of neuropsychiatry with an appointment as clinical professor of neurology and neuropathology at the New York Neurological Institute of Columbia University. At that time he was president-elect of the American Psychiatric Association. In 1932 he was elected president of the American Association for Research in Nervous and Mental Disease (Orton, 1966). However, despite his broad professional activities, his interest in dyslexia and his work in that area continued for the rest of his life.

Orton demonstrated a remarkable ability to select the major clinical features of dyslexia and also to determine the biological framework in which it should be studied. In the original descriptions of his first cases, he drew several major conclusions that have been proven correct over time: (1) vision was normal; (2) many of these children were ambidextrous; (3) there was a male preponderance in dyslexia; (4) there was a genetic predisposition within families and the high rate of similar disorders in the families of these patients; (5) there was frequently a delay in the acquisition and use of spoken language in dyslexic children; and (6) clumsiness was a complicating factor (Orton, 1937).

Chosen to give the annual Thomas E. Salmon Memorial Lectures in 1936, Orton presented a review of ten years of his research in the field of language disabilities (Orton, 1966). These lectures were published in his classic book *Reading, Writing, and Speech Problems in Children* (Orton, 1937).

In 1945 he reviewed his theories as follows:

The theory was offered that the special reading disability which serves as a serious handicap to academic advancement in many children may be explained as a failure in complete elision of memory records of the non-dominant hemisphere and as a persistence therefore of two more or less equipotenital records. . . . In other words, a physiological failure to establish the normal pattern of unilateral cerebral dominance in control of graphic language, reading, spelling and writing. To delimit this group of children with failures and delays in learning to read from those where other factors were operative, the term "strephosymbolia" was suggested. (Orton, 1966, 273)

Orton recognized that dyslexia may be neurologically based but that the treatment must be educational. His recommended training procedures showed remarkable insight (Cox, 1982;

Geschwind, 1982). They reflected and emphasized the fundamental problems of establishing associations between the visual symbol and its verbal counterpart and of establishing the appropriate sequencing of the auditory and written symbols, that is, the conversion of the spatially presented array into a temporal sequence. He worked closely with psychologist Anna Gillingham and teacher Bessie Stillman to develop a multisensory approach to teaching reading to dyslexic children. Clinical experiments in treatment were incorporated as an integral part of Orton's program of research in developmental delays and disorders in the acquisition of language. Extension of these investigations and wider experimental programs were carried forward at the Language Research Project of the New York Neurological Institute between 1932 and 1936 (J. L. Orton et al, 1975, 152).

It is likely that Orton, together with Gillingham, will be best remembered for his system of remedial training for dyslexic children. Of particular note, however, is Orton's statement:

No general formula can be given which will be applicable to all cases of any of the syndromes discussed (developmental alexia, special disability in writing, developmental word deafness, developmental motor speech delay, stuttering, and developmental apraxia). Each case of developmental delay forms an individual problem in which factors derived from the neurological status, the emotional reactions, the educational needs and the facilities for carrying on retraining must be evaluated and a program devised to conform to all of these. This point can scarcely be emphasized enough since we are all prone to search for a simplified and universally applicable formula, but no such general "method" can be defined for any of these syndromes and any attempt to apply such a blank prescription without thorough diagnosis of the individual case would assuredly lead to error and misguided effort. (Orton, 1937, 143–44)

Later he wrote:

Each child presents an individual problem, not only because of the diverse influence of a considerable number of environmental conditions but also because the relative part played by each of the major functions entering into the language faculty . . . varies markedly in different children as does the child's emotional reaction to his difficulty. (Orton, 1937, 157)

In his book he also stated:

It is suggested that these disorders in language development may derive from a comparable variation affecting the essential language areas of the brain and thus rest on a basis largely physiological in nature and not dependent upon defect or destruction of any part of the cortex. (Orton, 1937, 143)

The Orton Dyslexia Society, founded in his honor in 1949, is an international scientific and educational association concerned specifically with the widespread problem of developmental dyslexia. Its membership is open to all persons interested in the diagnosis and treatment of children and adults who have experienced difficulty in learning the skills of language in one or another of its forms.

The Samuel Torrey Orton Library, containing original manuscripts, case histories, research notes and treatment records of three thousand cases, is housed at the College of Physicians and Surgeons, Columbia University, a fitting tribute to the man and his work.

Lucius Waites
DALLAS, TEXAS

Sylvia O. Richardson
TAMPA, FLORIDA

REFERENCES

Cox, A. 1982. Programming for Teachers of Dyslexia. *Ann Dyslexia* 33:223–24.

Geschwind, N. 1982. Why Orton Was Right. *Ann Dyslexia* 33:13–33.

Hinshelwood, J. 1919. *Congenital Word-Blindness*. London: H. K. Lewis.

Orton, J. L., et al. 1975. Samuel T. Orton, M.D. Who Was He? *Bull Orton Dyslexia Soc* 25:145–63.

Orton, S. T. 1918. Some Observations on the Influence of Angle of Section on Measurements of Cortex Depth and on the Cytoarchitectonic Picture. *J Nerv Ment Dis* 47:241–48.

______. 1925a. The Pathology of the Hereditary and Familial Nervous and Mental Diseases. *Arch Neur* 13:96–115.

______. 1925b. "Word Blindness" in School Children. *Arch Neur Psych* 14:581–86

______. 1928. Specific Reading Disability — Strephosymbolia. *JAMA* 90:1095–99.

______. 1937. *Reading, Writing and Speech Problems in Children.* New York: W. A. Norton.

______. 1966. Some Studies in Reading Disability. Unpublished Address at Medical Convocation, University of Pennsylvania, 18 June 1945. In *"Word-Blindness" in School Children and Other Papers on Strephosymbolia (Specific Learning Disability-Dyslexia) 1925–1946*, 269–74. Ed. J. L. Orton. Pomfret, CT: The Orton Society.

______. 1989. *Orton's Reading, Writing, and Speech Problems in Children and Selected Papers*. Reprint of 1937 edition. Austin: Pro-Ed.

Waites, L. 1980. American Pioneers in the Topic of Word Blindness. In *Historical Aspects of the Neurosciences. Festschrift for Macdonald Critchley*. Ed. F. Clifford Rose and W. F. Bynum. New York: Raven Press.

LUDWIG PICK

LUDWIG PICK (1868–1944) (figure 1) was born on the last day of August, 1868, in Landsberg, Germany, where he spent his childhood. His father, Hermann Pick, managed a distillery in Landsberg. Ludwig was the oldest of seven children and was inspired by his maternal grandfather, Arthur Schönflies, a well-known mathematician. As a student, he developed a great interest in the natural sciences and was known for his memory and mathematical skills. He also became an excellent cellist and belonged to the school's drum and bugle corps. Physically he was of short stature, and the name of Little Ludwig, given to him by his school friends, stayed with him throughout life.

After finishing secondary school, Pick studied medicine at Heidelberg, Leipzig, Berlin, and Königsberg. He received his doctor of medicine degree in 1893 for his thesis on the etiology and pathology of thrombosis and began his career as a pathology assistant in a private women's clinic, the Leopold Landau Clinic in Berlin. The good education in pathology he received at Königsberg, combined with the in-depth knowledge of pathologic anatomy and histo-

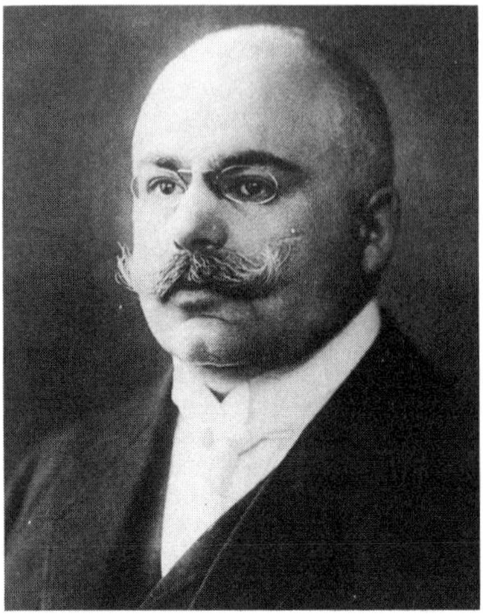

Figure 1. Ludwig Pick (1868–1944).

logical techniques gained through his associations with Ernst Neumann, Max Askanazy, and Coelestin Nauwerck, prepared him well for the directorship of the Microscopic and Pathologic Laboratory at the Landau Clinic.

In 1899 Pick entered Berlin University for postdoctoral work in pathologic anatomy. He became director of the Division of Anatomical Pathology of Friedrichshain Hospital in the city of Berlin in 1906 and in 1909 became full professor.

Pick's work led to significant contributions in the field of gynecology (Pick, 1907, 1908), and as a result he was widely recognized as a pioneer in gynecological pathology, accepting, for example, a guest lectureship in New York during the years 1913 and 1914. During World War I he served as a pathologist with the Third Army and in 1921 was made honorary professor on the Berlin Medical Faculty.

In 1914 Albert Niemann, a Berlin pediatrician, observed a female infant who died at age eighteen months after progressive deterioration associated with hepatosplenomegaly. At autopsy the spleen, liver, and other organs had a striking yellow-white color. This proved to be due to the presence of large cells that Niemann thought were consistent with Gaucher disease. In the years that followed, several similar cases identified as Gaucher disease were reported. During the years 1922 to 1927, Pick scrutinized these cases and, based on anatomical study, regrouped many of them into a new category called lipid cell splenomegaly (1927). Subsequently, Pick referred to this new syndrome as essential xanthomatosis (1933). As further reports appeared in the literature, these cases became more popularly known as Niemann-Pick disease. Pick, in collaboration with Max Bielschowsky, demonstrated central nervous system histological differences between Tay-Sachs and Niemann-Pick disease (Pick and Bielschowsky, 1927). He also concluded that the histological changes seen in both diseases were the outcome of metabolic disturbances. As a result of his accomplishments, Pick was invited as Dunham Lecturer at Harvard University and delivered a series of lectures there between 1931 and 1932.

Pick retired from the Pathological-Anatomical Institute, Municipal Hospital, Friedrichshain, in 1933 because of mandatory retirement regulations but remained as advisor to the Central Research Institute of the Berlin Health Office. After the Nazis came to power in Germany, he was forced out of his house, which he had built a short time earlier. He underwent several operations on both his eyes and consequently was bedridden for periods of time. The social contacts he had established over the years were broken in the precarious socio-political climate prevailing for Jews in prewar Germany. In March 1942 he was imprisoned in a Jewish hospital until he was sent to a concentration camp in June 1943. Eight and a half months later, on February 3, 1944, he died of pneumonia at the age of seventy-five. In the words of Franz Buechner who succeeded Pick at Friedrichshain, "The final destiny of this worthy man leaves a heavy impression upon our soul" (Gruber, 1968).

During his career, a period of forty years, Pick published over one hundred scientific papers. He was known as a master of morphopathology and histological analysis. He recognized the importance of speed in histological diagnosis, particularly the speed required in diagnosis for the patient waiting on the operating table. As a result, he developed several tissue-processing solutions. He also developed methods for preserving pathological specimens in jars for educational displays. His collection at the Friedrichshain Institute became world renowned, but unfortunately it was destroyed during the bombing raids on Berlin in 1945.

Pick's other major contributions included his work on the bacteriological properties of meningococci in cases of "acute stiff neck" (Pick, 1917). In addition, he studied congenital syphilis, especially with regard to the structure and growth of bone; with the help of roentgenograms he was able to correlate the pathological and radiological defects (Pick, 1928). In collaboration with Bielschowsky, he hypothesized that acute methanol intoxication caused ocular and central nervous system damage.

Pick was a hard worker. He personally conducted five to ten autopsies every day, including Sundays. During these autopsies, a small group of interested pathologists and clinicians surrounded the copper table. Folke Henschen, a student of Pick's from Sweden, recorded in his diary memories of the enthusiasm and vigor of Pick during these sessions. Pick was a kind person, willing to help and enlighten others with his knowledge. However, he knew that medical science is incomplete and perhaps must remain so in order to stimulate the pursuit of knowledge. During the second of his Dunham Lectures delivered at Harvard University (Pick, 1933), he recalled the words of the famous scientist, Karl Earnst von Baer:

> *Science is essential in its sources*
> *Boundless in extent,*
> *Infinite in structure,*
> *Unattainable in purpose.* (Pick, 1933)

Bala V. Manyam

Rhona S. Kelley

SPRINGFIELD, ILLINOIS

REFERENCES

Gruber, G. G.1968. Ludwig Pick. *Verh Dtsch Ges Path* 52:574–80.

Niemann, A. 1914. Ein unbekanntes Krankheitsbild. *Jahrb Kinderheilk* 79:1.

Pick, L. 1893. Beitrag zur Actiologic, Genese und Bedentung der hyalinen Thrombose. Med. Diss. Leipzig.

______. 1907. Über Meningokokken-Spermatocystitis. *Berlin klin Wschr* 30:31.

______. 1908. Die Komplementbindung als Ililfsmittel der anatomischen Syphilis-Diagnose. *Med Klin* 15:539.

______. 1917. Demonstration Mikroskop. Schnitte von petechialen Hautaffekten bei Meningokokken-Meningitis. Ebendort, S. 51.—Zur Patholog. Anatomie des infektiosen Ikterus. *Berlin klin Wschr* 19:4

______. 1927. Über die lipoidzellige Splenohepatomegalie Typus Niemann-Pick als Stoffwechselerkrankung. *Med Klin* 23:1483.

______. 1928. Über Ostteochondritis syphilitica im Kindsalter (Osteochondritis syphilitica tarda.) *Verh dtsch Path Ges* 23:248 .

______. 1933. II. Niemann-Pick's Disease and Other Forms of So-called Xanthomatoses. *Am J Med Sci* 185:601.

Pick, L., and M. Bielschowsky. 1927. Über lipoidzellige Splenomegalie (Typus Niemann-Pick) und amaurotische Idiote. *Klin Wschr* 6:1631.

BENJAMIN KNOX RACHFORD

"A CHILD IS NOT a little man." The shibboleth of Benjamin Knox Rachford (1857–1929) (figure 1) is quoted by modern pediatricians, although they are for the most part unfamiliar with the life and accomplishments of this pioneer child neurologist. Rachford was born in Alexandria, Kentucky, a small farming community across the Ohio River from Cincinnati, on November 28, 1857 (Lyon, 1929). His father and grandfather were physicians. Rachford received his primary education in Cincinnati and graduated in 1882 from the Medical College of Ohio in Cincinnati, garnering the Faculty Prize as well as the Joseph Ransohoff Prize for excellence in descriptive anatomy (Dreyfoos, 1929). After completing internship at the Commercial Hospital of Cincinnati in 1883, Rachford assumed his father's practice, who retired because of Parkinson's disease (Lyon, 1972).

Rachford's first paper described isolation of the source of a typhoid fever epidemic in a reservoir supplying Cincinnati (Rachford, 1888). He also led a commission that improved the safety of the city's water supply by moving the intake line far upstream from the sewer outflow.

In 1890 Rachford developed a new technique in the laboratory of Professor Johannes Gad of Berlin, which provided pure pancreatic secretions (Dreyfoos, 1929). He anastamosed a duodenal loop with an attached pancreatic duct to the "outer abdominal wall . . . so that it drained continuously to the outside" and found that fat digestion was optimum when equal mixtures of bile and 0.25 percent HCL were added to pancreatic juice (Rachford, 1891; Rachford and Southgate, 1895).

After establishing unassailable credentials in gastric physiology, Rachford limited his research to clinical medicine. He determined that 50 percent of his patients with chorea had anemia associated with tuberculosis. The remainder had rheumatic heart disease, rheumatism, scarlet fever, and hereditary etiologies (Rachford, 1893).

Rachford's observations on the etiology of migraine were unique and remain partially unconfirmed. He extracted proxanthine, a precursor to uric acid, exclusively from the urine of patients

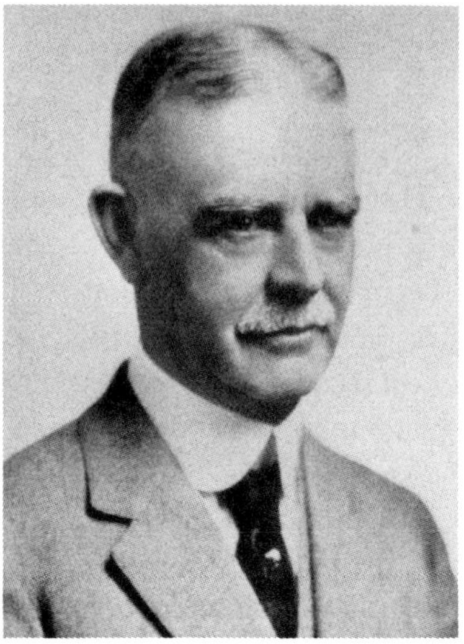

Figure 1. Benjamin Knox Rachford (1857–1929).

during attacks of migraine headaches. He claimed that autointoxication with proxanthine precipitated attacks (Rachford, 1905, 203), yet his carbonated "Siphon C" prescription, which contained lithium and sodium salicylate, was effective prophylactic therapy. Rachford's advice to avoid alcohol, cheeses, and coffee (Rachford, 1903) is still being given by doctors.

Rachford's view of neurosis was fully elaborated upon in his work, *Neurotic Disorders of Childhood*:

> *Neurotic . . . disease . . . is greatly increased by subjecting the immature nervous systems of young children to the almost constant strain and mental activity with which our social order has surrounded them. Teachers . . . of the young must be told that the nervous system of the child is not . . . of a little man; that it is structurally and functionally immature.* (Rachford, 1905, 112)

The child should "have plenty of exercise, fresh air and proper food" to avoid "early precocity" and adult neurosis (Rachford, 1905, 119).

Rachford's *Neurotic Disorders of Childhood* is a curious blend of personal observations, annotated quotations of other authors, and some opinions refuted by his contemporaries. The chapter on epilepsy contains a complex classification of developmental, organic, and toxic seizures; in contrast, one of his neurological contemporaries, William Spratling, had separated seizures into partial or generalized forms (Spratling, 1902). Rachford's classification of developmental epilepsy included generalized, hereditary, and reflex etiologies. Rachford believed that

> *the various ganglia of the brain or the motor cells of the cortex may . . . be changed by strong reflex irritation and discharge their nerve force under slight provocation. . . . One can understand how long standing reflex irritation from*

eye strain . . . may be a very strong exciting cause in the development of epilepsy. (Rachford, 1905, 238)

Continuous observations of epileptics before and after optical refraction amply demonstrated the worthlessness of eye glasses as an effective treatment for epilepsy (Peterson, 1902).

Rachford's *Diseases of Children* (1912) was a distinct improvement over his previous book due to the inclusion of clear photographs of patients and X rays. Vague and excessively lengthy sections were refined into pithy, practical statements. Both books presented the pathophysiology of disease in deference to the prevalent emphasis on anatomical pathology. Rachford devoted extensive sections to behavioral aspects of neurology in both books.

"Sleep is the physiological rest which the tired organism demands to repair the fatigue incident to the activity of cells, especially those of the nervous and muscular systems" (Rachford, 1912, 669). Rachford's description of night terrors aptly demonstrates the clarity of his observations:

A neurotic child, with his nervous system unusually excited by the incidents of the day, falls asleep and after an hour or two suddenly starts in his sleep with a cry of terror that alarms the household. . . . He is found apparently awake sitting up in bed . . . in a state of wild excitement, staring and pointing at some horrible, imaginary object . . . and after a few minutes of this agonizing fear, the attack spends its force . . . and the little patient falls back on the pillow and becomes quiet. (Rachford, 1912, 673)

His suggestions for treating insomnia are practical and and still effective:

The child should sleep in a well ventilated and not overheated room and the bed clothes be properly adjusted to the season of the year. . . . Mental excitement of all kinds, especially just before going to bed, should be avoided. . . . The use of medicine to promote sleep in children is rarely necessary. (Rachford, 1912, 677)

Rachford could also write with authority on topics removed from behavioral neurology. On Friedreich's ataxia, he observed that

the child initially walks with his legs apart in an awkward, unsteady manner . . . [and] *the leg is lifted carefully and brought down suddenly.*

Awkward, jerky sudden movements of the arm may be brought by asking the patient to pick up some object. (Rachford, 1912)

Rachford's strongest and most enduring contribution was his development of a university pediatrics department. His first effort to establish a separate children's ward was strenuously opposed by the administration of the Cincinnati General Hospital. They grudgingly recanted in January, 1898, after Rachford refused to sign death certificates of children not admitted to his ward. (Dreyfoos, 1929). In 1906, with the financial support of Mrs. Mary Emery and Mr. Charles Livingood, Rachford founded the Babies Milk Fund. Clinics distributed pure pasteurized milk at cost or for free to poor mothers. Nurses and pediatric house staff held well-baby clinics and instructed mothers upon proper infant care and nutrition. Rachford later integrated these clinics into the city's social services department (Lyon, 1972). In 1922 William Cooper Procter, president of the Procter and Gamble Company, invited Rachford to submit suggestions and plans for the construction of the Cincinnati Children's Hospital, which would include extensive research facilities, clinics, and the finest ward equipment (Dreyfoos, 1929). Thus Rachford was able to eventually establish a model for most academic departments of pediatrics. Rachford founded the Condon School to provide education to chronically ill children who had been formerly treated inadequately at home. Figure 2 shows a classroom that exemplifies Rachford's recommendations for providing sufficient opportunities for exercise and cooperation. Self-sufficiency was inculcated by having boys attend cooking classes and girls participate in shop courses (Fine, personal communication, 1989).

Rachford did not limit his professional activities to the sphere of Cincinnati. He was chairman of the Council of the American Pediatric Society from 1894 to 1901 and was elected its President in 1907 (Dreyfoos, 1929). During World I, Rachford exhausted his physical reserve. Too old to serve in the military, he urged his younger professors to enlist. He assumed their responsibilities and also most of the duties of dean of the medical school. His worsening health began to limit his activities and he relinquished chairmanship of the pediatrics department in 1927. He curtailed his practice in 1928 and died on May 5, 1929 (Dreyfoos, 1929). His

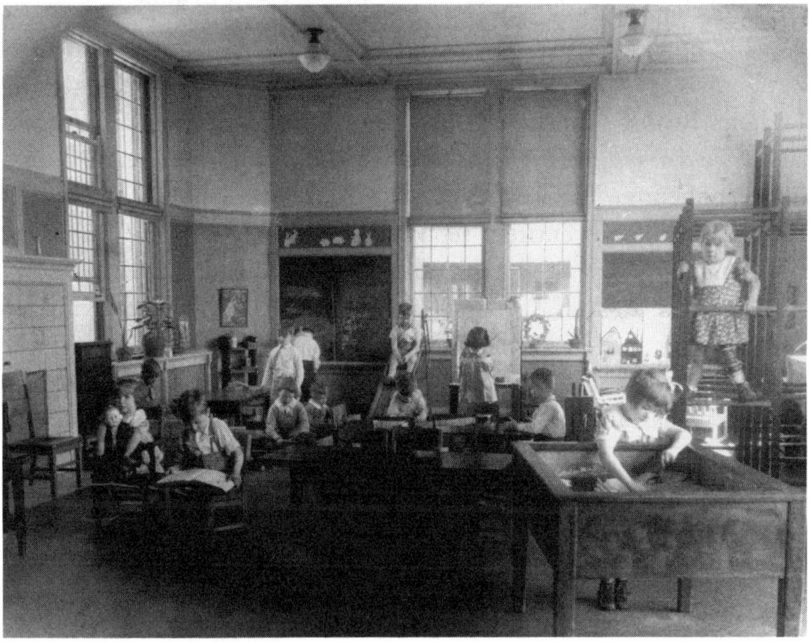

Figure 2. An elementary grade classroom at Condon School. Slides, a sand box, and other toys encouraged exercise and interpersonal relations.

partner, Dr. Max Dreyfoos, listed chronic nephritis as the cause of death (Ohio State Historical Society, 1929).

Rachford's inclusion in this volume is not based on a particular scientific or clinical contribution. He is, however, representative of a trend in pediatrics at the turn of the century in which there was an interest in the so-called "functional" rather than "organic" diseases of the nervous system. This was due to the influence of similar disorders being studied in adults by such luminaries as Jean Martin Charcot, William Gowers, Sigmund Freud, and Silas Weir Mitchell. It was, in part, a reflection of the larger age-old uncertainties concerning the origins of behavior, thought, and control of the body. It was also an indication of both the territorial discord between the evolving disciplines of psychiatry, pediatrics, and neurology, and a reflection of the quest of the young field of neurology for its domain as a specialty.

Most pediatric publications or treatises devoted solely to child neurology from this era contained chapters on these functional disorders, including sections on tics, habit spasms, headaches, chorea, and emotional problems. Thus, in Bernard Sach's *A Treatise on the Nervous Diseases of Children* (1895), Martin Thiemich and Jules Zappert's *Die Krankheiten des Nervensystems im Kindesalter* (1910) or Ludwig Bruns, August Cramer, and Theodor Ziehen's *Handbuch der Nervenkrankheiten im Kindesalter* (1912), extensive, detailed, and often confusing descriptions of these problems are encountered. At the same time, an entirely separate literature was being published by Rachford, as well as other, well known and respected pediatricians, such as Leonard Guthrie (1907) and Hector Cameron (1919) from England, and later Bronson Crothers (1926) in the United States. Rachford thus typified the early pediatric interest in one particular area of child neurology that is still quite perplexing and now is considered to overlap to some extent with child psychiatry and developmental pediatrics.

Edward J. Fine

Archie Fine

John S. Fine

BUFFALO, NEW YORK

REFERENCES

Bruns, L., A. Cramer, and T. Ziehen. 1912. *Handbuch der Nervenkrankheiten im Kindesalter*. Berlin: Karger Verlag.

Cameron, H. C. 1919. *The Nervous Child.* Edinburgh: Morrison & Gibb Ltd.

Crothers, B. 1926. *Disorders of the Nervous System in Childhood.* New York: D. Appleton.

Dreyfoos, M. 1929. Dr. Benjamin Knox Rachford. *J Med* (Cincinnati) 5:1–6.

Fine, J. 1989. Personal communication.

Guthrie, L. G. 1907. *Functional Nervous Disorders of Childhood.* London: Oxford University Press.

Lyon, R. A. 1929. The Medical Contributions of Dr. Benjamin Knox Rachford. *J Med* (Cincinnati) 9:6–12.

______. 1972. *Benjamin Knox Rachford*, 1–97. Cincinnati: Neiman Press, Education Horizons Publishers.

Ohio Historical Society. 1929. Death Certificate Archives. Columbus, OH.

Peterson, F. 1902. Epilepsy. *Trans Nat Assoc Study Epilepsy* 2:11–18.

Rachford, B. K. 1888. Etiology of the Present Typhoid Epidemic. *Cincinnati Lancet-Clin* 20:33–35.

______. 1891. The Influence of Bile on the Fat Splitting Properties of the Pancreatic Juice. *J Physiol* (Cambridge, England) 12:72–94.

______. 1893. The Etiology of Chorea. *Med News* (Phila) 62:429–33.

______. 1895. Comparative Anatomy of the Bile and Pancreatic Ducts in Mammals, Studied from the Physiological Standpoint of Fat Digestion. *Med* (Detroit) 1:1–11, 520–30.

______. 1896. A Child is Not a Little Man. *Cincinnati-Lancet Clin* 36:403–7.

______. 1903. Treatment of Migraine. *Med News* 83:630–34.

______. 1905. *Neurotic Disorders of Childhood.* New York: E. B. Treat.

______. 1912. *Diseases of Children.* New York: D. Appleton and Co.

Rachford, B. K., and F. H. Southgate. 1895. The Influence of Bile on the Proteolytic Action of Pancreatic Juice. *Med Rec* (NY) 48:878–90.

Sachs, Bernard. 1895. *A Treatise on the Nervous Diseases of Children for Physicians and Students.* New York: William Wood & Co.

Spratling, W. P. 1902. Epilepsy, its Etiology, Pathology and Treatment. *JAMA* 52:1126–30.

Thiemich, M., and J. Zappert. 1910. *Die Krankheiten des Nervensystems im Kindesalter*. Leipzig: F. C. W. Vogel.

BERNARD SACHS

BERNARD SACHS'S father, Joseph Sachs, was born in 1817 in Schweinfurt, Bavaria. While studying in Würzberg he fell in love with Sophia Baer; they eloped to Hamburg, set sail for Philadelphia in 1847, and found their way to Baltimore, where their sons Sam and Julius were born. After living in Boston for a time, the family returned to Baltimore where their red-headed identical twins were born on February 8, 1858; one of them was Barney Sachs (1858–1944) (figure 1). Sachs used, and preferred, this name throughout his life, but used Bernard professionally. His parents and siblings were obviously close, as his privately printed autobiography so touchingly demonstrates (Sachs, 1949).

Joseph Sachs moved his family to New York City in 1859,

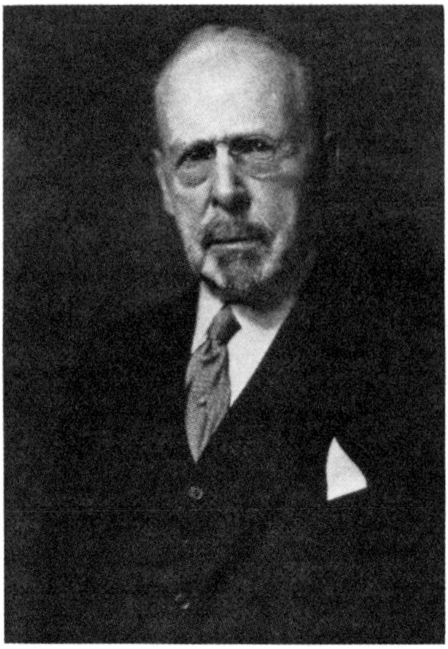

Figure 1. Bernard Sachs (1858–1944).

where he opened his own boarding school. In 1867 they moved to larger quarters, and both he and the school began to develop an impressive reputation. Bernard's twin was his constant companion until his death from scarlet fever at the age of five. Sachs himself had an early brush with death:

> *Just outside the back parlor there was a small porch (about eighteen feet from the stone pavement of the yard), and on this porch the twins were allowed to deport themselves. They were evidently well-behaved youngsters who would never dream of doing anything against the wishes of their parents; but one day, as the slightly older of the two, I climbed up on a chair, stood on it, looked over the railing, and fell to the yard below, fracturing my skull at the tender age of a little more than two years and three months. I can imagine the shock it must have been to that dear Mother; as I was told in later years. Professor Detmold, then Professor of Surgery at the College of Physicians and Surgeons, was called in. As though he had a premonition that the little patient was some day to devote himself to diseases of the brain, he resorted himself to a most extraordinary measure to bring the broken bones together. A leaden cap was molded and fitted to the head and the bones united promptly. . . . When I was able to walk again, [I] showed it off. . . . The result of Detmold's ingenious devise was admirable; nothing but a horizontal depression on the top of my head, and fortunately I escaped without any serious injury — no epilepsy, and I hope with a normal mental capacity.* (Sachs, 1949, 13)

His father's health failed and he sold the school and took the children to Germany in 1867, hoping to find a cure for his illness. Unfortunately, the elder Sachs's health continued to deteriorate, and he died two years later. Upon returning from Europe in 1869, Barney Sachs was enrolled in New York P.S. 35 for two years, then for a year at the Free Academy, later to become City College. During this period his mother developed severe diabetes and died in early 1872 at the age of fifty-two. Sister Emelie took over the household responsibilities, marrying within a few months and taking the brothers into her new home. Brother Julius had stayed behind in Germany to complete his Ph.D. at Göttingen, returning in 1871.

Sachs often publicly acknowledged his brother's role in shaping his career (Hausman, 1947). Julius opened his own school in New York City, naming it Sachs School, and Barney left City College for Sachs School in order to prepare for Columbia. This was a rich time for Sachs; he absorbed his brother's instruction in the classics, arts, and sciences, passing the Columbia entrance examination in June 1874. He decided to try for Harvard. Julius, though newly married, tutored his brother through the summer at Ithaca with his new bride. In early autumn, Sachs passed the examinations in Cambridge. His college years (1874–78) were devoted to a liberal arts curriculum, focusing more on science as time went on. He won the Bowdoin Prize for his dissertation on "A Comparison of the Fore and Hind Limbs of Vertebrates." William James taught Sachs's psychology course and had a determining influence in directing his career to the study of the mind. As it turned out, James's sight was failing, and, eager to read Wilhelm Wundt's new book, *Psychologie*, enlisted Sachs to read its German text to him. During this time, Sachs challenged himself to become a commencement speaker. He wrote an essay, "Goethe as a Man of Science," and submitted it under a pseudonym, for James was on the selection committee. He was an honor student and was elected to Phi Beta Kappa (Sachs, 1949).

After finishing college, he began his medical studies abroad. He visited Adrian Huxley in London and spent "a week in Paris to see the Exposition and to get my first look at gay Paris. I saw plenty. It was a great experience for an innocent lad of twenty." In October 1878 Sachs began his medical studies at Strasbourg in Alsace. Sachs found the medical faculty especially strong, recalling Heinrich Waldeyer (anatomy), Friedrich Goltz (physiology), Felix Hoppe-Seyler (pharmacologic chemistry), Adolph Kussmaul (medicine), Friedrich von Recklinghausen (pathology), and Wilhelm Freund (obstetrics and gynecology). Kussmaul was Sachs's most notable mentor, and the one whom he credited with teaching him the art of bedside diagnosis and the evaluation and treatment of the patient, not the case. Sachs described this experience years later (Sachs,

1942a): "While I was deeply interested in new procedures and laboratory methods, the guiding principle was that bedside observation was of the greatest importance." Sachs went to Berlin for one semester in 1881–82. There he was inspired by Rudolf Virchow's lectures and by Carl Westphal, who presented memorable lectures on mental disorders. Sachs returned to Strasbourg, preparing his doctoral dissertation in Goltz's laboratory on the influence of the spinal cord on the secretion of urine (Sachs, 1881). He received his medical degree on June 6, 1882.

After a summer vacation, Sachs went to Vienna for postgraduate training with the famous faculty at the Allgemeines Krankenhaus, and particularly with Theodor Meynert, who was to teach him brain anatomy. Sachs regarded Meynert as a great scientist, but as a teacher, unfortunately, "far from great." His time on rounds with Meynert in the psychiatry clinic was rewarding. Sachs later observed that Meynert and Westphal were great psychiatrists because they were also great neurologists. Sachs then went to the Salpêtrière in 1883, enjoying for several months the more dramatic presentations of Charcot. In the spring, he traveled to London to learn the views of Hughlings Jackson and found Jackson similar to Meynert — that is, hard to follow. However, he learned much from Jackson and placed him close to Kussmaul as an influence on his career. Sachs then returned to Vienna for a final winter. Meynert wrote *Psychiatrie* just as Sachs was returning to the United States, and Sachs translated it into English. It was a difficult task; apparently Meynert's German was as bad as his teaching. Ludwig Edinger later complemented Sachs for the translation, finding it easier to read than his native German!

In May 1884 Sachs returned to New York as a private assistant to Isaac Adler. Adler had a lasting impact in two areas. First, Sachs learned how not to treat assistants! Adler was harsh and unfair. Sachs took it upon himself thereafter to provide encouragement to those who studied with him. Second, Adler's family practice provided Sachs with his first two patients with amaurotic idiocy. Sachs noted, however, that Adler was true to form: "When I claimed the disease in question to be most unusual, Dr. Adler said, 'Nothing but an ordinary form of idiocy,' implying that it was absurd that a man who had been in practice less than three years should claim to have discovered a new disease" (Sachs, 1949).

In 1885 Sachs became an assistant to Edward Constant Séguin who had a "powerful influence" (Sachs, 1944). Sachs was appointed to the Polyclinic Hospital (1885), the Neurology Staff at the Montefiore Home (1888), and then as consulting neurologist at Mt. Sinai Hospital (1893). Sachs's own words best describe the status of neurology:

In the late seventies and early eighties of the last century, neurology had already made a distinct impression on medical science here and abroad . . . but general medicine as it does to this day (1942), tried to hold its child in check and to deny its rights. No private (voluntary) hospital had established wards for nervous diseases. The general medical attending was supposed to know it all. Discussing this question with Abraham Jacobi as far back as 1885, I asked him whether he realized that a knowledge of neurology has to be acquired and does not come by intuition. He pardoned my boldness and in spite of this frontal attack, we were good friends many years thereafter. (Sachs, 1942b, 292)

In order to fully understand Sachs's pursuits and his ability to have such an impact on neurology, some further information about his family is necessary. His brothers Julius and Samuel married sisters who were the daughters of Marcus Goldman. Samuel became a partner, forming Goldman, Sachs, & Co., a banking firm that grew to become international in scope. Brother Harry married Nellie Lorsch and became a special partner in Goldman, Sachs, & Co. Julius had a very illustrious academic career and, as pointed out by Abraham Flexner, was a very interesting personality and champion of secondary education (*N.Y. Times*, 1934b). Julius's son, Ernest Sachs (1879–1958), with guidance from his uncle Barney, became a distinguished professor of neurosurgery at Washington University in St. Louis and the founder of the Society of Neurological Surgeons (Denny-Brown, Rose, and Sachs, 1975). Bernard Sachs married Bettina M. Stein, daughter of Henry W. Stein of Frankfurt-am-Main, on December 18, 1887. They had two daughters, Alice and Helen. Alice married Jacob M. Plaunt and lived in Cincinnati. Helen married Nathan Straus, whose family owned R. H. Macy & Co. and Abraham & Straus. Straus was a state senator, active Democratic Party supporter, journalist, broadcaster, and real estate magnate (*N.Y. Times* 1961a, b, c). Sachs thus had time, financial backing, and, most important, the family and inner peace that allowed him to give so much to his chosen field of neurology. His portraits depict a man who exudes confidence.

Sachs's persistence as an early spokesman for neurology led to his receiving a commission to open one of the first neurological services at Mount Sinai Hospital in 1900. Sachs was to spend thirty-one years at Mount Sinai, becoming one of the New York City "triumvirate" with Charles Dana and Moses Allen Starr. In 1922 his brothers Samuel and Harry provided the financial backing to establish the expanded Mount Sinai wards in memory of their parents (Sachs, 1942a). Sachs retired in 1924.

Sachs published extensively on a wide variety of general neurological topics. His bibliography (Sachs, 1942b) attests to his special interests in neurological disorders in children. This interest is attributed to his family's prominent role in education (Meyer, 1942). In 1887, at the age of twenty-nine, Sachs presented his findings on amaurotic familial idiocy, first in July to the American Neurological Association and then in an article in the *Journal of Nervous and Mental Disease* (Sachs, 1887). This was followed by a series of nine additional articles over the next forty-two years that further defined the Tay-Sachs phenotype (Sachs, 1892, 1896a, b, 1898, 1903, 1910, 1928, 1929; Sachs and Strauss, 1910). The original article described the clinical and pathological picture. Sachs, taking the larger view, saw his patient as an important factor in understanding abnormal development and the pathology of mental illness. Sachs obtained help with the staining from Ira van Gieson. Herman Joseph Knapp (1831–1911) practiced ophthalmology in New York and Berlin (Evans, 1987); Sachs noted that Knapp saw his patient. Knapp presented the patient's initial findings at the seventeenth Heidelberg Ophthalmological Society meeting, first using the term "cherry red color" in describing the fovea. Knapp reported this as a benign finding in Heidelberg, but later realized the gravity of his later evaluations. By 1896 Sachs had accumulated nineteen patients with amaurotic idiocy and noted both their tendency to be Jewish and the role of consanguinity (Sachs, 1896a). After summarizing his concepts of the disease in 1910 for Osler's text, *The Principles and Practice of Medicine*, there was a hiatus in his writing on this disorder:

For years I was fairly satisfied with the belief that I had done all that could

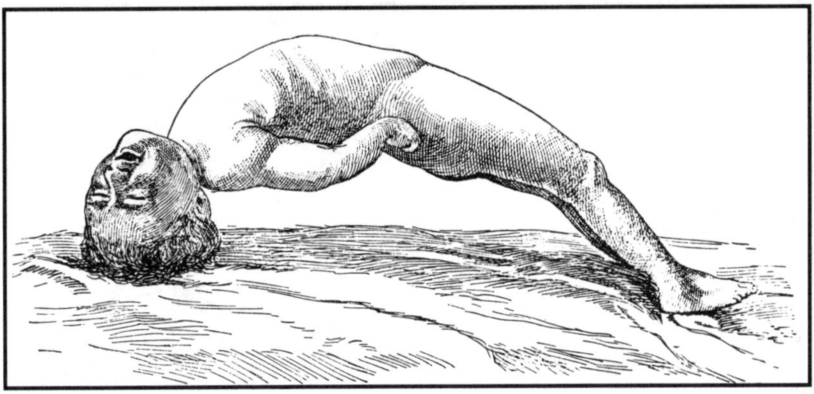

Figure 2. Sachs's clinical description of convulsions in children included this photograph. The accompanying text included an accurate description of the attack, causes, and approaches to treatment, as well as the potential dangers to the child of repeated attacks. Originally figure 38, p. 50, in *A Treatise on the Nervous Diseases of Children*, 1895.

be expected of me. Lo and behold! During the past decade, Epstein of Vienna, L. Pick and Bielschowsky in Berlin, corroborated by others, convinced me of the close relationship between this disease and Niemann-Pick disease; and after inspecting Pick's specimens in Berlin, I was convinced that in all these forms, a faulty lipid metabolism was the important underlying factor. (Sachs, 1944, 767)

Sachs also wrote studies on myotonia congenita (1886), intracerebral hemorrhage (1887), muscular dystrophies (1888 and later), and congenital syphilis (1896). He also wrote a number of papers on poliomyelitis and cerebral palsy. One paper, written with Frederick Peterson, reviewed 140 children with cerebral palsy and was one of the most widely quoted articles over the next forty years (Sachs and Peterson, 1890). Because of his interest in pediatrics, Dana suggested that he write a book on child neurology, which became *A Treatise on the Nervous Diseases of Children* (Sachs, 1895). This was the first pediatric neurology text and was translated into German in 1897 and later into Italian. This monumental work of more than six hundred pages demonstrated his wealth of information and broad experience in pediatric neurology; it remains a classic source for data on now uncommon conditions such as tetanus and diphtheritic neuropathy, and for information on the natural history of now more treatable diseases such as meningitis and hydro-

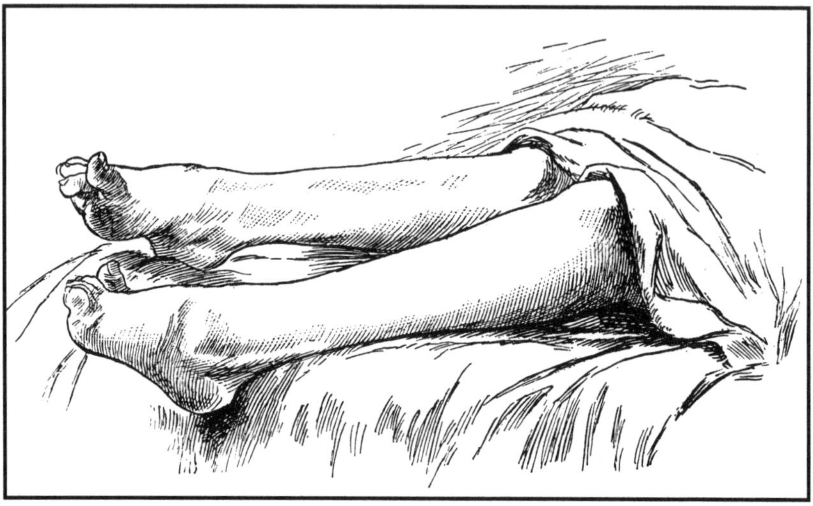

Figure 3. Friedreich's ataxia. Sachs reviewed the historical development towards recognition of this disorder, as well as recounting his own clinical experience. This illustration was taken from the work of Pierre Marie of the same disorder that accompanied other photographs of Sachs's own patients. Originally figure 93, p. 382 from *A Treatise on the Nervous Diseases of Children*, 1895.

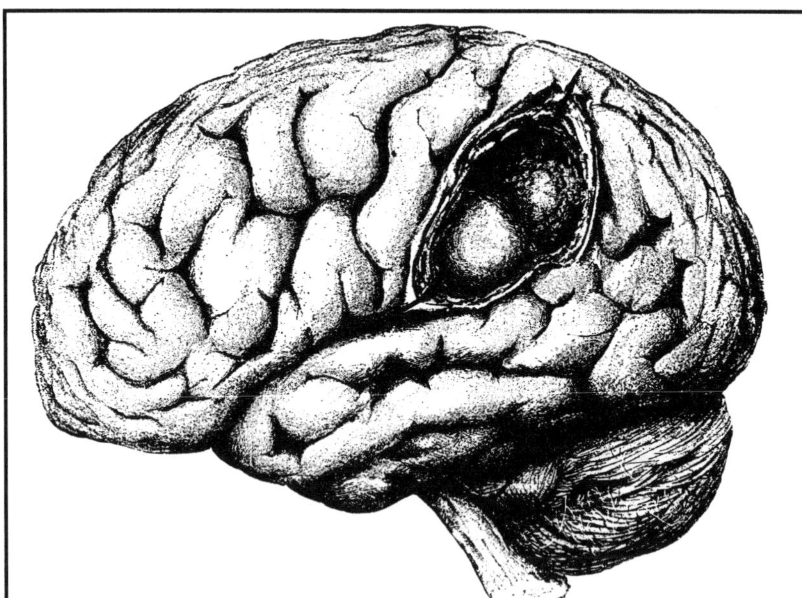

Figure 4. Sachs used the term cerebral palsy to describe a motor deficit and did not restrict its use to the perinatal period. The etiology of this hemorrhagic cyst was not clearly determined by Sachs, although he describes a "tumour" underneath (Sachs, 1895; originally figure 147, p. 546).

cephalus. Also discussed are some interesting therapies, including cannabis indicis for epilepsy (figure 2) and migraine, head wrapping for hydrocephalus, phrenic nerve stimulation for respiratory failure in diphtheritic neuropathy, and strychnine as an indispensable nervous system tonic. Also included are sections demonstrating several of the recently described genetic neurodegenerative and neuromuscular disorders, such as Friedreich's ataxia (figure 3) and Charcot-Marie-Tooth disease. Sachs also wrote one of the first comprehensive descriptions of tumors of the nervous system, which was accompanied by illustrations of both gross and microscopic examples (figure 4). The second edition was published in 1905, and more extensive revisions were incorporated with Louis Hausman (Plum and Jonas, 1973) in *Nervous and Mental Disorders from Birth Through Adolescence* (1926).

Sachs was deeply interested in science and advancing the frontiers of knowledge:

We were proud of those who had preceded us, eager to follow in their footsteps and to help American neurology in the fore-front of the scientific battle. . . . To those who may be inclined to have a slight sneer for the clinician and think him inferior to the laboratory worker, let me say as I have said elsewhere, all true scientific research in medicine stems from the bedside. The patient presents the problem, it is for the physician to study and solve it; and he can do much toward formulating these problems if he will wear his thinking cap at the bedside. (Sachs, 1944, 681)

Sachs practiced what he taught. Even in his last year, he wrote a scholarly article discussing the exciting issues on the frontiers of knowledge: Could infections (and not heredity) cause some congenital disorders? Will understanding the effects of acetylcholine give reason to clinical disorders of peripheral nerves? Should we use insulin shock for psychosis? Electrical (EEG) measurements for diagnosis? Radiation for hydrocephalus? Amazingly, this old man was incisive in picking out the "keepers" and cautioning where appropriate. He was enthusiastic to the end: "Pardon the young optimist. I would like to begin my career all over again" (Sachs, 1944).

Sachs was an organization man. He joined the American Neurological Association in 1886 and served as its president in 1894 and again in 1932. He was also twice president of the New York

Neurological Society and president of the New York Academy of Medicine. He was the prime motivating force and president of the First International Neurological Congress in Berne in 1931. He was then honorary president of the Second and Third (with Sherrington and Holmes) International Congresses of Neurology. He was awarded honorary memberships in the Moscow, Italian, and French neurological societies, the Royal Society of Medicine, and the Edinburgh Medico-Chirurgical Society (Sachs, 1949). In addition, he edited the *Journal of Nervous and Mental Disease* from 1886 to 1891.

Sachs maintained an interest in other areas of medicine including medical history (Sachs, 1944) and psychiatry. Adolph Meyer prepared a very erudite treatise on Sachs's relationship to psychiatry (1942). While enjoying the exchange of views with neurological psychiatrists, Sachs had several quarrels with the evolving psychoanalysts (Sachs, 1933) and regretted the emergence of psychiatrists without substantive neurological training. Freud responded: "Fortunately, I have not been hostile to organic neuropathology" (Sachs, 1944). But Sachs's critique, in a review of a new book on psychoanalysis, was more substantive:

The lawyer, knowing his case is weak, is apt to grow grandiloquent and to abuse opposing witnesses; that is what the psychoanalysts love to do; they hide behind unintelligible terms and accuse those who object to their pet theories, of ignorance, of complete misunderstanding, of malevolent opposition. . . . [The author] has attempted to establish an important relation between psychoanalysis and medicine and psychiatry, but we shall see that in doing this he has started from premises wholly unproven, and has made statements, often illogical, and generally misleading. We have the right to insist that the rules of logic be applied, as in all scientific investigations; and the psychoanalyst must either accept this condition or else abandon the claims of presenting sound scientific doctrine. . . . The future progress of psychiatry, especially in America, calls for far saner and safer leadership. . . . (Sachs, 1933, 725, 749)

He helped to found (and provided the name for) the Charaka Club, which was devoted to exploring history and the humanities in relation to medicine. This small group of about thirty included Dana, Silas Weir Mitchell, William Osler, Surgeon General John Shaw Billings, George L. Walton, and Harvey Cushing.

Sachs had many pursuits outside medicine. He did steady work for nine months and then took three months of "absolute relaxation." Sachs enjoyed traveling, mountain climbing, walking, and golf. The mountain climbing evolved from his student days in Europe, when he walked through (and over) the Alps to Italy! Sachs was also a public man; his name frequently appeared in the *New York Times* concerning his neurological pursuits, but he also made headlines as a crusader for many years for city sanitation, prevention of juvenile delinquency, and activism by physicians. A celebration of Sachs's career was held in 1942 and reported in the *New York Times*.

Sachs was able to accomplish many things, in large part because of his appreciation of divergence in the world and among his colleagues. This is perhaps best illustrated by his views concerning religion. He was raised a Reform Jew, and although drawn to Orthodox practices while in Germany as a child, remained of the Reform tradition. His Harvard years gave him Christian perspectives; he attended chapel daily. He wrote: "Whatever one's religious convictions may be, every cultured person should have the Old and New Testaments on the tip of his tongue without bragging of it" (Sachs, 1949, 20). Sachs had fond sentiments and appreciation for his heritage and education in Germany, but was deeply offended by the events of World War II. Speaking for his departed father, he said: "I think he would have been ashamed" (Sachs, 1949). Sachs was offered an honorary degree by the faculty at the University of Frankfurt but he declined

because I did not want to be the recipient of any honor from a university system that had completely ignored freedom of thought and freedom of speech even in strictly scientific inquiries. Racial persecutions are cruel, but the degradation of the once great German university system is a lasting disgrace to the entire nation. (Sachs, 1949, 52)

In 1903 Sachs befriended Benjamin Altman and later become his personal physician. Sachs advised Altman in securing porcelains and paintings and, while in Madrid in 1911, personally selected Velasquez's portrait of King Philip IV of Spain, representing it as the artist's best to Altman; it (and the rest of the Altman collection) is now in the Metropolitan Museum of Art in New York. Sachs later became a Trustee of the Altman Foundation. The president of B. Altman & Co. was Michael Friedsam, in whose name the Friedsam

Foundation was established. Sachs was able, through his association with B. Altman & Co., to establish and become the director of the first Pediatric Neurology Service at the New York Neurological Institute. Early in 1935 the Friedsam Foundation made a $100,000 grant to the Neurological Institute, which set aside the west half of the fifth floor (Elsberg, 1944, 120–21). Sachs directed the unit from 1935 to 1937; the initial staff was recruited from multiple disciplines (N.Y. Times, 1935a). The Division of Pediatric Neurology has continued its prominent role under Louis Casamajor (1881–1962) (Yahr, 1963), Sidney Carter (Schneider, 1990), and, currently, Darryl DeVivo.

Sachs had a prodigious career. He practiced for fifty-six years. He prided himself in personally recording the clinical histories of all his patients — some ten thousand by his estimate at the end of life. He was a pioneer of great importance in the growth of the fields of neurology and child neurology, and was the leading figure in American neurology at the time of his death (Hausman, 1942, 1947; Haymaker, 1970; Stumpf, 1981). He wrote 194 articles, worked for the government and for neurology, and founded child neurology in writings, funding, organizational tasks, and in spirit.

Sachs's wife, Betty, died September 28, 1940, at Quarry Lake, Valhalla (*N.Y. Times,* 1940). He subsequently married Rosetta Kaskel, who survived him. Sachs himself died after an illness of several weeks on February 8, 1944, at his home at the Plaza Hotel in New York City. Mayor La Guardia headed the list of twenty-two honorary pallbearers. After his death, Bernard Sachs was well remembered. Hausman commented that

Sachs saw and helped neurology in America pass from adolescence into vigorous manhood. We, who listened to his forceful convictions on so many occasions . . . are apt to forget that he belonged to the heroic age of neurology and psychiatry. (Hausman, 1947)

Sachs's son-in-law, Nathan Straus, described Sachs's character:

[T]he buoyant good spirits, the boundless generosity, and the complete selflessness of a unique personality. . . . In a long life I have not known any man, who combined to the same degree as Dad, gaiety with goodness, wisdom with tolerance. His friendliness, his kindness, his philanthropy, using the word in its finest sense, were not based at all on a sense of duty. He did good because

he enjoyed doing good. In him there was a joy of life, the happiness that comes of inner peace. And he sought always to help others achieve a like state. (Sachs, 1949, 20)

Some years after Sachs's death, with the growth of the specialty, the Child Neurology Society was founded. It was decided to invite a scientist to lecture who, though not a child neurologist, had contributed to the field. The first lectures of the society were given, and it was decided that the distinction of the speakers needed to be emphasized in some manner. In 1981 I had the privilege of introducing the lecturer and the idea that this lecture would be named in honor of Bernard Sachs. Unaware of the choir next door, I described Sachs as a "compassionate man, well loved and respected by his contemporaries. We can love him some more — and accept our heritage — by perpetuating this lectureship in his name." At that moment, the choir belted out a resounding "Hallelujah." Heeding this sign, the Executive Committee determined that the Bernard Sachs Lecture would continue, each year honoring a scientist who emulated Sachs's excellence and spirit.

David A. Stumpf
CHICAGO, ILLINOIS

ACKNOWLEDGMENTS

I am grateful to the New York Academy of Medicine for permission to use portions of my biography of Sachs (Stumpf, 1981), including the portrait.

REFERENCES

Denny-Brown, D., A. S. Rose, and A. L. Sahs. 1975. *Centennial Anniversary Volume of the American Neurological Association, 1875–1975*. New York: Springer Publishing.

Elsberg, C. A. 1944. *The Story of a Hospital: The Neurological Institute of New York, 1909–1938*. New York: Paul B. Hoeber.

Evans, P. R. 1987. Tay-Sachs Disease: A Centenary. *Arch Dis Child* 62:1056–57.

Hausman, L. 1942. Dr. Bernard (Barney) Sachs: Biographical Milestones. *J Mt Sinai Hosp* 9:258–60.

______. 1947. Bernard Sachs (1858–1944). *Proc Charaka Club* 11:231–38.

Haymaker, W. 1970. Bernard Sachs. In *Founders of Neurology*, 513–17. Ed. W. Haymaker and F. Schiller. 2d ed. Springfield, IL: Charles C Thomas.

Meyer, A. 1942. Historical Fragments on the Neurological and Psychiatric Specialties. Factors and Results in an Eminent Medical and Specifically Neurological Career. *J Mt Sinai Hosp* 9:213–48.

New York Times: Jan. 6, 1933a; Feb. 18, 1933b; Feb. 3, 1934a; Feb. 12, 1934b; May 10, 1934c; Jan. 25, 1935a; Mar. 3, 1935b; Nov. 15, 1935c; Sept. 30, 1940; Nov. 25, 1942; Feb. 9, 1944; Apr. 28, 1949; Sept. 14, 1961a; Sept. 15, 1961b; Sept. 16, 1961c.

Plum, F., and S. Jonas. 1973. Louis Hausman (1891–1972). *Trans Am Neur Assoc* 98:328–29.

Sachs, B. 1881. Ueber den Einfluss des Ruckenmarks auf die Harnsecretion. *Pflugers Arch ges Physiol* 25:299–322.

______. 1887. On Arrested Cerebral Development, with Special Reference to Its Cortical Pathology. *J Nerv Ment Dis* 14:541–53.

______. 1892. A Further Contribution to the Pathology of Arrested Cerebral Development. *J Nerv Ment Dis* 19:603–63.

______. 1895. *A Treatise on the Nervous Diseases of Children for Physicians and Students*. New York: Wood.

______. 1896a. A Familial Form of Idiocy, Generally Fatal, Associated with Blindness (Amaurotic Familial Idiocy). *J Nerv Ment Dis* 21:475–78.

______. 1896b. A Familial Form of Idiocy, Generally Fatal, Associated with Blindness (Amaurotic Familial Idiocy). *NY Med J* 58:697–703.

______. 1898. Die Amaurotische familiäre Idiotie. *Dtsch med Wschr* 24:33–35.

______. 1903. On Amaurotic Family Idiocy. A Disease Chiefly of the Gray Matter of the Central Nervous System. *J Nerv Ment Dis* 30:1–30.

______. 1910. Amaurotic Family Idiocy. *Mod Med (Osler)* 7:868.

______. 1928. *Amaurotic Family Idiocy (Tay-Sachs Disease)*. Philadelphia: Lea & Febiger.

______. 1929. Amaurotic Family Idiocy and General Lipoid Degeneration. *Arch Neur Psych* 21:247–53.

______. 1933. The False Claims of Psychoanalysts. *Am J Psych* 12:725–49.

______. 1942a. The First Neurological Division in New York City—At the Mount Sinai Hospital. *J Mt Sinai Hosp* 9:292–95.

______. 1942b. Bibliography. *J Mt Sinai Hosp* 9:262–70.

______. 1944. The Early Years and Rapid Development of Neurology in America and Its Relation to Medical Science. *J Mt Sinai Hosp* 10:678–83, 10:765–72.

______. 1949. *Barney Sachs, 1858–1944*. Privately printed. New York: Army Medical Library.

Sachs, B., and L. Hausman. 1926. *Nervous and Mental Disorders from Birth Through Adolescence*. New York: Paul B. Hoeber.

Sachs, B., and F. Peterson. 1890. A Study of Cerebral Palsies of Early Life, Based upon an Analysis of One Hundered and Forty Cases. *J Nerv Ment Dis* 17:295.

Sachs, B., and I. Strauss. 1910. The Cell Changes in Amaurotic Family Idiocy. *J Exp Med* 12:685–95.

Schneider, S. 1990. Sidney Carter. In *Founders of Child Neurology*. Ed. S. Ashwal. San Francisco: Norman Publishing.

Stumpf, D. A. 1981. The Founding of Pediatric Neurology in America. *Bull NY Acad Med* 57:804–16.

Yahr, M. D. 1963. Louis Casamajor (1881–1962). *Trans Am Neur Assoc* 88:299.

PAUL SCHILDER

PAUL SCHILDER (1886–1940) (figure 1) was born and educated in Vienna, receiving his medical degree in 1909. Although his primary interest would eventually lie in adolescent psychiatry, his writings span a wide variety of areas in both neurology and psychiatry. His most significant contribution to child neurology was his description of disseminated sclerosis (encephalitis periaxialis diffusa) based on observations made early in his career.

Schilder's first paper, on malignant gliomas of the sympathetic nervous system, was published in 1908 while he was still a medical student working as a neuropathology assistant to Gabriel Anton, who described the syndrome of cortical blindness (Schilder and Kassowitz, 1908). In the first three years after receiving his medical degree, Schilder published eight papers, including several analyzing athetoid and choreic movements.

It was during this time that he made his initial observations on encephalitis periaxialis diffusa, a disorder of acquired demyelination in childhood that would later bear his name. The first of several patients described by Schilder, a fourteen-year-old girl, came to his clinic on July 3, 1911, and died two and one-half months later on September 17. Seven months later, Schilder submitted a sixty-page paper with five figures and six full-page color illustrations to the most renowned German journal in neurology, the *Zeitschrift für die gesamte Neurologie und Psychiatrie.* Aside from his own extensive clinical and neuropathological observations, Schilder reviewed sixty-six related cases that had previously been published (Schilder, 1912). In his extensive discussion of these cases, he differentiated findings of his own patient, which he felt were indicative of a previously undescribed disease, especially the neuropathology. The clinical details of this case are interesting to review.

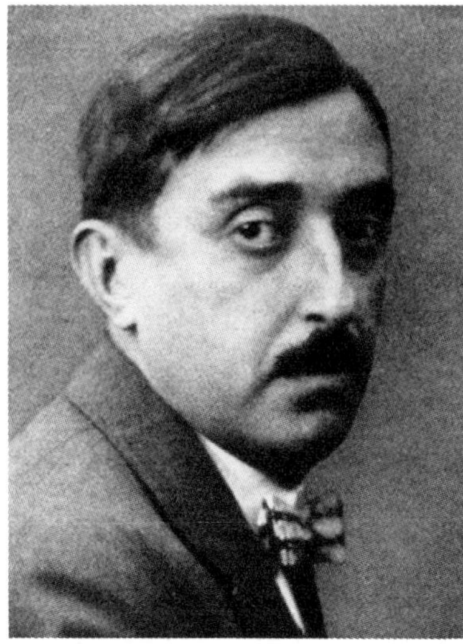

Figure 1. Paul Schilder (1886–1940).

The patient presented with an eight-week history of vomiting and visual loss and was diagnosed as having optic neuritis. Neurosurgical treatment, specifically puncture of the corpus collosum, was performed, and, two weeks later, she developed progressive lower and then upper extremity paralysis, lapsed into coma, and subsequently died from pneumonia. Neuropathologic examination revealed diffuse demyelination, sparing of the arcuate fibers with relative preservation of the axis cylinders, which were frequently surrounded by inflammatory cells. On this basis, Schilder termed the disorder encephalitis periaxialis diffusa.

This first case of Schilder's, because of the suggestion of inflammatory involvement, was ultimately considered by later writers to be similar to multiple sclerosis as originally delineated by Charcot and others. The following year, Schilder reported the case of another child whose disorder was familial and that was later considered the prototype for the genetically determined leukodystrophies (Schilder, 1913). This was followed by the report of Ernest Seimerling and Hans Creutzfeldt (1923) on a cerebral demyelinating disease in association with adrenal insufficiency and, a year later, by yet another report by Schilder of a patient with an encephalitic type of demyelinating process. This 1924 report by Schilder was ultimately considered to represent a third type of demyelinating process related to subacute infection (Schilder, 1924). In 1928 Max Bielschowsky and

Richard Henneberg proposed the term *leukodystrophy*, dividing the entities with diffuse sclerosis into either an exogenous inflammatory type or an endogenous, familial, progressive type. By 1934, twenty-two years after Schilder's index case, Leendert Bouman had tabulated more than one hundred cases in his monograph, *Diffuse Sclerosis (Encephalitis Periaxialis Diffusa)*. The studies of Ludo van Bogaert and Ivan Bertrand (1933), Ronald Norman (1947), J. Godwin Greenfield (1952), and Charles Lumsden (1955) all contributed to the reclassification of these disorders proposed by Charles Poser and Ludo van Bogaert in 1956 (Schumacher, 1975). In this classification, the "diffuse scleroses" were divided into three groups: (1) Schilder's cerebral sclerosis; (2) leukodystrophies; and (3) subacute encephalitis. Although he was unaware of it at the time, Schilder's three case reports served as the basis for classifying these disorders. This classification ultimately gained wide acceptance but now is being reexamined in regard to particular etiologies — for example, as lysosomal or peroxisomal disorders. This was particularly true for patients with X-linked adrenoleukodystrophy, who were for some twenty years referred to as having Addison-Schilder's disease. This disorder recently has been shown to be characteristic of a new group of neurometabolic disorders associated with peroxisomal dysfunction.

At Leipzig (1912–14), Schilder's interests clearly shifted toward psychiatry, and while there he published the first of many important papers and books in this field. Schilder was extremely productive at this time. Except for the World War I years of 1915 to 1917, Schilder published between one and twenty-four papers and books each year from 1909 to 1939 (Adler, 1965). These were balanced between neurology and psychiatry until 1934, after which work on psychiatry clearly predominated.

Following World War I Schilder returned to Vienna at the request of Wagner van Jauregg, who would later receive the Nobel Prize in medicine for his malarial treatment of syphilis. By 1925 Schilder had risen to the status of Professor Extraordinarus. He developed a close relationship with Sigmund Freud and became an active member of the Psychoanalytic Society. He used his knowledge of neuroanatomic localization and the behavioral manifestations of organic diseases derived from his observations on chronic epidemic encephalitis (of von Economo), general paresis of the insane (from his work with Wagner van Jaurreg), and polioencephalitis hemorrhagica superior (Wernicke's encephalopathy) to bridge the gap between neurology and psychiatry. What he considered his most important contribution to the medical literature, *Das Korperschema* was published in 1923. *The Image and Appearance of the Human Body* is a greatly expanded English version published in 1935, five years after he had come to New York as the director of the psychiatric division of Bellevue Hospital (Schilder, 1935). This work reflected his ongoing interest in the psychiatry of adolescence, particularly the value of art and its relation to the perception of body image. It was also in this year that he and his colleagues founded the Society for Psychotherapy and Psychopathology. Schilder served as the organization's first president and following his death in 1941, the society was appropriately renamed The Schilder Society in his honor.

One of Schilder's outstanding qualities, as recounted by Alexandra Adler, was his inspiring capability as a lecturer. Adler recalls a monthly meeting of the Vienna Society for Neurology and Psychiatry in which Schilder

> *electrified a soporific audience by starting his communication in a loud voice with these animated words: "A man runs naked through the streets shouting, 'The world has come to an end!'" After this, Schilder proceeded to elaborate on the symbolism in the delusions of the schizophrenic patient, the audience now in rapt attention.* (Adler, 1965, 848)

Throughout his distinguished career in psychiatry Schilder maintained an avid interest in neurology and the role of organic illnesses in psychiatric disorders of childhood. He fostered an attitude of thoroughness, insisting that each patient admitted to his psychiatric service also receive a thorough neurological and laboratory examination to exclude an identifiable organic basis for their psychiatric complaints. He placed great emphasis on the importance of the "soft neurological signs," working to bridge the gap between psychiatry and neurology (Schilder, 1931). Much of his later work resulted from psychiatric observation of children carried out in collaboration with his wife, Loretta Bender (of Bender-Gestalt fame).

Schilder was known for periods of deep introspection, and this propensity may well have contributed to his death, which was the result of being struck by an automobile as he crossed Times Square in New York. At the time of his death he had published numerous books and more than three hundred articles, including an autobiography (Schilder, 1940). For more than thirty years after his death, additional writings appeared, many as chapters in the publications of Loretta Bender.

The marriage of Paul Schilder, the neuroanatomical psychiatrist, with Loretta Bender, the behavioral psychiatrist, paralleled his life's work, which linked many aspects of child and adolescent neurology and psychiatry.

Warren A. Marks
FORT WORTH, TEXAS

Stephen Ashwal
LOMA LINDA, CALIFORNIA

ACKNOWLEDGMENTS

We must thank Ilsa von Braukitch for her assistance in the preparation of this sketch. Not only was she helpful with the acquisition of information, but as the granddaughter of Wagner von Jaurreg, she told some delightful stories about life in Vienna. She also kindly provided the photograph of Dr. Schilder from her grandfather's collection.

REFERENCES

Adler, A. 1965. The Work of Paul Schilder. *Bull NY Acad Med* 41:841–53.

Bouman, L. 1934. *Diffuse Sclerosis (Encephalitis periaxialis diffusa).* Bristol: John Wright and Sons.

Schilder, P. F. 1912. Zur Kenntnis der Sogenannten diffusen Sklerose (Über Encephalitis periaxialis diffusa). *Zeit ges Neur Psych* 10:1.

______. 1913. Zur Frage der Encephalitis periaxialis diffusa (sogenannte diffuse Sklerose). *Zeit ges Neur Psych* 15:359.

______. 1924. Die Encephalitis periaxialis diffusa (nebst Bemerkungen über die Apraxie des Lidschlusses). *Arch Psych Nervenkrankh* 71:327.

______. 1931. Organic Problems in Child Guidance. *Mental Hygiene* 15:480–86.

______. 1935. *The Image and Appearance of the Human Body: Studies in Constructive Energies of the Psyche*. London: Kegan, Paul, Trench, Trobner.

______. 1940. The Vita and Bibliographia of Paul Schilder. *J Crim Psychopathol* 2:221–34.

Schilder, P. F., and K. Kassowitz. 1908. Einige Verusche über die Feinheit der Empfindung bei bewegter Tastflache. *Pflugers Arch ges Physiol* 122:119–22.

Schumacher, G. A. 1975. The Demyelinating Diseases. In *Clinical Neurology*. Vol. 2. Ed. A. B. Baker and L. H. Baker. New York: Harper and Row.

FRIEDRICH SCHULTZE

THE SCIENTIFIC renaissance of the mid-nineteenth century left a permanent mark on medicine. The age that produced Albert Einstein, Charles Darwin, Sigmund Freud, and the Curies also produced neurologists such as Jean Martin Charcot, John Hughlings Jackson, Charles Sherrington, and Guillaume Duchenne. Germany contributed with Wilhelm Erb, Adolf Strümpell, and Nikolaus Friedreich. A perusal of German neurologic literature from 1880 to 1915 reveals many other names that have achieved eponymic immortality: Ludwig Edinger, Hermann Oppenheim, Carl Wernicke, and Adolf Wallenberg. A curious case is that of Friedrich Schultze — a wise academician who was a member of Germany's inner circle of neurologic intelligentsia and a close friend of Erb and Strümpell. His department at Bonn produced an enormous amount of clinical research and description, contributing heavily to the German neurologic literature. Indeed, Schultze was on the cutting edge of his specialty for half a century. Yet Schultze's name has somehow failed to achieve eponymic status. We know of no syndrome, common or arcane, anatomic feature, or phenomenon that bears his name.

Friedrich Schultze (1848–1934) (figure 1) was born in the town of Rathenow, in Brandenburg, Germany, the son of a well-known farmer and salesman. After a liberal education in the Brandenburg schools, he decided on a career in medicine, mostly from lack of a burning interest in anything else. He entered the University of Berlin in 1867, and was greatly influenced by Rudolf Virchow. He volunteered as a medic during the Franco-Prussian War (1870–71), caring for the wounded in a large military hospital in Berlin under the supervision of Heinrich Quincke. Schultze enjoyed the practical experience, but was glad to return to the scientific rigor and stimulation of the university, from which he graduated in 1871. He was studying basic physiology and preparing for his medical qualifying examinations in late 1871 when he was unexpectedly asked by the prominent clinician-scientist Professor Nikolaus Friedreich to join him as an assistant in Friedreich's medical clinic in Heidelberg. Under the influence of Friedreich and Erb, the University of Heidelberg was already a hub of neurologic investigation and clinical activity. Schultze eagerly accepted Friedreich's offer and moved to Heidelberg in 1872. There his considerable powers of observation and his boundless energy were put to work in neuropathological investigations, and his career in the neurosciences was launched. His lectures and demonstrations in pathologic anatomy achieved wide acclaim, and were increasingly attended by not only students, but also faculty members and practicing physicians from other hospitals and medical centers.

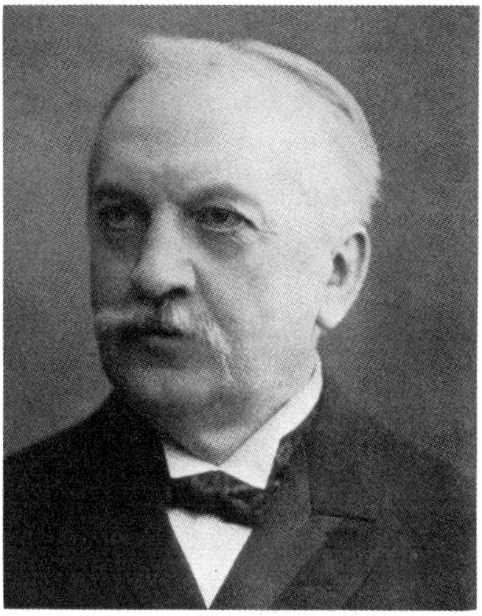

Figure 1. Friedrich Schultze (1848–1934).

Schultze is considered a founder of child neurology because of his significant clinical and pathological contributions to the understanding of poliomyelitis, porencephaly, syringomyelia and syringobulbia, meningitis, hydrocephalus, plumbism, muscular dystrophy, spinocerebellar degenerations, and many other conditions familiar to the child neurologist (Nonne, 1935; Schultze, 1894a, 1923).

Among his more prominent connections to pediatric neurology were his investigations, with Erb and others, in muscle diseases,

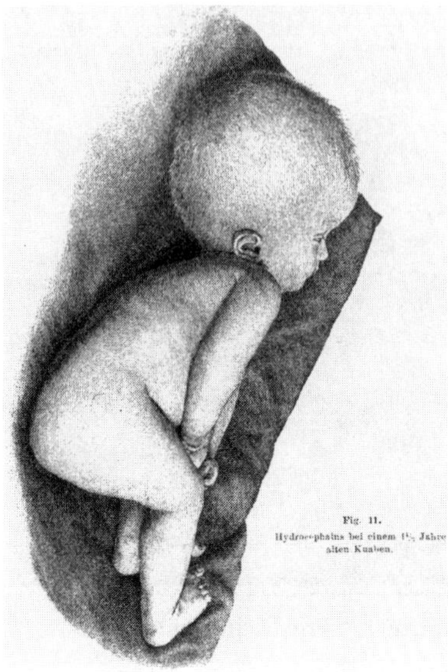

Figure 2. A 1 1/2-year-old child with hydrocephalus described by Schultze in his monograph *Die Krankheiten der Hirnhaute und die Hydrocephalie* (originally figure 11, p. 206).

published in a series of reports beginning in 1879 (Erb and Schultze, 1879; Schultze, 1886, 1895). The classification of localized and generalized muscle weakness, atrophy, and hypertrophy was poorly formulated at the time. The contributions of Schultze and his coworkers emphasizing clinical features, histopathology, and pathophysiology (the distinctions between neurogenic and myogenic weakness and atrophy), form a substantial part of the basis for modern classifications and diagnostic schemata, so important in current child neurology.

Schultze's investigations of peripheral nerve disorders included work on nerve injuries associated with delivery and hereditary neuropathy. In 1884 Schultze described three siblings who suffered from severe, predominantly motor, neuropathy (Schultze, 1884). However, because no other family members were affected, he was uncertain as to the exact etiology, and his notions about heredity were somewhat obtuse. It should be noted that the laws of Mendel, promulgated in the early 1800s, were only "rediscovered" and applied to human genetics in the waning years of that century. Schultze was probably not familiar with them. It is interesting, however, that his report was published two years prior to the reports of Charcot and Marie in France, and Tooth in England.

In 1901 Schultze published an extensive monograph entitled *Die Krankheiten der Hirnhaute und die Hydrocephalie*. This work of more than 250 pages was primarily devoted to child neurological problems such as meningitis, developmental abnormalities, and an extensive section on hydrocephalus (figure 2). Schultze provided numerous case histories, reviews of the literature, and many personal observations, as well as discussions of the pathology and how it related to clinical symptomatology. It also included, after

Quincke, a section on the performance of lumbar punctures in children, including technical aspects of performing these studies as well as their therapeutic uses.

Schultze also made significant contributions to the clinical and pathological phenomena of spinal cord diseases, notably tumors and syringomyelia (Schultze, 1894b). At the time, notions about the pathophysiology of syringomyelia largely involved congenital malformations. Schultze was among the first to recognize and argue forcibly that other causes existed, especially trauma. He noted hematomyelia in some newborns who expired and reasoned that syringomyelia might develop in children with similar lesions who survived.

Schultze moved to Bonn in 1888, where he continued his research until his death. In 1891, together with Erb, Strümpell, and Ludwig Lichtheim, Schultze founded and edited the *Deutsche Zeitschrift für Nervenheilkunde.* This was the predecessor of the current organ of the German Society for Neurology and the German Society for Neurosurgery, the *Zeitschrift für Neurologie.* He continued in this very influential editorship for over forty years.

Schultze had wide-ranging interests in other fields. Even while in medical school, his first publication was the humorous-satiric essay: "Unpolitische Fragen" ("Nonpolitical Questions"). He was active in civic affairs and promoting reforms in medical law, and proposed a common society for medicine, neurology, and pediatrics. He was a student of the Bible and Goethe. He was a consummate entertainer and host. Through his popular Hiking Society of Southwestern German Neurologists he convened friends for scientific discussions in the out-of-doors. Erb especially cherished these meetings (Nonne, 1935). Eventually, they were well attended by psychiatrists, ophthalmologists, and other physicians of diverse interests and specializations. At meetings and festivities Schultze was frequently the designated toastmaster, since he was consistently in good humor and never lacking an anecdote or thoughtful salutation. He was an active supporter of the theater and music, and a member of the city council of Bonn.

Schultze was remembered by his colleagues as the perennial generalist and the brilliant specialist, and as a pathologist who loved the clinic; his conclusions and recommendations in any case were always founded on solid knowledge of anatomy and pathology. This latter trait probably prevented any substantial interest in psychology and hypnotism. Although he admired Freud, he had a skeptical attitude toward the psychoanalysts' lack of objectivity in collecting data and reaching conclusions (Schultze, 1923).

He spent the closing years of his life with his devoted wife at home near the Rhine River, which he loved. He died on October 14, 1934, at the age of eighty-six, after a full life of clinical, academic, civic, literary, and humanistic achievement (Nonne, 1935).

Schultze's role appears to have been that of a contributor and a facilitator, or enabler, rather than that of a leader. He appears to not have been the sole or lead author of any article describing a new phenomenon, structure, or disease, a fact that has contributed to his relative obscurity in twentieth-century neurology, but which in no way diminishes his significant contributions.

Marvin P. Rozear

Thomas F. Platz

DURHAM, NORTH CAROLINA

REFERENCES

Erb, W., and F. Schultze. 1879. Eine Falle von Progressiver Muskelatrophie mit Erkrankung der grauen Vordersaeulen des Ruckenmarks. *Arch Psych* 9:369–88.

Nonne, M. 1935. Friedrich Schultze. *Dtsch Zeit Nervenheilk* 135:81–89.

Schultze, F. 1884. Über eine eigenthümliche progressive atrophische Paralyse bei mehreren Kindern derselben Familie. *Berl klin Wschr* 41:649.

______. 1886. *Über den mit Hypertrophie verbundenen progressiven Muskelschwund und aenliche Krankheitsformen*. Wiesbaden: J. F. Bergmann.

______. 1894a. Über die Friedreich'sche Krankheit and aenliche Krankheitsformen, nebst Bemerkungen über nystagmusartige Zuckungen bei Gesunden. Dtsch Zeit Nervenheilk 5:27–44.

______. 1894b. Differentialdiagnostik der Verletzungen der Cauda equina und Lendenanschwellung. *Dtsch Zeit Nervenheilk* 5:247–54.

______. 1895. Beiträge zur Muskelpathologie. *Dtsch Zeit Nervenheilk* 6:65–75.

______. 1896. Über Befunde von Haematomyelie und Oblongatablutung und Spattbildung bei Dystokien. *Dtsch Zeit Nervenheilk* 8:1–15.

______. 1901. *Die Krankheiten der Hirnhaute und die Hydrocephalie*. Wien: Alfred Holder.

______. 1923. Friedrich Schultze. *Medizin in Selbstdarstellungen*. 2:193–215.

WALTHER SPIELMEYER

OF ALL THE CHILDHOOD neurological disorders, the neuronal ceroid lipofuscinoses have clearly been associated with the greatest number of confusing eponyms. One of the traditional hurdles during most child neurology training programs is the ultimate confrontation and comprehension of the differences between the Batten-Mayou, Spielmeyer-Vogt-Sjögren, Jansky-Bielschowsky, Santavouri-Haltia, and Kufs subgroups of this cerebral degenerative condition. Among all these eponyms the contribution of Walther Spielmeyer (1879–1935) (figure 1) stands out. It was Spielmeyer's excellent clinical descriptions and correlative neuropathologic studies that were integral in separating these disorders from the unitarian concept of the amaurotic familial idiocies.

Born in Dessau, Germany, on April 23, 1879, Walther Spielmeyer was the youngest son in a large family. During his grammar school education, his teacher complained that he did not do well, and his piano lessons were curtailed in an effort to force him to devote more time to his studies. Young Spielmeyer considered other pursuits, including the ministry, but decided at an early age to study medicine (Cobb, 1953). His father died while he was in high school in Greifswald, but his mother made sure that he was able to continue his education. While in medical school in Halle he excelled in academics for the first time. He graduated in 1902, having written his dissertation on encephalitis (Hallervorden, 1935); Spielmeyer's teachers claimed that his graduation examination was unequaled in excellence.

While in Halle, he worked under Eduard Hitzig, from whom he learned neurophysiology, and under Karl Heilbronner, with whom he performed dissections of the central nervous system. He also was in contact with Gustav Aschaffenburg, the director of an asylum for mentally ill criminals. Because of this association, Spielmeyer decided to pursue psychiatry. Following graduation, Aschaffenburg recommended that Spielmeyer work with Carl Joseph Eberth in the pathology department at Halle, which he did for the next ten months. Aschaffenburg then recommended Spielmeyer to Alfred

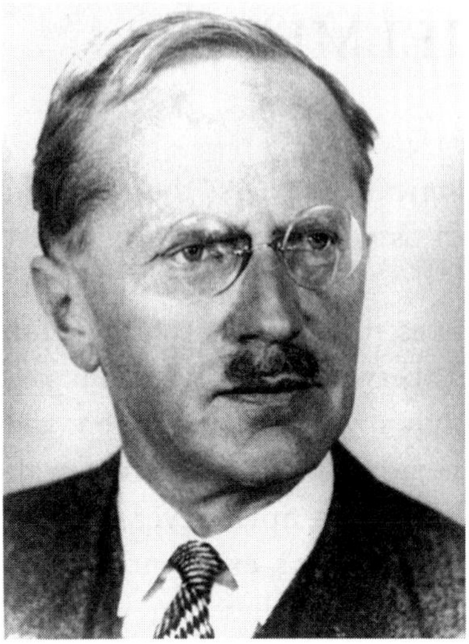

Figure 1. Walther Spielmeyer (1879–1935).

Hoche in Freiburg. There he entered psychiatry as a clinical assistant and continued there until 1912 (Cobb, 1953).

Even though his time with Eberth had been brief, it laid the foundation for his future dedication to pathology. While in Freiburg, Spielmeyer realized that he would not be productive as a clinical psychiatric researcher. This decision was partly based on his feeling that psychiatry was operating on an elemental level. So, while continuing in psychiatry, he also pursued histopathology. His first major work, *Technik der Mikroscopischen Untersuchung des Nervensystems*, was published in 1911 (Spielmeyer, 1911).

The entity recognized as Spielmeyer-Vogt disease, a form of neuronal ceroid lipofuscinosis, had its tangled beginnings in a web of diseases known as amaurotic familial idiocies. Prior to 1896, all diffuse cerebral degenerations were classified in the European literature as "cerebral sclerosis." In the 1890s, Warren Tay, an ophthalmologist, and Bernard Sachs, an American neurologist, described the disease of infancy that now bears their names, with Sachs proposing the term amaurotic family idiocy in an address before the New York Neurological Society meeting of 1896. Károly Schaffer, in 1902, examined the brains of several similarly afflicted infants and noted ballooning of the neurons (Schaffer, 1902).

Almost at the same time, Frederick Batten (1903) described two sisters, ages four and six years, with a striking macular degeneration of the retina and progressive cerebral impairment. Marmaduke Mayou, a London ophthalmologist, the following year described a similar disorder in three of seven children. In 1905 Heinrich Vogt described eight children with a similarly progressive neurological illness with visual impairment. That same year Spielmeyer published his first of several reports in the *Archiv für Psychiatrie und Nervenkrankheiten*. In his first years as a physician, Spielmeyer had encountered a family of four affected siblings following an oldest healthy child, and he noted that the affected children exhibited symptoms at the time of acquiring their permanent teeth ("zur Zeit der zweiten Dentition"). He recorded a clinical triad of epileptic attacks, rapidly progressive dementia, and loss of vision, postulating "luetische Infection des Vaters" (syphilitic infection of the father) (Spielmeyer, 1905). He noted the cortex as the site of primary involvement, with cells containing a granular, pigment-containing substance that distended the cell structure. In 1906 he amplified this early brief notation in an essay published in the *Neurologishes Centralblatt*, including drawings of typical cells as seen after applying the staining techniques of Max Bielschowsky and Franz Nissl (Spielmeyer, 1906). These pathologic observations were of major significance (Zeman, 1970). Until this time, the correlation and interpretation of neuropathologic findings in children with either retardation or cerebral degenerative diseases was quite confusing. Sachs, for example, attributed "arrested cerebral development" as the etiology in the children he described. In 1905, Károly Schaffer, after examining such patients, expressed the point of view that such neuronal swelling was due to a disease-specific cytopathologic process. This hypothesis was in part based on the previous studies of Nissl, who clearly showed specific neuronal changes upon toxin exposure, implying specific neurometabolic disturbances. Spielmeyer's observations of similar neuronal swelling and ballooning strongly supported Schaffer's hypotheses. These abnormal cell processes were known at that time as the Schaffer-Spielmeyer cell process. In fact, Spielmeyer later referred to these cells as a "pathognostic" nerve-cell alteration (1922). However, as Wolfgang Zeman indicated in his extensive review, Spielmeyer, who critically reviewed the literature on familial amaurotic idiocy (1923), also believed in a unifying concept of many of these disorders because of the presence of the abnormal lipid accumulations in these cell processes. Zeman pointed out that Spielmeyer did not recognize that the lipid accumulations did not correlate with the clinical symptoms or degree of neuronal atrophy. Had Spielmeyer realized the importance of this point, he might have deduced that different metabolic defects were present. It was not until the advent of specific biochemical analysis of these lipid accumulations that a major advance in the understanding of these disorders became possible (Zeman, 1970). However, Spielmeyer continued to write about these entities during his life, the last paper on this subject appearing in *Klinische Wochenschrift* in 1933.

As is well known, the early papers of Vogt and Spielmeyer were followed by Batten's descriptive essay of 1914, "Family Cerebral Degeneration with Macular Changes (So-called Juvenile Form of Family Amaurotic Idiocy)." Although clearly describing a different disorder than Tay-Sachs disease, the subtitle of Batten's paper created some obvious confusion. First, Batten was suggesting that his patients were a similar but older variant of infants with Tay-Sachs disease. Second, the same disorder known as Batten-Mayou disease in the English literature was recognized as Spielmeyer-Vogt disease in the European literature. The papers by Jan Jansky (1908) and Max Bielschowsky (1913) describing somewhat younger children with similar symptoms but without retinal changes, the so-called late-infantile form of neuronal ceroid lipofuscinosis, led to further uncertainties about classification of these diseases. The studies of Tage Sjögren in 1931 of 115 patients with "juvenile amaurotic idiocy," with most developing blindness in middle childhood, eventually resulted in this variant of neuronal ceroid lipofuscinosis that became known as the Spielmeyer-Vogt-Sjögren syndrome (Zeman, 1970).

In 1912 Spielmeyer left Freiburg at Emil Kraepelin's request to succeed Alois Alzheimer as director of the Anatomisches Laboratorium der Psychiatrischen und Nervenklinik in Munich. When he initially took the post, the clinic had a small staff, but within six months its ranks swelled to twelve. It was while in Munich, in 1914, that Spielmeyer married. His income was meager as laboratory director, so he held a consulting practice to make ends meet. It was at this laboratory that he began planning his textbook *Histopathologie des Nervensystems*. However, World War I delayed its publication by ten years, until 1922. This text was felt by many to be a milestone in neuropathology, explaining and amplifying the techniques of Nissl, Alzheimer, and others. In gratitude, Spielmeyer dedicated the book to Nissl.

Spielmeyer met his wife, Maria Romano Stark, a young woman of Polish origin, through mutual friends. He had previously seen her picture displayed in the home of Dr. Klarfeld and had fallen in love with the photograph. During their courtship, Maria was hospitalized in a tuberculosis sanitarium, and the two exchanged many letters. Many years passed before the birth of their only child, Ruth, in 1922, whom Spielmeyer adored. The family was close; they vacationed in Italy each summer to visit art galleries, and over Christmas vacations they skied in San Moritz or Galtur, Austria. Spielmeyer did not learn to ski until the age of forty-five but enjoyed it immensely. Maria Spielmeyer was a kind and gentle woman, fluent in many languages. Initially Jewish, she converted to Christianity, although later both became agnostics (Ruth Spielmeyer, personal communication).

During World War I, Spielmeyer was in charge of neurology at the Munich Military Hospital. Here he concentrated on peripheral nerve injuries and their regeneration. In 1917 he was offered a professor's chair of psychiatry at the University of Heidelburg, which he declined in order to work with Nissl in Munich; Spielmeyer and Nissl then collaborated for a year prior to Nissl's death in 1919. Walther Spielmeyer referred to that period as the most beautiful time in his life. Nissl's death followed Korbinian Brodmann's passing in 1918, and that of Alzheimer in 1916. Their deaths left Walther Spielmeyer as the leader of neuropathology in Germany.

At this time, students from all over the world came to study with him. He would review the work of his collaborators and students at least twice each day. He shared his knowledge freely and was tolerant of the lack of knowledge in his students, as well as the opinions of others. However, he could not abide sloppy work.

The work of the clinic soon outgrew its facilities, and in 1928 a new building was financed by the Rockefeller Foundation. Spielmeyer was then appointed director of the Hirnpathologishes Institute at the Deutsche Forshungsanstalt für Psychiatrie, following the death of Kraepelin in 1927. During these years, Spielmeyer's publications were many and diverse. His interests included vascular spasm and ischemic cell changes, the role of vascular spasm in epilepsy, encephalitis, experimental trypansomiasis, pertussis, and tuberous sclerosis. His laboratory coworkers included Lodwick S. Meriwether, Willibald Scholz, Harry M. Zimmerman, Julius Hallervorden, Hugo Spatz, and Houston Merritt. Spielmeyer had as many as 180 coworkers from 25 different countries in his laboratory. Of his laboratory, an American colleague wrote:

It seems odd, but whenever I listen to someone talk about neuropathology, I can immediately detect whether that person came from the Spielmeyer school, for anyone who studied there seems to be involved with thoroughness and keenness. (Scholz, 1961, 106)

In 1929 and 1931, he lectured in the United States, Brazil, England, the Netherlands, and Sweden. Such a tour was a rare honor at that time. He was also awarded the Achucarro Prize in Spain and the Erb Medal from the German Neuropsychiatry Society. He became coeditor of the *Zeitschrift für die gesamte Neurologie und Psychiatrie* in 1916, as well as editor of the *Zentralblatt für die gesamte Neurologie und Psychiatrie* beginning in 1921. He published his last major work, on the anatomy of psychosis, in a volume of Bumke's *Handbuch der Geisteskrankheiten* (Obituary, 1935). At the time of his death, he was editing a three-volume manuscript on neuropathology.

His work was notable for exclusion of any discussion about tumors of the nervous system, because, as he wrote, "davon verstehe ich nichts" (because I do not understand it). In fact, Willibald Scholz noted that if one wanted Spielmeyer to leave the room, they had only to bring up the subject of neoplasms (Scholz, 1961). Another idiosyncrasy was his sensitivity to noise. A standing joke in the laboratory was his reaction to a loud noise and his chastisement of the offender. Professionally, he was a perfectionist and retained an amazing knowledge of minute detail.

As a person, he was described as warm, jovial, and impulsive, but he could be polished and formal as well. He was devoted to his family and held frequent parties in his home, where he would invite guests to display their musical talent; then he sang with his daughter while his wife played the piano. At other times he would be host to professional musicians after concerts.

His final years saw the rise of Hitler's influence over Germany, which he found most disturbing. Initially optimistic, he later became an outspoken critic of Hitler. His wife and daughter left Germany in 1938, only to be separated because of Maria Spielmeyer's country of origin (Ruth Spielmeyer, personal communication). Maria Spielmeyer went to England, where she died in 1940. Their daughter, Ruth, came to the United States in 1939 and presently lives in New York City, where she practices psychiatry.

On February 6, 1935, Walter Spielmeyer died of pneumonia after a brief illness (Kilgour and William, 1935). In accordance with his wishes, he was buried after a quiet funeral at the Munich North Cemetery.

Bernadette M. Lange
LITTLE ROCK. ARKANSAS

REFERENCES

Batten, F. E. 1903. Cerebral Degeneration with Symmetrical Changes in the Maculae in Two Members of a Family. *Trans Ophthal Soc U.K.* 23:386–90.

______. 1914. Family Cerebral Degeneration with Macular Change (So-called Juvenile Form of Family Amaurotic Idiocy). *J Med* 7:444.

Cobb, S. 1953. Walther Spielmeyer. In *Founders of Neurology*, 214–19. Ed. W. Haymaker and F. Schiller. Springfield, IL: Charles C Thomas.

Hallervorden, J. 1935. Obituary. Walther Spielmeyer. *Klin Wschr* 14:590–91.

Kilgour, A. J., and H. W. William. 1935. Obituary. Walther Spielmeyer. *Am J Psych* 92:255–57.

Obituary. 1935. Walther Spielmeyer. *J Nerv Ment Dis* 81:724–25.

Sachs, B. 1896. A Family Form of Idiocy, Generally Fatal and Associated with Early Blindness (Amaurotic Family Idiocy). *NY Med J* 63:697–703.

Schaffer, K. 1902. Über einen Fall von Tay-Sachs'scher amaurotischer Idiotie mit Befund. *Wein klin Rdsch* 16.

Scholz, W. 1961. *Walther Spielmeyer und Sein Schulerkreis, 50 Jahre Neuropathologie in Deutschland, 1885–1935*, 87–107. Stuttgart: Springer-Verlag.

Spielmeyer, Ruth. Personal communication.

Spielmeyer, W. 1905. Über familiäre amaurotische Idiotien. *Arch Psych Nervenkrankh* 140:1038–39.

______. 1906. Über eine besondere Form von familiärer amaurotischer Idiotie. *Neur Centralbl* 25:51–55.

______. 1908. Klinische und anatomische Untersuchungen über eine besondere Form von familiärer amaurotischer Idiotie. *Hist Histopath Grosshirnrinde* (Jena) 2:193.

______. 1911. *Technik der mikroscopischen Untersuchungen des Nervensystem.* Berlin: J. Springer.

______. 1922. *Histopathologie des Nervensystems*. Berlin: J. Springer.

______. 1923. Familiäre amaurotische Idiotie. *Centralbl ges Opthal Grenzgebiete* 10:161–208.

______. 1929. Vom Wesen des anatomischen Prozesses bei der familiaren Idiotie. *J Psych Neur* 38:120–33.

______. 1933. Storungen des Lipiodstoff wechsels bei Erbkrankheiten des Nervensystem. (Am Beispiel der familiaren amaurotischen Idiotie). *Klin Wschr* 12:1273–76.

Zeman, W. 1970. Historical Development of the Nosological Concept of Amaurotic Familial Idiocy. In *Handbook of Clinical Neurology*. Vol. 10, 212–32. Ed. P. J. Vinken and G. W. Bruyn. Amsterdam: North Holland Publishing Co.

JAMES TAYLOR

JAMES TAYLOR (1859–1946) (figure 1) is remembered by most of the neurological world for his supportive role to two of the giants of British neurology, John Hughlings Jackson and William Gowers. However, Taylor himself made a significant contribution to child neurology by recognizing the need for a separate textbook on neurological diseases of children, and with the insights gained from years of experience, he wrote the first British textbook of child neurology (Taylor, 1905).

Taylor was born March 17, 1859, in Forres, Scotland. As an adult his first career was that of a bank clerk, but his interest in medicine lead to his enrollment at the University of Edinburgh, from which he graduated with an M.D. when he was thirty years old. After his graduation he was a resident physician at The Royal Hospital for Sick Children and The Royal Infirmary in Edinburgh.

In 1893, after a sojourn in Germany visiting neurological and ophthalmological clinics, Taylor was recruited by James Samuel Risien Russell, an Edinburgh graduate and friend, to the National Hospital in Queen's Square. While at the National Hospital, he joined the staff of both Queen's Hospital for Children at Bethel Green and Moorfields Eye Hospital. At these institutions he could pursue his two principal interests: the neurological diseases of children and diseases of the eye.

In 1895 Taylor published his best-known paper, a study of subacute combined degeneration and the two clinical subtypes of this disease (Taylor, 1895). In 1899 he helped William Gowers prepare the third edition of *Gowers' Manual of Diseases of the Nervous System*, the bible of British neurology and one of the most complete textbooks of neurology. In spite of the *Manual*'s completeness, Taylor recognized that neurology texts were deficient regarding neurological diseases that affect children. In 1905 he published his own textbook of child neurology, *Paralysis and Other Diseases of the Nervous System in Childhood and Early Life*. In his introduction, Taylor defended the need for "a work which deals with nervous conditions as they occur in young subjects." He asked:

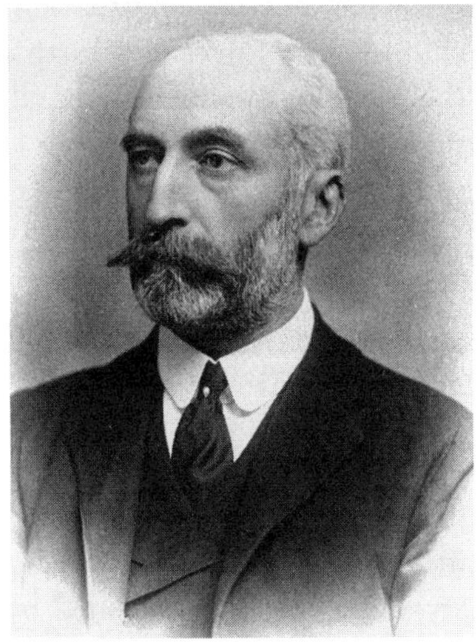

Figure 1. James Taylor (1859–1946).

Do such affections differ so materially from similar or identical diseases affecting adults that it is necessary or desirable to treat of them separately? Undoubtedly there are some points of distinction which justify such separate treatment. (Taylor, 1905)

The first point of distinction he offered was childhood hemiplegia, with its trophic changes and deformities that are not seen in adults. Frequently, there are also "superadded to the paralysis spontaneous movements of various kinds — choreiform, ataxia, athetoid, which are distinctly unusual in adults." Taylor continued:

Another point which will at once occur to the reflective is that whilst in the majority of cases of cerebral paralysis in the adult we are dealing with a diseased condition of the nervous system which is not primarily nervous, but is the result of atheroma and other diseases of vessels, in children such atheroma does not occur except in very rare instances; so that other causes have to be invoked — traumatism, acute inflammation, probably of toxic origin — to account for a condition of cerebral paralysis in the child which in the adult is usually the result of degenerative vascular diseases. (Taylor, 1895, 2)

Taylor then called attention to "the large class of diseases within children, the so called 'birth-palsies'." He insightfully recognized the contribution of structural malformation and maternal conditions as well a birth injury to these palsies. He concluded his justification of a separate text on child neurology by referring to the uniqueness of the inherited childhood neurodegenerative diseases and muscular dystrophies.

The book consists of 512 pages, contains few references and no bibliography, and is illustrated with photographs of patients and pathological specimens. The main sections of the book deal with infections of the central nervous system, especially polio, cerebral palsy, localizing signs in children with tumors, involuntary movements, and spinal cord and muscle diseases. "James Taylor's literary work was distinguished by an easy and graceful style, by wide knowledge and by strict adherence to facts" (Obituary, 1946a).

In 1905 at the age of forty-six, Taylor not only published his book but also married Elizabeth Marion. He met her at the Moorfields Eye Hospital while he was on staff there, and she was an ideal companion in a happy marriage that produced one daughter and lasted for over forty years (Obituary, 1946b).

Taylor received his appointment to Moorsfield's in 1899 and distinguished himself as an authority in neuroophthalmology. He held several important positions in the British Ophthalmological Society, including council member (1894–97), medical secretary (1897–1900), vice-president (1910) and honorary treasurer (1911–18). He was also elected president of the Neurological and Ophthalmological sections of the Royal Society of Medicine.

In 1924, at the age of sixty-five, Taylor resigned his post at the National Hospital but remained affiliated as a member of its Board of Managers. One year before Taylor's resignation, Macdonald Critchley had entered the National Hospital as a house physician. Critchley remembers Taylor as

> *a serious, dignified and rather taciturn man with a slight stoop; he wore a close-cropped beard. It was obvious that he was held in great respect by the other consultants, and they relied very much upon his judgement when academic (as opposed to clinical) problems arose. To us residents, he was rather remote.* (Critchley, 1988)

Taylor was a great admirer and close friend of Hughlings Jackson.

In 1925, after collecting and organizing Jackson's writings, Taylor published a number of his articles in a volume entitled *Neurological Fragments*. Included in that volume is a biographical memoir of Hughlings Jackson written by Taylor. With the editorial assistance of Gordon Holmes and F. M. R. Walshe, Taylor published more of Hughlings Jackson's important papers in a two-volume set, *Selected Writings of John Hughlings Jackson*, in 1931.

James Taylor's last scientific paper appeared in the *British Medical Journal* in 1945 (Taylor, 1945). He died one year later at the age of eighty-seven, having long outlived the famous neurologists who were his contemporaries, men such as William Gowers, Hughlings Jackson, David Ferrier, and Victor Horsley.

Gordon Holmes eulogized James Taylor as a man who

was on the whole reserved, but those privileged to enjoy {his} friendship found in it warmth, sincerity, and unassuming sympathy and readiness to help and advise. Outstanding features of his character were tolerance and practical common sense; that the latter distinguished his professional work was shown by the frequency with which he was consulted by fellow practitioners in search of advice in their own illnesses and those of their relatives. (Holmes, 1946, 969)

F. M. R. Walshe added to Holmes's tribute:

Perhaps, however, those of my generation may feel that his (Taylor's) major contribution to British neurology was the handing on of the tradition and the legend bequeathed by the great figures of the golden age of neurology in this country. (Walshe, 1946)

Paul Larson
TEMPLE, TEXAS

REFERENCES

Critchley, M. 1988. Personal communication. June 26.

Holmes, G. 1946. Obituary. *Brit Med J* 1:969.

______. 1954. *The National Hospital, Queen's Square, 1860–1948*. Edinburgh: Livingstone.

Jackson, J. H. 1925. *Neurological Fragments, with Biographical Memoir by James Taylor and Including the* Recollections *of Jonathan Hutchinson and Charles Mercier*. London: Oxford University Press.

______. 1931. *Selected Writings of John Hughlings Jackson*. Edited for the Guarantors of *Brain* by James Taylor with the advice and asistance of Gordon Holmes and F. M. R. Walshe. London: Hodder and Stoughton, Ltd.

Munk's Roll. 1955. *Archives of the Fellows of the Royal College of Physicians of London*, 398–99. London: Royal College of Physicians.

Obituary. 1946a. James Taylor. *Lancet* 1:945.

Obituary. 1946b. James Taylor. *Brit J Ophth* 30:497–98.

Taylor, J. 1895. On Nervous Symptoms and Morbidity in the Spinal Cord in Certain Cases of Profound Anemia. *Med-Chir Trans* 78:151–70.

______. 1905. *Paralysis and Other Diseases of the Nervous System in Childhood and Early Life*. London: Churchill.

______. 1945. Herpes Zoster and Chicken Pox. *Brit Med J* 2:385–86.

Walshe, F. M. R. 1946. Obituary. James Taylor. *Brit Med J* 2:67–68.

MARTIN THIEMICH

PEDIATRICS BEGAN TO develop as a separate specialty in Germany in the early nineteenth century with the opening of the Berlin Children's Clinic and Polyclinic in 1830 and the first children's hospital in Breslau in 1837. Within twenty to thirty years, most of the larger cities in Germany had such facilities, and they were quickly followed by the widespread appearance of academic centers for research and training in pediatrics. Foremost among the leaders of such centers were physicians such as Edward Heinrich Henoch, whose uncle, Moritz Romberg, was considered the founder of neurology in Germany; Otto Heubner, successor of Henoch at the Charité in Berlin, founder of the Children's Hospital in Leipzig (1891), and one of the major architects of German academic pediatrics; Otto Soltmann, director of the Children's Hospital in Breslau and Heubner's successor in Leipzig; and Adalbert Czerny, Soltmann's successor at Leipzig and one of the most inspiring teachers of pediatrics of his generation (Abt, 1959). A "descendant" of this tradition who trained and worked in Breslau and

Leipzig, and who coauthored the first German textbook of child neurology, was Martin Thiemich.

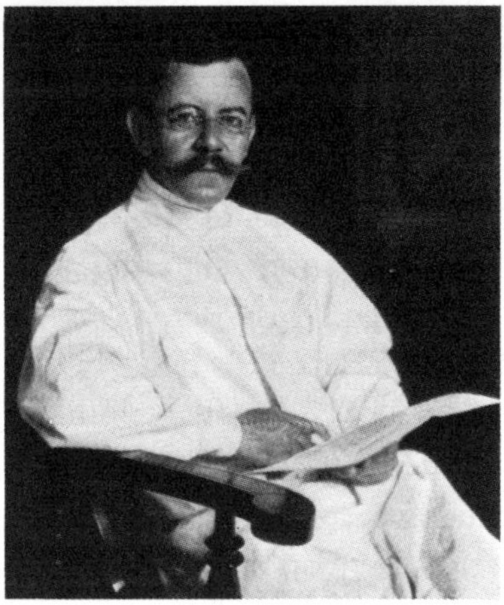

Figure 1. Martin Thiemich (1869–1921). From Weiser, "Martin Theimich," in *Das Leipziger medizinische Viertel* (Leipzig: Verlag von Alfred Lorentz, 1922).

Martin Thiemich (1869–1921) (figure 1) was born in Breslau, Germany. Little is known of his formal education, but he completed his medical studies in Breslau in 1894. He then worked as a clinical assistant in Czerny's clinic at the Children's University Hospital for several years and later served as a school physician from 1902 to 1907. Here he engaged in several studies of infant nutrition, examining several of the available infant formulas and their effects on growth (Thiemich, 1908). Thiemich moved to Magdeburg in 1908, working as physician to the Child Welfare Department until 1913. At that point he was asked to join the staff at the University of Leipzig, where he served as ordinary professor of pediatrics and eventually became director of the Children's University Hospital. As director, Thiemich was busy with administrative activities, concentrating on developing the pediatric service, and at the same time he worked towards developing a School of Nursing. He became intensely involved with many of the social, welfare, and political issues of the day, especially as they affected children. Thiemich, based on his earlier experiences, was very concerned about society's role in providing for the general care and nutrition of children. He worked diligently to bring such problems as the relatively high infant mortality rate in Germany to the public's attention. He argued against believers of social Darwinism, especially as it applied to children from impoverished families, and advocated greater public funding for infant nutrition. These problems were compounded by many of the hardships and relocations that occurred in association with World War I and the obvious effects they had on the health of children. While continuing in these efforts and maintaining his other clinical and administrative activities, Thiemich died on February 16, 1921, at the age of fifty-two.

Thiemich's inaugural presentation in Breslau (1901), "Über ploetzliche Todesfaelle im Kindesalter" ("About Fatalities in Childhood"), remains of topical interest today, as he presented the contemporary understanding of what is still a perplexing and poorly understood disorder, sudden infant death syndrome. This work concerned itself principally with sudden fatalities in early childhood, in which Thiemich examined the contradictions in popular theories of the day, such as laryngospasm, tracheal compression due to thymic hyperplasia, bronchiolitis, swallowing of the tongue, and aspiration of gastric contents. He emphasized the role of inadequate nutrition, due in part to improper milk intake, which he felt caused hyperexcitability of the nervous system and laryngospasm. Malnutrition was common and severe among Thiemich's patients, infant formulas as a substitute for breast milk were then far from being nutritionally complete, and hygienic conditions were poor, even in middle-class families. Infections such as gastroenteritis were common, and many of the infants with "sudden fatalities" probably suffered from severe electrolyte disturbances, especially hypocalcemia (Thiemich, 1900a). Thiemich's major concern, like many pediatricians of his time, was to combat the high rate of malnutrition by trying different feedings mimicking breast milk. One, proposed by Gustav Gaertner, known as "fat milk," was low in casein and thought to be less irritating to the gastrointestinal tract, and was tried by Thiemich (and Bernard Marfan) but was not of particular benefit (Thiemich and Papiewski, 1895–96).

It was at this time that Thiemich's interest in child neurology began to develop. He was particularly interested in the effects of malnutrition on the developing nervous system, especially intellectual and motor function. His study "Über Schaedigungen des Zentralnervensystems durch Ernaehrungsstoerungen im Saeuglingsalter" ("Concerning Affections of the Central Nervous System Due to Malnutrition in the Newborn and Infant") (1900b) found some evidence of spinal cord degeneration, particularly in the anterior horns, but was not specific to any known disease (Thiemich, 1898). He was also quite aware of the relation between malnutrition and problems such as mental retardation, seizures, and behavioral problems (Thiemich, 1911). In addition, Thiemich published works on several common problems of child neurology, including severe developmental disorders (Thiemich, 1900c), hysteria (Thiemich, 1903), toxic encephalopathies (Thiemich and Birk, 1907), psychological testing (Thiemich, 1910), and treatment of seizures (Thiemich, 1913).

One of Thiemich's major contributions to child neurology was his early neurophysiological studies using galvanic stimulation. He evaluated and mapped out the effects of such stimulation on cortical fields in animals, following the studies of previous investigators such as Otto Soltmann, Gustav Fritsch, and Eduard Hitzig (Thiemich, 1902). He observed that the onset of measurable cortical activity correlated chronologically with the time that infantile spasms and other forms of seizures appeared in children. Thiemich disagreed with Soltmann's hypothesis of "physiologic spasmophilia," in which the higher incidence of convulsions in childhood was considered to be the result of a lack of inhibitory cortical activities (Thiemich, 1906). Our current understanding of inhibitory and excitatory neurotransmitters and synaptic development certainly adds credibility to both their speculations. Thiemich correlated the onset of coordinated motor activities at three to four months of age (implying complex cortical activities) with the onset of seizures. He hypothesized a constitutional hyperexcitability of the nervous system rather than a lack of inhibition. He confirmed this hyperexcitability by demonstrating the "facialis phenomenon" (Chvostek sign), elicited by tapping the facial nerve and muscles below the cheekbone, to be more common in children with seizures or other disorders associated with hyperexcitability of the nervous system. He showed that galvanic stimulation of the median nerve in infants and children with seizures triggered muscle contraction at lower stimulus thresholds, suggesting greater excitability compared to normal children (Thiemich, 1900a). Thiemich also used these techniques to examine family members of epileptic children and found them to have greater excitability. He was thus the first to apply some form of quantitative and objective test of neurophysiological function to monitor the "excitability" of the nervous system in children.

Thiemich's major contribution to child neurology came in 1910 with his publication (together with Julius Zappert) of *Die Krankheiten des Nervensystems im Kindesalter* (*The Diseases of the Nervous System in Children*). This work first appeared, in part, as two sections in the

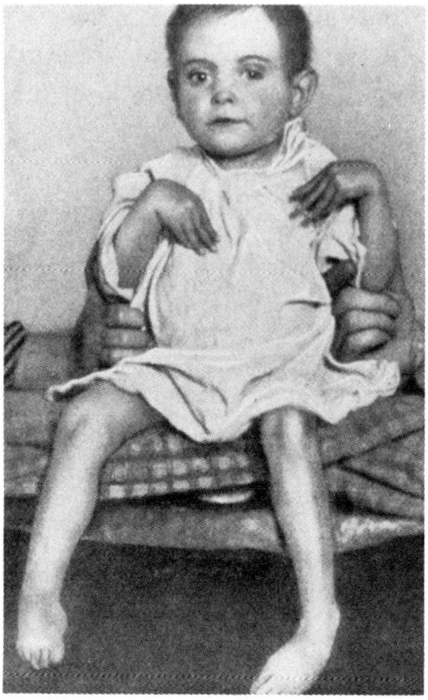

Figure 2. A four-year-old girl with tetany of all extremities with her upper limbs in the "begging" position. Originally figure 46, p. 168, from *Handbuch der Kinderheilkunde* (1910).

second edition of Pfaundler and Schlossmann's *Handbuch der Kinderheilkunde* (*The Diseases of Children*) (Thiemich and Zappert, 1910a) and that same year was issued as a separate monograph of 315 pages entitled *Die Krankheiten des Nervensystems* (*The Functional Diseases of the Nervous System*), with numerous photographs of children, charts, and detailed pathology. Thiemich wrote two of the six sections of this book (1910b). Both of these sections were translated into English and published in 1912 in Pflaunder and Schlossmann's book (Thiemich, 1912a, 1912b). The first, "Functional Diseases of the Nervous System," included discussions on convulsions, tetany, head nodding, chorea, neurasthenia, migraine, tics, hysteria, and psychoses. The second, "Diseases of the Meninges," reviewed diseases of the dura and pia mater; tuberculous meningitis; bacterial meningitis including those due to streptococci, influenza, and meningococci; and "serous" (viral) meningitis. Much of the first section dealt with Thiemich's interest in "hyperexcitability" of the nervous system and how it caused many of these functional nervous system diseases. He emphasized his major observation from earlier studies in which this "hyperexcitability" was transient and maximal during the acute illness, whether it was tetany or convulsions (figure 2). Thiemich disagreed with the prevailing view of Sydenham chorea, as expressed by Karl Bonhoeffer and William Gowers, among others, that the pathology of the disease was in the cerebellum; Thiemich thought it was "more or less diffuse and involving the entire central nervous system." The section on epilepsy included his comments on the correlation between age and type of seizures and a classification of childhood seizures, including grand and petit mal, focal or jacksonian, nodding epilepsy (salaam spasm), and epilepsia procursiva ("forced running"), which could be associated with some alteration of consciousness. A good example of the clarity and succinct style of Thiemich's thinking and writing is his section on childhood migraine:

According to our own experience, and the material in the Breslau Children's Hospital, hemicrania is exceedingly rare in childhood; but this may be due to local conditions. As migraine, probably more so than any other nervous disease, is produced by homologous inheritance, especially from the mother's side, we made a point, in taking the histories, to question the mothers in regard to their own previous diseases, and in innumerable instances were told that they had "head cramp" and all kinds of atypical attacks of headache; but rarely obtained a clear description of unilateral pain.

In view of this state of affairs, we shall have to content ourselves with merely stating the conflicting opinions, leaving the distinction between migraine and nervous headache to individual judgement. In typical cases, such as undoubtedly occur in older children, as shown, for example, by the trustworthy reports of Sachs, the disease is in every respect so like the migraine of adults that we are justified in omitting a more detailed discussion. (Thiemich, 1912a, 356)

Thiemich was an excellent and experienced clinician. For example, his observations about increased intracranial pressure illustrate his expertise in this section from "Diseases of the Meninges":

It is evident that increased intracranial pressure is most trustworthy as a guide in the diagnosis of meningitis when it is directly demonstrable and not deduced from other symptoms, which are themselves capable of various interpretations. This is possible in infants with sufficiently large anterior fontanelles. In fact the daily increasing bulging and tension of the fontanelle is one of the most reliable signs of meningitis in early life, and its value is still further enhanced by the fact that at this time it is difficult to establish other symptoms referred to or rely upon them on account of their ambiguity. Increased tension of the fontanelle, however, is indicative of meningitis only when the child is quiet and if moreover other causes, pneumonia, etc., can be excluded. We have seen a rigid, pulseless fontanelle notwithstanding severe depletion of fluids following diarrhoea in a case of sinus thrombosis, in a septic infant, without meningitis. (Thiemich, 1912b, 387)

This passage is followed by extensive discussions reviewing the current state of knowledge of the different known pathogenic organisms causing meningitis, their clinical presentation, and rare reported cases of survival. One other quote of interest to the modern child neurologist aware of the role of endotoxins and other agents released during infections that potentiate neurologic injury is the following speculation of Thiemich:

Finally of great theoretical interest is the fact now firmly established that in a number of affections (gastroenteritis, pneumonia, etc.), bacteria are demonstrable in the cerebrospinal fluid which may cause symptoms of cerebral irritation of more or less pronounced meningeal type merely by toxic action upon the cortical parenchyma without histologic changes of the meninges or of the superficial supportive structures. It is impossible to say how frequently this occurs or presents clinical symptoms. (Thiemich, 1912b, 426)

Thiemich and Zappert's book was probably the first complete text on child neurology to appear in Germany. Interestingly, it was soon followed by similar but more extensive books written not by pediatricians but by neurologists. The first was the exceptional *Handbuch des Nervenkrankheiten im Kindesalter (Handbook of the Nervous Diseases of Childhood)* published in 1912 by Ludwig Bruns, August Cramer, and Theodor Ziehen. The second, published the same year, was that of George Peritz, entitled *Die Nervenkrankheiten des Kindesalters* (*Nervous Diseases of Children*). The development of both pediatrics and neurology in Germany thus produced, within a two-year period, three comprehensive and thoughtful works in the field of child neurology, with Martin Thiemich being one of the main contributors.

Christine Fischer
HAMBURG, GERMANY

Stephen Ashwal
LOMA LINDA, CALIFORNIA

REFERENCES

Abt, I. 1959. History of Pediatrics. In *Brennemann's Practice of Pediatrics*. Vol. 1, 54–73. Ed. I. McQuarrie and V. C. Kelley. Hagerstown, MD: W. F. Prior.

Bruns, L., A. Cramer, and T. Ziehen. 1912. *Handbuch der Nervenkrankheiten im Kindesalter*. Berlin: Karger Verlag.

Peritz, G. 1912. *Die Nervenkrankheiten des Kindesalters*. Berlin: Fischers Medizinische Buchhandlung.

Thiemich, M. 1898. Über Ruckenmarks degeneration bei kranken Saeuglingen. *Mschr Psych Neur* (Berlin) 3:217–238.

______. 1900a. Über Tetanie und tetanoide Zustaende im ersten Kindesalter. *Jahrb Kinderheilk* (Wien) 1:99–120.

______. 1900b. Über Schaedigungen des Zentralnervensystems durch Ernaehrungsstoerungen im Saeuglingsalter. *Jahrb Kinderheilk* (Wien) 2:895–917.

______. 1900c. Über die Diagnose der Imbecilitaet im fruehen Kindesalter. *Dtsch med Wschr* 26:34–36.

______. 1901. Über ploetzliche Todersfaelle im Kindesalter. Inaugural speech in Breslau, October 22, 1900. *Vierteljahreschrift für Gerichtliche Medizin* (Berlin). 21:300–14.

______. 1902. Über die Funktionsfaehigkeit der motorischen Rindenfelder beim Saeugling. *Zeit klin Med* (Berlin) 45:226–36.

______. 1903. Über Hysterie im Kindesalter. *Jahrb Kinderheilk* (Wien) 58:881–94.

______. 1906. Über Spasmophilie im Kindesalter. *Med Klin Berlin* 2:430–33.

______. 1908. Die Physiologie der Kinderernaehrung. *Med Klin Berlin* 5:181–87.

______. 1910. Methoden zur Intelligenzpruefung beim Kind, speziell beim schwachsinnigen. Prager med Wschr 35:55, 70.

______. 1911. Die Bedeutung einer geordneten Saeuglings-und Kleinkinderfuersorge für die Verhuetung von Epilepsie, Idiothie und Psychopathie. In *Internationaler Kongress zur Fuersorge für Geisteskranke off. Ber.* Vol. 4, 461–63. Halle.

______. 1912a. Functional Diseases of the Nervous System. In *The Diseases of Children*, 295–385. Ed M. Pfaundler and A. Schlossmann. 2d ed. Philadelphia: J. B. Lippincott.

______. 1912b. Diseases of the Meninges. In The Diseases of Children, 386–427. Ed. M. Pfaundler and A. Schlossmann. 2d ed. Philadelphia: J. B. Lippincott.

______. 1913. Über die Behandlung der Kraempfe im fruehen Kindesalter. *Dtsch med Wschr* 39:537–40.

Thiemich, M., and W. Birk. 1907. Über die Entwicklung eklamptischer Zustaende in der spaeteren Kindheit. *Jahrb Kinderheilk* (Wien) 45:16–49, 204–30.

Thiemich, M., and W. Papiewski. 1895–96. Über die Ernaehrung magen-, darmkranker Saeuglinge mit Gaertnerscher Fettmilch. *Jahrb Kinderheilk* (Wien) 41:372–403.

Thiemich, M., and J. Zappert. 1910a. Funktionelle Erkrankungun des Nervensystems. In *Handbuch der Kinderheilkunde.* Vol. 4, 285–375. Ed. M. Pfaundler and A. Schlossmann. Leipzig: F. C. W. Vogel.

______. 1910b. *Die Krankheiten des Nervensystems im Kindesalter.* Leipzig: F. C. W. Vogel.

ALFRED TREDGOLD

ALFRED FRANK TREDGOLD'S (1870–1952) (figure 1) professional life was dedicated to the care of the mentally retarded. His activities encompassed medical care, pathological and clinical research, and social reform. His monument is his textbook, *Mental Deficiency*, which he personally guided through eight editions over a period of forty-four years.

Alfred Frank Tredgold was born on November 5, 1870, of a Lincolnshire branch of an old Cornish family (Tregol or Tragol). He studied at Durham University and the London Hospital, graduating in 1899. He was awarded several prizes and scholarships as an undergraduate, and his first published work appeared during this time, which was a study of the comparative anatomy of ribs in primates (Tredgold, 1897).

The year 1899 also marked Tredgold's marriage to Zoe Hanbury, the daughter of a barrister. This union, which endured almost half a century, proved both happy and fruitful, producing two daughters and one son. Roger Francis Tredgold, born in 1911, followed his father's footsteps, coauthoring the eighth edition of what had become the *Textbook of Mental Retardation.* Roger Tredgold continued as editor through the eleventh edition, which appeared in 1970. He also became a consultant in psychological medicine to University College Hospital.

Immediately following qualification, Tredgold took up the London County Council Research Scholarship in Insanity and Neuropathology. He was able to carry out microscopical work in the Claybury Pathological Laboratory under the supervision of

Frederick Walker Mott, FRS. At the turn of the century, this laboratory was the scene of considerable neuropathological research. Tredgold's distinguished contemporaries there included Charles S. Sherrington and Henry Head. His work also took him to the asylums administered by the London County Council. Subsequently, Tredgold wrote papers on the pathology of amentia, cerebral hemiatrophy, and disseminated sclerosis (Mott and Tredgold, 1899, 1900; Tredgold, 1903a, 1903b, 1904). Thus, his later clinical experience was built on firm neuropathologic foundations.

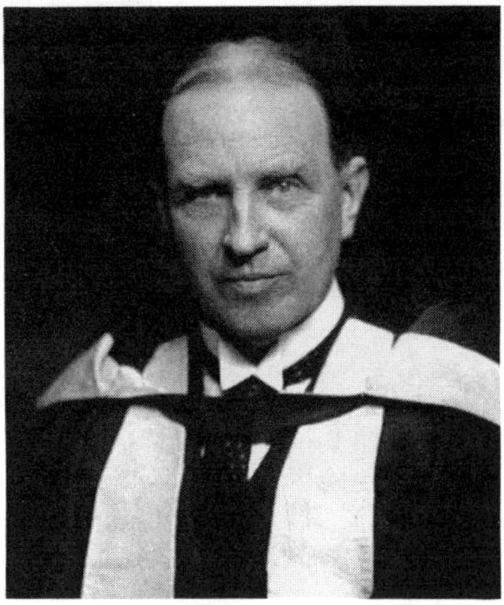

Figure 1. Alfred Tredgold (1870–1952).

When the scholarship expired, Tredgold was obliged to enter general practice in order to support his family. He entered into partnership with William Niall, paying two hundred and thirty pounds for purchase of the practice. Details of subsequent developments are not clear, but it would seem that the partners fell out, for Tredgold sought dissolution of the partnership and return of the purchase fee in 1903. The matter was settled eventually, to Tredgold's disadvantage, after proceedings before both the General Medical Council and the civil courts. The action attracted sufficient attention to be reported in the medical press, where an anonymous commentator suggested that the inexperienced Tredgold had been ill-advised (Mott and Tredgold, 1904).

Despite this setback, he was able to continue his research into mental retardation, and his reputation was such that he was appointed medical expert to the Royal Commission on the Feebleminded in 1905. The findings of this inquiry led to the enactment of the Mental Deficiency Act of 1913, which Tredgold vigorously and publicly supported. The act, subsequently described as "the charter" of the feebleminded (Tredgold, 1927a), attempted to provide comprehensive definitions of mental deficiency, and facilitated the placement of such individuals to special schools, training institutions, and asylums. Prior to this legislation, such matters had

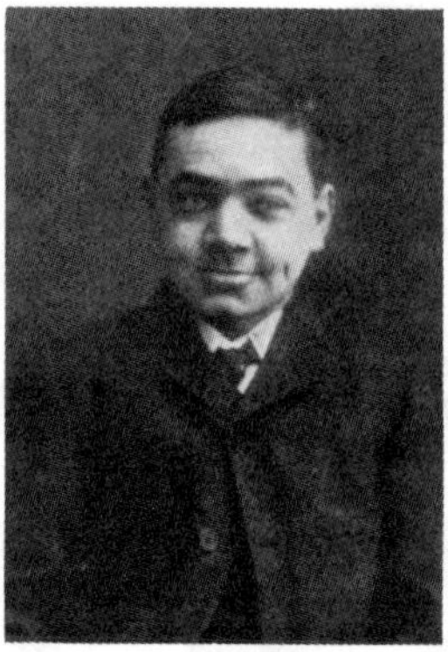

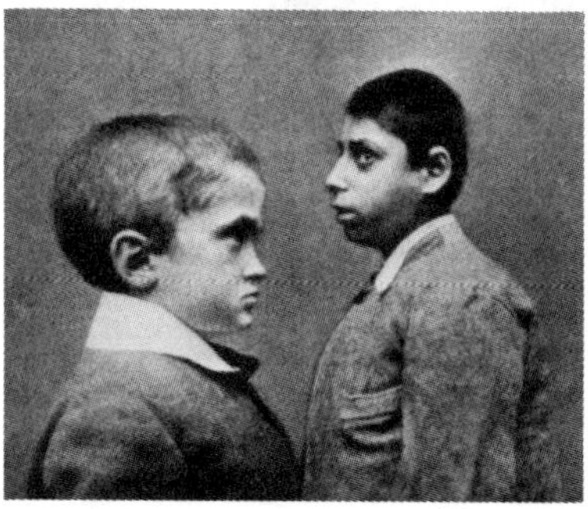

Figure 2. Tredgold's book *Mental Deficiency* contained numerous patient photographs. Figure 45 is that of a 21-year-old male followed for 6 years with "hypertrophy of the brain" and "mild feeblemindedness." Tredgold mentioned that his head circumference was 23-5/8″ (60 cm), height 5 feet and weight 9 stones (126 pounds) with features resembling acromegaly. Figure 46 illustrates two patients with hydrocephalus and microcephaly.

been dealt with under a number of acts, with less than ideal results.

Tredgold's magnum opus, Mental Deficiency (Amentia), first appeared in 1908, published simultaneously in London and New York. A handsome volume of 409 pages, it was divided into 20 chapters and 3 appendices, and illustrated with 29 plates. It was dedicated "To all those persons of sound mind who are interested in the welfare of their less fortunate fellow creatures." The subject of amentia is systemically approached, with opening chapters on incidence, causation, pathology and classification.

Clinical descriptions of the mentally deficient in general are followed by more detailed descriptions of progressively more impaired individuals, designated as the feebleminded, imbeciles, and idiots. Photographs accompany many of these descriptions (figure 2). A number of specific disorders are clearly recognizable, including Down syndrome ("Mongoloid amentia"), Tay-Sachs disease, microcephaly, megalencephaly ("hypertrophy of the brain"), hydrocephaly, hypothyroidism ("cretinism"), syphilis, and tuberous sclerosis. Interestingly, adenoma sebaceum is recognized as occurring in aments in general, but not specifically in tuberous sclerosis.

Tredgold's writing is clear, and bears the hallmark of an experienced and compassionate physician. Note, for example, his caveat regarding the examination of children:

[T]he child himself must be carefully examined. In doing this it is necessary to remember that many children, whether defective or sound, are nervous and ill-at-ease under examination, and I think that a large number of mistakes in diagnosis arise from the inspector's failure to gain the child's confidence. This should be the first concern, and the whole examination must be quiet and deliberate, but kindly and free from the slightest appearance of harshness. The child must, of course, be compared with his compeers in age and social position. (Tredgold, 1908, 139–40)

A celebrated chapter is the fourteenth, entitled "Idiots Savants." This has since been characterized as the first definitive treatment of the subject (Treffert, 1989). Tredgold began by noting the irregular, as well as defective, development of aments, and recognized that in certain individuals specific abilities may attain a "phenomenal" development in the face of generalized retardation. Cases of extraordinary facility with the special senses are described, such as the imbeciles able to identify clothing by its odor, or Langdon Down's patient "whose sense of touch was so delicate and fingers so deft that he could take a page of the *Graphic* and gradually split it into two perfect sheets, as one would peel a postage stamp off an envelope" (Tredgold, 1908, 271).

Other cases of artistic ability, remarkable memory, calculating ability, and mimicry are detailed, such as the case of the cretin Gottfried Mind (1768–1814), whose paintings of cats earned him the soubriquet of "Der Katzen Raphael." The centerpiece of the discussion is the case history, "The Genius of Earlswood Asylum." J. H. Pullen, born in 1835, suffered from profound deafness and had no formal education. He had little speech and was able to write and spell only the names of simple objects. He was inclined to moodiness and violent outbursts at times, and was confined to Earlswood Asylum in 1850.

Pullen was assigned to the carpentry shop and soon became an expert craftsman. In the course of almost sixty years he was enormously productive, accumulating drawings, furniture, and models of ships. He even illustrated the story of his life. His greatest work was the construction, over many years, of a model steamship, which he christened the *Great Eastern*. This was exhibited at the Fisheries Exhibition of 1883, where it won a medal for its designer and builder. The model contained well over a million parts, all manufactured by Pullen. Regrettably, the ship capsized at its first launch, but was subsequently rendered seaworthy.

Another of Pullen's constructions was "a monstrous human form about 13 feet high." By means of internal mechanisms, this fearsome, black-bearded, sword-brandishing effigy could be made to move its limbs or head, or protrude the tongue. As Tredgold stated, this was "calculated to strike terror into the heart of any juvenile beholder" (Tredgold, 1908, 277). Pullen was regarded by Tredgold as suffering from amentia secondary to sensory deprivation, and it was suspected that he suffered no intrinsic mental deficit.

Mental Deficiency concluded with a series of chapters on the legal, social, and rehabilitative aspects of mental retardation. Tredgold stressed the positive value of training for the mentally retarded and also argued strongly for the eugenic approach to prevention of amentia; nor does he neglect long-term care: "How illogical is the system which spends thousands upon the training of mentally defective children, and then turns them adrift to shift for themselves as best they can!" (Tredgold, 1908, 284)

Mental Deficiency was well received by contemporary reviewers, one of whom characterized the book as "a well got-up volume." It rapidly became established as the standard in the field, a position it maintained for many decades.

No doubt the success of *Mental Deficiency* was one factor that enabled its author to enter consultant practice in 1914. In the same year, Tredgold applied for fellowship of the Royal Society of Edinburgh, and was duly elected on the sixth of July. His supporters on that occasion included Edwin Bramwell, Sims Woodward, Sir James Barr and Sir T. S. Clouston (Duncan, 1989).

The outbreak of war in August 1914 found Tredgold, a member of the volunteer movement since 1905, anxious to serve his country. The War Office had no use, it seems, for a neurologist in the Royal Army Medical Corps, and thus Tredgold served as a combatant. Holding a major's commission, he landed at Suvla Bay in the Gallipoli Campaign in 1915 as a battalion adjutant. Following the evacuation of Gallipoli, he was transferred to Egypt and the Sinai, where he served until dysentery and cholecystitis forced his repatriation. He continued to serve as a commander of a territorial depot until the end of the war, when he returned to consultant practice.

In 1919 Tredgold was awarded the M.D. by Durham University. Two years later he became a member of the Royal College of Physicians of London; he was elected a fellow in 1929. In the 1920s Tredgold's reputation was well established, and he held many appointments to institutions for the mentally deficient, in addition to membership in lay societies and his appointment as consultant neurologist to the Royal Surrey County Hospital.

In 1927 he was invited to deliver the annual Galton Lecture to the Eugenics Society, (Tredgold, 1927b). This honor recognized his long commitment to the "eugenic ideal," which had been a constant theme in his contributions to the literature (Tredgold 1909, 1911, 1912a, 1912b, 1920, 1921, 1926, 1927c, 1927d, 1930).

Tredgold saw the application of eugenic principles as essential to the progressive evolution of humanity. He reiterated his view that heredity was the underlying cause of most mental deficiency, and that a "neuropathic diathesis" was the basis for such inheritance. Such a diathesis was supposed to be due to impairment, or devitalization, of the germ cell. Tuberculosis or alcoholism could exert such an influence. The expression of such a diathesis was believed to be modified by environmental factors, hence the advisability of special training.

Tredgold did not believe that simple Mendelian inheritance could explain the observed patterns of mental deficiency in families. He did believe, however, that carriers existed, and that they were responsible for keeping mental disease alive in the community. Thus, the mating of carriers with the healthy was seen as "the greatest danger to the race." The suggested solution to this problem was education. Tredgold saw no role for enforced sterilization as practiced in other parts of the world, but rather sought to prevent propagation by banning the marriage of defectives. He hoped that the eugenic ideal "should have the quality of a sentiment and emotion, like the religious and aesthetic sentiments which had been so widely diffused and had achieved so much" (Tredgold, 1927b).

In 1928 the Department of Psychological Medicine at University College Hospital had grown to the extent that a separate section devoted to "child guidance" was required. Alfred Tredgold was by this time the senior authority in this field in England, and accepted the position of specialist physician and lecturer to the medical school. He continued in this position until mandatory retirement in 1935, when he was appointed consulting physician. This did not mark the end of his active professional life, however. Tredgold continued to lecture at an annual course for school medical officers arranged by the Central Association for the Care of the Mentally Defective, and, of course, he was engaged in the continual revisions of his textbook.

Aged sixty-eight at the outbreak of World War II, Tredgold was clearly not in a position to repeat his role in the 1914–18 conflict. His contribution to the war effort instead took the form of a *Manual of Psychological Medicine for Practitioners and Students* (Tredgold, 1943). Like all his publications, this was a clearly written, practical guide. Although criticized for some unorthodoxies, the book won sufficient acceptance to run through two more editions, one posthumously.

Zoe Tredgold died in 1947, and Alfred Tredgold's health began to decline. He lost the sight in one eye as a consequence of glaucoma, and suffered a gradual decline in his remaining vision. In 1951 he finally gave up work after suffering a stroke. The last year of his life was occupied in the preparation of the eighth edition of his textbook (coauthored with his son), and in tending his garden. He died on September 17, 1952.

Perhaps the finest tribute to Alfred Tredgold, the compassionate physician, is that of an anonymous obituarist: "It was said of him that no parent who visited him came away without feeling comforted and happier. . . . We of his generation think well of him" (Obituary, 1951).

Marc C. Patterson
ROCHESTER, MINNESOTA

REFERENCES

Duncan, W. 1989. Personal communication.

Mott, F. W., and A. F. Tredgold. 1899. Hemiatrophy of the Brain and Its Effects upon the Cerebellum and Spinal Cord. Brain 22:634–36.

______. 1900. Hemiatrophy of the Brain and Its Results on the Cerebellum, Medulla and Spinal Cord. Brain 23:239–63.

______. Niall v. Tredgold. 1904. *Lancet* 2:559–60.

Obituary. 1952. A. F. Tredgold, MD, FRCP. *Brit Med J* 2:726–27.

Tredgold, A. F. 1897. Variations of Ribs in the Primates, with Especial Reference to the Number of Sternal Ribs in Man. *J Anat Physiol* 31:288–302.

______. 1903a. Insanity in Imbeciles. *J Ment Sci London* 49:19–36.

______. 1903b. The Pathology of Insanity. In *Archives of Neurology*. Vol. 2. Ed. F. W. Mott. London: Macmillan Co.

______. 1904. Disseminated Sclerosis: An Account of the Microscopical Examination of Three Cases with Some Observations on the Pathogenesis of the Disease. *Rev Neur Psych Edinburgh* 2:497–527.

______. 1908. *Mental Deficiency (Amentia)*. London: Bailliere, Tindall and Cox.

______. 1909. The Feeble-Minded: A Social Danger. *Eugenics Rev Lond* 1:97–104.

______. 1911. Eugenics and the Future Progress of Man. *Eugenics Rev Lond* 3:94–117.

______. 1912a. Some Medical Aspects of Eugenics. *Med Press Circ* 44:110–12.

______. 1912b. Marriage Regulations and National Family Records. *Eugenics Rev Lond* 4:74–90.

______. 1920. The Problem of Degeneracy. In *Annual Report, 1918*, 547–62. Washington, D.C.: The Smithsonian Institution.

______. 1921. Inheritance and Educability. *Eugenics Rev Lond* 13:339–50.

______. 1926. The Place of Inheritance in Preventive Medicine. *Med Press Lond* n.s. 72:91–94.

______. 1927a. The Abandoned Mental Deficiency Bill. *Brit Med J* 1:77–78.

______. 1927b. Mental Disorder in Relation to Eugenics. *Brit Med J* 1:386.

______. 1927c. Mental Disease in Relation to Eugenics. *Lancet* 1:526–28.

______. 1927d. Mental Disease in Relation to Eugenics. *Eugenics Rev London* 19:1–11.

______. 1930. Note on Sterilization of Mental Defectives. *Ment Welfare* 11:9–14.

______. 1943. *Manual of Psychological Medicine for Practitioners and Students*. London: Bailliere, Tindall and Cox.

Treffert, D. A. 1989. An Unlikely Virtuoso, Leslie Lemke and the Savant Syndrome. *Sciences* (Jan./Feb.):28–35.

HEINRICH VOGT

THE LATE NINETEENTH and early twentieth centuries were an important epoch in the history of neurology. Insight into neurological diseases became possible with the tools of neuroanatomy and neuropathology. In particular, newly discovered tissue-staining methods allowed detailed studies of the brain parenchyma. A wealth of new information on neurological syndromes and their associated pathology was published in many medical and neurological journals. Neurology flourished in Germany at this time, where clinical departments and laboratories attracted physicians from all over the world. It was also during this era that neuropathology became a subspecialty and neurology became more independent but not yet separated from psychiatry. Many articles on child neurology were published in international journals by French, English, and German authors. Among these authors, Heinrich Vogt can be regarded as one of the better-known German neurologists who contributed much to the field of child neurology in the early years of his academic career.

Heinrich Vogt (1875–1957) (figure 1) was born in Regensburg (Scheminsky, 1958). He was raised in a Protestant family and his father was a school teacher. Vogt spent his first years in school in Regensburg and later moved to Augsburg where he graduated from one of the most prestigious Latin gymnasiums in Bavaria, the gymnasium of St. Stephan. Nothing is known about Vogt's academic record, because all school documents were destroyed in 1944 by the disastrous Augsburg bombing. He began medical school in Munich, moved to Heidelberg, and finally graduated from the University of Göttingen. He then returned to Heidelberg and received his doctorate from the University of Heidelberg with his thesis "Paralyse des Nervus Facialis im Anschluß an Otitis media acuta" ("Facial Nerve Palsy after Acute Otitis media") (Vogt, 1899). To his fellow students and teachers, he was known as studious and scientifically oriented, and was destined for a promising academic career. The famous Heidelberg surgeon, Dr. Vincenz Czerny, who sat on Vogt's medical thesis committee in Heidelberg, remarked: "Heute noch unser Schüler, morgen bereits unser Lehrer" (Today one's student, but tomorrow one's teacher) (Scheminsky, 1958).

After receiving his doctorate, Vogt moved to Göttingen, worked at the Anatomy Institute, and was a resident under Professor August Cramer, head of Psychiatry at the University of Göttingen. Vogt spent little time in clinical psychiatry and became a staff member of the Heil und Pflegeanstalt Langenhagen, a large state hospital for the mentally retarded and epileptic near Göttingen. There Vogt began his systematic studies of patients with progressive mental deterioration, or "idiocy," a term commonly used at that time for progressive neurodegenerative disease.

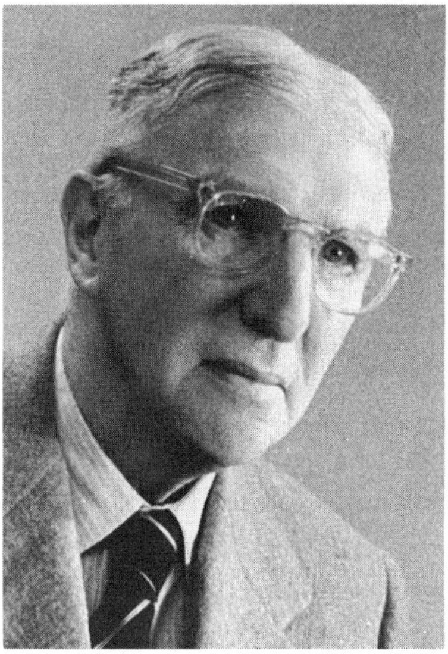

Figure 1. Heinrich Vogt (1875–1957).

Little effort had previously been undertaken on behalf of these patients, for the mentally retarded children locked up in large, understaffed state institutions were of little interest to academically oriented clinicians. Psychiatric patients, on the other hand, were cared for in well-staffed university hospitals and attracted much more attention and interest from the medical profession. Vogt was greatly influenced by the work of Désiré Bourneville (1880) and Alois Alzheimer (1904). Alzheimer's neuropathological studies of "idiocy" and his attempt to correlate the clinical picture with anatomical findings, that is, to divide clinical syndromes by their pathological characteristics, were of great importance to Vogt's work.

Vogt intensively studied several patients with progressive mental deterioration and noticed a peculiar form of "inherited amaurotic idiocy," (Vogt, 1905a) which was different from that described earlier by Warren Tay in 1881. He reviewed all known cases similar to those reported by Bernard Sachs and Tay and compared age of onset, early symptoms, progression of the disease, and inheritance pattern. He described with the accuracy of an astute clinician the cases of three families. In the first family, two of six members were affected; in the second, two out of two members; and in the third, two of ten cases were affected. The clinical course in all of them was remarkably similar (Vogt, 1905a). Visual disturbances were the first symptoms, followed by a decline of intellectual alertness. Other more subtle symptoms were followed by a progressive downhill course that resulted in seizures and loss of reading, writing, and speaking abilities. Social skills declined, a spastic quadriparesis followed, and the patients ultimately died in a vegetative marantic state.

Vogt compared previously published cases with those he found at Langenhagen (Freud, 1893). He separated the patients with amaurosis and progressive mental decline into two groups. First, an early familial infantile form that progressed rapidly from the age of six to twelve months until death. The second, a juvenile form, showed familial occurrence but with slower progression, yet early manifestations of the disease were similar. The onset in this form occurred around age six in previously developmentally and intellectually normal children with the onset of visual disturbances and then a decline of intellectual, motor, and social skills. The first group of patients were of Jewish background without any neurological problems in nonaffected members. The second had an increased incidence of epilepsy, meningitis, and cerebral malformations, as well as a history of heavy alcohol abuse on the paternal side.

Vogt announced the pathological findings at the end of his paper which was soon to be published but a month later in November, 1905, at a meeting in Karlsruhe, Walther Spielmeyer reported the characteristic neuronal inclusions of the disease (Spielmeyer, 1905) that Vogt had described before Vogt had a chance to publsih his paper. Rightfully, both author's names should serve as the eponym for this disease, which is one of the neuronal ceroid lipofuscinoses, although Vogt deserves to have his name placed before Spielmeyer's. Vogt-Spielmeyer disease, or juvenile amaurotic familial idiocy, should be the correct name, instead of Spielmeyer-Vogt disease.

In 1907 Vogt was named Professor of Psychiatry in Göttingen. Two years later, he moved from Göttingen to Frankfurt am Main and became director of the Department of Psychiatry in the

Senckenberg Institute at the University of Frankfurt, which, at that time, was chaired by Ludwig Edinger.

Vogt had gained a considerable reputation among his colleagues Constantin von Monakow, Otto Binswanger, and Alois Alzheimer. He had published articles on various child neurology topics and, together with Walter Weygandt (1906), edited a journal for the research of juvenile imbecility (*Zeitschrift für Erforschung des Schwachsinns*), which can be regarded as a forerunner of the current child neurology journals. His main interests in writing were on cerebral malformations (Vogt, 1905b, 1906a, 1906b, 1908a, 1911), childhood epilepsy (Vogt, 1907a, 1908b, 1908c, 1910a, 1915), tuberous sclerosis (Vogt, 1905c, 1907b, 1908d, 1910b), and the institutional care of epileptics and the developmentally retarded (Vogt, 1908c, 1909b, 1912). He was asked by Monakow to review the Zurich cases of cerebral malformations and he published a comprehensive and detailed study in the Anatomical Institute's bulletin. Vogt was studying these various conditions because he was searching for the morphological substrate of the clinical syndrome of idiocy. He found it in the abnormal inclusions of the ganglia cells of the disease that bears his name, in the neurons of tuberous sclerosis patients and in the abnormal cytoarchitecture of cerebral malformations. Vogt's second major contribution in this regard is that he is credited with the first report linking together the triad of mental retardation, adenoma sebaceum, and seizures in tuberous sclerosis (1907b).

In 1907 Vogt was asked to deliver the principal address on epilepsy at the annual meeting of the Psychiatric Society. In 1910 his book entitled *Epilepsie im Kindesalter* was published. He wrote a chapter on inherited defects of developmental disorders of the brain in Max Lewandowsky's *Handbook of Neurology* in 1912 and in 1915 he also wrote a chapter on epilepsy in the *Handbook of Psychiatry*. Vogt left academic neurology and Frankfurt in 1911 and became director of a neurological sanatorium, the Nerotal, in Wiesbaden. He remained there from 1911 until 1925. His last publication on the subject of neurology was on war injuries of the nervous system.

In 1925 Vogt left Wiesbaden and settled in Bad Pyrmont where he opened a private practice in balneology (the science of the therapeutic uses of bathing). A change in his medical career had occurred. He devoted the remainder of his life to research and academic work on medical hydrology. He founded the first research institute on medical hydrology in Breslau and became its first chairman. He edited a balneology journal and a handbook on balneology. Vogt lost almost everything after World War II when Breslau became part of Poland. He moved back to Bad Pyrmont, worked in his private practice, and died in Bad Pyrmont on September 24, 1957.

Heinrich Vogt had a remarkable medical career. Today his balneological studies are well known and regarded as pioneer work (Scheminsky, 1958). When he died, surprisingly no obituary appeared in any neurological journal. Vogt left academic neurology early in his medical career, although he had established himself as a well-known and respected neurologist. His reasons for leaving remain unclear. Those who knew him could give no clue. Vogt himself never talked about this to his students and residents.

Vogt's contributions to child neurology are as important as those that he made later in his career to medical hydrology. His textbook on childhood epilepsy, the chapter on epilepsy in the *Handbook of Psychiatry*, as well as his writings on cerebral malformations and tuberous sclerosis, were among the most comprehensive reviews of these topics in his time.

Vogt advocated the establishment of juvenile courts. These courts were to be staffed with teachers, social workers, and educators to serve as consultants in court procedures concerning retarded juvenile delinquents (Vogt, 1912). He felt strongly that society had a humanitarian obligation to care for the disadvantaged. This was in contrast to a public trend that regarded the handicapped as being a burden on society, a trend which found its criminal highlights with the Nazi euthanasia program in World War II.

Vogt certainly would be much better known in neurology if he had remained in the field and his inclusion as a founder of child neurology is certainly appropriate. His last university position in neurology was in Frankfurt. The directorship of the Senckenberg Institute in the Department of Psychiatry's neuropathological laboratory was a prestigious university post, once headed by Alzheimer. His reasons for leaving Frankfurt to become chief of a neurological sanatorium in Wiesbaden are not known. Wiesbaden was a balneological center, much frequented by Germans and Europeans. It was there that his medical career took its turning point. Nevertheless, his early recognition of one of the forms of neuronal ceroid lipofuscinoses, his clinical studies of childhood epilepsy, and his clinical and neuropathological investigations of tuberous sclerosis are major contributions to the field of child neurology.

Harold Reich
AUGSBURG, GERMANY

Adolf Weindl
MUNICH, GERMANY

ACKNOWLEDGMENTS

I am indebted to Professor A. Ewers and Dr. J. Wiesner of the private Vogt Institute in Bad Soden for their help and advice.

REFERENCES

Alzheimer, A. 1904. Einiges über die anatomischen Grundlagen der Idiotie. *Centralbl Nervenheilk Psych* 27:497

Bourneville, D. M. 1880. Contribution à l'étude de l'idiotie. Sclérose tubéreuse des circonvolutions cérébrale, idiotie et épilepsie hemiplégique. *Arch neur* 1:81–91.

Freud, S. 1893. Über familiäre Formen von cerebraler Diplegie. *Neur Centralbl* 15:16.

Spielmeyer, W. 1905. Über familiäre amaurotische Idiotien. *Arch Psych Nervenkrankh* 140:1038–39.

Scheminsky, F. 1958. Heinrich Vogt. *Zeit angew Bäder-Klimaheilk* 5:1–11

Tay, W. 1881. Symmetrical Changes in the Region of the Yellow-Spot in Each Eye of an Infant. *Trans Ophth Soc U. K.* 1:55–57.

Vogt, H. 1899. *Die Paralyse des Nervus facialis im Anschluß an Otitis media acuta.* Heidelberg: Inaugural Dissertation.

______. 1905a. Über familiäre amaurotische Idiotie und verwandte Krankheiten. *Mschr Psych Neur* 18:161–71, 310–57.

______. 1905b. *Über die Anatomie, das Wesen und die Entstehung mikrocephaler Mißbildungen, nebest Beiträgen über die Entwicklungsstörungen der Architektonik des Zentralnervensystems.* Wiesbaden: J. F. Bergmann.

______. 1905c. Über einen Fall von kongenitalen Adenoma sebaceum. *Mschr prakt Derm* 10:5.

______. 1906a. Zur Pathologie und pathologischen Anatomie der verschiedenen Idotieformen. Teil 1: Familiäre Idiotie. *Mschr Psych Neur* 22:403.

______. 1906b. Der Mongolismus. *Zeit Erforsch jugendl Schwachsinns* 2:1.

______. 1907a. Die klinische Gruppierung der Epilepsie. *Allg Zeit Psych* 64:421.

______. 1907b. Zur Diagnostik der tuberösen Sklerose. *Zeit Erforsch jugendl Schwachsinns* 2:1

______. 1908a. Über die Idotie und einige anatomische Fragestellungen zu ihrer Erforschung. *Münch med Wschr* 55:1559.

______. 1908b. Epilepsie und Schwachsinnszustände im Kindesalter. *Arch Kinderheilk* 48:321.

______. 1908c. Fürsorge für Idioten, Epileptiker und geistig Minderwertige. Dritter Intern. Kongreß für Irrenpflege (Wien). *Dtsch med Wschr* 34:2101.

______. 1908d. Zur Pathologie und pathologischen Anatomie der verschiedenen Idiotieformen. Teil 2: Tuberöse Sklerose. *Mschr Psych Neur* 24:106.

______. 1909a. Über Fälle von Jugendirresein im Kindesalter. *Allg Zeit Psych* 66:542.

______. 1909b. Pathologie und pathologische Anatomie der Idiotie. 2: Tuberöse Sklerose. *Mschr Psych Neur* 25:123.

______. 1909c. Zur Diagnostik der tuberösen Sklerose. *Zeit Erforsch jugendl Schwachsinn* 2:1.

______. 1910a. *Epilepsie im Kindesalter mit besonderer berücksichtigung erzieherischer, unterrichtlicher und forensischer Fragen.* Berlin: S. Karger.

______. 1910b. Jugendliche Lügnerinnen. *Zeit Erforsch jugendl Schwachsinnes* 3:394.

______. 1911. Familiäre amaurotische Idiotie, histologische und histopathologische Studien. *Arch Kinderheilk* 51:1.

______. 1912. Die angeborenen Defekte und Entswicklungsstörungen des Gehirnes. In *Handbuch der Neurologie.* Vol. 3. Ed. Max Lewandowsky. Berlin: J. Springer.

Vogt, H., and A. Fredenthal. 1912. *Becker sowie Polligkeif Das Jugendgericht Frankfurt am Main* Berlin: J. Springer.

______. 1915. Epilepsie. In *Handbuch der Psychiatrie.* Vol. 1. Ed. Gustav Aschaffenburg. Leipzig and Wien: Deuticke.

The Growth and Recognition of Child Neurology as a Separate Entity

THE MIDDLE TWENTIETH CENTURY

1940 – PRESENT

OVERVIEW

IN 1923 JUST 10 PERCENT of American physicians were specialists; by 1940 the number had increased to 20 percent, and by 1985 to 88 percent (Halpern, 1988, 2). Similar trends reflecting an increase in subspecialization were also occurring worldwide. Pediatrics differs from the majority of medical specialties, which have scientific and technical innovation as their origins. Most specialties developed from the treatment of diseases of specific organ systems, for example, neurology, ophthalmology, and otolaryngology; or from the use of very specific technologies, such as radiology or anesthesiology. In contrast, pediatrics' evolution was strongly influenced by ideological currents and social reform movements outside the medical profession (Halpern, 1988, 9).

The emerging speciality of pediatrics tended to imitate older, more established specialties in regard to its development. Late nineteenth-century pediatric consultants built their reputations for expertise in children's disease and infant feeding through appointments in foundling homes, children's hospitals, and medical colleges. They used their prestige to attract private patients. Later they attended the child and infant welfare clinics and participated in the child hygiene movements. Within a short period of time delivery of health care was transferred from a free government service to fee-for-service practice. As noted by Sydney Halpern:

Routine medical supervision of well babies and children became an established professional service during the third and fourth decade of the twentieth century. Its creation placed physicians in a fundamentally new relation to the American family. Specialists now counseled parents on the parameters of normal child development and dispensed advice on proper methods of child hygiene and training. They examined healthy youngsters on a periodic basis, frequently during infancy and at regular intervals through the remainder of childhood . . . . But never before had there existed a discrete professional service monitoring the growth and development of individual children. Nor had professional advice to parents been so systematically organized. (Halpern, 1988, 13)

This growth in the demand for pediatricians occurred in conjunction with the rapid growth of academic pediatrics. In 1922 only ten American medical schools had full-time salaried posts in pediatrics. By 1947 forty-six schools had at least one full-time pediatric professor and by 1959 there were over seven hundred professors of pediatrics in academic positions.

Pediatric subspecialties began to develop in the 1930s and 1940s, more than half a century after the organization of pediatrics itself. Pediatrics developed before the modern era of medical science and outside the medical school system. In contrast, subspecialties such as child neurology developed within the framework of academic departments of medical schools and universities. Pediatrics derived its impetus from social-based reform spurred by issues of social and public health. The subspecialties, however, developed from scientific and technical advances and innovations. By 1986 the American Board of Pediatrics had established subspecialty board certification in cardiology (1960), hematology and oncology (1973), nephrology (1973), neonatal and perinatal medicine (1974), endocrinology (1976), diagnostic laboratory (1984), immunology (1984), critical care medicine (1985), and pulmonary disease (1985) (Halpern, 1988, 110).

PEDIATRICS

The progress in pediatrics in the past five decades has clearly been extraordinary and only some of the major advances can be highlighted. What is striking is the transition between the appearance of new technology, its rapid use for understanding disease, and its almost immediate application to therapy. Secondly, the global interchange of scientists and clinicians interested in pediatric problems, frequently with governmental support, has accelerated these phenomenona.

Many of the specific viral agents causing pediatric infectious diseases, such as hepatitis, coxsackie, and echovirus, were discovered during the 1940s. One of the major advances was that by John Enders, Thomas Weller, and Frederick Robbins, who first grew polio virus in tissue culture (1949). This led to the isolation of many different viral pathogens but, more importantly, was instrumental in the future development of vaccines such as the inactivated (1954) and live attenuated (1962) polio virus vaccine, the live attenuated measles vaccine (1963), and the rubella vaccine (1966). The role of specific viral agents as pathogens of many childhood disorders was established, as was the concept of viral-induced fetal teratogenesis when maternal rubella infection was shown to cause congenital cataracts (1941). The introduction of sulfonamides and penicillin was followed by a veritable explosion of newer and more potent antibiotics whose effectiveness was enhanced by advances in pharmacology, microbiology, and bacterial genetics. Tuberculosis could now be effectively treated with the introduction of streptomycin (1944), para-aminosalicylic acid (1946), isoniazid (1951), and rifampin (1965).

Of fundamental importance and long-term significance were the extraordinary advances in genetics. It is hard to believe that it was only in 1956 that Joe Tjio and Albert Levan showed conclusively that there were only forty-six chromosomes in man, and that in 1959 Jerome LeJeune and his Parisian colleagues described Trisomy 21, the chromosomal defect in Down Syndrome. It is now estimated that approximately 10 percent of patients with developmental retardation have major chromosomal defects. This estimate will surely increase over the next several decades. The first karyotyping of amniotic fluid cells was reported in 1966 and the following year Cecil Jacobson and Robert Barter suggested its use in genetic counseling for both chromosome analysis and cell culture techniques to test for enzyme deficiencies causing metabolic disorders. Recombinant DNA technology has led to the antenatal diagnosis of thalassemia, sickle cell disease, Duchenne muscular dystrophy, and other disorders, by the use of restriction fragment-linked polymorphism techniques.

Therapeutically, this technology has led to the production of human growth hormone, insulin, somatostatin, and interferon. The mapping of the human genome will ultimately change the approach to the diagnosis and treatment of many pediatric diseases.

Over the past several decades, neonatology has become a strong, hospital-based, technology stimulated, and labor-intensive subspecialty that has had a dramatic effect on all areas of pediatrics and is, in part, responsible for the creation of pediatric intensive-care units for older chlidren. Both have had a substantial impact on the salvaging of very young patients' lives as well as the victims of acute injury and other serious medical problems. They have also created an important role for the pediatrician, that of medical management of post-surgical care.

One of the early advances in the care of the newborn was the discovery of the cause of erythroblastosis fetalis (1939) and the identification of the Rh system of red blood cell antigens (1940). Alfred Hart performed the first successful exchange transfusion in 1925, and in 1946 Louis Diamond and colleagues introduced the technique of umbilical vein catheterization. Later, specific immune gammaglobulin was used to prevent this disorder. Retrolental fibroplasia was recognized by Theodore Terry (1942) and its relation to excessive and prolonged oxygen exposure was suggested by Dame Kate Campbell (1951). Respiratory distress syndrome was described as a specific pathologic entity in 1953 and a deficiency of pulmonary surfactant was believed responsible for this disorder. Several practical advances included the development of the APGAR score by Virginia Apgar (1952), the use of phototherapy for treatment of hyperbilirubinemia (1958), the development of sophisticated ventilators for the management of respiratory diseases in the 1970s, the introduction of hyperalimentation, and, more recently, the use of extracorporeal membrane oxygenation. Neonatal screening programs were established for phenylketonuria in the 1960s and later for hypothyroidism (1974).

Metabolic disorders described in the past forty years are too numerous to review, as they span many entities. The primary idea of specific gene-mediated enzyme deficiencies associated with either structural or functional changes in mitochondria, lysosomes, peroxisomes, and other cell constituents has led to the discovery not only of many new diseases but the realization that phenotypic expression can be due to more than one type of enzyme abnormality. Likewise, disease expression has been shown to be related to tissue or organ-specific enzyme deficiencies, making both diagnosis and the engineering of specific treatments much more complex than initially anticipated.

Pediatric cardiology and cardiovascular surgery have made enormous strides since the end of World War II. André Frédéric Cournand performed the first cardiac catheterization in infants in 1949. Surgical milestones included the first ligation of a patent ductus arteriosus (1938) and the first successful ventriculoseptal defect closure (1955), followed over the next thirty years by increasingly more complex surgical procedures leading to cardiac transplantation. These were all made possible by using profound hypothermia, prolonged circulatory arrest, the membrane pump oxygenator, and advances in transplantation immunology. In the past decade cardiac ultrasound has, for the most part, replaced angiography for the evaluation of congenital heart disease in children.

The fields of hematology, oncology, and immunology hold a unique place in pediatrics. The therapeutic advances during the past forty years have allowed more optimistic treatment goals. Also recognized as important is the general application of the therapeutic model of nationwide multicenter clinical trials that has been pioneered by those working in the fields of chemotherapy and radiation oncology. Many of these advances can be traced to the investigations of Sidney Farber and his colleagues, who showed that the folic acid antagonist, Aminopterin, induced remission in childhood leukemia (1948). In hematology many milestones have been recorded. Thomas Cooley described thalassemia in 1925 and later stressed the genetic implications of this disorder and its usefulness as a model for other pediatric diseases. Iron deficiency anemia and congenital aplastic anemia and their clinical consequences were both reported in the 1930s. Linus Pauling recognized the changes in the structure of hemoglobin that ultimately led to the understanding of sickle cell disease (1949). Over the next decade other disorders were described such as folic acid responsive megaloblastic anemia, glucose-6-phosphate deficiency, and chronic granulomatous disease of childhood. Major advances were made in the treatment of hemophilia, and bone marrow transplantation has been successful in the treatment of immunodeficiency syndromes, Wiskott-Aldrich syndrome, and aplastic anemia. Clinical immunology began with the recognition of several new diseases, including agammaglobulinemia (1952), transient hypogammaglobulinemia of infancy (1956), and DiGeorge syndrome (1965). Two clinical milestones that have had profound impacts are the development of transplantation immunology and the creation of monoclonal antibodies. Transplantation of kidneys (1960s), livers (1970s), and hearts (1980s) in children have achieved high rates of long-term acceptance, due in large part to the availability of improved immunosuppressive agents and better understanding of the mechanisms of tissue rejection and tolerance. The development of monoclonal antibodies for immunodiagnosis, tumor imaging, and the evaluation and treatment of infection and other diseases has and will continue to profoundly change the way children are evaluated and treated.

One of the major therapeutic advances over the past forty years has been the use of corticosteroids for the treatment of many different pediatric diseases. A sampling of these diseases includes myasthenia gravis, polymyositis, cerebral edema, asthma, isoimmune thrombocytopenia, collagen vascular diseases, nephrotic syndrome, hepatitis, allergic and hypersensitivity reactions, skin diseases such as eczema, inflammatory eye disorders, and adrenal insufficiency.

The problems and issues in public health and social welfare have changed during the past fifty years. The large-scale studies of water fluoridation in the late 1940s led to its widespread use for prevention of dental caries. At the same time, Benjamin Spock's *Common Sense Book of Baby and Child Care* (1946) made available to millions of families the collective wisdom of generations of pediatricians. It also created a new industry. Parents now have access to a wide variety of books, magazines, and videotapes on all aspects of pediatrics. More serious problems were also brought to the attention of the pediatric community and to the public. The battered child syndrome, a term used by Henry Kempe in 1961, now seems epidemic in many communities. Recognition of the Sudden Infant Death Syndrome in the 1960s was initiated by a series of papers in the 1940s and 1950s by Jacob Werne and Irene Garrow, who disproved suffocation as the cause of this problem. Newer concerns associated with maternal smoking, substance and alcohol abuse, the effects of higher divorce rates, and the lack of access to health care for many children has created problems of an immense nature without straightforward solutions.

At the turn of the century there were perhaps fifty physicians in the United States whose careers were solely devoted to the care of children. Now, there are over ten thousand members of the American Academy of Pediatrics. The growth of the specialty in many other areas of the world has been as strong. This growth in the United States was stimulated by the formation in 1931 of the Society for Pediatric Research and the National Science Foundation in 1950. The National Institute of Child Health and Human Development was established in 1961 and the journal *Pediatric Research* began publication in 1967.

NEUROLOGY

By the 1940s knowledge gained in the neurosciences was considerable. One would suspect, however, that those practicing neurology or engaged in research would have been quite impressed by the dramatic and diverse advances that followed. This is best exemplified by the Nobel Prize being awarded to neuroscientists twenty-five times since 1944. In fact, it is generally agreed upon that neurology, and subsequently child neurology, truly became independent disciplines only in the past several decades.

Investigations of brain cytoarchitecture were greatly enhanced by electron microscopy. Also of importance were the cortical ablation studies by John Fulton and others in determining frontal lobe function. One of the major landmarks in the neurosciences was the elucidation of the role of inhibitory and excitatory neurotransmitters in synaptic transmission. Although the concept of chemical neurotransmission had been proposed by Otto Loewi in 1921, the delineation of the specific neurotransmitters has been relatively recent. Determination of the synaptic pathways and regional content of the different neurotransmitters has led to better understanding of their regulatory function of behavior, learning, memory, coordination, and consciousness.

Prior to 1940 the field of neuroendocrinology was virtually nonexistent, but over the past fifty years discoveries in this area revolutionized our understanding of the interaction between the nervous system and somatic growth and function. Although details are too numerous to cite, major accomplishments include: the identification and partial characterization of many of the pituitary hormones, recognition of hormonally mediated feedback, discovery of the hypophysial portal system, and the phenomena of neurosecretion. Over the past twenty-five years, amino acid sequences of these agents have been delineated and now radioimmunoassays measure and genetic engineering techniques produce several of these hormones.

The dividends for years of research in neurochemistry were realized as entirely new categories of diseases were reported. In many areas neurochemistry supplanted neuropathology, particularly as different forms of lipid, glycogen, and mucopolysaccharide disorders were elucidated. The recognition of lysosomal and mitochondrial dysfunction, for which Christian de Duvé won the Nobel Prize in 1974, helped clarify the progressive nature of many of these conditions. The realization that specific enzyme deficiencies could be expressed in varied clinical presentations widened the search for such disorders in patients of different age groups with an array of neurological symptoms. Genetic counseling programs were introduced as assays for these enzyme deficiencies were found, allowing both prenatal screening and fetal diagnosis. Attempts at replacement therapy by use of liposomes or bone marrow transplantation have yet to reverse or ameliorate neurological progression of these conditions. As recombinant DNA technology is applied, specific treatments presumably will become available.

Many advances occurred in the fields of neurophysiology and epilepsy. Alan Hodgkin, Andrew Huxley, and John Eccles shared the Nobel Prize in 1963 for their investigations of the physiology of the nerve action potential. In 1964 Hiroyuki Matsumoto and Cosimo Ajmone-Marsan described the paroxysmal depolarization shift and in 1968 David Prince described the presence of inhibitory post-synaptic activity at the periphery of seizure foci. In 1959 Charles Symonds suggested that gamma-amino-butyric acid might serve as a natural anticonvulsant and since then its role as an inhibitory neurotransmitter has been established. Under the guidance of Henri Gastaut, a commission of the International League Against Epilepsy met in 1964 and developed a new classification of epilepsy. This was modified by an international commission appointed by the World Federation of Neurology and several other groups and the new classification was published in 1970. Among the anticonvulsants introduced, many continue to be effective, such as mephenytoin (1947), primidone (1954), carbamazepine (1954), ethosuximide (1960), diazepam (1968), and sodium valproate (1973). Surgical treatment of epilepsy was proven beneficial by Wilder Penfield and Herbert Jasper from Montreal in the 1950s and by Murray Falconer and his colleagues in England in the 1960s. The use of depth electrode and telemetry techniques by neurosurgeons and neurologists has, over the past two decades, enhanced patient selection for such surgical treatment.

Research in behavioral neurology and higher cortical functions advanced in many directions. The early studies of James Papez were instrumental in our current understanding of temporal lobe and hippocampal function (1937). Later, Heinrich Klüver and Paul Bucy showed how bilateral temporal lobectomies in monkeys effected emotional and cognitive function. James Olds and Peter Milner investigated the effects of self stimulation of the limbic system in rats. Their studies suggested that this area was important in the regulation of emotions and behavior (1954). The differential split-brain functions of the two hemispheres were derived from Roger Sperry's psychological investigations of patients who had undergone sectioning of the corpus callosum (1974). The importance of amphetamines, opioid peptides and other pharmacologic agents continued to be studied and were clinically important as they led to the development of sedatives, tranquilizers, CNS stimulants, muscle relaxants, and analgesic agents. The concepts of neural plasticity and regeneration of the brain altered basic concepts of developmental neurobiology.

The clinical therapeutic gains since 1940 have also been dramatic. Treatment of myasthenia gravis and Parkinson's disease are perhaps the most notable. Other contemporary neuropharmacological triumphs included the use of a variety of dopamine blocking agents for the treatment of affective and tic disorders and the treatment of depression with medications that blocked norepinephrine uptake or inhibited monoamine oxidase activity. Such advances had another and more profound effect: it became clear that many emotional disorders were genetically or organically determined. The separation between neurology and psychiatry began to lessen.

Antibiotic therapy lowered the morbidity and mortality of acute central nervous system bacterial infections. Also impressive was the reduction in mortality of general paresis by 94 percent and tabes dorsalis by 86 percent between 1916 and 1954. In neurovirology, several other milestones are worth noting, including the development in the 1970s and 1980s of antiviral chemotherapeutic agents against herpes simplex encephalitis. Another important event was the identification of several different slow virus infections of the nervous system, such as subacute sclerosing panencephalitis (1933), Kuru disease (1957) and Creutzfeldt-Jakob disease (1968). Also of importance was the reduction in the incidence of subacute sclerosing panencephalitis by the introduction of measles vaccine and of the encephalopathy associated with pertussis infection by immunization. Another and more recent notable phenomenon is the evolving recognition of the neurological complications of acquired immunodeficiency syndrome (AIDS).

Among the most practical and far-reaching achievements have been those made in neuroradiology. Myelography, discography, and percutaneous angiography were introduced in the late 1940s and early 1950s. These advances now seem of less importance compared to the development of computer tomographic scanning, positron emission, magnetic resonance and ultrasound imaging, interventional radiology, and radiation therapy.

A better understanding of many acute neurological disorders has created an important role for neurology in the emergency room and intensive care unit. The role of the brainstem reticular formation and the work of Fred Plum and Jerome Posner summarized in *Stupor and Coma* (1966) and the introduction of the Glasgow Coma Scale by Graham Teasdale and Bryan Jennett (1974) focused much interest on the causes, methods of evaluation, and treatment of such patients. The concept of brain death, introduced by P. Mollaret and M. Goulon in 1959, gained further credence after the Harvard brain death criteria were published in 1968. In an age of organ transplantation, the objective and impartial diagnosis of brain death by neurologists has been critical in avoiding many difficult ethical issues. The use of computer tomographic scanning, intracranial pressure monitoring, rapid diagnosis of toxic and metabolic encephalopathies, and attempts at cerebral protection have provided both diagnostic and therapeutic challenges to the current generation of practicing neurologists.

Within a decade after the end of World War II, the need for rebuilding and restructuring clinical, research, and training programs in neurology prompted both private and governmental assistance. In the United States this began through the efforts of many volunteer organizations such as the National Foundation for Infantile Paralysis, the National Multiple Sclerosis Society, the Muscular Dystrophy Association, the United Cerebral Palsy Association, the Myasthenia Gravis Foundation, and the National Epilepsy League. Funding for the study of neurology dramatically increased after the founding of the National Institute of Neurological Disease and Blindness (1951), which later became the National Institute for Neurological Diseases and Stroke (1968), and is now the National Institute of Neurological Disorders and Stroke (Tower, 1975). Because of the tremendous increase in support for research and training, the number of residency positions in adult neurology rose from 32 in 1947 to 1444 in 1988. The American Board of Psychiatry and Neurology, which had been established in 1934, developed further subspecialty certification in child psychiatry (1959) and child neurology (1968). The American Academy of Neurology, organized in 1948 with 52 charter members, had grown to 5670 members by 1988. Among the many new journals started, *Neurology*, sponsored by the American Academy of Neurology, began publication in 1951 and the *Annals of Neurology* in 1977.

CHILD NEUROLOGY

In the early part of this century, medical schools began to introduce full-time salaried professorships and specialized research units that later became incorporated into clinical training programs. In the United States, subspecialty clinics were initiated by pediatric departments between the 1920s and 1940s, as were specialized laboratory services. By creating subspecialty clinics and wards, pediatric departments stimulated interest in clinical research as the number of patients with similar conditions became large enough to categorize and study. Clinicians were now able to propose new methods of diagnosis and treatment and soon attracted more patients by referrals from other pediatricians and families of patients. This environment helped create the framework for the growth of many pediatric subspecialties. For example, advances in developmental neurobiology, epilepsy, and neurometabolic diseases drew attention to the differences between pediatric and adult patients with neurological disorders. By the 1950s academic departments were able to support full-time faculty engaged in both clinical and research activities in child neurology. Young investigators moved to other departments and set up their own programs. Subspecialty careers were given a tremendous boost beginning in the 1950s when the National Institutes of Health provided large numbers of research and training grants.

Several factors stimulated the development of child neurology. On the clinical side were the advances in diagnostic testing, such as electroencephalography, neurodiagnostic imaging, and electromyography. Child neurologists, rather than pediatricians, were trained and became responsible for interpreting and applying data acquired through use of these techniques to pediatric patients. They were perceived as having particular expertise by their pediatric and adult neurology colleagues as well as the parents of these children. As this technology became more widespread and was used to evaluate almost every brain disorder, the advice and consultation of child neurologists was sought more frequently. Although electroencephalography is perhaps the best example of how this special training promoted the field of child neurology, advances in muscle histology and recognition of many new neuromuscular diseases illustrate another aspect of this growth. Over a brief period of thirty years, pediatric neuromuscular disease became a distinct and complex field, and child neurologists were increasingly called upon to evaluate children with such disorders. Among the physicians who contributed to this field are John Walton, Raymond Adams, Victor Dubowitz, Sven Brandt, Ingrid Gamstorp, and Randolph Byers.

Another factor that stimulated the growth of child neurology relates to the treatment of epilepsy. To adequately treat seizure disorders, a sophisticated knowledge of electroencephalography was needed, as well as a comprehensive understanding of the pharmacology and toxicology of the medications used for treatment. Again, child neurologists were most suited to provide acute and chronic care for such patients, and because of the high incidence of this disorder, it became a management problem of a fairly large magnitude. It is safe to say that a significant portion of most child neurologists' clinical activities is related to the care of children with epilepsy. Several founders included in this section who made important contributions in the field of electroencephalography and epilepsy include William Lennox, Samuel Livingston, Cesare Lombroso, Jean Aicardi, and Peter Tizard.

In the hospital setting, child neurology consultations became more desirous, particularly for evaluating the serious neurological complications of diseases usually treated by pediatricians, such as bacterial meningitis and toxic and metabolic encephalopathies. Child neurologists in many centers assumed primary responsibility for the care of such severely ill children as well as those with other acute neurologic disorders; they were also willing and available to provide long-term care after hospital discharge. As pediatric intensive care became more centralized in tertiary care facilities, the volume of patients and demand for active child neurology services to participate in the care of such patients increased.

One of the major social and educational trends occurring since the end of World War II was the continued shift towards a society based on information processing and sophisticated technology. The value of higher education became increasingly apparent to parents desirous of their children's success. At the same time, schools were becoming more responsible for their students and required medical input to evaluate those with learning, attention deficit, and behavioral disorders. Child neurologists were soon asked to evaluate many such children who were having school-related problems, to rule out seizures, and to see if medication was indicated. As this coincided with the significant increase in fundamental knowledge about the nervous system, parents, school officials, and to an increasing extent pediatricians, sought this type of consultation. The advent of the use of central nervous system stimulants and other medication to treat depressive or aggressive behavioral disorders further stimulated these referrals. In addition, many of those interested in child neurology took an active role in this particular educational, political, and medical arena. Macdonald Critchley, Ronald MacKeith, and Neil Gordon are among many of the founders who had a strong interest in such developments.

Child neurologists also became more involved in the evaluation and care of the mentally retarded child. Historically, it is worth recalling that in the nineteenth and early twentieth century, those interested in the field of psychiatry played an active role in the evaluation and care of such children primarily because of the foundation set by Philippe Pinel, Jean Esquirol, and Jean Itard in France. However, with Sigmund Freud the advent of psychoanalytic theory clearly shifted psychiatry away from interest in the mentally retarded child, a gap that was eventually filled by child neurologists. Contributions in neuropathology supporting the organic and medical model for understanding the problems of such children were made by many, including Bernard Alpers, Ronald Norman, Dorothy Russell, J. Godwin Greenfield, Ludo van Bogaert, Gilles Lyon, and Paul Yakovlev.

This generation of pediatric neurologists who followed Frederick Batten, Bernard Sachs, and Bronson Crothers was also self-taught and came from both pediatrics and adult neurology. They practiced pediatric neurology on a part-time basis, still seeing children or adults depending on their primary field of interest. They organized epilepsy and cerebral palsy clinics and also served in some capacity in state institutions for the mentally disabled. Many obtained appointments in academic pediatric departments and subsequently organized and headed child neurology divisions. Examples of such individuals include Douglas Buchanan, Sidney Carter, David Clark, Philip Dodge, Neil Gordon, Bengt Hagberg, Thomas Ingram, Gilles Lyon, Ronald MacKeith, Johannes Melchior, Paul Sandifer, and William Wyllie. The next generation of child neurologists were already involved in more formal training programs. By the 1960s they obtained some degree of formal training early in their professional career and had exposure to a wider variety of patients in the more concentrated environment of an academic setting. Symposia and special sections were held at many of the national meetings of both the principal pediatric and neurological organizations. Still, their training was not formalized until official board certification was established. In the United States, formal training programs were initiated by the National Institute of Neurological Disease and Blindness, which began funding in 1957. Eleven years later the American Board of Psychiatry and Neurology began certification in neurology and psychiatry with special competence in child neurology.

During the 1960s and 1970s, federal support for training and research fueled an incredible increase in the number of formally trained child neurologists. By the mid 1970s most medical schools had pediatric neurologists on their faculty engaged in teaching, research, training, and caring for children with an ever-widening spectrum of neurological disorders. Within a short time, pediatric neurologists were setting the standard of care for many of the common neurologic disorders of childhood. Currently there are 74 child neurology training programs in the United States, offering 86 first-year positions, and as of 1990 there were 731 board-certified child neurologists.

As the number of pediatric neurologists in many countries increased, it become obvious that separate professional societies representing their own political, medical, and academic interests were desirable. Such societies were established in Japan (1961), Scandinavia (1962), England (1971), the United States (1972), Belgium (1978), China (1985), and many other countries. Typical of the growth of these societies is that of the Child Neurology Society in the United States, which increased from 223 members in 1972 to 924 members in 1990, and the Japanese Society of Child Neurology growing from 150 members in 1961 to approximately 2600 current members. The European Federation of Child Neurology Societies (EFCNS) was established from the Oxford Club meeting of 1970, organized by Ronald MacKeith, and attended by some 30 pediatric neurologists. The EFCNS, which now has more than 400 members, created many regional societies, including the Dutch (Netherlands), Eastern European (Czechoslovakia, USSR), French (Belgium, France, Italy, Luxembourg, North Africa, Portugal, Spain), German (Germany, Switzerland), Scandinavian (Denmark, Finland, Norway, Sweden), United Kingdom, and Eastern Mediterranean (Israel, Turkey) groups. In 1973 the International Child Neurology Association was founded with an international membership and now contains approximately 500 members.

Another example of the dramatic growth of child neurology is the number of journals now devoted to this field. A list of some of these includes: *Developmental Medicine and Child Neurology* (1958; formerly the *Cerebral Palsy Bulletin*), *No To Hattatsu* (1969; *Brain and Development*), *Neuropediatrics* (1969; formerly *Neuropadiätrie*), *Pediatric Neurosciences* (1975; formerly *Child's Brain*), *Shoni No Noshinkei* (*Nervous System in Children*; 1976), *Brain and Development* (1979), *Pediatric Neurology* (1985), and the *Journal of Child Neurology* (1986).

The 1990s have been designated the "Decade of the Brain" by the United States government. As we enter this last decade before the beginning of a new millennium, it is remarkable to reflect on the changes that have occurred in pediatrics, neurology, and child neurology. One hundred years ago pediatrics was in its infancy and child neurology a gleam in the eye of a few physicians. Today there are over four thousand child neurologists. (Please see the list at the end of the Introduction for references.)

RAYMOND ADAMS

RAYMOND DELACY ADAMS (figure 1) was born on February 13, 1911, in Portland, Oregon. His father's family came originally from Canterbury, England, and his mother was of Swiss and French ancestry. No previous members of the family had pursued medical careers. Adams completed an undergraduate degree at the University of Oregon in 1932, and began work in the Graduate School of Experimental Psychology at the university in 1933. While working on a doctorate in psychology he became interested in experimental sensory physiology. This interest in neurophysiology, fostered by Edwin Conklin and Robert Seashore, led Adams to enter Duke University Medical School, where he received his medical degree in 1936. Although he had originally intended to return to the study of psychology, he spent the next two years as a medical house officer at Duke University Hospital, first as an intern and then as an assistant resident in medicine. It was during this medical training that Adams developed a lifelong interest in neurology, which was encouraged by Robert Graves, then chief of neurology at Duke University. Alan Gregg, who was vice-president of the Rockefeller Foundation and a close friend of Stanley Cobb, persuaded Adams to take a three-year Rockefeller fellowship for the study of neurology. The first year of this fellowship was a residency in neurology at the Massachusetts General Hospital (MGH),

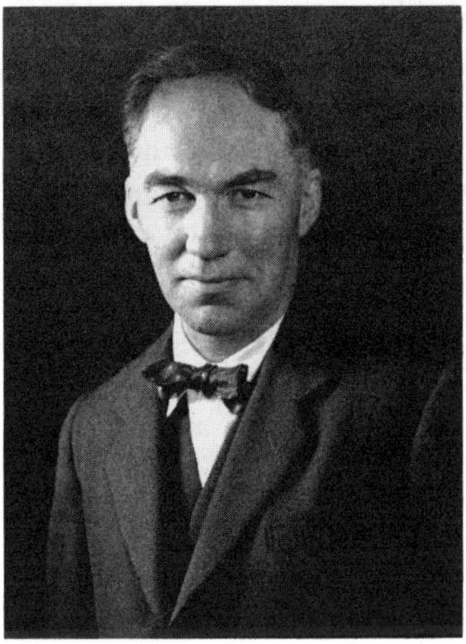

Figure 1. Raymond Adams at the time he became Bullard Professor of Neuropathology in 1954.

while the second year was under the tutelage of Stanley Cobb, former chief of the Harvard Neurological Unit at the Boston City Hospital and then chief of the Psychiatric Unit at the Massachusetts General Hospital. Adams spent the third year of his fellowship as a fellow in psychiatry at Yale University in the Institute of Human Relations. During these years, he met Charles S. Kubik, chief of neurology at the MGH, whose critical mind and interest in neuropathology significantly influenced Adams in his future neurological studies.

After spending a year in the private practice of Eugene Cohn, Adams returned to psychiatry at Duke University. He was offered a position with Houston Merritt, who was then acting director of the Neurological Unit at the Boston City Hospital. Derek Denny-Brown had been nominated to succeed Tracy Putnam as director of the Neurological Unit, but when war broke out in 1939 Denny-Brown joined the British army (Byrne, 1964). In 1941 Harvard Medical School secured the release of Denny-Brown from British military service, which allowed him to work at the Boston City Hospital. Following the arrival of Denny-Brown, Adams worked for the next ten years primarily in the Mallory Institute of Pathology at the Boston City Hospital, both in general pathology and in neuropathology. In 1944 Adams replaced Houston Merritt as chief assistant to Denny-Brown, and in 1945 he served for one year as acting director of the Neurological Unit during Denny-Brown's recall to active military service.

During his years at the Boston City Hospital, Adams devoted much effort to the clinical and neuropathological study of diseases that affected the nervous system. His first paper, entitled "The Arnold-Chiari Malformation," published in the *New England Journal of Medicine* in 1941, anticipated his later interest in brain morphology and his interest in child neurology (Adams, Schatzki, and Scoville, 1941). His other research at this time included the study of the neuropathologic changes of Hemophilus influenza infection in children (Adams, Kubik, and Banner, 1948), hereditary stenosis of the aqueduct of Sylvius as a cause of congenital hydrocephalus (Bickers and Adams, 1949), and neurologic changes seen in liver disease and hepatic coma (Adams and Foley, 1953).

Along with his extensive work in neuropathology during this time, Adams was a lecturer in neurology at the Tufts Medical School in Boston and a neurological consultant to the Pratt Diagnostic Hospital and to the Floating Hospital for Infants and Children. From 1944 to 1951 Adams acquired extensive clinical experience in child neurology. He realized that there were significant gaps in the study of clinical child neurology during this time, with only a few neurologists such as Frank Ford and Douglas Buchanan dedicated to the study of this field. From 1949 to 1951 Adams served as chief of the Neurologic and Psychiatric Services at the New England Center Hospital in Boston. He also continued as assistant pathologist at the Mallory Institute at Boston City Hospital.

In 1951 Adams succeeded Charles S. Kubik as chief of the neurology service at the Massachusetts General Hospital. Expertise in child neurology in New England at this time was very limited and only a few physicians — for example, Bronson Crothers, Randolph Byers, and Adams — had substantial experience with the neurological diseases affecting infants and children. Adams continued to see pediatric neurological cases during this period, but realized that it was important to begin training others in the practice of pediatric neurology. In 1954 he became the Bullard Professor of Neuropathology at Harvard Medical School. Shortly thereafter, Adams and Allan Butler, chief of the Children's Medical Service at the Massachusetts General Hospital, established the Child Neurology Service at the latter institution, choosing Philip Dodge, a resident in neurology, to develop the service. Since 1956 two of the seven residents in neurology selected each year at MGH are committed to the study of child neurology. The support for child neurology continued. In 1956 the Joseph P. Kennedy, Jr. Foundation donated funds to renovate the top three floors of the Burnham Building at MGH, with these floors designated as laboratories and work areas for the study of child neurology (Castleman Crockett, and Sutton, 1983). With this expansion, the Child Neurology Service at MGH became the first endowed division in the country. Adams's work in child neurology and study of the diseases associated with mental retardation were also instrumental in the development of the Eunice Kennedy Shriver Center for Mental Retardation, located on the grounds of the Fernald State School in Waltham, Massachusetts. Dr. Hugo Moser, who had been a resident in neurology at MGH, was instrumental in setting up the neurochemistry division at the Shriver Center and later became its director. This center, established in 1959, was the first of twelve federally funded centers in the United States for the study of mental retardation.

Adams continued to pursue a variety of clinical interests that included not only child neurology but all aspects of neuropathology. His interest in muscle disease culminated in the important textbook *Diseases of Muscle*, edited by Adams, Denny-Brown, and Carl Pearson, and first published in 1953. Further work in his study of diseases of muscle continued with the collaboration of a succession of research fellows at the MGH, including Sir John Walton, Carl Pearson, and Bryon Kakulas. Adams has published more than 240 articles dealing with a remarkable array of topics: neurological complications of liver disease, experimental allergic neuritis, metabolic diseases affecting the nervous system, alcoholic cerebellar degeneration, hydrocephalus, cerebrovascular disease, and central nervous system infections. He did additional work on nutrition and alcoholic neurological diseases with the collaboration of Maurice Victor, with whom he wrote an outstanding textbook of general neurology, *Principles of Neurology*, first published in 1977. He also studied hypoxic encephalopathy, and with James Lance described the syndrome of intention myoclonus following severe hypoxia (Lance and Adams, 1963). Adams made yet another major contribution to child neurology when he and Gilles Lyon coauthored another excellent book, *Neurology of Hereditary Metabolic Diseases of Children*, published in 1982. This book, which remains one of the most complete neurological texts concerning inborn errors of metabolism, categorized metabolic diseases according to age of presentation and clinical signs, distinguished metabolic problems from other neurological diseases of childhood, and provided a practical guide for laboratory tests of hereditary metabolic encephalopathies. Adams's list of publications includes many articles important to the study of child neurology. These include seminal studies on the Arnold-Chiari malformation, congenital cysts of the spinal meninges, the clinical and pathological aspects of encephalitis and influenzal meningitis, acute necrotizing hemorrhagic encephalopathy, hereditary aqueductal stenosis, congenital muscular dystrophy causing arthrogryposis multiplex congenita, the acute encephalopathies in infants and children, childhood spinal cord tumors, neurological diseases associated with varicella, the neuropathology of Zellweger syndrome, N 5, 10–methylenetetrahydrofolate reductase deficiency as a cause of homocystinuria, and the neuropathology of posthemiplegic athetosis.

When asked what he considered to be his most important contribution to child neurology, Adams felt it has been his fostering the development of the child neurologist-neuroscientist. He considered it important that young academic physicians have a strong background in clinical neurology and to use information learned about the function of the nervous system, including physiology, psychology, and pathology, to expand the field of child neurology. Adams noted that the most enjoyable aspect of his life in academic neurology was working with a wide variety of young scholars interested in the many diseases that affect the nervous system. He encouraged trainees to study the pediatric aspects of muscle disease and of neuroimmunology and supported the work of researchers such as Mary Efron, Vivian Shih, and Harvey Levy in the study of disorders of amino acid metabolism that affect functioning of the nervous system. Other Massachusetts General Hospital neurology trainees, such as Guy McKhann, Hugo Moser, and Edwin Kolodny, continue to make significant contributions to the study of inherited metabolic disorders affecting neurological function.

Concerning his interest in neuropathology, Adams was most proud of his support of Paul Yakovlev, whom Adams was able to bring to the Warren Museum at Harvard Medical School. While at Harvard, Yakovlev developed the methodology of whole brain serial sectioning that enabled him to study the morphology of a host of brain malformations. This support for morphological studies of mental retardation continued with the work of Verne Caviness and Roger Williams at the Massachusetts General Hospital.

Adams's second wife, a graduate of the American University of Beirut, was also a physician. He has four children: one of his daughters has a Ph.D. in biochemistry, and a son has worked as an educator of learning disabled children. Another daughter is married to a neuropathologist. Adams has nine grandchildren, one of whom has a Ph.D. in neurobiology, while another is completing medical school at Duke University.

Adams continued as the Bullard Professor of Neuropathology at the Harvard Medical School and chief of the Neurology Service until 1978. He then became the Bullard Professor of Neuropathology Emeritus and, until recently, served as director of the Eunice Kennedy Shriver Center for Mental Retardation and director of the Kennedy Research Laboratories at the Massachusetts General Hospital and the Walter F. Fernald School in Waltham. Adams is considered by his colleagues to be a remarkable clinician with a unique ability to synthesize a complex array of data and arrive at a correct diagnosis. Students and house officers throughout the years attest to Adams's superlative skill as a teacher of clinical neurology and neuropathology, especially in the realm of clinicopathological correlation. He has maintained active ties internationally, working extensively in neuropathology at the University of Lausanne in Switzerland and the American University of Beirut in Lebanon. He has received honorary medical degrees from schools in six countries. The outstanding contributions of Raymond Delacy Adams to child neurology were recognized in 1985 when he received the Hower Award from the Child Neurology Society.

Edward M. Kaye
BOSTON, MASSACHUSETTS

REFERENCES

Adams, R. D., D. Denny-Brown, and C. Pearson (eds.). 1953. *Diseases of the Muscle*. New York: Paul Hoeber.

Adams, R. D., and J. M. Foley. 1953. The Neurological Disorder Associated with Liver Disease. Metabolic and Toxic Diseases of the Nervous System. *Res Nerv Ment Dis* 32:198.

Adams, R. D., C. S. Kubik, and F. J. Banner. 1948. The Clinical and Pathological Aspects of Influenzal Meningitis. *Arch Ped* 63:354, 408.

Adams, R. D., and G. Lyon. 1982. *Neurology of Hereditary Metabolic Diseases of Children*. Washington, D.C.: Hemisphere Press.

Adams, R. D., R. Schatzki, and W. B. Scoville. 1941. The Arnold-Chiari Malformation. *NEJM* 225:125–31.

Adams, R. D., and M. Victor (eds.). 1977. *Principles of Neurology*. New York: McGraw-Hill Publishing Co.

Bickers, D. S., and R. D. Adams. 1949. Hereditary Stenosis of the Aqueduct of Sylvius as a Cause of Congenital Hydrocephalus. *Brain* 72:246.

Byrne, J. J. 1964. *A History of the Boston City Hospital: 1905–1964*. Boston: Sheldon Press.

Castleman, B., D. C. Crockett, and S. B. Sutton. 1983. *The Massachusetts General Hospital, 1955–1980*. Boston: Little Brown and Co.

Lance, J. W., and R. D. Adams. 1963. The Syndrome of Intention or Action Myoclonus as a Sequel to Hypoxic Encephalopathy. *Brain* 86:111–36.

JEAN AICARDI

JEAN FRANÇOIS MARIE AICARDI (figure 1) was born in 1926 and is a native of Rambouillet, France. He studied at the Paris Medical School and was appointed Interne des Hôpitaux de Paris in 1951. During his "internat" years, he took a keen interest in neurology at the Hôpital de la Salpêtrière under Raymond Garcin, and in child neurology at the Hôpital des Enfants Malades in Paris.

There was actually no child neurology in postwar France. It was not until 1952 that the first French unit of child neurology opened in the Hôpital des Enfants Malades. It evolved from a special unit designed for the care of children with poliomyelitis into a full neurological service under the direction of Stéphane Thieffry, who was the first pediatrician in France to dedicate himself entirely to child neurology. Thieffry's unit attracted neuropathologists, electroencephalographers, and some young French pediatricians of worth who were interested in neuropediatrics, among whom the most outstanding were Gilles Lyon and Jean Aicardi.

In the early 1950s, Aicardi was preparing his thesis on convulsive disorders in the first year of life and was impressed and fascinated by the works of Henri Gastaut. He first met Gastaut, as well as Joseph Roger, in 1960 in Marseille on the occasion of a symposium on infantile spasms. Their ideas, as well as those of Collette Dreyfus-Brisac, a pioneer in the field of electroencephalography in childhood, and Jean Bancaud, who, together with Jean Talairach and their coworkers, developed stereoelectroencephalography and stereotactic neurosurgery of epilepsy, were to play a significant part in the development of Aicardi's thinking in the field of epileptology.

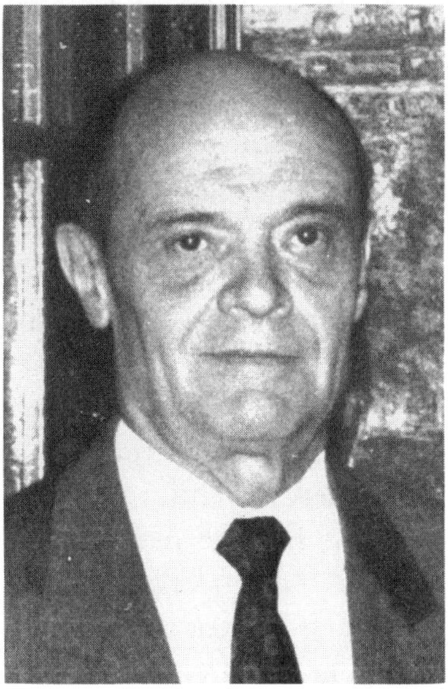

Figure 1. Jean Aicardi.

A deciding event of Aicardi's life was his visit to Harvard Medical School and the Children's Hospital Medical Center in Boston as a research fellow in 1955–56. Not only did he have the opportunity to increase his knowledge of child neurology and meet personalities such as Charles Janeway, William Lennox, and Cesare Lombroso, but, above all, he discovered the dynamic and rigorous style of American research, a process that he adopted for his own.

Returning to Paris, Aicardi became the pediatrician of the Department of Infantile Surgery at the Hôpital des Enfants Malades, where he remained until 1964 while continuing his interest in child neurology. He then worked as an assistant to Thieffry from 1964 to 1979 in the Department of Child Neurology at the Hôpital Saint Vincent de Paul. In 1968 he joined the Institut National de la Santé et de la Recherche Médicale (INSERM) and still belongs to this organization as a research director. He returned with his team to the Hôpital des Enfants Malades in 1979 to create and run a new unit of child neurology, of which he is still in charge.

In 1970 Aicardi was invited to Oxford, England, by the late Ronald MacKeith in order to participate in the first meeting of the European Study Group in Child Neurology, an exclusive group of The Spastics Society, an organization that has played an important role in the development of child neurology in Europe. This group became the European Federation of Child Neurology Societies in 1973 and has branches in most European countries.

Aicardi has been actively involved in the development of the French-speaking branch of the European Federation, of which he has served as general secretary. This branch includes Belgium, France, Italy, Luxembourg, North Africa, Portugal, and Spain. He is currently its president, and is also a member of the Council of the International Child Neurology Association, as well as a member of many scientific societies in Europe, America, and Australia. He was awarded the Cornelia de Lange Medallion from the Dutch Society of Child Neurology in 1985 and the Hower Award from the American Child Neurology Society in 1986. Through his work, he has become known throughout the world. His scientific relations with foreign colleagues have turned into solid friendships, and a great number of patients and students have come to him from all parts of the world.

Although Aicardi keeps himself up-to-date on all the basic aspects of neuroscience, he has always remained a clinician while collaborating closely with electroencephalographers, neuroradiologists, neurosurgeons, pathologists, and biologists. His scientific works include more than 250 original papers, to say nothing of many guest lectures and papers he has given at international meetings or congresses. Approximately one-half of his works deal with childhood epilepsy, while many are devoted to brain malformations, progressive encephalopathies, and to almost every aspect of child neurology — for example, acute encephalitis (Aicardi et al, 1977). Childhood epilepsy has, however, always consumed a great deal of Aicardi's activity. He published the results of more than twenty-five years of work and thought in this field in a significant book, *Epilepsy in Children* (Aicardi, 1986).

Jean Aicardi was among the first to be concerned with epilepsy in the first year of a child's life, particularly infantile spasms. As early as 1957, he made the distinction between cryptogenic and symptomatic forms of infantile spasms, a distinction that has important prognostic implications (Thieffry and Aicardi, 1959). This concept was to be applied to a variety of other childhood epilepsies. He and his team continued to study this disorder, especially the etiology, prognosis, and treatment with ACTH or corticosteroids. Extension of this work led him to study the so-called epileptic encephalopathies, particularly Lennox-Gastaut syndrome (Chevrie and Aicardi, 1972) and the myoclonic epilepsies of childhood (Aicardi and Chevrie, 1971), of which he contributed to the nosological clarification. He also described a cryptogenic myoclonic epilepsy and an early myoclonic encephalopathy.

His works on status epilepticus (Aicardi and Chevrie, 1970) and febrile convulsions (Aicardi and Chevrie, 1976) showed the potential role of prolonged motor epileptic seizures, whatever their etiology, even if febrile convulsions are most often involved, in the genesis of some acquired encephalopathies in childhood, especially acquired hemiplegia. He participated actively in studies on the prophylaxis and emergency treatment of febrile convulsions and status epilepticus.

In the field of the epilepsies with partial seizures, Aicardi supplemented the knowledge of benign epilepsy of childhood with rolandic spikes, and showed that the form of epilepsy with occipital spike-wave complexes suppressed by eye-opening was not a homogeneous entity with an always-favorable outcome. He also described an atypical partial benign epilepsy, which is often mistaken for Lennox-Gastaut syndrome although certain electroclinical features and prognosis completely differentiate each from the other (Aicardi and Chevrie, 1982).

Working on progressive encephalopathies, Aicardi's main purpose has always been to go beyond the post-mortem diagnosis obtained from neuropathologic data. Because many of these diseases are genetic disorders, he used clinical, electrophysiological, and biochemical features, as well as electron microscopic and biochemical data from muscle, skin, or conjunctival biopsies in order to establish an early diagnosis, often making genetic counseling or prenatal diagnosis possible (Arsenio-Nuñes, Goutières, and Aicardi, 1981).

Among progressive encephalopathies he was interested especially in neuronal ceroid lipofuscinoses, infantile neuroaxonal dystrophy (Castelein and Aicardi, 1979), mitochondrial encephalomyopathies and Rett syndrome (Hagberg et al, 1983). Andreas Rett had described this syndrome in Vienna in 1966, but this description had strangely gone unnoticed. Work by Aicardi and his colleagues beginning in 1980 permitted its rediscovery, and, in collaboration with Rett and European and American workers, international studies have enhanced our understanding of this disorder. It is now suspected that Rett syndrome, which exclusively affects females, represents approximately 30 to 35 percent of progressive encephalopathies in girls. More than seven hundred cases have been published. This disease begins between six and thirty-six months of age with intellectual regression and severe behavioral disorders. Afterwards, loss of purposeful hand use, microcephaly, epileptic seizures, ataxia, as well as a pyramidal syndrome appear in the course of the next two to three decades. The etiology is still unknown, but Rett syndrome is likely to be a genetic disorder linked to the X chromosome. Two other new progressive encephalopathies were described by Aicardi. The first is a familial encephalopathy with calcifications of the basal ganglia and chronic cerebrospinal fluid lymphocytosis (Aicardi and Goutières, 1984). The second is an ataxia with ocular motor apraxia mimicking ataxia-telangiectasia (Aicardi et al, 1988).

The most important contribution of Aicardi in the field of brain malformations was the description in 1965, and again in 1969, of a new morbid entity known at present as Aicardi syndrome, of which more than two hundred cases have been published (Aicardi, Chevrie, and Rousselie, 1969). Symptomatology of this syndrome includes in a female infant, or at least in a subject with two X chromosomes: infantile spasms, funduscopic lesions known as *choroidal lacunae*, modified hypsarrhythmia with suppression-burst activity and a split-brain pattern, costo-vertebral malformations, corpus callosum agenesis, intraventricular heterotopias, and often cystic abnormalities of the choroid plexus. The only pathogenic hypothesis compatible at the moment with the available data is that of a dominant mutation occurring de novo on an X chromosome, a mutation precociously lethal for the male conceptus. This mutation might be located on the short arm of an X chromosome.

Jean Aicardi has also studied the clinical and radiological features, as well as the possible genetic etiology, of several other brain malformations, notably Walker-Warburg syndrome (Bordarier, Aicardi, and Goutières, 1984), Joubert syndrome, the syndrome of absence of the septum pellucidum with porencephalies, and the syndrome of the pseudomonoventricle due to a malformation of the septum pellucidum with frontal horn agenesis.

This short essay can hardly convey the extent of Jean Aicardi's knowledge and capacity for work. His passion for child neurology has always allowed him to continue his scientific investigations despite countless difficulties. He is currently writing a new book that promises to be a personal survey of every field of child neurology.

Jean-Jacques Chevrie
PARIS, FRANCE

REFERENCES

Aicardi, J. 1986. *Epilepsy in Children*. New York: Raven Press.

Aicardi, J., et al. 1988. Ataxia-Ocular Motor Apraxia: A Syndrome Mimicking Ataxia-Telangiectasia. *Ann Neur* 24:497–502.

Aicardi, J., and J. J. Chevrie. 1970. Convulsive Status Epilepticus in Infants and Children. A Study of 239 Cases. *Epilepsia* 11:187–97.

______. 1971. Myoclonic Epilepsies of Childhood. *Neuropädiatrie* 3:177–90.

______. 1976. Febrile Convulsions. Sequelae and Mental Retardation. In *Brain Dysfunction in Infantile Febrile Convulsions*, 247–57. Ed. M. A. B. Brazier and F. Coceani. New York: Raven Press.

______. 1982. Atypical Partial Benign Epilepsy of Childhood. *Dev Med Child Neur* 24:281–92.

Aicardi, J., J. J. Chevrie, and F. Rousselie. 1969. Le syndrome spasmes en flexion, agénésie calleuse, anomalies choriorétiniennes. *Arch fran péd* 26:1103–20.

Aicardi, J., and F. Goutières. 1984. A Progressive Familial Encephalopathy in Infancy with Calcifications of the Basal Ganglia and Chronic Cerebrospinal Fluid Lymphocytosis. *Ann Neur* 15:49–54.

Aicardi, J., et al. 1977. Acute Measles Encephalitis in Children with Immunodepression. *Ped* 59:232–39.

Arsenio-Nuñes, M. L., F. Goutières, and J. Aicardi. 1981. An Ultramicroscopic Study of Skin and Conjunctival Biopsies in Chronic Neurological Disorders. *Ann Neur* 9:163–73.

Bordarier, C., J. Aicardi, and F. Goutières. 1984. Congenital Hydrocephalus and Eye Abnormalities with Severe Developmental Defects: Warburg's Syndrome. *Ann Neur* 16:60–65.

Castelein, P., and J.Aicardi. 1979. Infantile Neuroaxonal Dystrophy. *Brain* 102:727–48.

Chevrie, J. J., and J. Aicardi. 1972. Childhood Epileptic Encephalopathy with Slow Spike-Wave: A Statistical Study of 80 Cases. *Epilepsia* 13:259–71.

Hagberg, B., et al. 1983. A Progressive Syndrome of Autism, Dementia, Ataxia, and Loss of Purposeful Hand Use in Girls: Rett's Syndrome: Report of 35 Cases. *Ann Neur* 14(4):471–78.

Thieffry, S., and J. Aicardi. 1959. Les spasmes en flexion du nourrisson. 36 observations. Etude critique. *Sem Hôp Paris* 34:1167–78.

BERNARD ALPERS

BERNARD ALPERS (1900–1981) (figure 1) represented the unusual amalgam of investigator, clinician, neuropathologist, neurologist, neuropsychiatrist, and teacher. He was professor of neurology and chairman of the Department of Neurology at Jefferson Medical College from 1939 until his retirement in 1966. He was president of the American Association of Neuropathologists, president of the American Neurological Association, and president of the American Board of Psychiatry and Neurology. He was also the author of two neurological texts and more than 160 scientific papers.

Alpers was born on March 14, 1900, in Salem, Massachusetts, into a Jewish family of modest means. He was one of seven children, and early perception of family needs established a work ethic that he maintained throughout his life. A graduate of Harvard College, he chose medicine over the rabbinate but continued scholarly study of the Torah throughout his life. He received his medical degree from Harvard Medical School in 1923 and a doctor of science degree in medicine from the University of Pennsylvania in 1930. As a student at Harvard Medical School he developed an interest in pediatrics and in neurology, but ultimately his interest in the nervous system influenced his career choice. While a medical student, he spent two years as an extern at Boston Psychopathic Hospital. This experience introduced him to psychiatry and served as a source of material for four papers on cerebrospinal fluid chemistry and physiology, his first publications, which appeared in 1924 and 1925. He spent his first two years after medical school in training at the Philadelphia Orthopedic Hospital and Infirmary for Nervous Disease. From 1925 to 1928 he was a Commonwealth Fellow in Neuropsychiatry at the Graduate Hospital of the University of Pennsylvania and at the Philadelphia General Hospital. His publications during this period included papers on Friedreich's ataxia (Alpers and Waggoner, 1929) and the neurological complications occurring during pregnancy (Alpers and Palmer, 1929).

At this time, the relation between neurosurgery and neuropathology was forever altered by the monograph on gliomas by Percival Bailey and Harvey Cushing. As a result of this publication, in 1928 at the urging of Francis Grant, Alpers was awarded the Francis Clark Traveling Fellowship in Neurosurgery for the purpose of studying neuropathology in Europe. He was then to return to the University of Pennsylvania to establish a neuropathology laboratory with Charles Frazier's neurosurgical service.

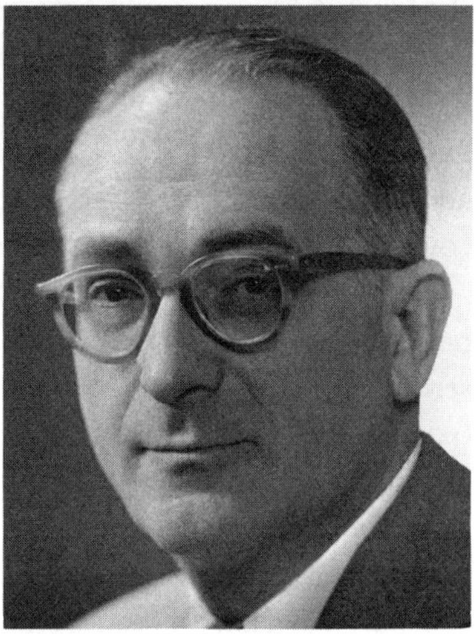

Figure 1. Bernard Alpers (1900–1981).

Alpers spent 1928 and 1929 in Madrid studying with Pio del Rio Hortega and in Hamburg-Friedrichsberg in the laboratory of Professor Alfons Jakob. While in Jakob's laboratory he examined an unusual case of infantile encephalopathy, which he reported at the American Neurological Association meeting in 1930. The paper was entitled "Diffuse Progressive Degeneration of the Gray Matter of the Cerebrum." It was subsequently published in full as a detailed clinical and pathological report (Alpers, 1931a). This condition, subsequently known as Alpers disease, represented a progressive gray matter degenerative disease of infancy in which cerebral degeneration was not a lesion of the white matter but a primary disease of the cortical gray matter. Thirty years later, Alpers reviewed the disease again and concluded that it constituted a clinical and pathological entity (Alpers, 1960). Subsequently, other authors have suggested the condition to represent a spongiform encephalopathy of probable heterogeneous metabolic, biochemical, or viral etiology.

Upon his return from Europe, Alpers established the Neuropathology Laboratory in the Department of Neurosurgery at the University of Pennsylvania. During the next eight years as director of that laboratory, Alpers, in conjunction with Charles Frazier, Francis Grant, and other medical associates, published a series of pioneering studies on brain tumors including papers on oligodendrogliomas (Kwan and Alpers, 1931), ganglioneuromas (Alpers and Grant, 1931), adamantinomas (Frazier and Alpers, 1931), brainstem gliomas (Alpers and Watts, 1935; Alpers and Yaskin, 1939),

Rathke's Cleft tumors (Frazier and Alpers, 1934) and parasellar tumors. During this same period he published papers in experimental neuropathology dealing with the origin and development of giant cells (Alpers, 1931b) and the functions of the glia (Cramer and Alpers, 1932), studies that anticipated the ultrastructural discoveries that came decades later.

Alpers continued to be interested in the interaction between pediatrics and neurology, and between 1933 and 1939 published a series of papers on the pathologic background of cerebral diplegia (Alpers and Marcovitz, 1938), the role of intrauterine infection and intoxication in cerebral birth injuries (Alpers and Patten, 1936), the factor of hemorrhage in cerebral birth conditions (Patten and Alpers, 1933), hemiatrophy of the brain (Alpers and Dear, 1939), and on the participation of neuroglia in the formation of myelin in the prenatal infantile brain (Alpers and Haymaker, 1934). These pathological studies of cerebral birth conditions led him to state:

Trauma at birth has too long occupied a hallowed place in the explanation of many of these conditions. That it suffices for the explanation of the etiology in some cases there is little room for doubt, but we question very much whether its importance is as great as has hitherto been supposed. There are too many cases in the group under discussion in which there was no history or proved suggestion of trauma at birth and in which labor was not only short but easy. So too was the favored explanation of anoxemia at birth. There are many instances in which anoxemia is not demonstrable. The occurrence of subarachnoid hemorrhage at birth presupposes trauma, which is often not demonstrable in these cases; besides, the role of subarachnoid hemorrhage in the production of these disorders is obscure and as yet unproved. (Alpers and Patten, 1936, 145)

It is difficult to see how from a pathological standpoint hemorrhage confined to the subarachnoid space can cause cortical changes which are associated with cerebral birth conditions. We are inclined to discount the influence of such hemorrhage in the production of such clinical syndromes. It seems possible that the condition in some, possibly in many, of the cases under consideration had its beginning in utero long before birth occurred. (Patten and Alpers, 1936, 759)

He stated further from his studies,

Probably only a small percentage of cases of convulsions or mental deficiency are due to brain damage associated with the process of birth, but in obscure cases of convulsions birth injury is often blamed in the absence of adequate proof. (Alpers and Berry, 1960, 282)

In 1939 Alpers became head of the Department of Nervous and Mental Diseases at Jefferson Medical College in Philadelphia. Several months later, he established an independent Department of Neurology and a Laboratory of Neuropathology there; he remained chairman of the department until his retirement in 1966. In this position, he stimulated and fascinated students and residents with his ability to correlate the anatomical, neuropathological, and clinical presentation of neurological conditions. His knowledge of the history of his patient's problems was exhaustive and he was a meticulous examiner at the bedside. His residents learned their neurology at the bedside and during his daily 6:30 a.m. patient rounds. Patients were often awakened by these early morning rounds, and then found themselves involved with him in a discussion of the literary merits of a book he found at the bedside. He was an avid Red Sox baseball fan, and it was said that if Ted Williams had had a good game, morning resident rounds were a piece of cake.

Medical students were treated to his weekly neurological lectures in the "pit," the former surgical amphitheater of the Jefferson Medical College Hospital, which was made famous by the painting "The Gross Clinic" by Thomas Eakins. Both in his lectures and at the bedside, he "ridiculed long lists of differential diagnostic possibilities and emphasized that, based on collective data, clinical problems deal entirely with pertinent possibilities and not with a long list of all possibilities." During the 1940s, 1950s, and 1960s, Alpers published extensively on the problems of sciatica, cerebrovascular disease, vertigo, cerebral aneurysmal syndromes, metastatic diseases of the brain, and the normal and diseased anatomy of the Circle of Willis. Alpers was fluent in Hebrew, German, Spanish, and French. This linguistic ability made available to him much of the world's medical literature and contributed to the exhaustive literature reviews that accompanied his medical publications (Alpers, 1945, 1958).

Bernard J. Alpers was a shy man. At times this was misinterpreted as a type of aloofness; however, those who took the time to know him found him to be an extremely warm, humorous, generous man who cared greatly about the well-being of his students, residents, and colleagues. He impressed his students with the necessity for thoroughness and patience in medicine, qualities that he himself continually manifested. He had an unassuming manner and was easy to approach, a characteristic that endeared him to his students and colleagues.

In 1959 the graduating class from Jefferson Medical College presented the college with Alpers's portrait, a tribute reserved for the most respected and beloved of professors. The portrait was hung with due ceremony in the college and thereafter it was said that "Dr. Alpers studiously avoided the corridor where it was displayed. He said he wasn't prepared to walk through a corridor and find himself staring down from a wall."

Following his retirement in 1966 from the chairmanship of the Department of Neurology, he continued to practice medicine and spend time with his wife, Lillian, also a physician. He continued to be an avid reader and student of the Torah, the Commentaries, and of comparative Semitic literature. He also reflected on his teaching days and the problems of getting caught up in the relentless schedule of academic and clinical neurology. He spoke of his need "to flee to some refuge like home, which seemed the best of all pleasures." Indeed, his wife and his three sons were his refuge.

In 1979, in his wry way, he commented on his beloved Red Sox and on the political scene, "Ah, those Red Sox. I sent a telegram to St. James Carter asking him to get two starting pitchers for the Red Sox, suggesting that if he could help them win a pennant he would turn the country around."

Dr. Alpers died at the age of 81 in 1981. He was a consummate physician, investigator, and teacher, and his contributions to child neurology have been substantial. He was honored by his students and by his colleagues, and was respected as a true friend and a gentle man.

Stuart B. Brown
MIAMI, FLORIDA

☙ REFERENCES

Alpers, B. J. 1931a. Diffuse Progressive Degeneration of the Gray Matter of the Cerebrum. *Arch Neur Psych* 25:469–505.

______. 1931b. Origin and Development of Giant Cells in Gliomas. *Arch Neur Psych* 25:281–98.

______. 1945. *Clinical Neurology*. Philadelphia: F. A. Davis.

______. 1958. *Vertigo and Dizziness*. New York: Grune and Stratton.

______. 1960. Progressive Cerebral Degeneration of Infancy. *J Nerv Ment Dis* 130:442–48.

Alpers, B. J., and R. G. Berry. 1960. Cerebral Birth Injuries. In *Injuries of the Brain and Spinal Cord*, 255–84. Ed. S. Brock. 4th ed. New York: Springer.

Alpers, B. J., and R. B. Dear. 1939. Hemiatrophy of the Brain. *J Nerv Ment Dis* 89:653–71.

Alpers, B. J., and F. C. Grant. 1931. The Ganglioneuromas of the Central Nervous System. *Arch Neur Psych* 26:501–23.

Alpers, B. J., and W. Haymaker. 1934. The Participation of Neuroglia in the Formation of Myelin in the Prenatal Infantile Brain. *Brain* 57:195–205.

Alpers, B. J., and E. Marcovitz. 1938. Pathologic Background of Cerebral Diplegia. *Am J Dis Child* 55:356–82.

Alpers, B. J., and H. D. Palmer. 1929. The Cerebral and Spinal Complications Occurring During Pregnancy and the Puerperium. *J Nerv Ment Dis* 70:465–84.

Alpers, B. J., and C. A. Patten. 1936. Cerebral Birth Conditions. *Am J Dis Child* 52:144–67.

Alpers, B. J., and H. W. Waggoner. 1929. Extraneural and Neural Anomalies in Friedreich's Ataxia. *Arch Neur Psych* 21:47–60.

Alpers, B. J., and J. W. Watts. 1935. Mesencephalic Gliomas. *Arch Neur Psych* 34:1250–73.

Alpers, B. J., and J. C. Yaskin. 1939. Gliomas of the Pons. *Arch Neur Psych* 41:435–59.

Cramer, F., and B. J. Alpers. 1932. The Functions of the Glia in Secondary Degeneration of Spinal Cord. *Arch Path* 13:23–55.

Frazier, C. H., and B. J. Alpers. 1931. Adamantinoma of the Craniopharyngeal Duct. *Arch Neur Psych* 26:905–65.

______. 1934. Tumors of Rathke's Cleft. *Arch Neur Psych* 26:501–23.

Kwan, S. T., and B. J. Alpers. 1931. The Oligodendrogliomas. *Arch Neur Psych* 26:279–321.

Patten, C. A., and B. J. Alpers. 1933. Cerebral Birth Conditions with Special Reference to the Factor of Hemorrhage. *Am J Psych* 12:741–68.

ANDRÉ-THOMAS

ALTHOUGH CHILD NEUROLOGY'S heritage is considered international in scope, it is almost universally agreed that the unique area of neonatal neurology evolved from the remarkable contributions of a series of French pediatricians and neurologists, originating from the time of Charles Michel Billard and François Valleix. Billard is remembered for his *Traité des maladies des enfans nouveaux-nés et à la mamelle* (1828), one of the earliest pediatric treatises that dealt extensively with newborn diseases. Valleix is credited with publishing the first complete monograph solely devoted to the newborn infant, the *Clinique des maladies des enfants nouveaux-nés* (1838). In the latter part of the nineteenth century, Jules Parrott described syphilitic pseudoparalysis in the newborn (1872), as well as writing several works related to the diseases of the brain in infancy. Aside from the studies of Otto Soltmann and the work of Albrecht Peiper that began in 1912, there was an unusual hiatus before it was appreciated how little was known about the neurological function of the newborn. Primarily because of the extensive investigations of André-Thomas (1867–1961) (figure 1), and later his colleagues, we can say that the modern era of neonatal neurology began.

Born in Paris, the city which he never left, and proud to say that he survived three wars, André-Thomas was married and had a son and two grandchildren. He died at the age of ninety-four, still physically and intellectually active. He felt he had lived too long because he had survived the death of his only son, who died accidentally in 1960. His wife, who suffered much from cervical arthritis, died at the age of ninety.

André-Thomas has been described as taciturn, having a silent, reserved character, but he was also known to have had a good sense of humor. He was a hard worker, curious, and always trying to understand the problems of medicine in more depth. He had a true research spirit. He was adamant that his name be written with a dash between his first and last name (André-Thomas). There was apparently a physiologist working in Paris and publishing at the same time, who also had the name André Thomas. André-Thomas insisted on the dash to avoid the confusion caused by their similar names.

André-Thomas lived frugally, not having the financial means to live otherwise. He never had a car. He rarely took a vacation and almost never left France. His sole exercise was his frequent long walks, which he truly enjoyed. Until the age of eighty-four, he continued his long walks, describing himself as a "foot soldier." His greatest pleasure was going to the circus to admire the choreography of the acrobats. He was always astonished by and paid particular attention to their equilibrium. In a way, one suspects that he was combining "business with pleasure" because he had a lifelong interest in the function of the cerebellum. Another one of his favorite pastimes was painting with water colors.

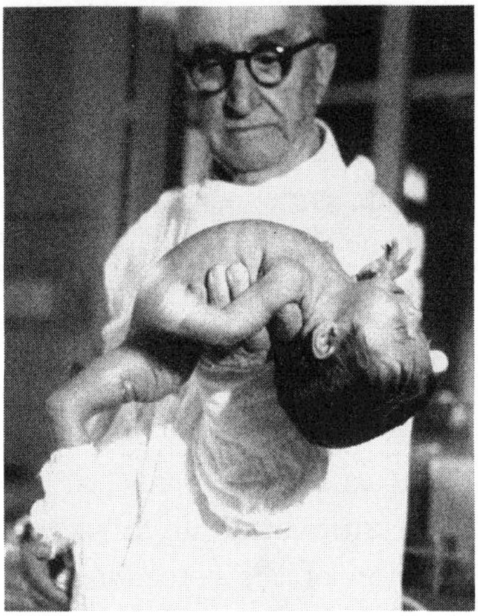

Figure 1. André -Thomas (1867–1961) in 1952 examining a hypotonic infant in horizontal suspension.

Even though he was an outstanding student and had excellent training with the famous neurologist, Jules Dejerine, André-Thomas was not accepted by the Assistance Publique de Paris as a "médecin des hôpitaux" and consequently not into the mecca of French neurology, the Salpêtrière. His bitterness regarding this remained with him throughout his lifetime. He therefore was forced to begin a private practice at the Hôpital Saint Joseph, a private institution where he was in charge of outpatient services. During this period (1901–32), he trained many neurologists, such as Roma Amyot from Montreal, with whom he maintained a close friendship and personal correspondence for more than twenty-five years. In 1932, after twenty-one years of service, he was required to relinquish this position but remained in contact with patients, thanks to his former students and colleagues, such as Dr. Huc at the Hôpital Saint Joseph, and later Etienne Sorrel at the Hôpital Trousseau.

In 1905, when André-Thomas was thirty-eight, he was admitted to the French Neurology Society where he was venerated by prestigious neurologists, such as Georges Guillain and Raymond Garcin, who admired his clinical spirit and applied his findings to the care of patients. Because of these contacts, he was able to engage in some research at the Salpêtrière. In 1917, at the age of fifty, the direction of his research was greatly influenced by the seriously wounded soldiers he saw and cared for. He began to study, in depth, cerebral and spinal injury correlating anatomic verification with functional recuperation. This period was very productive and stands out in three investigative areas that subsequently became classic and fundamental in André-Thomas's work. These areas are the continuation of his earlier interest in equilibrium and the function of the cerebellum (André-Thomas, 1940); investigations on the axial musculature and its innervation (André-Thomas and Ajuriaguerra, 1948); and finally, perhaps as a prelude to his later studies on the newborn, his interest in studies on muscle tone (André-Thomas and Ajuriaguerra, 1949).

André-Thomas's wide-ranging and erudite contributions spanning over sixty years probably could have been predicted from the quality of his thesis on the anatomical, clinical, and physiological studies of the cerebellum (André-Thomas, 1897). It should be remembered that the early experimental studies of Luigi Rolando (1809, 1825, 1830) and the later partial ablation studies of Luigi Luciana (1891) laid the foundation for the modern studies of cerebellar function (McHenry, 1969). At about the same time, clinical descriptions of the numerous brainstem and cerebellar syndromes were being delineated (Dejerine, 1914). In the first quarter of the twentieth century, the studies of Victor Horsley and Edward Albert Sharpey-Schäfer, Charles Sherrington, and Robert Bárány further contributed to knowledge of the cerebellum. However, it was the studies of Gordon Holmes (1904, 1922) in England and André-Thomas in France, based in part on their World War I studies of head injuries, that were fundamental in correlating the clinical and pathological functions of the cerebellum. With Grainger Stewart, Holmes devised the standard clinical tests of cerebellar function that are used today in the neurological examination (McHenry, 1969). The studies of André-Thomas during this period helped elucidate the mechanisms controlling equilibrium and movement, as well as the importance and limitations of the labyrinthine and vestibular systems in their control. He also demonstrated the contribution of muscle proprioceptive input in the overall integrative activities of the cerebellum (André-Thomas, 1925). Many of these descriptive studies were based on careful and repeated clinical examinations of patients with vascular lesions, abscesses, tumors, injuries, or atrophy, which were verified by postmortem examination. This work led to a comprehensive picture of the afferent and efferent cerebellar pathways and to a better understanding of the cerebro-cerebellar, spino-cerebellar, and vestibulo-cerebellar systems (Ajuriaguerra, 1955). Earlier with Dejerine, he had published their classical clinical study of a family with olivo pontocerebellar atrophy (1900) and in 1905 he recognized a form of generalized atrophy of the cerebellum (Ajuriaguerra, 1955).

Another area of special interest to André-Thomas was that of the autonomic nervous system. An example of this was his description of the celiac reflex in which deep epigastric compression may activate sympathetic activity, which could be detected by an increase in the radial pulse (Ajuriaguerra, 1955). The opportunity to examine patients wounded during the World War I allowed André-Thomas to study several conditions systematically, particularly "goose bumps," that is, pilomotor reflex activity. His analyses of the topographical distribution of this reflex were of use in further developing clinical methods for localizing the site of nerve injury. He also completed exhaustive studies on vasomotor, temperature, and sweating reflex actions and their cutaneous distributions, as well as their reactions to externally applied stimuli in other areas of the body. These observations were extended in his studies of "répercussivité," in which he expressed his belief in a higher integrative action among the autonomic nervous system, emotions, behavior, and responses to external stimuli.

André-Thomas's studies of muscle tone were of practical importance. Rather than focusing on an illusive definition of tone, he defined its characteristics in both the normal state and in various pathological conditions. He stressed the importance of the relation between agonist and antagonist muscles in his work on nerve injury, and collaborated with Etienne Sorrel and Mme Sorrel-Dejerine in their research on obstetrical paralysis (1943). He also examined the importance of muscle relaxation during normal voluntary movement and emphasized the close integration of agonist contraction and antagonist relaxation in such activities. His studies on muscle tone in patients with polio emphasized the importance, not just of the deficit seen in the agonist muscles, but also of the action of the antagonist muscles. This work was of significant value, as it contributed to improved methods of physical therapy in these patients.

Because of his influential followers, André-Thomas was finally admitted to the French Academy of Medicine in 1938. He was seventy at this point and said somewhat maliciously that it was because they finally judged him to be inoffensive. In 1955 he received official recognition when the Society of Neurology celebrated his fiftieth-year jubilee. He was then eighty-seven and was very touched by the celebration.

After World War II, at an age when all his colleagues were retired, André-Thomas became interested in the newborn infant. Because of his background in adult neurology, and because he was aware of the lack of data about the neurological examination of the newborn, André-Thomas devoted the remainder of his life to the study of the development of the newborn and infant.

He published many detailed observations as he visited the various newborn and infant units in Paris. He was invited by his admiring colleagues, who were now chiefs of these units at the Hôpital Saint-Joseph, the Hôpital Sainte-Anne, and the Hôpital Baudelocque, which contained the high-risk newborn and premature unit of Alexandre Minkowski.

Because he had retired and had no official position, André-Thomas's work consisted of brilliant observations that, unfortunately, could not be continued as long-term developmental studies. He always found great satisfaction in working with newborns and infants. He once said: "Les deux enfances se touchent, la deuxième joue à la poupée avec la première." This is an excerpt from a letter sent to Dr. Roma Amyot in 1947, which roughly means that the child in the old man becomes increasingly present, taking pleasure in playing with the child of infancy.

One of the contributors to this sketch, Suzanne Saint-Anne Dargassies, began working with André-Thomas in 1949, and together they published the monumental work that summarized their vast knowledge about the neurology of the newborn and infant, *Etudes neurologiques sur le nouveau-né et le jeune nourrisson* (André-Thomas and Saint-Anne Dargassies, 1952). Two years later, with Yves Chesni and Saint-Anne Dargassies, André-Thomas published the illustrated *Examen neurologique du nourrisson*, a landmark work that was subsequently translated into English and published in 1960 as *The Neurological Examination of the Infant* (André-Thomas, Chesni, and Saint-Anne Dargassies, 1955, 1960). Paul E. Polani had already introduced André-Thomas to the English-speaking world (Polani, 1959) and the following year wrote the foreword to the English translation of this work.

A few years later, in association with Mme Suzanne Autgaerden, André-Thomas published another important work, *Psycho-affectivité des premiers mois du nourisson* (André-Thomas and Autgaerden, 1959). After his death in 1961, his last book on the development of motor activity from fetal to postnatal life, entitled *La locomotion de la vie foetale à la vie post-natale*, was published (André-Thomas and Autgaerden, 1963).

André-Thomas's application of his life's experience to the studies of tone, equilibrium, and reflex activity created a framework for his analysis and development of the neurological examination of the newborn. Emphasizing the differences in regional brain development of the newborn, he analyzed the patterns of acquisition for many of the developmental reflexes that compose the neonatal neurological examination of today. In particular, his studies of the stepping reflex, equilibrium, active and passive tone, and locomotion defined the normative patterns of these responses in infants. In other studies, he compared these responses to those seen in infants with brain injury or developmental malformations, such as anencephaly, microcephaly, and dysraphic conditions (André-Thomas, 1954; André-Thomas and Gruner, 1954). The extension of these findings with his other collaborative studies in the premature infant developed a foundation for our current understanding of the neurodevelopmental function of such young infants.

André-Thomas was Dejerine's best student (Dejerine and Thomas, 1902). He inherited from Dejerine a will for hard work, objectivity, a profound understanding of the science of symptomatology, and a remarkable knowledge of the anatomical pathology of the nervous system. His work was more analytical than synthetical. His observations were, at times, too long, detailed, and laborious, but were always filled with information and instruction. He was very concerned with details, wishing to neglect nothing for those interested in learning. One can find a complete description of the nature and importance of his contributions to the field of child neurology in the papers by Julian de Ajuriaguerra (1955), Chesni (1955), and Saint-Anne Dargassies (1960).

André-Thomas's contribution to child neurology was his monumental work on the clinical examination of the newborn and infant. Even today, with all our modern technology and methods, his insights and knowledge guide the thoughtful clinician. He has made a great contribution to the well-being of infants. He was never so admired as after his death, a phenomenon that frequently occurs with great men.

Bernard Lemieux
SHERBROOKE, QUEBEC, CANADA

Suzanne Saint-Anne Dargassies
PARIS, FRANCE

REFERENCES

Ajuriaguerra, J. de. 1955. L'oeuvre scientifique du Dr. André-Thomas. Livre jubilaire du Dr André-Thomas. *Rev neur* 93(1):1–28.

André-Thomas. 1897. *Cervelet étude anatomique, clinique et physiologique.* Paris: G. Steinheil.

______. 1925. Pathologie du cervelet et troubles de la réflexivité. In *Nouveau traité de médecine*. Paris: Masson et Cie.

______. 1940. *Equilibre et équilibration.* Paris: Masson and Cie.

______. 1954. Le nouveau-né normal et l'anencéphale. *Presse méd* 42:885–86.

André-Thomas and J. de Ajuriaguerra. 1948. *L'Axe corporel. Musculature et innervation. Etude anatomique, physiologique et pathologique*. Paris: Masson.

______. 1949. *Etude sémiologique du tonus musculaire*. Vol. 1, 52. Paris: Flammarion.

André-Thomas and S. Autgaerden. 1959. *Psycho-affectivité des premiers mois du nourisson.* Paris: Masson.

______. 1963. *La locomotion de la vie foetale à la vie post-natale*. Paris: Masson.

André-Thomas, Y. Chesni, and S. Saint-Anne Dargassies. 1955. *L'Examen neurologique du nourrisson*. Paris: La Vie médicale.

______. 1960. *The Neurological Examination of the Infant.* Ed. R. C. MacKeith,

P. E. Polani, and E. Clayton-Jones. London: The Medical Advisory Committee of the National Spastics Society.

André-Thomas and J. J. Dejerine. 1900. L'atrophie olivo-ponto-cérébelleuse. *Nouv Icon Salpêtrière* 12:330.

André-Thomas and L. Gruner. 1954. Un microcéphale réduit aux formations axiales archaïques. Etude anatomo-clinique. *Ann méd* 55:35–57.

André-Thomas and S. Saint-Anne Dargassieus. 1952. *Etudes neurologiques sur le nouveau-né et le jeune nourrisson.* Paris: Masson and Cie.

André-Thomas, E. Sorrel, and Mme Sorrel-Dejerine. 1943. Paralysie obstétricale du membre supérieur. Type radiculaire supérieur (c^5C^6) *Rev neur* 75:57–73.

Chesni, Y. 1955. La sémiologie nerveuse de l'enfant dans l'oeuvre d'André-Thomas. Livre Jubilaire du Dr André-Thomas. *Rev neur* 93(1):93–100.

Dejerine, J. J. 1914. *Sémiologie des affections du système nerveux.* Paris: Masson et Cie.

Dejerine, J. J., and A. Thomas. 1902. *Traités des maladies de la moëlle épinière.* Paris: J. B. Baillière.

McHenry, L. 1969. *Garrison's History of Neurology.* Springfield, IL: Charles C Thomas.

Polani, P. E. 1959. Neurological Examination of the Newborn According to the Work of Prof. André Thomas. *Cerebral Palsy Bull* 5:19–22.

Rémillard, Guy. 1930–1957. Personal correspondence of André-Thomas to Roma Amyot.

Saint-Anne Dargassies, S. 1960. Neurologic Development of the Infant. The Contributions of André-Thomas. *World Neur* 1:71–77.

SVEN BRANDT

SVEN MOZART BRANDT (figure 1) was born on April 9, 1913, in Frederiksberg, Denmark. His father was general consul in Cairo and, after a short time, Sven and his mother returned to Denmark, where he went to school in Copenhagen. He passed his student examination in 1931 and began studying medicine at the University of Copenhagen. The undergraduate, preclinical, and clinical studies at the university were combined into a program extending over seven to eight years, and Brandt graduated in 1939 and decided to continue his clinical education.

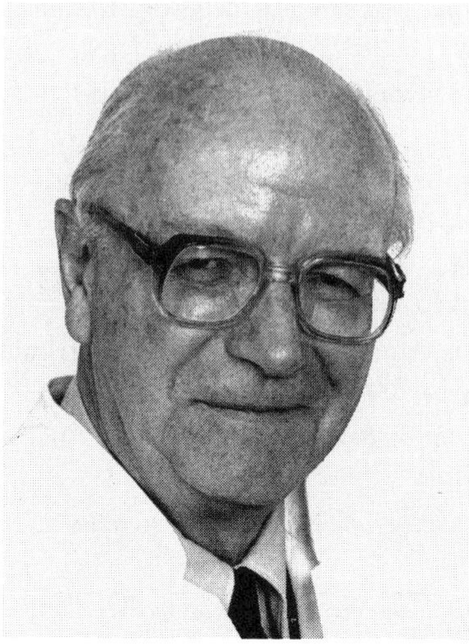

Figure 1. Sven Brandt at the time of his retirement in 1983.

At an early stage in his career, Brandt became interested in neurology and particularly in the neurology of children. This was stimulated among other factors by his connection with Knud Krabbe (Krabbe's disease) who inspired him to continue training in these fields. Brandt qualified in two medical disciplines, neurology and pediatrics, an exceptional and unusual accomplishment in Danish medical education. His training was mainly done in Aarhus, where he worked closely with Professor Bent Anderson in the Department of Pediatrics.

Early in his career he started work on his thesis, which was a careful clinical study of Werdnig-Hoffmann's disease. During his appointment to the pediatric department at the Aarhus University Hospital, he was confronted with four patients in whom the diagnosis of amyotonia congenita and Werdnig-Hoffmann infantile progressive muscular atrophy were being considered. These four patients prompted his continued interest in this disorder. He then contacted all the clinical departments in Denmark where such patients could possibly be admitted and collected his original material for his thesis, which he completed in 1948 and defended in 1950 (Brandt, 1950). The most important conclusion from this work is as follows: "It has not been possible through study of the literature or by means of Danish material of hospitalized children to confirm the existence of any well-characterized disease corresponding to the 'amyotonia congenita' described by Oppenheim in 1900." Another conclusion was that "muscular flabbiness is a rather common symptom in a number of morbid conditions in childhood — of widely variable character." His contribution was so important that it is still quoted frequently in the world literature of child neurology.

In 1947 Brandt traveled with a group of Danish pediatricians to New York to attend the International Pediatric Congress. During that stay he became acquainted with several pediatric neurologists in the United States. This contact resulted in a return visit with his family to the United States the following year to the Institute of Neuropsychiatry at the University of Illinois and with Frederick and Erna Gibbs in Boston to study neurophysiology and electroencephalography in children.

Brandt's stay in the United States was quite beneficial, because he traveled widely and met numerous leaders in the fields of pediatrics and child neurology, including those interested in cerebral palsy, such as Winthrop Phelps, William Lennox, Bronson Crothers, and Meyer Perlstein.

When he returned to Denmark after his sabbatical in the United States, his interest in child neurology focused on the areas of pediatric electroencephalography and cerebral palsy. He was on a committee responsible for planning the treatment of cerebral palsy in Denmark and in 1949–50 became the director of the Cerebral Palsy Clinic connected with the Ortopaedisk Hospital and Samfundet og Hjemmet for Vanfre (The Society and Home for Disabled Persons). In 1950 Brandt received his Doctor of Medicine degree from the University of Copenhagen for his work *Werdnig-Hoffmann's Infantile Progressive Muscular Atrophy*. At almost the same time he was asked to affiliate with the Queen Louises Children's Hospital by the late Professor Oluf Andersen. There he practiced pediatric neurology and, together with his wife Helgan, started the first Danish Pediatric Neurophysiology/Electroencephalography laboratory. He was a leader in this field and made many valuable contributions to it (Brandt, Brandt, and Vollmond, 1961; Brandt and Brandt, 1955). His wife, a pharmacologist by training, had always supported Sven's work and, when the EEG unit was established, she became the principal technician. They worked closely together in this area until continuation of the Queen Louises Children's Hospital work could no longer be maintained. In the meantime, a new clinic for cerebral palsy and pediatric neurology was opened by the Society for the Disabled. When this hospital was taken over by the Rigshospitalet in 1977, Brandt was appointed pediatric neurologist in the Department of Pediatrics of the University Hospital, Rigshospitalet. It was around this time that Brandt made several additional contributions to the field of pediatric neurology, including a paper on myoclonic encephalopathy associated with neuroblastoma (Brandt et al, 1974), juvenile lipidoses (Brandt et al,

1977), and the neurologic findings in glutaric aciduria (Brandt et al, 1978).

In addition to his engagement in professional work, Brandt was also active in the membership of different subcommittees and working groups responsible for the care of children with cerebral palsy, EEG technician training, and the problems of children who were handicapped or had disabilities. He was also very musical and, in his younger years, had considerable doubt as to whether he should enter medicine or choose a career as a professional musician. His favorite instrument was the cello, which he played excellently; he was a member of a number of small chamber groups.

Besides his dissertation, Brandt published about eighty papers, mainly on pediatric neurology. Among his lectures, he is well remembered for a paper on the history of child neurology, delivered in 1977 at the First International Congress of Child Neurology, entitled "The Parentage of Child Neurology." Interestingly, this was only the third attempt to record some of the historical trends of the evolution of this subspecialty, the others being that of Abraham Levinson in 1949 and Mynie G. Peterman in 1957. Brandt's opening remarks reflect his sense of honesty, humor, and integrity — and the same dread feeling that permeates all modern physicians: that the explosive growth of scientific knowledge has escaped our ability to comprehend and utilize what is known:

Let me begin by expressing my gratitude to the president for his invitation to me on this special occasion. The only motivation, I suppose, must be my age and my lifelong interest as well as bedside experience in neurological disorders in the growing human being. Let me admit that personally I feel myself seriously outdated today by the younger generation. For a 62-year-old, basic knowledge within important paraclinical sciences like biochemistry, immunology, physiology and other disciplines is developing so fast that he has only one quality left to which he may cling in order to survive: his general experience and his clinical memory and flair. (Brandt, 1977, 3)

To culminate a distinguished career, Brandt was also recognized as a Knight of the Order of Dannebrog (Dannebrogsordenen). Brandt worked for many years on the Medical Council of The Spastics Society in Denmark but, more recently, has devoted his time to music and family life. He is quite fortunate that one of his sons is a professional musician, so his musical talent has been passed on to the next generation, as will his contributions to the field of child neurology.

Johannes C. Melchior
COPENHAGEN, DENMARK

REFERENCES

Brandt, S. 1950. *Werdnig-Hoffmann's Infantile Progressive Muscular Atrophy.* Copenhagen: Munksgaard.

______. 1977. The Parentage of Child Neurology. In *Topics in Child Neurology,* 3–7. Ed. M. E. Blaw, I. Rapin, and M. Kinsbourne. New York: Book Division of Spectrum Publications.

Brandt, S., and H. Brandt. 1955. The Electroencephalographic Patterns in Young Healthy Children from 0 to Five Years of Age. *Acta Psych Neur Scand* 30:77–80.

Brandt, S., H. Brandt., and K. Vollmond. 1961. EEG Response to Photic Stimulation in 120 Normal Children. *Epilepsia* 2:313–17.

Brandt, S., et al. 1974. Encephalopathia Myoclonica Infantilis (Kinsbourne) and Neuroblastoma in Children. A Report of Three Cases. *Dev Med Child Neur* 16(3):286–94.

Brandt, S., et al. 1977. Juvenile Neurolipidosis of Bernheimer-Seitelberger's Type. Histopathological and Biochemical Findings. *Acta Neur Scand* 56(6):587–602.

Brandt, S., et al. 1978. Glutaric Aciduria in Progressive Choreo-athetosis. *Clin Genet* 13(1):77–80.

Levinson, A. 1949. Notes on the History of Pediatric Neurology. In *Victor Robinson Memorial Volume: Essays on the History of Medicine.* Ed. S. R. Kagan. New York: Froben.

Peterman, M. G. 1957. Pediatric Contributions to Neurology. *JAMA* 165:2161.

DOUGLAS BUCHANAN

IN NAMING HIM its first Hower Award recipient, the Child Neurology Society recognized the role of Douglas Buchanan (1901–1983) (figure 1) in the emergence of child neurology as a specialty. Few would disagree that the full-time practice of child neurology and the establishment of special training programs in the United States began with three or four individuals, one of whom was Douglas Buchanan. Over some forty years he combined the skillful evaluation of his patients with great insight into their neurological conditions, communicating this knowledge in a highly stimulating fashion to medical students and in depth to a succession of residents and fellows from 1936 to 1970, at least fifteen of whom carry on his tradition in this country and abroad. The University of Chicago School of Medicine gave him its highest honor, the Gold Key award, in 1970. Yet he was even prouder that every medical school class for a decade or more chose him to administer the Oath of Hippocrates. He did this in an especially moving way, with an emphasis on the continuity of medicine across the millennia.

Douglas Buchanan was born in Glasgow on January 14, 1901, one of three children of a singing master. He spoke of his childhood awe of the famous surgeon William Macewen, whose home and offices were up the street, and identified this as one of the early roots of his interest in medicine. He took his degrees from the University of Glasgow (M.A. 1922, B.Sc. 1922, M.B., Ch.B. 1925). In the years 1923–25 he was Barbour Fellow in Physiology of the Nervous System at the University of Glasgow. He carried this interest in basic physiological research to a five-year postdoctoral period at Trinity College, Cambridge, where he was simultaneously investigator for the Medical Research Council project on vision and lecturer on physiology of the nervous system. From 1929 to 1931 he was resident physician at the National Hospital for Nervous Diseases in Queen's Square, London. He often spoke of his experiences in those years, emphasizing the case demonstrations and other activities of the then junior consultant, S. Kinnier Wilson, who at fifty years of age had just been appointed full physician in 1928 (Holmes, 1954). Kinnier Wilson's slow rise, Buchanan's attachment to him, and Buchanan's leaving England may all be related to the fact that both men were Scots and therefore possibly subject to bias in that time and place.

The opportunity for Buchanan to leave London came in the form of an inquiry from Paul C. Bucy of the University of Chicago. Bucy, who was studying at Queen's Square, received a letter asking him to look for a child neurologist. He approached Buchanan, who expressed interest and soon thereafter received a formal invitation. In his autobiography, Percival Bailey states that his dream of a unified neurological service at the University of Chicago was frustrated by men in power, including the professor of pediatrics, who "imported a neurologist [from] outside our organization. . . " (Bailey, 1969, 233). Since Bucy was Bailey's junior colleague at the time, this comment probably reflects Bailey's difficult administrative position rather than contradicting Bucy's clear recollection. In any case, Buchanan arrived in Chicago in 1931 and remained there, rising to become professor of pediatrics and neurology at the University of Chicago. He was also consulting neurologist to the Children's Memorial Hospital, Chicago, until 1963. One measure of Buchanan's esteem by his colleagues was his election within the general faculty of the university to its highest level of executive responsibility, the Committee of the Council of the Faculty Senate. Formal retirement came at age sixty-five, at which time he sat for a portrait. Through the invitation of his successor, Robert Y. Moore, he continued to see patients and teach for another fifteen years. Buchanan did make a trial return to London in 1973–74, admitting only to failing "to find a place to stay," but he did encounter other problems, including the beginning of the long terminal illness of his beloved wife, Marian, whom he had married in London in 1930. She died several years before he did. In 1976–77, he

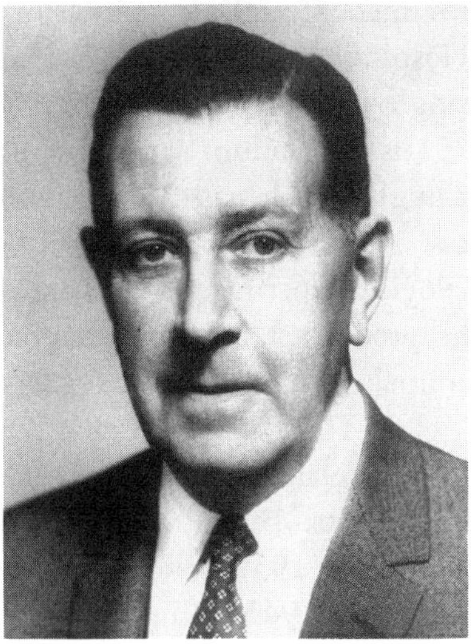

Figure 1. Douglas Buchanan (1901–1983) at the time of his retirement from the University of Chicago.

resumed attending responsibilities at the University of Chicago Hospitals when called upon to assist during a transitional period, single-handedly providing an adult neurology consultation service.

His curriculum vitae and published works show us one side of Douglas Buchanan's contributions, with their breadth and focus on case reports. Although he published only two papers reporting physiological experiments (Buchanan and Garven, 1926; Buchanan, 1929), he proudly stated in later years that he had studied experimental animals for a long time before approaching patients (Schulman, 1988). Three case presentations with published abstracts appeared from England and nine from Chicago (1932–42), covering a variety of subjects. Buchanan was first author of three papers (Buchanan and Bucy, 1932; Buchanan and Walker, 1941; Buchanan, Walker, and Case, 1942). Nine chapters and reviews appeared from 1938 to 1958, dealing with, among other topics, seizures (Buchanan, 1946), the motor unit (Buchanan 1950, 1958), and demyelinating diseases (Buchanan, 1955).

A number of the papers concerned intracranial tumors of childhood, an interest that culminated in his classical monograph on this subject (Bailey, Buchanan, and Bucy, 1939). Bailey and Bucy were the consulting neurosurgeons to Children's Memorial and in the early years transferred patients to the University of Chicago Hospital for surgery. The one hundred patients grouped by type of tumor in the book were first seen mostly at Children's Memorial. Buchanan collected almost all of the cases, but due to his dislike of writing and dissatisfaction with the product, did not put them into publishable form. Bailey suggested to Bucy that the latter write the text using Buchanan's materials. The histories of the cases are marked by great clarity and economy of expression despite the use of repetition for emphasis. These features were so characteristic in Buchanan's history-taking and clinical presentations that one suspects that Bucy was frequently able to incorporate portions of Buchanan's clinical notes unaltered. One such case, describing obstruction of the aqueduct of Sylvius, exemplifies the synthesis of clinical and pathological material that permeates this book.

The child was in many ways the most remarkable of the whole series. She stayed in the hospital for 517 days and during 507 days she was fed three times a day by nasal tube. During 509 days of this time the child lay in bed as if quietly resting, with her eyes open, but there was absolutely no evidence of any response to the human voice, and her condition could best be described as a state of suspended animation. During one period sleep-studies were carried out by Dr. N. Kleitman, and he concluded that she did show signs of rhythmic sleep. This we had found also from ordinary observation, since at times her eyes would close and the pupils would contract. Her temperature regulation was grossly disturbed during the entire period, ranging anywhere from 36 C. to 40 C. Her strange condition could not be accounted for by the hydrocephalus. Examination of the cerebral cortex demonstrated only the usual changes seen with hydrocephalus, which even in this severe stage are not incompatible with an alert mentality. (Bailey, Buchanan, and Bucy, 1939, 250)

Interestingly, error is candidly noted in reporting this case. Although the ventriculogram showed the tumor to be in the left lateral ventricle, "the right lateral ventricle was opened at operation and the tumor had to be removed through the septum lucidum." The tumor in this patient was described as a polar spongioblastoma. Perhaps the only aspects of Buchanan as the physician and clinical observer that this book does not convey are the quickness and sureness with which he could see the details of a child's neurological dysfunction and the special twinkle in his eye as he recounted details of current or past cases.

There were persisting rumors of, and apparently initial efforts toward, a *Textbook on Neurological Diseases in Childhood.* Buchanan would sometimes take out and show one of his many manila envelopes containing case reports and illustrations, presumably meant for this book (which he listed as "in progress" in his curriculum vitae). He received an honorary M.D. from the University of San Carlos de Guatemala in 1956, the home school from 1964 to 1971 of at least one former trainee. He was a member of a National Institutes of Health study section and its chairman from 1968 to 1971. In addition, he was a long-time member of the Physiological Society of Great Britain, the British Psychological Society, the American Neurological Association, the American Pediatric Society, and the Chicago Neurological Society, serving as president in 1956.

Although Buchanan's patients always received his best medical attention and most were devoted to him, his practice had features that we associate more with his time and place of origin than modern Chicago. Outpatients at Children's Memorial Hospital, scheduled for his weekly afternoon sessions, were seen in a manner reminiscent of Charcot's and S. Kinnier Wilson's demonstrations. These patients, entirely new to him, were brought into an amphitheater filled with the interns and residents of that hospital. The University of Chicago intern or resident sat aside at a small desk making notes in the medical record (Schulman, 1988). Buchanan took the history, examined the patient, spoke extemporaneously, and dictated a prescription that the resident also wrote out. This continued throughout the afternoon. If requested, inpatients were sometimes seen as well. At the University of Chicago Hospital, patients waited in examining rooms for long periods while he reviewed charts, discussed cases, and took all of the students and residents present for coffee. Families were generally given only the barest information about their child's situation and were not encouraged to ask questions. Much of the mechanics of caring for his many patients was done in private and outside of hours, by correspondence and telephone, as became evident during his time in England. Buchanan made a rule of always making a diagnosis. The change in diagnosis that sometimes occurred during subsequent visits might give the impression of error or indecision. However, the diagnoses were plausible at the stage when made. Particularly when a child with a progressive syndrome was followed for a long time, the changing neurological picture was reflected in a sequence of diagnoses, reflecting his commitment to specific diagnosis even at the risk of temporary error. This approach was integral to Buchanan's extremely effective style of teaching; he also believed that it was a comfort to the family.

Buchanan had an extraordinary memory, both for patients and publications. One of his joys was the challenge of frequently meeting new clinical problems in child neurology that he had never seen before. In his seventh decade, he was as excited as any young physician to make a correct diagnosis and back it up with an obscure reference. Presented one day with a history and examination of what sounded like banal mental retardation in a young woman, he led the way to a distant adult floor of the hospital. On meeting her in the corridor, he seemed to shake her hand and then turned, beckoning us to follow, as always with his right index finger. He marched straight to the medical library, straight to a particular stack, and taking a volume from the shelf, opened it to an article on Rubinstein-Taybi syndrome. He handed the volume to the senior resident who had evaluated and presented the patient, tapped the page, and said "You'll write a note, won't you?" On that occasion the glee was hidden, but not the lesson.

Douglas Buchanan's natural element was clinical teaching in the format of case presentation and discussion. This made him a popular discussant at meetings. But his career is epitomized by the teaching conferences that he held weekly at the University of Chicago for decades. They differed from his outpatient sessions in being designed purely for teaching. He would search out a case for days if necessary, or fabricate one that he thought suitable by using a child who could be convincingly "modified." Illustrative materials, usually books and articles, never projection slides, were brought along and shown. Although these sessions began at 9 a.m. on Saturday, the amphitheater was always filled. These presentations were primarily for medical students. If Buchanan was not himself responsible for the exceptionally high output of neurologists from this medical school, he surely provided the first clinical stimulus for most. His clinical skill and knowledge, his scholarly devotion to history, and the great warmth of his personality combined to form the essence of this inspiring physician-teacher.

Nicholas J. Lenn
CHARLOTTESVILLE, VIRGINIA

ACKNOWLEDGMENTS

The author is indebted to Drs. David Clark, Paul Bucy, and especially Sidney Schulman, who shared materials and recollections.

REFERENCES

Bailey, P. 1969. *Up from Little Egypt*. Chicago: The Buckskin Press.

Bailey, P., D. N. Buchanan, and P. C. Bucy. 1939. *Intracranial Tumors of Infancy and Childhood.* Chicago: University of Chicago Press.

Buchanan, D. N. 1929. Meskalimausch. *Brit J Med Psych* 9:67–88.

______. 1946. Convulsions in Infancy and Childhood. *Med Clin North Am* 30(1): 163–72.

______. 1950. Some Disorders of the Motor Unit in Infancy and Childhood. *Med Clin North Am* 34(1): 147–64.

______. 1955. The Demyelinating Diseases. In *Clinical Neurology*, 1075–1106. Ed. A. B. Baker. New York: Hoeber-Harper.

______. 1958. Spinal Nuclear Amyotrophy and Other Causes of Flaccidity in Infancy. In *Clinical Neurosurgery*. Vol. 3. Ed. R. G. Fisher. Baltimore: Williams and Wilkins.

Buchanan, D. N., and P. C. Bucy. 1932. Athetosis. *Brain* 55:479–92.

Buchanan, D. N., and H. S. D. Garven. 1926. Chronaxia in Tetany. *J Physiol* 62:115–28.

Buchanan, D. N., and A. E. Walker. 1941. Vascular Anomalies of the Spinal Cord in Children. *Am J Dis Child* 61:928–32.

Buchanan, D. N., A. E. Walker, and T. J. Case. 1942. Pathogenesis of Chorea. *J Ped* 20:555–75.

Holmes, G. 1954. *The National Hospital, Queen's Square*. Edinburgh: E. & S. Livingstone.

Schulman, S. 1988. Personal communication.

RANDOLPH BYERS

RANDOLPH KUNHARDT BYERS (1896–1988) (figure 1) was a key figure in the development of child neurology at Boston Children's Hospital during the half-century or so that began shortly after the establishment of a neurologic division under Bronson Crothers in 1920. His career continued well beyond the period of establishment of an independent department and the Bronson Crothers Professorship in 1962. From 1951 to 1962 Byers headed the neurology service, turning his attention full time to the neurology of children and relinquishing his private practice of general pediatrics. Since the late 1920s his real fascination was clearly the neurologic disorders of children. He was greatly influenced by his mentor and colleague, Bronson Crothers, but he was significantly self-taught and built upon his strong base as an active pediatric generalist. He was not formally trained in neurology. As he recalled:

I never undertook neurologic training for registration by the Board of Neurology and Psychiatry because one of its requirements at that time (1930s) was a two-year stint as an intern-resident in a residential psychiatric hospital. This seemed to me beside the point and too demanding. In the lack of neuroanatomic and neuropathologic training, I've always suffered, but have enjoyed myself.

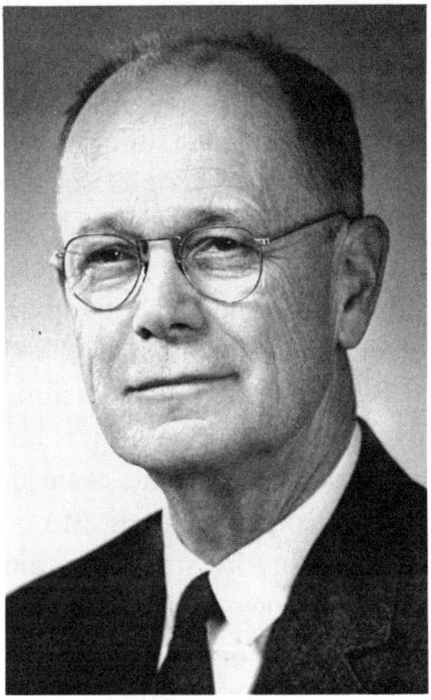

Figure 1. Randolph Byers (1896–1988).

In what might be termed the "Boston School of Child Neurology" during the half-century dominated by Crothers and Byers, the influence of general pediatrics was stronger than in other centers such as Baltimore, Chicago, and New York, where the pioneers were neurologists first and foremost. The pediatric background clearly influenced the approach of Crothers and Byers to the field, and both tended to think and write more broadly about the child and family in the management of neurologic problems. Such titles in Byers bibliography as "Cerebral Palsy Nursery Schools" (Berenberg, Byers, and Meyer, 1952), "The Doctors Responsibility in the Prevention of Postnatal Diseases of the Brain" (Byers, 1957) and "To Tap or Not to Tap" (Byers, 1973) exemplify this point of view. In addition, Byers, unlike Crothers, was much more involved in the diagnosis and management of acute disease, and the strong influence of the general pediatrician was apparent in his interest in all aspects of the study of lead poisoning, diphtheria-pertussis-tetanus (DPT), encephalopathy, and other conditions. Byers and Crothers were thus "in step" with the pediatrics of the era and, quite literally, in step with each other. An amusing series of anecdotes revolve around Bronson Crothers's compulsion to walk in step with a companion. This habit was fully accepted by Byers, who not only accommodated Crothers but adopted it as his own. Problems arose when they were joined by a third person in the line of march, which required a hop and a skip to re-order the arrangement. Certain pediatric residents, aware of this, would purposefully alter their step repeatedly in the course of a long walk down the connecting corridors of the old Boston Children's Hospital. From a slight distance behind, the entire procession was marked by repeated hops and skips as Crothers and Byers repeatedly corrected their steps to accommodate the outsider.

Byers's important contributions to many aspects of lead intoxication began when he was an intern at the Massachusetts General Hospital in 1921 and came under the influence of Joseph Charles Aub, George Richards Minot, and Risinkoff, who were actively engaged in the studies of biologic characteristics and toxicity of lead. His own first contribution on the subject, written in 1943 with psychologist Elizabeth Lord, was "Late Effects of Lead Poisoning on Mental Development," remains topical today (Byers and Lord, 1943). It gave the first insight into the deleterious effect of otherwise neurologically silent lead intoxication, a subject of current public health interest. The acute encephalopathy of lead intoxication attracted his attention, including treatment of the acute ingestion with chelating agents when they became available (Byers and Maloof, 1954), and the application of population-screening methods to determine children at risk (Kopito, Byers, and Shwachman, 1967). In 1959 he reviewed his experience with forty-five cases, which included the warning that treatment was dangerous if the gastrointestinal tract contained lead. Today, due in significant measure to his interest in the subject, acute symptomatic lead encephalopathy is uncommon, and the chief issues of concern are the effect of lead burden on the developing fetus and of low-lead body burden on the more subtle aspects of intellectual performance.

Byers's 1948 study of diptheria pertussis tetanus (DPT) encephalopathy continues to have an input on modern practice, but, due to distortion in a litigious society looking for malpractice claims, its current influence is unfortunate (Byers and Moll, 1948). Byers and Moll were able to collect fifteen cases in the ten-year period prior to 1948 in which an encephalopathy with seizures ensued within forty-eight hours of a DPT injection, usually leaving significant neurologic residual. This paper called attention to the need for a less toxic vaccine, largely satisfied by careful control of the alum-precipitated toxoid. The incidence of serious adverse reactions in the Boston area and elsewhere shortly became less frequent as compared with the incidence implied by the Byers and Moll study. Parenthetically, the DPT paper was followed in two years by an account of thirty-five cases of pertussis admitted to Boston Children's, six of which had neurologic sequellae (Byers and Rizzo, 1950).

Byers retained the continuing interest of Crothers's service in the chronic encephalopathies of children. Both he and Crothers were heavily committed to the tonic neck reflex as a method of assessment and prognosis, and his review of the subject in 1938 remains a scholarly exposition of the basis of the phenomenology (Byers, 1938). His paper on the evolution of hemiplegia in infancy pointed out the necessary differentiation of the flaccid arm of the neonatal hemiplegia from brachial plexus injury and the value of careful assessment of the leg, which may show no more than increased range of passive movement about the ankle (Byers, 1941). In 1955 he reviewed the Boston Children's experience in twenty-three patients who had neonatal kernicterus and emphasized the age-related variation in the clinical expression of this disorder and the frequency of deafness (a confounding issue in judging mentation), as well as choreoathetosis and impaired upward gaze as the triad of signs that characterized the chronic encephalopathy (Byers, Paine, and Crothers, 1955). His philosophy of concern for the child under pressure to recover or achieve was a continuing theme of his approach and his statement, "The dependent position of the child puts him at the mercy of a series of tyrants who have almost unlimited power over him." In this he included parents, of course, but also people such as grandparents, who influence parents, as well as later in life, "teachers, social workers, ministers and police [who] tend to usurp the tyranny."

Over the years, Byers turned his attention to a variety of subjects, and each paper makes a clinical point; for example: "Infantile Muscular Atrophy," written with Betty Banker, called attention to the wide spectrum of age of onset and the direct effect on longevity (Byers and Banker, 1961), the expression of steroid myopathy in children (Byers et al, 1962), a classic description of the clinical problem and risk factors of dural sinus thrombosis (Byers and Hoss, 1933), the diagnosis of acute hemorrhagic leukoencephalopathy and the value of corticosteroid treatment (Byers, 1975).

Byers established the first formal training program in child neurology at Boston Children's Hospital. This initiative came late in his career, and trainees were few in number; but they included individuals who have responsible positions today, such as Peter Berman, University of Pennsylvania; Arthur Rose, Downstate Medical Center, New York; William McLean, Bowman Gray; and Richard Ross, the University of Florida at Gainesville. His influence as a teacher by precept and example continued well beyond his "retirement," and both adult and child neurology trainees of the Longwood Neurological Program during the first decade of its existence all profited from his wisdom and extensive experience. This extended to staff and included a major contribution to the post-professorial education of his successor, the author of this essay.

My best summary of Randy Byers is to quote the last paragraph from the Memorium written for the *Harvard Alumni Bulletin*:

From my perspective, the memory that tends to overshadow his other contributions and accomplishments is the recollection of a gentle and understanding person. This influenced all his relationships, as physician, teacher and colleague. It was easy to become very fond of him and many people did. Over the years I learned that he held some sharp and insightful opinions about certain of his colleagues but they were usually kept to himself. He personified the best of old school Boston medicine and will be remembered as a truly gentle man.(Barlow, 1988)

Charles F. Barlow
BOSTON, MASSACHUSETTS

REFERENCES

Barlow, C. F. 1988. Memorium: Randolph K. Byers (1896–1988). *Harvard Med Alum Bull* 62:67–68

Berenberg, W., R. K. Byers, and E. Meyer. 1952. Cerebral Palsy Nursery Schools. *Quart Rev Ped* 7:27–33.

Byers, R. K. 1938. Tonic Neck Reflexes in Children. *Am J Dis Child* 55:696–742.

______. 1941. Evolution of Hemiplegias in Infancy. *Am J Dis Child* 61:915–27.

______. 1957. The Doctor's Responsibility in the Prevention of Postnatal Diseases of the Brain. *Ped Clin North Am* 4:1013–32.

______. 1959. Lead Poisoning: Review of the Literature and Report on 45 Cases. *Ped* 23:585–603.

______. 1973. Commentary: To Tap or Not to Tap. *Ped* 51:560–61.

______. 1975. Acute Hemorrhagic Leukoencephalitis: Report of 3 Cases and Review of the Literature. *Ped* 56:727–35.

Byers, R. K., and B. Q. Banker. 1961. Infantile Muscular Atrophy. *Arch Neur* 5:140–64.

Byers, R. K., and G. M. Hoss. 1933. Thrombosis of the Dural Sinuses in Infancy and in Childhood. *Am J Dis Child* 45:1161–83.

Byers, R. K., and E. E. Lord. 1943. Late Effects of Lead Poisoning on Mental Development. *Am J Dis Child* 66:471–94.

Byers, R. K., and C. Maloof. 1954. Treatment of Lead Poisoning by Calcium Disodium Versenate in Children. *Am J Dis Child* 87:559–69.

Byers, R. K., and F. C. Moll. 1948. Encephalopathies Following Prophylactic Pertussis Vaccine. *Ped* 1:437–57.

Byers, R. K., R. S. Paine, and B. Crothers. 1955. Extrapyramidal Cerebral Palsy with Hearing Loss Following Erythroblastosis. *Ped* 15:248–54.

Byers, R. K., and N. D. Rizzo. 1950. A Follow-up Study of Pertussis in Infancy. *NEJM* 242:887–91.

Byers, R. K., et al. 1962. Steroid Myopathy. *Ped* 29:26–36.

Kopito, L., R. K. Byers., and H. Shwachman. 1967. Lead in Hair of Children with Chronic Lead Poisoning. *NEJM* 276:949–53.

SIDNEY CARTER

IN 1976 THE FOURTH national meeting of the Child Neurology Society convened in Monterey, California, bringing together the majority of the country's child neurologists. The third annual Hower Award, established by an Ohio family to commend excellence in child neurology, was awarded to Sidney Carter (b. 1912) (figure 1). During the awards banquet his long-time associate, Neils Low, asked the neurologists in the audience trained by Dr. Sidney

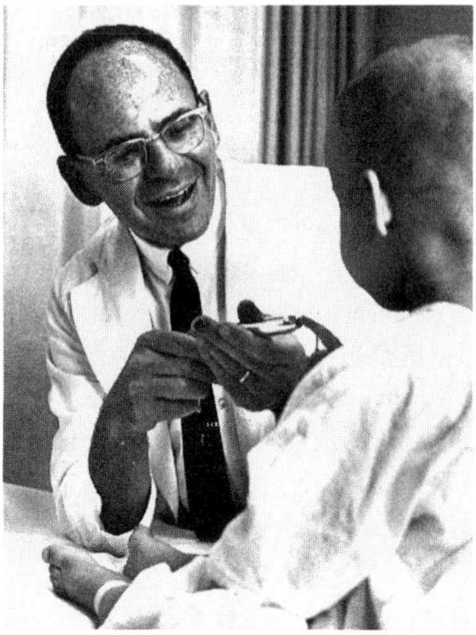

Figure 1. Sidney Carter examining a child at the Neuropsychiatric Institute, Columbia University.

Carter to stand. Nearly one-half of the audience rose. The contributions of Sidney Carter were made obvious by the number of standing physicians and their unabashed enthusiasm toward their former mentor. Sidney Carter was not only instrumental in training many child neurologists but also established guidelines for virtually all subsequent training programs, initiated federal funding for training programs, and established the credentialing process for certification of child neurologists.

He was born in Boston, Massachusetts, on December 8, 1912, and grew up in Winthrop, Massachusetts, a New England shoreline community north of Boston. His father was a small businessman, and his mother ran the home. He attended local public schools, graduating from high school during the Great Depression. He had two brothers, one seven years his junior who grew up to be a distinguished rabbi, while another younger brother died of meningitis during infancy. Sidney Carter entered Dartmouth College in 1930; it was with difficulty that his father raised $400.00 for that first year's tuition. He met expenses by working odd jobs throughout college. Following graduation in 1934, he entered Boston University School of Medicine, graduating in 1938. Many years later he recalled that a basic scientist, Leroy Conel, piqued his interest in neuroembryology, and his first obstetrical delivery as a senior medical student was an infant with a meningomyelocele. Carter interned at St. Mary's Hospital in Waterbury, Connecticut, where he briefly considered becoming an obstetrician. During 1939 and 1940, he was a psychiatric resident at Westboro State Hospital, Westboro, Massachusetts. The following year he became a neurology resident at Boston City Hospital.

At that time, Boston City Hospital was run jointly by faculty medical teams from Boston, Harvard, and Tufts universities. The neurological unit was directed by Harvard. In 1928 a grant from the Rockefeller Foundation supplied funding to develop a specific neurological teaching and research unit. Tracy Jackson Putnam was director from 1934 until 1940, when he left to head the Neurological Institute of Columbia-Presbyterian in New York. Subsequently, H. Houston Merritt became acting director of the neurology service. Merritt was already well-known for his research on cerebrospinal fluid and in 1938, along with Putnam, reported the first animal studies on the anticonvulsant properties of sodium diphenylhydantoinate (Merritt and Putnam, 1938).

H. Houston Merritt was a dynamic clinician, an established researcher, and an excellent poker player who was idolized by his residents. Nonstop Sunday rounds were made at several hospitals to review the residents' most interesting and difficult consults. The uniqueness of this neurology service and its extraordinary teachers acting as role models presumably reinforced Carter's selection of a neurologic career. Perhaps earlier familial and personal events initiated Carter's interest in neurology. During high school, Sidney Carter's cousin married the dynamic and much admired neurosurgeon, Leo M. Davidoff, eponymically known to child neurologists for the Dyke-Davidoff-Masson syndrome (hemiparesis secondary to contralateral cerebral atrophy associated with compensatory unilateral skull overgrowth). Personal tragedies, the deaths of his brother due to meningitis and his mother, who succumbed to a brain tumor during his senior year in medical school, may have influenced his decision to become a neurologist.

In addition to Merritt, a teacher who later became a close friend, the Boston City faculty included Raymond Adams, already knowledgeable in neuropathology, whose meticulous neurologic examinations contrasted sharply with Merritt's clinical intuitiveness. In 1943 Derek Denny-Brown arrived from England to become director of the Neurology Service at Boston City Hospital. Sidney Carter was the last chief resident of Merritt's at Boston City Hospital and the first chief resident of Denny-Brown. In December 1943 physicians of the Boston City Hospital were mobilized to England and worked at the Seventh General Army Hospital during the turbulent days of World War II. In England, Carter was assistant chief of the Neuropsychiatric Section and neurological consultant to both army casualties and British civilians who had the misfortune to collide with U.S. Army jeeps and who made subsequent claims against the United States. In 1945 he became chief of the Neuropsychiatric Section of the 116th General Hospital in Nuremburg, Germany. During this assignment, he was responsible for the neurological care of Nazi war criminals standing trial in Nuremburg for crimes against humanity.

He returned to Boston in 1946, where he was offered a fellowship at the Boston City Hospital, but decided on a fellowship with his former professor, Houston Merritt, who had moved to New York to run the neurological unit at Montefiore Hospital. In 1948 Merritt was appointed director of neurology at Columbia-Presbyterian's Neurological Institute in New York City and Sidney Carter, Daniel Sciarra, and Melvin Yahr followed Merritt to the Neurological Institute. Sidney Carter became assistant attending neurologist at the Columbia-Presbyterian Medical Center (College of Physicians and Surgeons of Columbia University). In 1951 he was appointed by Merritt as chief of the Pediatric Neurology Service at the Neurological Institute.

The Pediatric Neurology Service at the Neurological Institute developed in the 1920s under the direction of Bernard Sachs. After his retirement, the second director of the Pediatric Neurology Service was Louis Casamajor. Casamajor decided to retire in 1951, somewhat prematurely, because of progressive deafness. At this time, the pediatric neurology service consisted of six beds on 4 West at the Neurological Institute. These beds were occupied by profoundly impaired children with chronic encephalopathies or degenerative neurological disorders. Carter had slowly gravitated to this service because of a developing interest in child neurology and began making rounds with Casamajor. However, his appointment by Houston Merritt to become director of the service was neither sought nor anticipated.

Following this appointment, however, child neurology showed rapid growth. This was due to Carter's interest and willingness to do consults at Babies Hospital as well as attending multiple teaching rounds there. By 1956, Rustin McIntosh, the eminent director of Babies Hospital, felt that housing children at the Neurological Institute was inappropriate and allowed the Pediatric Neurology Service to transfer its beds to Babies Hospital at Columbia-Presbyterian Medical Center. Child neurologists were simultaneously not only given the opportunity to diagnose, investigate, and treat neurological disorders as consultants, but would also manage pediatric medicine. This was a monumental decision by McIntosh and his staff to embrace the then novel concept that child neurologists could manage both pediatric and neurological problems. Subsequently, this plan became the prototype for university-based child neurology services throughout the country.

Discussions between Pearce Bailey, director of the then National Institute of Neurological Disease and Blindness in Bethesda, Maryland, Merritt, Carter, Philip Dodge, and David Clark led to the federal funding of training fellowships for child neurologists in 1957. This was prompted by the belief that World War II had stunted the development of neurology as a specialty and left the country short of neurologists. Prior to this, there had been no hospital funding for the training of pediatric neurologists. As a result of discussions with Bailey, Merritt, and McIntosh, Carter established his program in child neurology, receiving support for two fellows for each year of a three-year program. Carter organized the original training program, modeling it essentially after the three-year adult training program, with one year spent in learning the fundamentals of neurology on the adult service, one year of neurodiagnostic training, and one year spent on the child neurology service, as opposed to the traditional neurology residency of a second supervising year on the adult service. Fellows coming into this program had already completed a pediatric residency. By the mid-1960s, it was not clear which specialty, neurology or pediatrics, should absorb child neurology. Dialogue developed between members of the American Board of Pediatrics (Randolph Byers of Harvard and Ralph Platou of Tulane) and the American Board of Psychiatry and Neurology (Frank Forster of the University of Wisconsin and Carter). Based on the necessity for formal training in neuroanatomy and neurophysiology for pediatric neurologists, obviously lacking in the pediatric residency, these discussions led to the development of certification in 1967 by the American Board of Psychiatry and Neurology with a designation of Special Competence in Child Neurology. Carter neglected to apply for the Special Competence certificate until later, receiving certificate No. 39 in 1969.

Carter rose rapidly in the academic ranks at Columbia. From 1950 to 1955, he was assistant professor of neurology at the College of Physicians and Surgeons, Columbia University. Between 1955 and 1960 he was an associate professor of clinical neurology. From 1960 to 1962, he was professor of clinical neurology and from 1962 to 1978, he was the Dwight David Eisenhower United Cerebral Palsy Professor. In 1978 he became Professor Emeritus of Neurology and Pediatrics and the Sidney Carter Professorship in Pediatric Neurology at the College of Physicians and Surgeons of Columbia University was established. The first and current Sidney Carter Professor is Darryl C. DeVivo, formerly of Washington University.

During his tenure, Carter was recognized for his clinical and didactic skills. Patient referrals clustered in the greater New York metropolitan area, but by the 1960s, his diagnostic acumen generated international referrals. These patients were shared with medical students, pediatric, and neurology residents, and child neurology fellows. The most difficult diagnostic problems became the clinical basis for a monthly nocturnal meeting in the library on the fourteenth floor of the Neurological Institute. Amidst beer and pretzels the evening culminated in a clinicopathological case conference discussed by residents, fellows, neuropathologists, child neurology faculty (Abe Chutorian, Arnold Gold, Jim Hammill, Niels Low), and visitors (Isabelle Rapin, Joe French, Al Aron). The neurology residents and fellows held a noncompeting monthly Friday evening social club, known as the Marchiafava-Bignami Society, to which faculty were invited.

Early publications by Carter emphasized treatment of epilepsy (Merritt and Carter, 1950; Yahr et al, 1952; Ransonoff and Carter, 1954) and the introduction of new anticonvulsants (Carter, Sciarra, and Merritt, 1950; Sciarra et al, 1954). Later collaborations with colleagues and child neurology fellows covered a wide range of clinical topics such as tumors (Bray, Carter, and Taveras, 1958; Chutorian et al, 1964), and cerebrovascular disease (Gold, Ransonoff, and Carter, 1964; Hilal et al, 1971). Fellows were encouraged to analyze the enormous experience of the Columbia-Presbyterian hospitals. Many of these diverse studies, especially the long-term neurological complications of infectious disease, continue to be widely referenced and remain familiar to child neurologists (Weiss and Carter, 1959; Aron, Freeman, and Carter, 1965). Approximately eighty journal articles were contributed by Carter and his collaborators. In addition, Carter was responsible for editing the neurology section of Nelson's *Textbook of Pediatrics*, which eventually was published as a monograph entitled *Neurology of Infancy and Childhood* in collaboration with Arnold Gold (1974).

The neurological community also recognized Carter's attributes and demanded his energies. From 1958 to 1966, he was director of the American Board of Psychiatry and Neurology, becoming president in 1965. He was a member of the Board of Trustees of the American Academy of Neurology from 1959 to 1963, and was president from 1969 to 1971. In addition, he was president of the American Neurological Association from 1978 to 1979. Thus, Carter was president of all three major neurological organizations: the American Board of Psychiatry and Neurology, the accrediting organization for neurologists and psychiatrists; the American Academy of Neurology, the largest society of neurologists; and the American Neurological Association, the oldest of the neurological associations.

In 1978 Sidney Carter left Columbia University to become chief of neurology at Blythedale Children's Home in Valhalla, New York, where he has remained active in treating chronic neurological illnesses in children and teaching pediatric neurology to orthopedic, pediatric, and neurology residents from a number of New York-area medical schools.

In 1945 Sidney Carter married Elizabeth Marion Crosby, an American army nurse stationed in England. After moving to New York City, they settled in Yonkers, New York. Three sons were born, Jeffrey, Jonathan, and Jeremy. These youngsters were probably the most acute observers of a director of an active teaching program who also maintained a busy neurological practice. Continuous demands required a caring physician to see patients during early morning hours, lunch times, and after hours. Rounds frequently could not be completed until late at night. None of his sons chose medicine as a career.

Carter's unique contribution to the development of child neurology as a specialty can be extracted from this brief biography. He separated child neurology into an independent service with its own beds with responsibility for total care, both pediatric and neurological, by the child neurologist. He was successful in developing a federally funded fellowship to train child neurologists and established a three-year training protocol similar in basic sciences, neurodiagnostic techniques, and clinical neurology to the adult training program. He arranged for the credentialing of child neurologists by the American Board of Psychiatry and Neurology, thus establishing child neurology as a semi-independent neurologic specialty. Additionally, he maintained the respect of adult neurologists by his personal involvement in the politics of all the major neurological associations and the National Institutes of Health.

He believed strongly that it was necessary to train child neurologists for academic settings so they would ultimately train both pediatric and neurology residents. Most training programs continue this approach in developing child neurologists, although in recent years larger numbers of graduates are establishing themselves as community-based clinicians.

These accomplishments are recognized not only by the many child neurologists who trained at the Neurological Institute under the direction of Carter, but by child neurologists throughout the country. Many younger neurologists, acting as Board examiners for the first time, have had an opportunity to be a coexaminer with Carter. It was not unusual for them to remark that they had never had a more caring, concerned, or considerate examiner of a neurology candidate. Fellow examiners, trained at the Neurological Institute, would generally simply look at each other and smile. They were already well aware of Sidney Carter's kindness and the high esteem he held for fellow creatures in distress, whether they were physicians undergoing a stressful examination, children with serious neurological problems, or their grieving parents.

A few questions still remain unanswered among Carter's former fellows. Did Sidney ever win a pot in Merritt's weekly poker game? Why white socks, even with a tuxedo? These humorous personal mysteries remain, but his contributions to the development of child neurology are obvious to the neurologic, pediatric, and greater medical communities.

Sanford Schneider
LOMA LINDA, CALIFORNIA

ACKNOWLEDGMENTS

Gratefully, I acknowledge the contributions of those who shared their thoughts on Dr. Carter for this chapter: Peggy Ferry, M.D. (University of Arizona); Arnold Gold, M.D. (Columbia University); Melvin Greer, M.D. (University of Florida); and James Schwartz, M.D. (Emory University).

REFERENCES

Aron, A. M., J. M. Freeman, and S. Carter, 1965. The Natural History of Sydenham's Chorea. *Am J Med* 38:83–95.

Bray, P. F., S. Carter, and J. M. Taveras, 1958. Brainstem Tumors in Children. *Neur* 8:1–7.

Carter, S., D. Sciarra, and H. H. Merritt. 1950. Phenylacetylurea in the Treatment of Convulsive Seizures. *Dis Nerv Sys* 11:139–41.

Carter, S., and A. P. Gold. 1974. *Neurology of Infancy and Childhood.* New York: Appleton-Century-Crofts.

Chutorian, A. M., et al. 1964. Optic Gliomas in Children. *Neur* 14:83–95.

Gold, A., J. Ransonoff, and S. Carter. 1964. Vein of Galen Malformation. *Acta Neur Scand* (Suppl.) 2:40.

Hilal, S. K., et al. 1971. Primary Cerebral Arterial Occlusive Disease in Children. Part 1: Acute Acquired Hemiplegia. Part 2: Neurocutaneous Syndromes. *Rad* 99:71–94.

Merritt, H. H., and S. Carter. 1950. Anticonvulsant Drugs. *Med Clin North Am* 34:341–50.

Merritt, H. H., and T. J. Putnam. 1938. A New Series of Anticonvulsant Drugs Tested by Experiments on Animals. *Arch Neur Psych* 39:1003–15.

Ransonoff, J., and S. Carter. 1954. Hemispherectomy in the Treatment of Convulsive Seizures Associated with Infantile Hemiplegia. *Proc Assoc Res Nerv Ment Dis* 34:176–95.

Sciarra, D., et al. 1954. Clinical Evaluation of Primidone (Mysoline), New Anticonvulsant Drug. *JAMA* 154:827–29.

Weiss, S., and S. Carter. 1959. Course and Prognosis of Acute Cerebellar Ataxia in Children. *Neur* 9:711–21.

Yahr, M. D., et al. 1952. Evaluation of Standard Anticonvulsant Therapy in 319 Patients. *JAMA* 150:663–67.

DAVID CLARK

A STUDENT OF BOTH Douglas Buchanan and Frank Ford, David Barrett Clark (b. 1913) (figure 1) has become the consummate clinician and teacher. He was born in Glen Ellyn, Illinois, now a suburb of Chicago, but at that time a small rural community. The family's Scottish heritage is evident in his father's observation that "we could be characterized as being poor but respectable, except for the fact that if I must be poor I'm damned if I'll be respectable." Clark began college as a veterinary student at Michigan State College. While preparing sections of rabbit cerebral cortex for a histology course, he became fascinated with the nervous system. Realizing after two years of veterinary school that he was more interested in human medicine, Clark was able to pursue premedical courses while still in the veterinary program.

He entered the University of Chicago Graduate School of Medicine after a lengthy correspondence with the dean about whether a veterinary student should ever be admitted to any medical school. The neuroscience program at Chicago provided a unique environment in the 1930s. As an anatomy student, Clark had contact with such famous neuroscientists as Heinrich Klüver and C. Judson Herrick. Clark was awarded the William H. Wilder Fellowship in Anatomy, which carried an annual stipend of $400. This sum paid Clark's tuition but left nothing on which to live. Clark and one other student were hired by the anatomist George William Bartelmez to maintain his monkey colony. Bartelmez carefully pointed out that he needed someone to look at the food budget very carefully. So, for a year the monkeys (and Clark) thrived on hamburgers, fresh eggs, and green vegetables. He obtained his Ph.D. in anatomy in 1939 with his dissertation entitled "The Human Spinal Cord Twenty Years After Total Transection."

David Clark spent the war years working on the neuropathology of war gases as a research assistant to Steven Polyak. During this time he also developed a close personal and professional relationship with Douglas Buchanan, which was to last until Buchanan's death over forty years later. Though Buchanan's primary appointment was at the University of Chicago, he was also the attending physician in charge of the neurological services at Children's Memorial Hospital, where he conducted a weekly clinic and ward rounds, often accompanied by Clark. From 1942 through 1946 Clark had his own part-time affiliation with the Children's Memorial Hospital as its neuropathologist, reflecting his developing interest in neuropathology. Clark resumed his medical studies after the war, earning his medical degree from the University of Chicago in 1946 and interning in pediatrics from January through June of 1947. During this time he met and subsequently married an attractive pediatric attending physician, Barbara Kenyon, who shared his love of animals, especially horses. In characteristic style, David first proposed to "Major Barbara" late one night at the bedside of a young patient with large subdural hematomas.

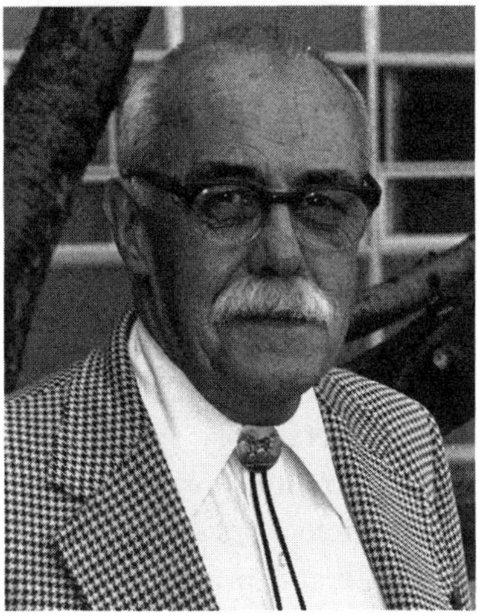

Figure 1. David Clark.

In July 1947 Clark began an internship in medicine at Johns Hopkins Hospital, followed by a year of neurology residency. During the academic year 1950–51, he went to London as the Fulbright Lecturer in Neurology, National Hospital, Queen's Square, and worked with J. Godwin Greenfield. This important experience left enduring memories. Almost forty years later, on teaching rounds, he still illustrates clinical principles with stories about how the neurologists at the National Hospital approached similar clinical problems.

On his return from England, Clark thrived at Johns Hopkins, rising in the ranks from instructor to associate professor. His close relationship with his mentor, Frank Ford ("The Judge"), can be seen in the thirty-two references to Clark in Ford's classic textbook *Diseases of the Nervous System in Infancy, Childhood, and Adolescence* (Ford, 1966). The atmosphere at Johns Hopkins, with its emphasis on clinical expertise, was to Clark's liking. Clark became widely known for his discerning analysis of cases on the ward and his virtuoso performances in the clinical pathological conferences (CPC). In his hands the CPC is both exciting and instructive. Clark reasons his way through the differential diagnosis aloud, explaining in detail why the clinician should accept or reject each possible explanation for the patient's signs and symptoms, arriving at the correct diagnosis with an almost uncanny knack. Because of his retentive memory, he is especially good at recalling clinical details and is seldom fooled twice by the same clinical entity. He can be an especially daunting visiting professor. With expertise in both clinical neurology and neuropathology, he has often surprised his hosts by reinterpreting the clinical story, the radiologic films, and the pathologic slides to demonstrate that his diagnosis is at least plausible and probably correct, while theirs is neither. An accomplished raconteur, he usually manages to entertain while he instructs.

In the late 1950s, Clark was one of the original child neurology consultants to Pearce Baily, who was then director of the National Institute of Neurological Diseases and Blindness. Clark was among the small group of advisors instrumental in the development and organization of the National Collaborative Perinatal Project. The project was intended to be a relatively small and carefully crafted prospective study designed to identify the causes of major neurological deficits in young children but was later expanded to include sixty thousand pregnancies.

An energetic and colorful teacher, Clark was especially popular with the students and house staff at Johns Hopkins. One of his major concerns was the extent to which the interns controlled patient care. Clark argued that first-class training for interns should not result in second-class care for their patients. His earlier experiences in both Chicago and London had convinced him that control of patient care by the attending physician was essential to good house staff training. Throughout his years at Johns Hopkins, neurology was not a separate department, but a division within the Department of Medicine. Indeed, during his long and distinguished career at Johns Hopkins, Frank Ford never had admitting privileges. The inability to form a Department of Neurology in the face of vigorous opposition from the Departments of Medicine and Pediatrics became an intractable problem. He chafed under the reins of the Department of Pediatrics, which was staffed with colleagues who wanted to care for children with neurologic disorders, but who often seemed uninterested in the nuances and complexities of neurologic diagnosis and treatment.

In 1965 Clark accepted appointment as the first professor and chairman of the Department of Neurology at the newly organized medical school of the University of Kentucky in Lexington. William Willard, who was both dean of the College of Medicine and vice-president of the Medical Center, had a reputation for recruiting outstanding chairpersons and giving them the freedom to develop their own programs. An additional advantage was the school's location in the center of the American thoroughbred industry, for by this time the Clarks had progressed from horse lovers to breeders.

The new department started with a faculty of three neurologists, including the chairman. In forming a new department, Clark was able to establish traditions that reflected values developed at the University of Chicago, the National Hospital at Queen's Square, and Johns Hopkins. Neurology became a unified service covering both adults and children. The special problems of diagnosis and treatment of neurologic disease in different age groups were not ignored, but the emphasis was upon elucidating pathogenic patterns and developing diagnostic methods applicable to all patients with neurologic disorders. Clinical teaching was stressed, and woe to the house officer who tried to hide a patient with neurologic disease from the chief! Clark had mastered the technique of late evening strolls through the wards. Unannounced, he would appear on the ward to ask the nurses (all known to him by first name) "What's up?" He would then proceed to any patients with neurologic complaints, even those on other services. Nurses were familiar with his late-night telephone inquiries about patients and his rapid appearance at the first hint of trouble. Clark became a favorite of the residents and students. They appreciated his ability to rationalize a complicated differential diagnosis and his willingness to do this at any hour. His amusing stories also enlivened the long evenings at the hospital.

The zenith of the week's teaching was the Tuesday evening conference. From 7 to 9 p.m., the house staff briefly presented the most difficult neurologic patients they could find. Clark would then retake the history, do the examination, and announce his diagnosis. Only then were any laboratory or biopsy data presented and a final diagnosis made. A weekly audience of fifty to seventy-five residents, students, faculty, and community neurologists would usually attend. They came to see if the professor could be topped (he seldom was) and to learn more about neurology.

Neurologic illnesses were not seen as isolated events, separate from the rest of the patients' lives. Adopting the pattern he had observed at the National Hospital, Queen's Square, Clark hired his own social worker, who was appointed to the faculty, made daily ward rounds with the service, and became an integral part of the department. Many of the department's Appalachian patients were impoverished and unable to travel into Lexington on any regular basis. Clark persuaded the U.S. Public Health Service to provide a three-year demonstration grant to enable him to take the university neurologists into the mountains. He set up periodic clinics in small mountain towns and staffed them with the local public health nurses, and a team of doctors, students, and social workers from the university. As a result, in 1972, the Commonwealth of Kentucky assumed responsibility for funding biweekly regional neurology clinics (Baumann and Leonidakis, 1979).

The accent on clinical teaching and patient care did not signify neglect of such goals as training neurologic investigators and advancing knowledge. Clark continued his interests in the pathology of congenital and perinatal neurologic disorders and in the neurologic complications of congenital heart disease, which were begun at Johns Hopkins (Ford and Clark, 1956; Tyler and Clark, 1957a, 1957b, 1958a, 1958b; Clark and Anderson, 1961; Clark, 1967). Involved in the controversy over the relation between birth control pills and stroke, he eventually testified to the existence of this relation before a Congressional committee.

Another area of interest was subacute sclerosing panencephalitis, which was endemic in rural Kentucky. Clark participated in both immunologic investigations and a partially effective trial of amantadine therapy (Haslam and Gerson, 1971; Haslam, McQuillen, and Clark, 1969; Robertson, Clark, and Markesbery, 1980). Clark never limited his purview to child neurology. He has maintained an interest in the pathology of the senile dementias and has encouraged the development of an Alzheimer's disease research group in the department (Cook, Schneck, and Clark, 1981).

Clark has preferred oral to written communication. While he published relatively few articles, he has continued an active program of guest lectures. He has been invited to London as the Teal Lecturer at the Royal College of Physicians in 1967; to Birmingham as the Sir Leonard Parsons Lecturer in 1973; to Oxford as the Litchfield Lecturer in Residence, Oxford University, in 1976; to London as the MacKeith Lecturer, British Society of Child Neurologists, in 1980; and as the Visiting Professor, Royal Society of Medicine, in 1985; and at the Royal Alexandra Hospital for Children in Sydney, Australia, in 1973 and 1979. He gave the Douglas Reye Memorial Lecture to the International Congress of Child Neurology in Sydney in 1979. For his many contributions to child neurology, Clark received the Hower Award from the Child Neurology Society in 1979. He has been active in the training and certification of neurologists, especially child neurologists. He has served as director of the American Board of Psychiatry and Neurology (1967 to 1979) and a member of the AMA Residency Review Committee for Psychiatry and Neurology (1966 to 1974). Few of the hundreds of neurologists whom he has worked with will ever forget him. Soft spoken and smiling, he gives the impression of both knowing and liking you while insisting you solve apparently impossible clinical puzzles.

David Clark has made a unique and important contribution to child neurology as a distinct discipline with a unique body of knowledge. To his colleagues, his outstanding qualities are kindness and an extraordinary clinical insight. He is warm and compassionate with both patients and their families. Added to this is his painstaking attention to the details of history and examination, coupled with a careful and critical separation of fact from supposition. Certainly this approach is part of his legacy from his colleagues at Queen's Square. He brings to clinical neurology a degree of insight and breadth of knowledge that is uniquely his.

Robert J. Baumann
LEXINGTON, KENTUCKY

Herbert M. Swick
MILWAUKEE, WISCONSIN

☙ REFERENCES

Baumann, R. J., and M. G. Leonidakis. 1979. Extending Neurologic Services to Rural Children. *Neur* 29:1298–1300.

Clark, D. B. 1967. Brain Abscess and Congenital Heart Disease. *Clin Neurosurg* 14:274–87.

Clark, D. B., and G. W. Anderson. 1961. Correlation of Complications of Labor with Lesions in the Brains of Neonates. *J Neuropath Exp Neur* 20:275–78.

Cook, R. H., S. A. Schneck, and D. B. Clark. 1981. Twins with Alzheimer's Disease. *Arch Neur* 38:300.

Ford, F. R. 1966. *Diseases of the Nervous System in Infancy, Childhood, and Adolescence*. 5th ed. Springfield, IL: Charles C Thomas.

Ford, F. R., and D. B. Clark. 1956. Thrombosis of the Basilar Artery with Softening in the Cerebellum and Brain Stem Due to Manipulation of the Neck. *Bull Johns Hopkins Hosp* 98:37–42.

Haslam, R. H. A., and K. Gerson. 1971. Subtle Immunologic Abnormalities in Four Boys with Subacute Sclerosing Panencephalitis. *NEJM* 285:78–82.

Haslam, R. H. A., M. P. McQuillen, and D. B. Clark. 1969. Amantadine Therapy in Subacute Sclerosing Panencephalitis. *Neur* 19:1080–86.

Robertson, W. C., D. B. Clark, and W. R. Markesbery. 1980. Review of 38 Cases of Subacute Sclerosing Panencephalitis: Effect of Amantadine on Survival. *Ann Neur* 8:422–34.

Tyler, H. R., and D. B. Clark. 1957a. Incidence of Neurological Complications in Congenital Heart Disease. *AMA Arch Neur Psych* 77:17–22.

______. 1957b. Cerebral Vascular Accidents in Congenital Heart Disease. *AMA Arch Neur Psych* 77:483–89.

______. 1958a. Loss of Consciousness and Convulsive Disorders in Patients with Congenital Heart Disease. *AMA Arch Neur Psych* 79:506–10.

______. 1958b. Neurologic Complications in Patients with Coarctation of the Aorta. *Neur* 8:712–18.

CYRIL COURVILLE

☙ CBC MEANS "complete blood count" to most physicians, but beginning in the early 1930s physicians, especially neurologists and neurosurgeons in the greater Los Angeles area, began to recognize these letters as referring to Cyril Brian Courville (1900–1968) (figure 1), physician, neurologist, neuropathologist, writer, editor, researcher, and professor of neurology.

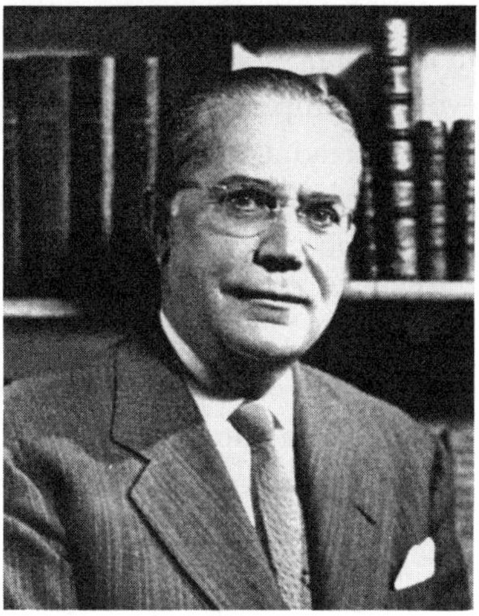

Figure 1. Cyril Courville (1900–1968).

Interest in diagnosis, treatment, and research into diseases of the nervous system were slow to develop in Southern California and did not begin to bloom until about 1920 when Carl Rand began to limit his practice to neurosurgery, and Samuel Ingham, who trained in neuropsychiatry at the University of Pennsylvania, set up practice in Los Angeles. These men inspired and trained many young physicians during the next half-century. Among the first of these was Courville (Breuer, Lomax, and Marshall, 1983).

Courville, "Cy" to his friends, was born in 1900 in Traverse City, Michigan, into a middle-class Seventh-Day Adventist home. He was an excellent scholar, receiving his baccalaureate degree from Emanuel Missionary College (now Andrews University) in Berrien Springs, Michigan. He entered the College of Medical Evangelists (now the School of Medicine at Loma Linda University) in California at age twenty-one and graduated in 1925. He interned at the Los Angeles County General Hospital (LACGH) for fifteen months and then became a resident there under Carl Rand, chief of the Neurosurgery Service. In 1927 he went to the Peter Bent Brigham Hospital in Boston to work under Harvey Cushing as a voluntary assistant. His industry, keen powers of observation, and devotion to detail helped him absorb a great deal of neurological information in a relatively short time. In a letter dated August 16, 1927, to Edward Risley, dean of his medical school, he wrote: "This is a very interesting and important line of my work for I am learning to do absolutely careful and accurate examinations upon which the success of neurological diagnosis depends." Years later, when I was a resident under Courville, the results of this early training were still apparent and we residents were required to record all positive and negative findings. As a result, our reports were never less than five and often seven or more single-spaced pages in length. In fact, our reports often evoked complaints from referring physicians — they didn't have time to read all that!

While in Boston, Courville came under the influence of Percival Bailey, who was studying the histology of brain tumors removed by Harvey Cushing. Admiration for Bailey aroused Courville's interest in neuropathology, and on his return to California he began a residency in this field at the LACGH. This choice eventually brought him international recognition as scientific articles flowed from his pen — as many as twenty-four in a single year (1936).

One of Courville's early interests was in suppurative infections of the central nervous system, an interest he shared with Johannes M. Nielsen, with whom he often collaborated, jointly authoring over a dozen papers in that area. Many of these papers dealt with the complications of otitis media, mastoiditis, and sinusitis in childhood (Courville and Nielsen, 1934, 1935). Courville recognized that many of these cases were associated with the development of focal Jacksonian seizures; that spread of infection occurred by several routes, including retrograde venous extension into the sinuses; and that the cerebral lesions were toxic, thrombotic, or infectious in nature.

Gradually his interest and curiosity began to center on anoxic and traumatic brain insults. This led to his major contributions to pediatric neurology — the causes, pathological changes, and clinical results of anoxia and trauma of the central nervous system in the fetus, newborn, and infant — and was the motivation for a monograph, *Cerebral Palsy* (1954), and three books: *Commotio Cerebri* (1953a), *Cerebral Anoxia* (1953b), and *Birth and Brain Damage* (1971), finished two weeks before his death in 1968 and published posthumously by his wife. This last book was probably his most important contribution, because it synthesized and correlated all his earlier work with that of other researchers in a clarification of the causes and results of perinatal insults to the brain. His goal was emphasized by his statement in the epilogue:

But the most important desired effect of a monograph such as this will be to stimulate the obstetricians to make a new and sustained drive to study the causes and preventions of the episodes of perinatal anoxia in an effort to prevent the ruined lives of cerebral paralytics, the epileptics and the mental defectives who survive the curse of perinatal anoxia. (Courville, 1971)

Thus his emphasis on the sequelae to perinatal cerebral anoxia and injuries led to better understanding of the pathogenesis of the lesions found in brain-injured infants and children. This knowledge resulted in changes in obstetrical and pediatric practice that have effectively reduced the morbidity resulting from some of these problems. His studies of cerebral palsy also helped to clarify understanding of these conditions.

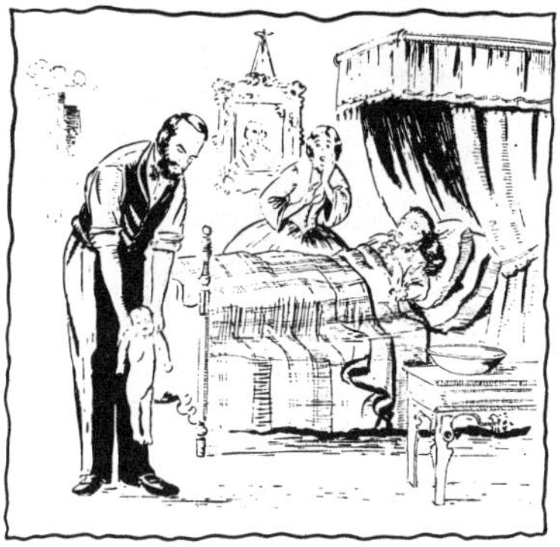

Figure 2. Courville's works were usually annotated with a comprehensive historical introduction. This photograph is from his book *Cerebral Anoxia* (originally figure 5, p. 36) and depicted techniques of resuscitation in the section on anoxia of the newborn.

Courville's books were interesting in that they usually included a succinct but thorough historical review of the subject (figure 2), as well as diagrams that summarized in a clear-cut way the analysis of his extensive neuropathological experiences. His books *Cerebral Anoxia* and *Birth and Brain Damage* were replete with photographs of illustrative neuropathologic specimens accompanied by occasional drawings that elucidated the proposed pathophysiological mechanisms (figure 3).

While Courville's consideration of anoxia was particularly oriented toward the "future" of the neuron, the brain, the patient, and society, his interest in craniocerebral injuries directed some of his research "backwards" in time to the sources of head injury in primitive cultures, earlier civilizations, and in mythology, where stones, rocks, clubs, swords, spears, axes, and similar weapons were used to fight wars, settle disputes and commit crimes of violence. He began collecting weapons, and artifacts such as skulls, helmets, and illustrative "case histories" of famous and infamous head injuries. This extensive and intriguing collection is held at Loma Linda University. Courville's interest in history, folklore, and mythology was evidenced by the frequent references in his writings to pertinent incidents from these sources. His books and monographs often de-

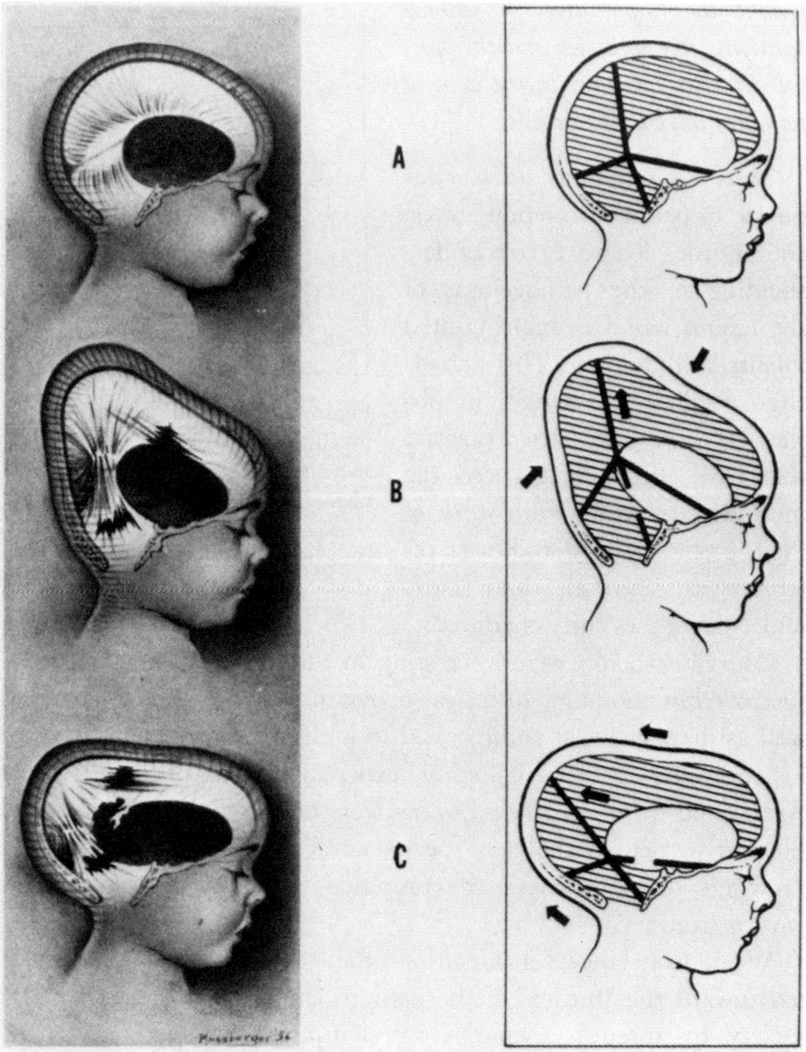

Figure 3. Based on his extensive neuropathologic experience with the newborn, Courville frequently included diagrams to demonstrate the pathogenesis of different types of birth injuries, such as those involving tentorial tears, as published in *Birth and Brain Damage* (originally figure 3, p. 26).

voted an early chapter to an historical review of that particular condition. Overshadowing the collection of artifacts mentioned above, however, was his personal library, a collection of books that covered neurology, neuropathology, neurosurgery, and the broad range of his other interests. After his death in 1968, his library with its thousands of volumes was acquired by the Medical Library of the University of California, Irvine (Thomas and Cooper, 1978).

Courville's reputation as a neuropathologist was nurtured by his association with the Los Angeles County General Hospital, where access to clinical cases and pathological specimens was unexcelled. Nearly 50,000 autopsies were performed during his forty years of tenure. In 1934, soon after the hospital moved into more modern facilities, Courville established the Santiago Ramon y Cajal Laboratory of Neuropathology. These quarters were a welcome change from the cramped space in which he had worked as a neuropathology resident and where he recalled "the warm association which existed between my knees and a steam radiator" under the thirty-inch shelf on which hospital charts, notes, slides, and specimens vied for his attention. In the new laboratory the Neuropathology Service blossomed, and so did its director's research activities and writing of scientific papers.

As the flow of brain specimens through the Ramon y Cajal Laboratory increased, regular weekly brain-sectioning sessions were held on Thursday afternoons, conducted by both Nielsen, with his special interest in cortical localization, and Courville, with his interest in tumors and trauma. The orientation was toward both morbid anatomy and clinicopathologic investigation. These sessions were attended by students, residents, neurologists, neurosurgeons, psychiatrists, and other interested physicians, some of whom drove sixty or more miles to attend these sessions and the neurology conferences held the same evenings. In the latter meetings the neurology residents would present interesting or puzzling neurological and neurosurgical patients to a prestigious group of clinicians presided over by Samuel Ingham, and including Courville, Nielsen, Carl Rand, George Thompson, Elinor Ives, Karl Von Hagen, Clemson Marsh, Emil Selitz, Eugene Ziskind, Clarence Olsen, Frank Anderson, Albert A. Marinacci, Kenneth Abbott, Edwin Amyes, R. Raney, Aidan Raney, Cullen W. Irish, and Philip Vogel (who later, with Joseph Bogen, revived the cerebral commissurotomy for the treatment of intractable seizures). It was from the study of a series of these patients that Roger Sperry received the Nobel Prize for Physiology in 1981. In these discussions Courville's keen insight and careful attention to details gave his opinions much weight, but, as has been said of another famous neurologist, he was "occasionally wrong, but never in doubt." These meetings were educational, entertaining, and sometimes exciting, as illustrated by the time a patient with "stiffman syndrome" staggered, lost his balance, and fell, ending up on the lap of Elinor Ives.

Although Courville was an excellent clinician and diagnostician, his real love was his writing. As an editor of the *Bulletin of the Los Angeles Neurological Society*, he often almost literally "composed, edited and carried" the new volume to the printer. His energy and productivity resulted in over twenty books and monographs and 330 articles on scientific, historical, biographical, and other subjects related to medicine but especially to the study of the nervous system. Much of his scientific writing was pertinent to pediatric practice, especially his last book, *Birth and Brain Damage*, which contains a complete bibliography of his works. His early interest and writings on cerebral infections, the effect of anoxia on the brain, birth injuries, brain tumors in children, and cerebral palsy helped to spur the development of pediatric neurology in the western United States.

Hans Berger's surface recording of the electrical potentials of the brain attracted Courville's interest early in the 1940s, and in the next few years two "electroencephalographs" were constructed under his direction by Lester C. Dale, an electronic wizard at the White Memorial Hospital. The first instrument had two channels, and the second, four, permitting it to be used clinically. It provided surprisingly dependable tracings that were relatively free of machine artifacts. Dale, with his son-in-law George Rathbun, next built an eight-channel machine, which was the mainstay of the newly formed Department of Electroencephalography. For a few years this instrument was better than any that were commercially available. Courville, on the basis of his interest in and knowledge of neuroanatomy, neuropathology, and clinical neurology, became adept at EEG interpretation. He wrote only two papers on this subject (1949), but he trained his residents in these skills, and during the 1950s a large number of the tracings done in Los Angeles were read by his former resident, Leslie B. Mann; and when I finished my residency I established the Neurodiagnostic Laboratory on the Loma Linda campus of the medical school. The EEG became and remains a very useful tool in pediatric neurology, primarily in the care of children with epilepsy.

Courville's interest in the degenerative diseases of the nervous system led him to study and write about the neuropathological changes in multiple sclerosis (1959, 1963, 1964, 1965). He noted that some of the features of the lesions were similar to those seen in venous thrombosis and for a time tried treating patients with heparin. Results were first encouraging, then equivocal, and finally disappointing, as have been so many new treatments for this unpredictable disease.

Another of Courville's interests was forensic neurology, and he contributed a chapter entitled "Forensic Aspects of Trauma to the Central Nervous System and Its Membranes" to the book *Legal Medicine*. In 1964 he published *Forensic Neuropathology; Lesions of the Brain and Spinal Cord of Medico-Legal Importance*. Frequent references to the legal aspect are found in many of his writings, including *Commotio Cerebri*, *Cerebral Anoxia*, and *Cerebral Palsy*. His reputation as an expert witness grew as a result of this work, and he frequently testified in court, where he was often a star witness. On one occasion he was asked to examine the brain of an aged western movie star and commented in court about the severe cerebral atrophy and its possible effect on competence to make a will. Another occasion was referred to by William Frederick Norwood, Ph.D., in his preface to *Birth and Brain Damage*:

He received acclaim in the public press when called as a consultant in 1963 after fighter Davey Moore received a fatal blow in the ring. Dr. Courville described the kind and location of the blow that would produce the concussion he discovered. Ringside observers thought there was no such blow, but a careful study of the motion picture film revealed precisely the cause of the injury as described by Dr. Courville.

Although medicine "flavored" most of Dr. Courville's activities, he was involved in many other areas. He was an excellent artist, with skills ranging from "chalk talks" to oil painting to sculpture. He illustrated his lectures to medical students and to lay groups with blackboard sketches, which helped to make him the respected teacher he was, and added interest to subjects that might otherwise have been dull. His oil paintings were reminiscent of the old masters and rivaled them in quality. He also had an interest in music, stimulated in part by his marriage to a talented musician, Margaret Farnsworth, in 1939.

Since he was a highly disciplined individual and also an energetic student of the Civil War, it is not surprising that he was intrigued by military matters. Prior to World War II he was involved in the establishment of the 47th General Hospital, the White Memorial Hospital Army Reserve unit, which was later activated and sent to the South Pacific. While still a major he developed a medical cadet corps for the training of medical personnel. This unit was adopted by the Seventh-Day Adventist Church because of its noncombatant status, making it possible for Adventist youth to enter the medical corps as "conscientious cooperators." The training book for this program was edited by Courville and contained his picture with a group of officers.

Courville taught at the Loma Linda University School of Medicine for over forty years, beginning in 1926 (Macpherson et al, 1966). He was appointed professor of neurology in 1933 and thirty-three years later the title Distinguished Service Professor was conferred upon him. He was active in many professional groups including the American Neurological Association, the American Academy of Neurology, the American Association of Neuropathology, the American Academy of Forensic Science, the American Association of Cerebral Palsy, and the American Association for the Advancement of Science. He personally organized the Harveian Society to foster interest in research and scholarly pursuits. He was also important in the organization of the Los Angeles Society of Neurology and Psychiatry, and in the establishment of its publication, the *Bulletin of the Los Angeles Neurological Society*, to which he was a frequent contributor, a coeditor with J. M. Nielsen for many years, and a member of the editorial board until 1966, when he was made emeritus editor.

Recognition is especially due Cyril Brian Courville for his excellent contributions to the development of child neurology, especially in the areas of birth injuries, cerebral anoxia, cerebral palsy, and suppurative lesions of the central nervous system.

Guy M. Hunt
LOMA LINDA, CALIFORNIA

REFERENCES

Breuer, F. A., E. M. R. Lomax, and L. H. Marshall. 1983. *History of the Human Brain*. Los Angeles: UCLA Publication Service Department.

______. 1953a. *Commotio Cerebri*. Los Angeles: San Lucas Press.

Courville, C. B. 1953b. *Cerebral Anoxia*. Los Angeles: San Lucas Press.

______. 1954. *Cerebral Palsy*. Los Angeles: San Lucas Press.

______. 1964. *Forensic Neuropathology; Lesions of the Brain and Spinal Cord of Medico-Legal Importance*. Mundelein, IL: Callaghan and Company.

______. 1971. *Birth and Brain Damage*. Pasadena: Church Press.

Courville, C. B., and J. M. Nielsen. 1934. Intracranial Complications of Otitis Media and Mastoiditis; Statistical Study with Survey of 10,000 Necropsies. *Acta Oto-Laryng* 21:1960.

______. 1935. Cerebral Manifestations Following Acute Otitis Media in Infancy and in Early Childhood, with Particular Reference to the Occurrence of Jacksonian Convulsions, Conjugate Deviation of the Head and Eyes, and Hemiplegia. *Am J Dis Child* 49:1–27.

Macpherson, W. W., et al. 1966. Cyril Brian Courville. *Med Arts Sci* 24:139–42.

Thomas, M. L. M., and W. C. Cooper. 1978. *Catalogue of Works in the Neurological Sciences Collected by Cyril Brian Courville, M.D. Representative of Clinical Neurology, Neuroanatomy, and Neuropathology with Particular Reference to Head Trauma*. Irvine: The University of California.

MACDONALD CRITCHLEY

ALTHOUGH MANY OF THOSE involved in the formative stages of child neurology came from diverse professional backgrounds, some, such as Macdonald Critchley (b. 1902) (figure 1), had early taken a special interest in the subject. His first appointment in London was as a house physician to the Hospital for Sick Children, Great Ormond Street, a delightful contact that he maintained in one form or another throughout his later career. His chiefs at Great Ormond Street were Sir George Still (also consultant to Kings College Hospital), Sir Robert Hutchison, and Frederick Poynton, all pediatricians. For years there was no neurologist on the staff of the Hospital for Sick Children. During this period and after Critchley

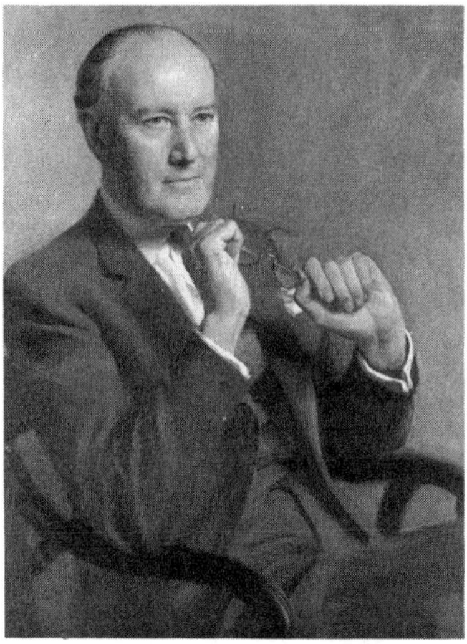

Figure 1. Photograph of the painting of Macdonald Critchley by Norman Hepple.

became a neurologist, he gave occasional lectures at the hospital and sometimes saw patients there. Later, after the staff neurologist, Paul Sandifer, had died, Critchley was invited to serve as a temporary consultant neurologist. This occurred just after Critchley's retirement from the National Hospital and National Health Service in 1965. Thus, Critchley both began and ended his hospital career in London at the same place, the Hospital for Sick Children, Great Ormond Street.

Born and reared in Bristol, Macdonald was somewhat of a child prodigy. His unusual literary talent became apparent when he won the *Daily Mail* competition at the age of eleven. Shortly afterward, he founded and edited the school magazine at Christian Brothers Colleges. By fifteen he had won a university place but, because of his young age, he spent an extra year in the study of Greek.

Critchley's studies at Bristol University and Medical School were interrupted by World War I. Driven by patriotic zeal when he was too young to enlist, he managed through a complicated series of maneuvers to serve in both the Royal Air Service and Royal Army. Following his return to Bristol University, he won a First Class Honours degree at the age of twenty-three. After serving as a house physician at the Bristol General Hospital for six months, he moved to London for further training.

Neurological training followed at the Maida Vale Hospital (1923–24) and over the subsequent three years at the National Hospital, Queen's Square. It was during this period that his medical writing began and that his interest in child neurology first became apparent. Because of his previous training at Great Ormond Street, he was alert to the problems of children, and, as he advanced in his neurological studies he was quick to discern those special facets of pediatric neurological disorders that differentiated them from the adult. Such differences were carefully analyzed and emphasized in at least a dozen of his early papers, about half of which were written while he was still a house officer. As with most other neurologists of the previous generation, Critchley's observations on children in these early papers have helped establish that background of knowledge that now demarcates the field of child neurology. Two examples are worth special comment. In a study of tuberous sclerosis, Critchley and Charles Earl analyzed the clinical findings in twenty-nine patients and were probably the first to point out its possible confusion with autism (Critchley and Earl, 1932). In another study, on the muscular dystrophies, he emphasized the many transitional forms, the fact that these could occur in members of a single family, and the association of the dystrophies with such other anomalies as scleroderma, optic atrophy, hereditary cerebellar ataxia, and mental retardation (Critchley, 1950).

Critchley's earlier studies were notable, not only for their keen clinical analysis and emphasis on childhood differences, but also for their exhaustive reviews of the literature. In retrospect, it was not surprising that he obtained staff appointments at both the National and Kings College hospitals at the early age of twenty-eight. I have been able to identify over twenty of his earlier papers that dealt with the neurological disorders of childhood, reviewing such topics as Leber's optic atrophy (1928), congenital neurosyphilis (1929), post-diptheric chorea (1924), brain tumors in children (1925), migraine (1933), and reflex epilepsy (1933).

Critchley's outstanding career as a teacher and lecturer was clearly augmented by his great command of the English language and his ability as an actor. He informed me on one occasion that he had considered the stage as a career at one early point and certainly he delighted in his membership in the Garrick Club of London. The club takes pride in its historical past, and my wife and I thoroughly enjoyed his hospitality there. His ability to hold his audience was phenomenal, as he made every presentation a fascinating experience. It was this highly developed talent, as well as his knowledge of French and German, that made him a popular lecturer and visiting neurologist in Europe before World War II.

Before the onset of the war, Critchley volunteered for the Royal

Navy and served for nearly seven years with the rank of surgeon captain. Thus, he was one of the very few who served in all three branches of the British military. Following his demobilization in May 1946, he returned to the National Hospital, where he remained until retiring from the active staff in 1965. He then continued in private practice until the age of eighty-four. Whereas before World War II, Europe and London had been Critchley's stage, the whole world became his stage following it. I first saw him in San Francisco (Medical School of the University of California) for a six-week period in 1951 and three other times since then for shorter periods. This peripatetic tendency, as well as his remarkable ability to present even esoteric neurology with great éclat, inevitably led to his election in 1965 as president of the World Federation of Neurology. He served in this capacity for the maximum term of eight years.

A second and more important aspect of Critchley's contribution to child neurology developed in this latter period and was the product of his interests in the higher functions of the brain — the use of language and written symbols in communication and the various disorders of such functions. Critchley's expertise in this field became world renowned. Although he published three early papers on mirror-writing, the bulk of his papers and books on developmental dyslexia did not come until later. The story is an interesting one, and I quote from one of his letters:

The dyslexia story . . . began dramatically in 1961. The ophthalmologists invited me to deliver the prestigious Doyne Memorial lecture in Oxford, and I chose as my topic "Inborn Reading Disorders of Central Origin." The lecture theater was packed to overflowing. . . . I realized that most of those present were either teachers or educational psychologists.

It became clear to me that there was a great scepticism, even hostility, on the part of teachers, the Ministry of Education, and educational psychologists to the concept of a specific developmental dyslexia. With a few notable exceptions, few neurologists, paediatricians or even paediatric neurologists were interested in the subject. General practitioners, too, were not concerned — unless one of their own children happened to be a poor reader.

Pressure groups of parents began to be set up, and slowly it began to be accepted that dyslexia existed and could be alleviated by special teaching techniques.

In 1964 I published my Developmental Dyslexia, *which was the first serious book on the subject in the U.K. It had great popularity and in 1970 I brought out* The Dyslexic Child. . . .

As President of the World Federation of Neurology I instituted a research group on Dyslexia. . . . We arrived at a definition of developmental dyslexia. However, educational psychologists in particular directed a steady stream of criticism at it. In 1978 Eileen [Mrs. Critchley] and I published Dyslexia Defined, *in which we suggested a longer and less vulnerable definition.*

Working with me, Eileen and I saw a steady stream of dyslexic children. We were able to study them thoroughly and make careful, detailed records. By the time I retired at the age of 84, I had seen 3,500 cases.

I wrote many papers on the subject. . . . The last three of them were more factual. Two appear in my Citadel of the Senses . . . *The third is in . . .* The Handbook of Clinical Neurology. *This sets out my most important observations.* (Critchley, 1989)

Critchley's pioneer work in the field of developmental dyslexia was recognized in America as well as in Great Britain, and in 1974 he was given the Samuel T. Orton Award.

A third aspect of Critchley's practice should be noted with respect to his work in the field of child neurology. His tact in handling retarded and dyslexic children and their families was superb. His verbal and acting ability again made him outstanding in this respect. Even more important, however, was his sympathetic understanding of the problem and its many social implications.

This sketch of Critchley would not be complete without at least a brief summary of the degrees, titles, and honors that were bestowed upon him. It would require two pages to list them all. They include the Order of the Commander of the British Empire; four honorary medical degrees; Correspondent Etranger, Académie Nationale de Médecine de France; Honorary Fellow, Royal Society of Medicine; and honorary membership in over thirty other national neurological societies around the world. In addition, he was president of the International League Against Epilepsy, the Association of British Neurologists, and the Harveian Society, and vice-president of the Royal College of Physicians. He was dean of the Institute of Neurology, Queen's Square, founding editor of the *Journal of the Neurological Sciences*, assistant editor of *Brain*, founder of the Migraine Trust, and held twenty-five distinguished lectureships. Although now almost ninety, quietly retired in Somerset, and nearly blind, his mind is still active and, with the help of his wife, Eileen, he is still writing, including one of the biographical sketches for this volume.

Robert B. Aird
SAN FRANCISCO, CALIFORNIA

ACKNOWLEDGMENTS

I gratefully acknowledge the help of Eileen Critchley in preparing this biographical sketch.

REFERENCES

Critchley, M. 1924. Post-Diphtheritic Chorea. *Brit J Child Dis* 21:188.

______. 1925. Brain Tumors in Children. *Brit J Child Dis* 22:251.

______. 1933. On Reflex Epilepsy. *Ann London Country Council Rep* 933:4.

______. 1950. The Muscular Dystrophies. *Practitioner* 164/980:118–21.

______. 1961. Inborn Reading Disorders of Central Origin. *Trans Ophth Soc* 81:459–80.

______. 1964. *Developmental Dyslexia*. London: W. Heinemann.

______. 1970. *The Dyslexic Child*. London: W. Heinemann.

______. 1985. Specific Developmental Dyslexia. In *Handbook of Clinical Neurology*. Vol. 46, 105–21. Ed. J. A. M. Fredericks. Amsterdam: Elsevier.

______. 1986. *Citadel of the Senses and Other Essays*. New York: Raven Press.

______. 1989. Personal communication.

Critchley, M., and E. A. Critchley. 1978. *Dyslexia Defined*. London: W. Heinemann.

Critchley, M., and C. J. C. Earl. 1932. Tuberous Sclerosis and Allied Conditions. *Brain* 55:311–46.

Critchley, M., and F. R. Ferguson. 1933. Migraine. *Lancet* 1:123.

Ferguson, F. R., and M. Critchley. 1928. Leber's Optic Atrophy and Its Relationship with the Heredo-Familial Ataxias. *J Neur Psych* 9:120.

______. 1929. A Clinical Study of Congenital Neurosyphilis. *Brit J Child Dis* 26:163.

PHILIP DODGE

PHILIP ROGERS DODGE (b. 1923) (figure 1) was born in Beverly, Massachusetts, and raised in New England. Most of his early years were spent either in Beverly, then a quiet, largely blue-collar town along the coast north of Boston (a region known locally as the North Shore) and in Lawrence, then a bustling mill town during the heyday of the large woolen mills in many towns north of Boston. During his youth, Dodge worked in a large variety of jobs to supplement his family's modest income.

Dodge remained in New England to receive his undergraduate education at the University of New Hampshire and Yale University. He attended medical school at the University of Rochester, where he received his M.D. in 1948. During his medical training at Rochester, Dodge worked as a research assistant in experimental neuroanatomy and neurosurgery with Wilbur Smith, who first kindled Dodge's interest in the nervous system. Dodge served as an intern in medicine at the Strong Memorial Hospital in Rochester and then returned home to train in Boston in neurology and neuropathology in the Neurology Services of the Harvard Medical School at the Boston City Hospital with Derek Denny-Brown and at the Massachusetts General Hospital with Raymond D. Adams. Dodge's continuing interest in neuropathology was fostered further by the tutelage and stimulation of Benjamin Castleman and Edward P. Richardson, Jr., at the Massachusetts General Hospital.

Dodge served in the U.S. Army as chief of the neurology services in Tokyo, Hawaii, and Kentucky in the early 1950s. During his service in Japan (1950–51), he had many interactions with Japanese neurologists, and, typical of all of Dodge's interactions, then and now, warm relationships developed and were to grow over the next thirty years. Interestingly, his work in the army in Tokyo included active participation in neurosurgery; indeed, he participated in approximately seven hundred surgical procedures related to injuries of the brain and spinal cord. Dodge's early work in experimental neurosurgery in Rochester served him well during this period. During his tenure in Fort Campbell, Kentucky, he was head of psychiatry as well as neurology, and put to good use

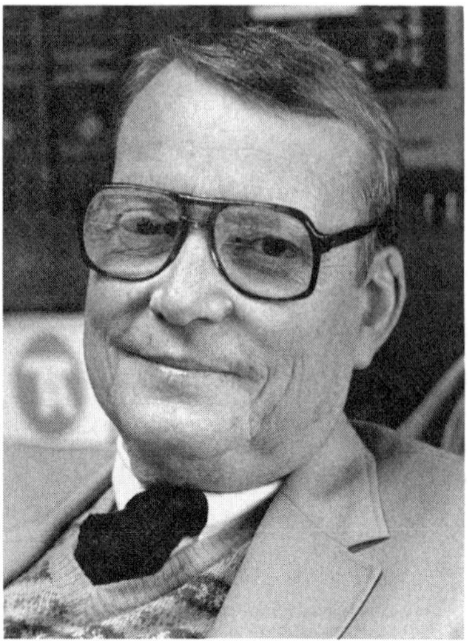

Figure 1. Philip Dodge.

the interest in psychiatric disease previously stimulated at the Massachusetts General Hospital by his interaction with Mandel E. Cohen.

After his service in the army, Dodge returned to Boston in 1956 to join the faculty of the Harvard Medical School and the staff of Raymond D. Adam's famous neurology service of the Massachusetts General Hospital. Indeed, at this time Dodge was keeping a promise to Adams, who, six years before had recognized Dodge's great potential and asked whether he would be willing to develop a program at Massachusetts General specifically dealing with the neurology of children. Dodge indicated that he would be willing but had a commitment to the military, to which Adams replied: "Fine, and when you extricate yourself from the military, get in touch with me." This conversation, in keeping with many of Adams's crucial administrative decisions, took place in the parking lot of the Boston City Hospital.

In the years following his return to the Massachusetts General Hospital in 1956, Dodge developed and refined his interest in child neurology, and from 1956 to 1967 he created at Massachusetts General Hospital a pediatric neurology service that enjoyed an international reputation. Fellows from around the world came there to learn from Dodge and then returned home to begin pediatric neurology in their own countries. Dodge's pediatric neurology service trainees during that period are now heads of divisions of child neurology or chairmen of departments of neurology or pediatrics. Indeed, these graduates of Philip Dodge's pediatric neurology service are leaders at medical schools located in essentially every major region of the United States and abroad.

While at the Massachusetts General Hospital from 1956 to 1967, Dodge had a major influence not only on his own fellows but on scores of pediatric house officers and Harvard medical students. He was a tireless teacher who made himself available at all hours. A common experience for a pediatric house officer at the Massachusetts General was to find Dodge walking through the wards of the Burnham building late in the evening, inquiring about interesting and difficult cases, and spending hours helping the house officer work through the complicated issues. On the other side of the coin, Dodge always had the knack of making the seemingly most mundane case interesting, uncovering new kernels of information and leaving behind several "pearls." A testimonial to the impact Dodge had during those years is the fact that a large number of outstanding pediatric house officers at Massachusetts General later followed him to St. Louis.

Dodge's impact on his child neurology fellows at Massachusetts General was huge and was experienced in many ways. All of us recall the famous Friday afternoons when he saw outpatients in his office in the Burnham building. After evaluating the patients and presenting them to him, each of us had the opportunity, really the privilege, to watch him examine the child, so very skillfully. Perhaps most impressive was the manner in which Dodge interacted with the parents of the child with neurological disease — his empathy, sensitivity, and remarkable insight into the impact of the disorder on every aspect of the couple's lives. We learned how to be physicians from the quintessential physician.

In 1967 Dodge went to St. Louis and Washington University as professor and head of the Edward Mallinckrodt Department of Pediatrics and as medical director of the St. Louis Children's Hospital. Under his leadership, the Department of Pediatrics at Washington University and St. Louis Children's Hospital attained preeminence in this country and abroad. Teaching and research programs flourished, and the best of medical care was delivered to all who came to that institution (figure 2). Careers of young faculty members developed in an atmosphere of collegiality, as Dodge constantly protected the time of everyone, except his own. He could be discovered at all hours, whether it be at 7 p.m. on a weekday, on a Saturday afternoon, or a Sunday morning. In considerable part as a consequence of Dodge's efforts, many of his faculty have assumed positions of leadership in academic pediatrics and pediatric subspecialities.

Dodge's warmth and personal goodness is exemplified by the

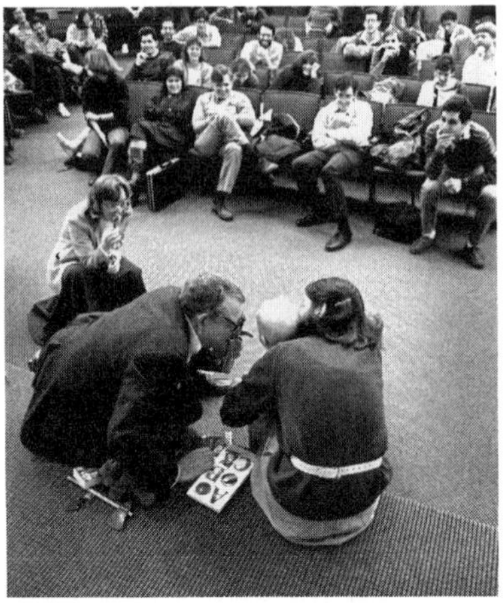

Figure 2. Philip Dodge during one of his very popular sessions with second-year Washington University medical students on the neurological examination of the infant.

frustrating experience of attempting to converse with him as one walked with him through the Children's Hospital, especially when the custodians and housekeeping personnel were working. Dodge greeted every one of them by name and asked about their family members by name. Their warm responses showed their appreciation for his caring, his sensitivity, and his understanding. Dodge, it seems, was forever giving to everybody. Perhaps these characteristics and their contagiousness were the main reasons that he could establish such a congenial department among such a large group of active, ambitious, intellectually aggressive young faculty.

Despite his commitment to protect the time of his faculty (one of whom once said that he couldn't understand how "such a cream puff with such a big and sensitive heart" could put up such a vigorous fight to protect his faculty), Dodge assumed a role of leadership at many levels in pediatrics and in neurology. He served on a large number of national scientific advisory committees, including the National Advisory Child Health and Human Development Council, and was chairman of the Mental Health Commission of the State of Missouri. He is a member of virtually every national and international pediatric and neurology society, and has served on editorial boards of the *Journal of Pediatrics, Pediatric Research*, *Neurology*, and *Developmental Medicine and Child Neurology*. Among the numerous awards granted to him, Dodge received the prestigious Hower Award of the Child Neurology Society in 1978.

Over the years Dodge has contributed approximately 150 publications to the medical literature. An attempt to review these in any detail would result in a veritable textbook of pediatric neurology. Any collection of representative examples should include his studies of the neurologic complications of fluid and electrolyte abnormalities. His work in this area includes both clinical (Crawford and Dodge, 1959) and experimental (Dodge, Crawford, and Probst, 1960; Hogan et al, 1983) studies. He described the major features of myasthenia gravis (Millichap and Dodge, 1960), and myotonic dystrophy (Dodge et al, 1965) in children. His review of congenital neuromuscular disorders with its discussion of the approach to the hypotonic infant provided a framework that is employed by most child neurologists today (Dodge, 1961). He described many of the major clinical features of the battered child syndrome before the topic became a popular one (Dodge, 1962). His description of acute toxic encephalopathies in children and their multifactorial etiologies (Lyon, Dodge, and Adams, 1961) set the stage for the description a few years later of Reye syndrome. He demonstrated the value of transillumination to child neurologists (Dodge and Porter, 1961), in keeping with his frequent teaching that careful analysis of the patient with relatively simple tools was the key to correct diagnosis.

His studies of subdural effusion in children taught us the multiple etiologies of this condition, the importance of underlying brain injury in the determination of prognosis, the mechanisms of reaccumulation of fluid, the effective therapies, and, particularly, the criteria for determining the appropriate intervention (Rabe, Flynn, and Dodge, 1962, 1968; Rabe, Young, and Dodge, 1964). He presented a classic exposition (Swartz and Dodge, 1965) of the neurology and neuropathology of bacterial meningitis in children, the likely pathogenetic mechanisms involved in the various neuropathologic states, and the relative frequency of hearing impairment as a sequela of acute bacterial meningitis (Dodge et al, 1984). He described an interesting collection of his patients who exhibited a nonprogressive syndrome of intellectual deficits, other neurologic features, and, notably, excessively rapid growth in childhood (Sotos et al, 1964). That syndrome now bears the name of his colleague in endocrinology, Juan Sotos. Among his other particularly astute clinical observations were the descriptions of unilateral pupillary dilation during and immediately following seizures and transient blindness following often relatively mild head injury in children (Griffith and Dodge, 1968).

Dodge contributed a large number of clearly written reviews and chapters in books. Most included original material that, as he would say, he "never found the time to write up." Included among these are marvelous discussions of pediatric cerebrovascular disease, myelitis and myelopathies, head injury, and diffuse nonbacterial inflammatory disorders of the nervous system. Surely a classic among these is his description of the neurologic examination of children in the several editions of Thomas W. Farmer's *Textbook of Pediatric Neurology*. Finally, his book *Nutrition and the Developing Nervous System*, written in collaboration with Arthur L. Prensky and Ralph D. Feigin, is widely recognized as a classic work (1975). When Dodge elected to devote his time to his research and teaching and to retire as chairman of pediatrics in St. Louis, he was promptly asked by the director of the National Institute of Child Health and Human Development to serve as a special assistant to review major aspects of the extramural mental retardation and developmental disabilities programs of that Institute. Not surprisingly, Dodge deferred his own plans and served 60 percent of the next year in that capacity. At the time of this writing he has returned to the Division of Child Neurology at Washington University to contribute, as only he can, to the research, service, and teaching activities.

At a testimonial to Philip Dodge on the occasion of his retirement from the chair of pediatrics at Washington University, which was attended by former trainees and faculty from all over the country, I said the following words about him, words that express the feelings of all who have been touched by him:

He has given to me in many ways over the years. . . . He's been a father, a counselor, and a trusted friend. . . . He has gently directed my career at crucial times with a wisdom that is remarkable. . . . He has been there to give — whether it's the evening at the end of a difficult day or a Saturday afternoon or the middle of the night at a time of personal crisis. . . . I've been very fortunate to have been here with him. . . . Phil, it's a privilege to be able to tell you publicly how much you have meant to me and to thank you very, very much.

Philip Dodge's impact on child neurology as a discipline and on all of us has been enormous.

Joseph J. Volpe
ST. LOUIS, MISSOURI

REFERENCES

Crawford, J. D., and P. R. Dodge. 1959. Complications of Fluid Therapy in Patients with Neurologic Disease: With Special Emphasis on Water Intoxication and Hypertonic Dehydration. *Ped Clin North Am* 6:257–79.

Dodge, P. R. 1961. Congenital Neuromuscular Disorders. *Res Publ Assoc Nerv Ment Dis* 38:479–533.

______. 1962. *Medical Implications of Physical Abuse of Children: Protecting the Battered Child.* Vol. 21, 23–25. Children's Division, The American Humane Society Publications.

Dodge, P. R., J. D. Crawford, and J. H. Probst. 1960. Studies in Experimental Water Intoxication. *Arch Neur* 3:513–29.

Dodge, P. R., et al. 1965. Myotonic Dystrophy in Infancy and Childhood. *Ped* 35:3–19.

______. 1984. Prospective Evaluation of Hearing Impairment as a Sequela of Acute Bacterial Meningitis. *NEJM* 311:869–74.

Dodge, P. R., and P. Porter. 1961. Demonstration of Intracranial Pathology by Transillumination. *Arch Neur* 5:594–605.

Dodge, P. R., A. L. Prensky, and R. D. Feigin. 1975. *Nutrition and the Developing Nervous System.* St. Louis: C. V. Mosby.

Farmer, T. W. (ed.). 1964. *Pediatric Neurology.* New York: Hoeber Medical Division Harper and Row Publishers.

Griffith, J. F., and P. R. Dodge. 1968. Transient Blindness Following Head Injury in Children. *NEJM* 278:648–51.

Hogan, G. R., et al. 1983. The Incidence of Seizures after Rehydration of Hypernatremic Rabbits with Intravenous or Ad Libitum Oral Fluids. *Ped Res* 18:340–45.

Lyon G., P. R. Dodge, and R. D. Adams. 1961. The Acute Encephalopathies of Obscure Origin in Infants and Children. *Brain* 84:680–708.

Millichap, J. G., and P. R. Dodge. 1960. Diagnosis and Treatment of Myasthenia Gravis in Infancy, Childhood, and Adolescence: A Study of 51 Patients. *Neur* 10:1007–14.

Rabe, E. F., R. E. Flynn, and P. R. Dodge. 1962. A Study of Subdural Effusions in an Infant with Particular Reference to the Mechanisms of Their Persistence. *Neur* 12:79–92.

______. 1968. Subdural Collections of Fluid in Infants and Children: A Study of 62 Patients with Special Reference to Factors Influencing Prognosis and the Efficacy of Various Forms of Therapy. *Neur* 18:559–70.

Rabe, E. F., G. F. Young, and P. R. Dodge. 1964. The Distribution and Fate of Subdurally Instilled Human Serum Albumin in Infants with Subdural Collections of Fluid. *Neur* 14:1020–28.

Sotos, J. F., et al. 1964. Cerebral Gigantism in Childhood: Syndrome of Excessively Rapid Growth with Acromegalic Features and a Nonprogressive Neurologic Disorder. *NEJM* 271:109–16.

Swartz, M. N., and P. R. Dodge. 1965. Bacterial Meningitis: A Review of

Selected Aspects. I. General Clinical Features, Special Problems and Unusual Meningeal Reactions Mimicking Bacterial Meningitis. II. Special Neurologic Problems, Postmeningitic Complications and Clinicopathological Correlations. *NEJM* 272:725–31, 842–48, 898–902, 954–60, 1003–10.

VICTOR DUBOWITZ

VICTOR DUBOWITZ (b. 1931) (figure 1), a pioneer in the classification and histochemical diagnosis of congenital myopathies, did not originally intend to become a pediatrician. While awaiting appointment as a doctor on a South American cruise ship in 1957, he took advantage of a temporary opportunity to relieve a house officer at Queen Mary's Hospital for Children, a comprehensive children's hospital with a chronic care facility in Carshalton, Surrey. The departing resident outlined the responsibilities of the service, indicating that there was no need to look in on the children with muscular dystrophy unless an acute problem developed. Dubowitz's curiosity was piqued, and he set out immediately for their ward, little realizing he was inaugurating a distinguished career in investigating the neuromuscular disorders of childhood.

Dubowitz was born on August 6, 1931, in Beaufort West, South Africa. By his teens, he could not decide whether to enter medicine or chemical engineering. He opted for medicine at the University of Cape Town and, because of his interest in science, elected to take an extra year obtaining a bachelor's degree in physiology. He was fascinated by neurophysiology, extensively studying the works of John Fulton, John Zachary Young, and Santiago Ramon y Cajal. Following graduation in 1954, he interned at the Groote Schuur Hospital at the University of Cape Town in surgery and medicine and decided to become a general practitioner.

To broaden his medical background, he moved to London in 1956 and accumulated experience in many medical specialties, including emergency medicine, ophthalmology, dermatology, obstetrics, gynecology, and endocrinology. His initial association with

Queen Mary's Hospital for Children, intended to be temporary, continued for two and one-half years. His research interests were stimulated by the fact that information on childhood myopathies, particularly muscular dystrophy, was very limited. While serving as a senior house officer, he simultaneously became a research fellow at the Postgraduate Medical School of Hammersmith Hospital in London under the supervision of Tony Pearse, an early member of the new science of histochemistry. Dubowitz and Pearse applied new techniques in oxidative and glycolytic histochemistry to the delineation of fiber types in human muscle and the chronic changes in muscular dystrophy and other myopathies (Dubowitz and Pearse, 1960a, 1960b).

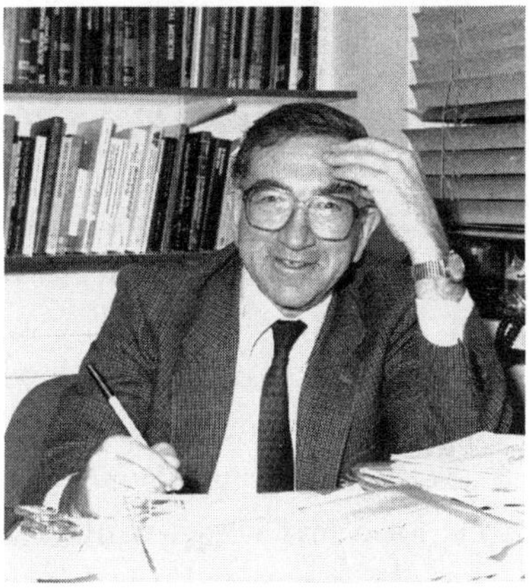

Figure 1. Victor Dubowitz.

In 1960 Dubowitz was awarded a doctorate in medicine from the University of Cape Town for his thesis, "Progressive Muscular Dystrophy in Childhood." That year he was appointed lecturer in clinical pathology at the National Hospital for Nervous Diseases in Queen's Square. By 1961 he had returned to the pediatric field as a lecturer in child health at the University of Sheffield under R. S. Illingworth. In 1965 he was awarded a Ph.D. from the University of Sheffield with his thesis entitled "A Histochemical Study of Enzymic Differentiation in Mature and Developing Human and Animal Muscle and Its Clinical Applications" (Dubowitz, 1965a, 1965b). That same year he was promoted to senior lecturer in child health at the University of Sheffield, as well as consultant pediatrician. During 1965–66 he spent a year as research associate at the Institute of Muscle Disease at Cornell University Medical College in New York. In 1972 he accepted the position of chairman of the department of pediatrics and neonatal medicine of the Institute of Child Health at the Royal Postgraduate Medical School of the University of London. He rapidly established a muscle clinic and research facility, which in 1975 blossomed into the Jerry Lewis Muscle Research Centre, with a capital grant from the Muscular

Dystrophy Association of America and a grant from the British Muscular Dystrophy Group with active support from John Walton.

Dubowitz entered into a unique collaboration in the late 1950s. Lilly Sebok completed her medical degree at the University of Melbourne and was sent for postgraduate endocrinology training to London, where she met and married Victor Dubowitz. She was born in Budapest of Viennese and Hungarian parents; the family emigrated to Australia following World War II. Following their marriage, she continued her endocrine research but, after their move to Sheffield, she was hired as a temporary locum as pediatric registrar for a few weeks while awaiting transfer of her grant. She subsequently continued in this position for five years, beginning a lifelong commitment to neonatal research. Victor Dubowitz had already become interested in estimating neurological maturity of the newborn by clinical features and nerve conduction velocity studies, and they both became interested in estimating gestational age on the basis of the clinical examination. Their collaboration resulted in a landmark paper (Dubowitz, Dubowitz, and Goldberg, 1970), which initiated the estimation of gestational age by the combined neurologic and external examination now known as the Dubowitz Score. This method of clinical assessment for determining gestational age is now widely used in neonatal medicine throughout the world. It is certainly common, when determining fetal age, for a pediatrician to state that he/she is "Dubowitzing" the patient. Their continued collaboration has resulted in further studies on the developing nervous system, including clinical electrophysical and imaging aspects, culminating in a monograph on neurological assessment of the newborn infant (Dubowitz and Dubowitz, 1981) and a color atlas on brain lesions (Dubowitz, 1990), bringing together their integrated clinical and investigative approach.

Victor Dubowitz's pioneering work on the application of histochemical techniques to the study of muscle has recently gained new momentum with the application of a new generation of immunocytochemical methods to the study of normal and diseased muscle (Dubowitz, 1989).

Dubowitz's research has resulted in eight books and over two hundred scientific publications. An important contribution was *The Floppy Infant*, first published in 1969, which did much to improve the clinician's ability to diagnose a specific disorder rather than simply accepting an infant as being hypotonic and weak. His book with Michael Brooke, entitled *Muscle Biopsy: A Modern Approach* (1973) was a landmark in the introduction of modern histochemical techniques into the routine processing and assessment of muscle biopsies. In 1978, the encyclopedic *Muscle Disorders in Childhood* was published and was acclaimed by clinicians.

The international recognition of their work has allowed the Dubowitz family extensive world travel. They have enjoyed touring with their four sons, combining university lectures with camping adventures. Three of their sons are now physicians; the youngest, the only maverick, is a budding architect.

Multiple honors have recognized Victor Dubowitz's contributions to children. He has been invited to lecture at major universities throughout the world and was named as the Royal Society of Medicine Foundation Visiting Professor in 1986, delivering a series of lectures throughout the United States. In 1988 he delivered the Bernard Sachs lecture to the Child Neurology Society. He continues to contribute actively to understanding the childhood myopathies by his careful clinical observations and scientific studies. He is currently embarking on a prospective study of myoblast transfer as a potential therapy of animal and human dystrophy.

Sanford Schneider
LOMA LINDA, CALIFORNIA

REFERENCES

Dubowitz, L. M. S, V. Dubowitz, and C. Goldberg. 1970. Clinical Assessment of Gestational Age in the Newborn Infant. *J Ped* 77:1–10.

Dubowitz, V. 1965a. Enzyme Histochemistry of Skeletal Muscle. I. Developing Animal Muscle. *J Neur Neurosurg Psych* 28:516.

______. 1965b. Enzyme Histochemistry of Skeletal Muscle. II. Developing Human Muscle. *J Neur Neurosurg Psych* 28:519.

______. 1969. *The Floppy Infant*. Clinics in Developmental Medicine, No. 31. London: Spastics International; Heinemann Press.

______. 1978. *Muscle Disorders in Childhood.* London: W. B. Saunders.

______. 1989. *A Colour Atlas of Muscle Disorders in Childhood.* Chicago: Wolfe Medical Publications Year Book.

______. 1990. *A Colour Atlas of Brain Lesions in the Newborn*. London: Wolfe Medical Publications.

Dubowitz, V., and M. H. Brooke. 1973. *Muscle Biopsy: A Modern Approach*. London and Philadelphia: W. B. Saunders.

Dubowitz, V., and L. M. S. Dubowitz. 1981. *The Neurological Assessment of the Pre-Term and Full-Term Newborn Infant*. Clinics in Developmental Medicine, No. 79. London: McKeith Press/Basil Blackwell; Philadelphia: J. B. Lippincott.

Dubowitz, V., and A. G. E. Pearse. 1960a. Reciprocal Relationship of Phosphorylase and Oxidative Enzymes in Skeletal Muscle. *Nature* 185:701–2.

______. 1960b. Oxidative Enzymes and Phosphorylase in Central Core Disease of Muscle. *Lancet* 2:23–24.

FRANK FORD

FRANK RODOLPH FORD (1892–1970) (figure 1) was born in Baltimore as a result, to put it in his own words, "of two diametrical opposite strains of heredity." As noted in John Chambers's reminiscence (1971), Ford's maternal Scotch-Presbyterian stock furnished him with emotional control, endurance, pious fortitude, resignation, kind-heartedness, true charity, and stability of character, the latter at times manifesting itself as pig-headedness. His father's wealthy Virginia family, predominantly of English origin, endowed him with the antithesis, characterized by fertility of mind, readiness of wit, intellectual exuberance, volatility of spirit, and a dominating personality.

Ford's early schooling was in Baltimore, but after his family moved to Virginia, he attended a local school and finished high school at the Boys Latin School in Baltimore. Here he was regarded as an excellent student, finishing second in his class. After completing his undergraduate studies at Johns Hopkins University, he remained there and graduated from medical school in 1920. Ford served as a house officer in psychiatry under Adolph Meyer; this service complimented his interests in neurology, neuroanatomy, and neuropathology, to which he fortunately had an ex-

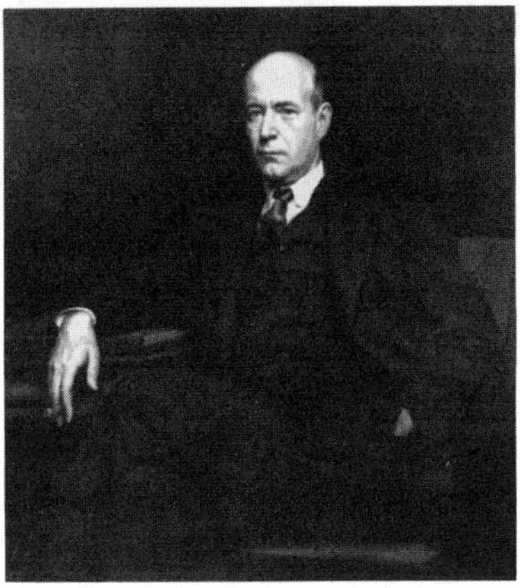

Figure 1. Frank Ford (1892–1970).

cellent exposure under Meyer. He then began a period of training in clinical neurology under Foster Kennedy at Bellevue Hospital in New York. There is one anecdote about Ford during this period as related by John Chambers that typified his character:

He observed that the various neurological consultants who made daily rounds had what to him was a rather annoying habit. Only the first consultant who saw the patient would leave a detailed clinical note; those who examined the patient later simply concurred with the original impression. In order to glean all the knowledge that might ensue from having the independent views of several expert neurologists, Dr. Ford simply removed each consultation note from the chart, replacing them only at the time of the patient's discharge. (Chambers, 1971, 98)

After his return to Hopkins in 1923, Ford became a house officer in neurology, which was then still under internal medicine. His emergence as a brilliant clinical neurologist was followed by his appointment as head of neurology, a position he held from 1932 to 1958. During this period he worked closely with Walter Dandy and was very active in medical student and resident teaching. As noted by Arthur King, one of Ford's student's and house officers, neurology in the 1930s in the United States had little student appeal. Neuroanatomy was presented in a rather confused manner; physiology was in a state of flux; pathology ignored the field entirely, and the current textbooks of neurology were so unimaginatively written that they were a cure for insomnia (King, 1971). But, as King remarked:

Suddenly in the third year of medical school, we students were exposed to a man who was a chain smoker, appeared in ruffled clothing, spoke with a slight lisp, had a pixie-like twinkle in his eyes and so great an economy of movement, he appeared almost constantly bored. Miraculously, however, he made the elucidation of clinical neurologic problems simple, readily understandable and enjoyable. While he pointed out the student's lack of under-

standing of the anatomy and physiology of the central nervous system, he quickly imparted his belief to the students that there was hope for improvement. In fact, he indicated a little attention to detail might even make us good diagnosticians. It didn't take long for us to learn that the "game" of medicine for Dr. Ford was to locate and define the pathologic process. (King, 1971, 103)

King had more to say about Ford's style and philosophy of teaching as well as his sense of humor:

Dr. Ford never sought to lecture to the gallery or to become a "popular teacher." His style was quiet, informal, simple and concise, with a minimum of display and histrionics. He cast his pearls of wisdom to the class and the students choosing to pick these up were given freely of many more, while those who didn't so indulge were passed over without regret or remorse. His remarks were interspersed between the ever-present cigarette or cigar. Most of us recall Dr. Ford enjoyed an obscure brand of Puerto Rican cigarette, known as El Toro, and the potency of this was astounding. Dr. Ford was very generous with his smokes, and affably and benignly, he would offer an unsuspecting student a chance to relax and have a smoke. Like a smiling spider, Dr. Ford lay quietly in wait for his victim. While the class could hardly contain itself, Dr. Ford would witness the sequence of events in a calm and detached manner. (King, 1971, 104)

One of Ford's closest associates at Hopkins was Dr. Frank Walsh, who recalled Ford's regular participation in the well-known Saturday morning neuro-ophthalmology conferences:

The Wilmer Institute owes much to Dr. Ford. Until he retired from active practice, less than a year ago, for more than thirty years Dr. Ford was always present at the Saturday Morning Conferences. As most of you know, this clinic in the Wilmer Institute begins at 10:30. At approximately five minutes before starting time, Dr. Ford would appear, usually having been chauffeured by his wife Louel, though on occasions he arrived by taxi and his droll stories about taxi drivers were either amusing or amazing. His pattern after arrival never varied; he would walk across the lecture room, deposit his hat on the radiator, thence go to his front row seat on the aisle. There he was available for quiet greetings or questioning, and completely relaxed proceeded to take a long cigar from a pocket, light it, and await the appearance of the first patient. Immediately he gave complete attention to the history as presented, and in many instan-

ces he already had observed significant abnormalities as the patient walked or was wheeled into the room. All became aware that the chronology of symptoms and signs registered almost automatically in his mind. His memory of cases, names and writings was phenomenal. It was my practice first to obtain audience participation and carefully to avoid obtaining Dr. Ford's comments until all others had finished their discussion. When I asked Dr. Ford to evaluate the situation, his answer was directed to me in a low voice and only those close to him could hear his remarks. I would summarize what he had said. This exercise became completely routine. In his discussion Dr. Ford always placed his comments into one of three categories: First, when he was completely sure of the principal diagnosis, he stated this in few words; second, when several probabilities existed, he gave an appropriate explanation of each; third, when the diagnosis was completely obscure, he prefaced his observations by "I do not know." This self discipline was a prominent feature of Dr. Ford's personality. When his diagnosis was certain, that is category one, he would willingly indicate the reasons leading to that conclusion. One soon learned that to argue against his unqualified diagnosis was utterly without merit. When the diagnosis fell into category two or category three, Dr. Ford was at his best as a teacher and it was then that his subtle humor often lightened the occasion. (Walsh, 1971, 105)

Ford's unusual ability to arrive at the most suitable diagnosis with a minimum of effort was apocryphal. It was often said by many of his colleagues that they would prefer to have the "Judge's" opinion, after he simply walked past the door of a patient's room, than that of most any other consultant after the performance of a lengthy and complex examination.

As recounted by the senior author of this sketch who trained under Ford:

He relied on a precise, carefully assessed history and on observation for almost all his diagnosis. He had refined observation to the point where he elicited physical signs only to clear up a critical point or two. Incredible experience gave him an ability and assurance in evaluating signs and symptoms that I saw equalled by Sir Charles Symonds, but never excelled.

On one occasion we were were shown a young woman whose complaint was of vomiting and unsteadiness. She was grossly ataxic, vomiting almost constantly, but had no other real localizing signs. She had had a posterior fossa exploration, which was negative. The neurosurgeons were diagnosing multiple sclerosis. Dr. Ford listened quietly, watched the demonstration of her signs, leaned forward and asked, "Do you have any numbness around your mouth?" "No, sir," was the answer. The patient was removed — he was meticulous about such matters — he looked at the young neurosurgeon and said, "She has a tumour in the floor of the fourth ventricle." When the negative exploration was quoted, he said simply, "Did you split the vermis?" The answer was, of course, no, and a week later he was proven right.

He would only rarely explain himself to a large group. Tackled alone, he pointed out that patients with such severe brainstem involvement from multiple sclerosis almost invariably had circumoral sensory disturbances, relatively rare, especially bilaterally, in tumor.

He used little in the way of examining tools beyond his powers of observation. He never carried an examining bag, and I rarely saw him use a percussion hammer or a tuning fork. Sensory examination was, for him, restricted to pinprick, and for this he used a large finishing nail, which he sharpened a bit. He held that the usual pin was far too sharp, and gave misleading answers. He did carry a series of wires, about four inches long, tipped with red and blue, red and white, and a large and small white head. He used these for visual fields, and was a past master at confrontation fields. It was one of these few points on which he and Dr. Walsh differed, Walsh holding that standard perimetry was necessary, Ford often proving him wrong. (David Clark, personal reminiscence, 1990)

Despite the fact that Ford was averse to travel, attended no national meetings, and infrequently published papers, he was widely regarded as one of the foremost neurologists of his time and one of the premier child neurologists in the United States. Early in his career he developed an interest in what was then considered "developmental neurology" and in 1927 he published his first book, *Birth Injuries of the Nervous System*. This work was actually coauthored with Bronson Crothers and Marian C. Putnam, the latter two contributing the section on cord birth injuries. The first part of this 164–page monograph contained Ford's section on "Cerebral Birth Injuries." This ran to 75 pages, contained some 136 references, and consisted of Ford's analysis of the literature of the previous 50 years on different aspects of perinatal birth injury. Added to this were additional comments by Ford, based on observations of 200 children with bilateral spastic paralysis seen at the Harriet

Lane Home outpatient clinic and 100 autopsied cases of hydrocephalus. The material is worth reading today, as most of what was stated was succinct and superbly written. In his concluding remarks on the literature of cerebral diplegia, Ford had this to say:

Thus, five principal theories have been advanced to account for cerebral diplegia; that it is due to asphyxia, to meningeal hemorrhage, to an arrest of development resulting from prematurity, to a degenerative process in utero, and to a congenitally defective development of the brain. (Ford, 1927, 23)

Because Ford's comments reflected the general consensus of the time, it is interesting, from a current perspective, to realize that the concept of subependymal and periventricular hemorrhage had not yet been introduced.

Because he was so systematic in his record keeping and was referred many complex patients to evaluate, Ford accumulated a vast amount of clinical material that formed the basis of his monumental *Diseases of the Nervous System in Infancy, Childhood and Adolescence.* This was first published in 1937 and consisted of 950 pages. His work went through 6 revisions; the last, 1500 pages in length, was sent to the publisher shortly before his final illness. The fourth and fifth editions were translated into Italian, Spanish, and Polish. As related by Guy McKhann:

At other centers, Neurology was heavily under the influence of European schools, the German School of Neuropathology and the British School of Neurophysiology. Here, as exemplified in his textbook, Dr. Ford gave a straightforward presentation—a definition and etiology, the pathological anatomy, the salient clinical features, the diagnosis, the prognosis, and treatment. Where necessary, Dr. Ford told the reader with a brief case history, "This is how the case presented to me." (McKhann, 1971, 108)

Ford's book was encyclopedic. It represented years of concentrated effort and collection of case material, with all phases of the manuscript being completed by him, including the typing (Harvey, 1976). Although not recognized by many of Ford's colleagues at Hopkins, his book actually followed a series of works that, over the previous forty years, was defining the field of child neurology. These included the works of Bernard Sachs (1895), James Taylor (1905), Martin Thiemich and Jules Zappert (1910), Ludwig Bruns,

August Cramer, and Theodor Ziehen (1912), Georg Peritz (1912), Albrecht Peiper (1912), and Bronson Crothers (1926). However, as summarized by Lawson Wilkens, the famed Hopkins endocrinologist who reviewed Ford's book in the Hopkins alumni journal:

He has broken away from the purely anatomical classification under which the neurological diseases were grouped as diseases of the brain, of the spinal cord, of the peripheral nerves, or as general diseases of the nervous system. Instead, Dr. Ford has brought the multitude of conditions into significant perspective to each other by an etiological classification. Under this scheme he discusses in separate chapters (1) the prenatal or congenital defects of the nervous system, (2) the heredofamilial or degenerative diseases, (3) the infections of the nervous system, (4) the toxic and metabolic disorders involving the nervous system, (5) the vascular lesions and circulatory disorders of the nervous system, (6) tumors and (7) injuries of the nervous system by physical agents. Chapters are given also to the epilepsies and paroxysmal disorders of the nervous system, the diseases of the autonomic nervous system, and the diseases of muscles. At the beginning of each chapter, as an introduction to the particular etiological division of nervous disorder, the author gives a general discussion of the group and a sub-classification of the various diseases included. This sub-division is on an anatomical basis. These classifications and discussions add greatly to the value of the work and enable the reader for the first time to see not only the well-known classical neurological diseases but the newer, less familiar variations in proper relationship. (Wilkens, 1937, 101)

Ford's legacy as a teacher is hard to describe since, in the accepted sense, he had no pupils. He never had a residency training program. He never had a fellow. He never even had a bed service in a children's hospital.

Yet he did have pupils — many of them. His method of teaching was first to decide if he liked you. If he didn't, the relationship, always courteous, went no further. But if he did, he spared no effort. His method was to come into the clinic, sit down, light a match on the NO SMOKING sign, get his cigar to drawing well, then catch your eye and say, "Doctor, come over here and talk to me. Don't you think that . . . well, perhaps the peroneal nerve is usually involved after the tibial, instead of before it, in leprous neuropathy." When you got up you knew more about leprous neuropathy than you had thought there was to be known. Next day he would hand you three or four slips of paper with key references typed on them. He acted on Chaucer's injunction — "and gladlie teeche!" (David Clark, personal reminiscences, 1990)

David Clark
LEXINGTON, KENTUCKY

Stephen Ashwal
LOMA LINDA, CALIFORNIA

REFERENCES

Bruns, L., A. Cramer, and T. Ziehen. 1912. *Handbuch der Nervenkrankheiten im Kindesalter*. Berlin: Karger Verlag.

Chambers, J. W. 1971. Frank Rodolph Ford. *Johns Hopkins Med J* 128(2): 97–99.

Ford, F. R. 1937. *Diseases of the Nervous System in Infancy, Childhood and Adolescence*. Springfield, IL: Charles C Thomas.

Ford, F. R., B. Crothers, and M. C. Putnam. 1927. *Birth Injuries of the Nervous System. Part I — Cerebral Birth Injuries. Part II — Cord Birth Injuries.* Baltimore: The Williams and Wilkins Company.

Harvey, A. M. 1976. Frank Ford. In *Adventures in Medical Research: A Century of Discovery at Johns Hopkins,* 401. Baltimore: The Johns Hopkins University Press.

King, A. B. 1971. Dr. Ford as Seen by Former Students and House Officers. *Johns Hopkins Med J* 128(2): 103–4.

McKhann, G. M. 1971. Speaking of Dr. Ford for the Field of Neurology. *Johns Hopkins Med J* 128(2): 108–9.

Peritz, G. 1912. *Nervenkrankheiten des Kindesalter.* Berlin: Fischer's Medicin Buchhandlung.

Sachs, B. 1895. *A Treatise on the Nervous Diseases of Children for Physicians and Students*. New York: Wood.

Taylor, J. 1905. *Paralysis and Other Diseases of the Nervous System in Childhood and Early Life*. London: J & A Churchill.

Thiemich, M., and J. Zappert. 1910. *Die Krankheiten des Nervensystems im Kindesalter*. Leipzig: F. C. W. Vogel.

Walsh, F. B. 1971. Dr. Ford as he Appeared to His Colleagues. *Johns Hopkins Med J* 128(2): 105–7.

Wilkens L. 1937. Book Briefs: *Diseases of the Nervous System in Infancy, Childhood and Adolescence*, by Frank R. Ford. The Johns Hopkins Alumni Magazine, 101.

YUKIO FUKUYAMA

CHILD NEUROLOGY IS CURRENTLY a very active and well-represented discipline in Japan, with several thousand members participating in the Japanese Society of Child Neurology. Unlike its development in Europe, England, Scandinavia, and the United States, where maturation proceeded over a period of one hundred years, child neurology rapidly evolved in Japan in the early 1950s. This development coincided with the separation of adult neurology from internal medicine and the declaration of pediatrics as an independent specialty. Neurology was actually introduced in Japan at the turn of this century by the combined efforts of German physicians who were invited to teach at the Tokyo Imperial University, and later, by several Japanese physicians who trained in Germany and France under such luminaries as Hermann Oppenheim, Wilhelm Erb, and Jean Charcot (Aki, 1980). However, it was during the period of rebuilding after World War II that the importance of neurology was more clearly recognized, as was the need to separate this discipline from psychiatry. With the efforts of Shigeo Okinaka, the Japanese Society of Neurology was established in 1960, and clinical adult neurology expanded rapidly. At the same time, the influence of American medicine was beginning to be felt in Japan, especially in the field of pediatrics, where subspecialties were emerging as the future trend for the care of children. Thus, at the major universities, the need to develop subspecialty programs was appreciated and eventually they were established. Apart from this, another group of physicians, who traditionally had been involved with the care and research of children with psychiatric and neurological disorders, saw the need for organizational development. In 1960 they formed the Society of Pediatric Psychiatry and Neurology. Amidst all these changing, and perhaps conflicting, trends over the past thirty years, Yukio Fukuyama (b. 1928) (figure 1) has been actively involved in the direction and development of child neurology.

Yukio Fukuyama was born in Takachino-machi in Miyazaki Prefecture in May 1928. He was raised in Kumamoto, where he lived until he graduated from high school in 1948. He entered Tokyo University, and, as a medical student, was much influenced by Shigeo Okinaka, professor of medicine and founder of neurology in Japan. He received his M.D. in 1952, and, after a one-year internship, began training in pediatrics at the University of Tokyo Hospital. From 1954 to 1957 he attended the graduate school of medicine where he engaged in clinical research in pediatric neurology under the late Tadao Takatsu. Takatsu, the father of pediatric specialties in Japan and head of the department, recognized Fukuyama's great promise and asked him to specialize in child neurology and implement its development, as he felt it was one of the most important pediatric specialties. Fukuyama initially devoted much effort in establishing pediatric electroencephalography in the Department of Psychiatry and pediatric electromyography in the Department of Physiology at the University of Tokyo. He initiated a study group of child neurologists at the University of Tokyo, together with his colleagues Masataka Arima, Masamichi Nagahata, and several other young investigators. During the early 1960s, this study group was very active in both clinical and research activities. The outpatient child neurology clinic was always extremely busy, seeing many patients with intractable neurological diseases who were referred for further consultation and assessment. Fukuyama had instituted a policy that, when the clinic was completed, case conferences, journal clubs, and research meetings were held until late in the evening.

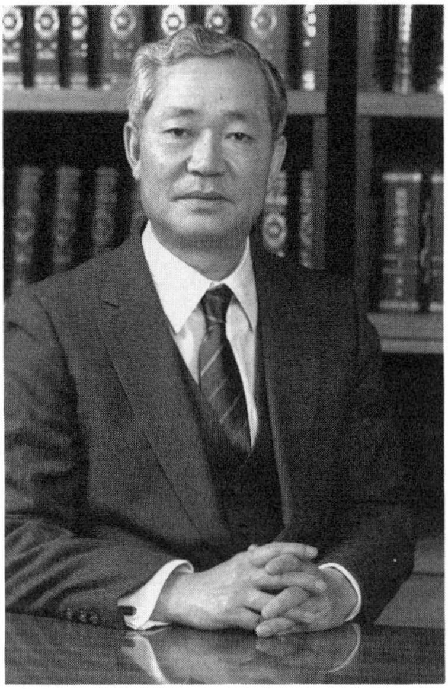

Figure 1. Yukio Fukuyama.

Fukuyama's major scientific contributions to child neurology are very extensive. He is known for his excellent studies on infantile spasms, febrile seizures, benign infantile convulsions, and neuromuscular disorders. In 1960 he described a unique type of congenital muscular dystrophy, which is now well known as the Fukuyama type of congenital muscular dystrophy (FCMD) (Fukuyama, Kawazura, and Haruna, 1960; Fukuyama, Osawa, and Suzuki, 1981). His clinical study of 215 children with infantile spasms, in which he reviewed the clinical, electroencephalographic, etiologic, and pathogenetic aspects of this disease, deserves to be considered as a classic (Kurokawa, Goya, and Fukuyama, 1980).

Fukuyama has also written on Leigh's syndrome (Kamoshita, Mizutani, and Fukuyama, 1970), the role of immunizations in infantile spasms (Fukuyama, Tomori, and Sugitate, 1977), acute fulminant myoglobinuric polymyositis (Fukuyama, Ando, and Yokota, 1977), treatment of seizures (Fukuyama et al, 1963), mitochondrial myopathies (Suzuki and Fukuyama, 1983), Moya Moya disease (Fukuyama and Umezu, 1985), neurologic complications of Kawasaki disease (Hirasawa, Awaya, and Fukuyama, 1985), and childhood multiple sclerosis (Fukuyama and Hirano, 1985), among many other subjects. Aside from his lecture on the history of child neurology in Japan (Fukuyama, 1984a), he has written more philosophical works about the potential future of child neurology in Japan (Fukuyama, 1984b). He has also edited or written numerous books in the field of child neurology. These include *The Fundamentals of Child Neurology* (Fukuyama, 1979), *Neurological Examination in Children* (Fukuyama, 1980a), *Clinical Electroencephalography in Children* (Fukuyama, 1980b), and *An Atlas of Clinical Child Neurology* (Fukuyama, 1986). Another of his literary interests is a series of compendiums on epilepsy that he has put together, in which he collected and summarized the world's literature in this field from 1945 to the present. The fifth edition of *Epilepsy Bibliography* was published in 1985.

In 1961 the Japanese Society of Child Neurology (JSCN) was established by Takatsu, with Fukuyama regarded as the most important founding member. He was promoted to associate professor of pediatrics at the University of Tokyo in 1964 and assisted Takatsu, who served as president of the Eleventh International Congress of Pediatrics, held in Tokyo in November 1965. Fukuyama then moved to the newly created National Children's Hospital in 1965 as director of the Division of Neurology, and in 1969 was appointed professor and chairman of the Department of Pediatrics at Tokyo Women's Medical College. That same year, he succeeded Takatsu as chairman of the Board of Trustees of the JSCN. He began publication of *No To Hattatsu*, which was the Japanese edition of the journal *Brain and Development*, the official journal of JSCN. He later established *Brain and Development* as an international journal in 1979, served as its editor-in-chief, and improved the quality and reputation of this publication. In addition to these two journals, Fukuyama has served as an editorial member of *Acta Paediatrica Japonica* (Tokyo), *Clinical Neurology* (Tokyo), *Folia Psychiatrica et Neurologica Japonica* (Tokyo), *Congenital Anomalies* (Nagoya), *Indian Journal of Pediatrics* (New Delhi), *Epilepsy Research* (Amsterdam), and *Pediatric Neurology*.

In 1983 the Twenty-Fifth Annual Meeting of the Japanese Society of Child Neurology was celebrated. Fukuyama was honored there, and gave a special lecture entitled "A Quarter-Century of the Japanese Society of Child Neurology," which was later published in *Brain and Development*. This is an interesting paper, because it traces the development of child neurology in Japan (Fukuyama, 1984a).

Fukuyama has presided over and organized many domestic as well as international meetings, including the Ninth Annual Meeting of the Japanese Chapter of the International League against Epilepsy in 1975, the Nineteenth Annual Meeting of the JSCN in 1977, the First and Second International Symposia on Developmental Disabilities (1977 and 1979), and the Sixth Annual Meeting of the Japan Association of Medical Genetics (1983). Thus the present stature of child neurology in Japan derives largely from the contributions that Fukuyama has made over the past thirty years in the areas of clinical care, research, and administrative responsibilities.

At the Third International Congress of Child Neurology in Copenhagen (1982), Fukuyama was elected the fourth president of the International Child Neurology Association (ICNA) following John Stobo Pritchard from Canada, Niels Low from the United States, and Ritske le Coutre from the Netherlands. He served until 1986, devoting himself to creating the Asian Oceanic Association of Child Neurology, with the Conference on Child Neurology being successfully held in Taipei in 1983 and the second in Jakarta in 1987. Now, as Congress president, he is organizing the Joint Convention of the Fifth International and Third Asian Oceanic

Child Neurology Congress in Tokyo (November 1990). I believe this will be one of the most important events, not only of his life, but also in the history of child neurology in Japan.

Shigehiko Kamoshita
TOKYO, JAPAN

REFERENCES

Aki, M. 1980. The History of Neurology in Japan, with Special Reference to Its Postwar Period. In *Historical Aspects of the Neurosciences*, 451–62. Ed. F. C. Rose and W. F. Bynum. New York: Raven Press.

Fukuyama, Y. (ed.) 1979. *The Fundamentals of Child Neurology* (in Japanese). Tokyo: Shindan To Chiryosha.

Fukuyama, Y. 1980a. *Neurological Examination in Children* (in Japanese). Pediatrics Book Series No. 12. Tokyo-Osaka-Kyoto: Kanehara.

______. 1980b. *Clinical Electroencephalography in Children* (in Japanese). Tokyo-Osaka-Kyoto: Kanehara.

______. 1984a. A Quarter-Century of the Japanese Society of Child Neurology. *Brain Dev* 6:109–18.

______. 1984b. Perspectives of Child Neurology — Present and Future (in Japanese). *Japan J Ped Med* (Tokyo) 16:305–8.

______. 1985. *Epilepsy Bibliography. Books and Monographs (1945–1984)*. 5th ed. Tokyo: Kyowa Hakko Kogyo Co..

______. 1986. *An Atlas of Clinical Child Neurology* (in Japanese). Tokyo: Shindan To Chiryosha.

Fukuyama, Y., T. Ando, and J. Yokota. 1977. Acute Fulminant Myoglobinuric Polymyositis with Picornavirus-like Crystals. *J Neur Neurosurg Psych* (London) 40:775–81.

Fukuyama, Y., et al. 1963. Medical Treatment of Epilepsies in Childhood. A Long-Term Survey of 801 Patients. *Epilepsia* 4:207–24.

Fukuyama, Y., and Y. Hirano. 1985. Multiple Sclerosis and Related Conditions in Childhood (in Japanese). *Clin Neur* (Tokyo) 24:1221–23.

Fukuyama, Y., M. Kawazura, and H. Haruna. 1960. A Peculiar Form of Congenital Progressive Muscular Dystrophy (in English). *Paed Univ Tokyo* 4:5–8.

Fukuyama, Y., M. Osawa, and H. Suzuki. 1981. Congenital Progressive Muscular Dystrophy of the Fukuyama Type: Clinical, Genetic and Pathologic Considerations (in English). *Brain Dev* (Tokyo) 3:1–29.

Fukuyama, Y., N. Tomori, and M. Sugitate. 1977. Critical Evaluation of the Role of Immunization as an Etiological Factor of Infantile Spasms (in English). *Neuropaed* (Stuttgart) 8:224–37.

Fukuyama, Y., and R. Umezu. 1985. Clinical and Cerebral Angiographic Evolutions of Idiopathic Progressive Occlusive Disease of the Circle of Willis ("Moya Moya" Disease) in Children (in English). *Brain Dev* (Tokyo) 7:21–37.

Fukuyama, Y., M. Osawa, and H. Suzuki. 1981. Congenital Progressive Muscular Dystrophy of the Fukuyama Type: Clinical, Genetic and Pathologic Considerations (in English). *Brain Dev* (Tokyo) 3:1–29.

Hirasawa, K., Y. Awaya, and Y. Fukuyama. 1985. Neurological Complications in Kawasaki Disease (in Japanese). *Japan J Ped Med* (Tokyo) 17:784–90.

Kamoshita, S., I. Mizutani, and Y. Fukuyama. 1970. Leigh's Subacute Necrotizing Encephalomyelopathy in a Child with Infantile Spasms and Hypsarrhythmia. *Dev Med Child Neur* (London) 12:430–35.

Kurokawa, T., M. Goya, and Y. Fukuyama. 1980. West Syndrome and Lennox-Gastaut Syndrome: A Survey of the Natural History (in English). *Ped* 65:81–88.

Suzuki, H., and Y. Fukuyama. 1983. A Histological Study of Mitochondrial Myopathy in Patients with Partial Pyruvate Dehydrogenese Complex Deficiency (in Japanese). *No To Hattatsu* 15:290–300.

INGRID GAMSTORP

BORN IN LUND, Sweden, in 1924, Ingrid Gamstorp (figure 1) trained in child neurology in the United States and went on to become an internationally acclaimed child neurologist. Author of numerous articles and a major pediatric neurology textbook she is besk known for her pioneering investigations in pediatric neuromuscular disorders (Gamstorp, 1963, 1967).

Gamstorp received her initial medical training in Lund. While studying to become a pediatrician, she was assigned to work in a pediatric unit in Kristianstad, Sweden. It was there that she encountered the first patient with what she termed "adynamia episodica hereditaria," also known as familial hyperkalemic periodic paralysis. Because of excellent Swedish church records going back to the late seventeenth century, she was able to locate and personally examine two large families, most of whom still lived in the area around Kristianstad. Her study of the 138 members of these two families led to a landmark monograph on the disorder, pub-

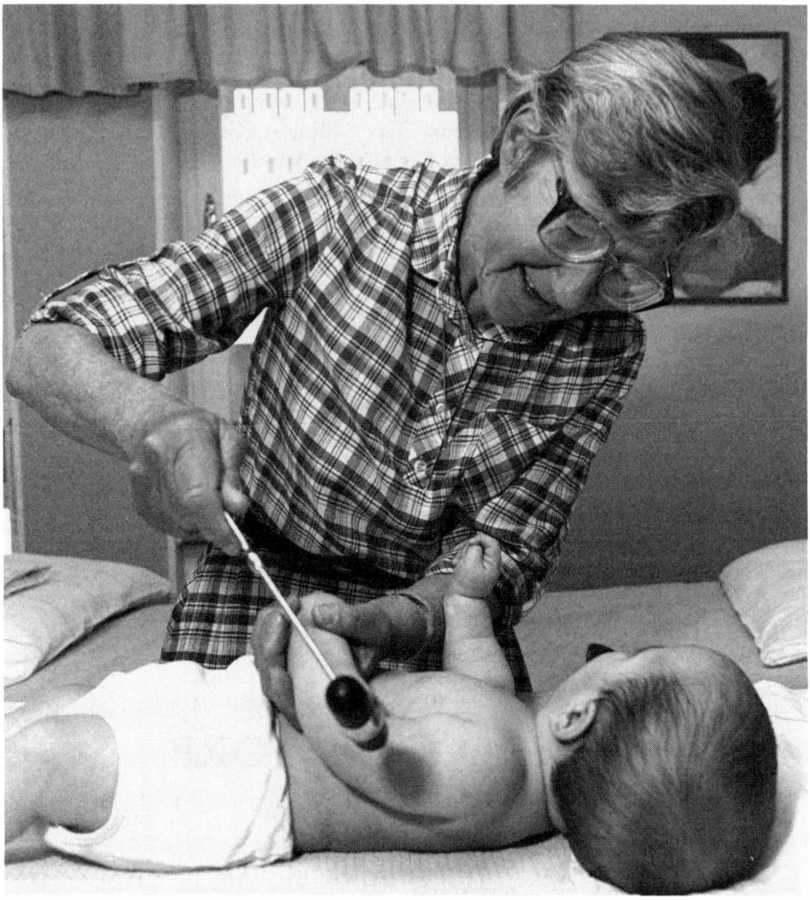

Figure 1. Ingrid Gamstorp.

lished as a thesis in 1956 (Gamstorp, 1956). Working with these families stimulated her interest in neurology, which in Sweden was then considered primarily a branch of internal medicine. She subsequently trained with Gunnar Wohlfart, a neurologist known worldwide for his work on neuromuscular disorders, and later studied electromyography with Fritz Buchtal.

In 1958 Gamstorp received a Jerry Lewis Fellowship in Neuromuscular Disorders to study in the United States. She spent two months at the University of Utah, followed by two years at the Massachusetts General Hospital. While there she received training in neurology, pediatric neurology, neuropathology, and clinical neurophysiology with a number of prominent neurologists, including Raymond Adams, Philip Dodge, Robert Schwab, and Edward P. Richardson. She developed close friendships with her new American colleagues and continues to correspond and meet with them.

In 1961 she returned to the Department of Pediatrics in Lund to practice and teach the relatively new specialty of pediatric neurology. In 1967 she was named head of the Department of Pediatrics in Jonkoping, and in 1972 she moved to Uppsala to assume a professorship in pediatric neurology.

Perhaps because of her international training and travels, Gamstorp was instrumental in founding the International Child Neurology Association in 1973 and served as its secretary-treasurer from 1976 to 1980. Always an advocate for her patients, she spoke out forcefully on issues when she felt the child's best interests were not being served.

Ingrid Gamstorp was first and foremost a clinician. I first met her when she came to Portland, Oregon, in the early 1970s to address the Portland Pediatric Society. When she made rounds at the university we were all impressed with her astute diagnostic skills, as well as her kind and gentle manner with children.

In 1970 she wrote the first edition of her major textbook, *Pediatric Neurology*, noting in the acknowledgments that

the diseases affecting the nervous and muscular system in infancy, childhood, and adolescence have grown in importance mainly because of their often handicapping effect on the young individual; they play an increasing role for all physicians dealing with infants and children. (Gamstorp, 1970, 5)

The text is one of the few organized according to symptoms, making it an ideal early reference for the house officer interested in neurological disorders of children. Sensibly and clearly written, the book is amply illustrated with pictures of handsome blond Swedish children. Chapter Two on the neurologic examination is vintage Gamstorp:

Throughout childhood, the best results are obtained if the neurologic examination is done as a game and a competition between child and examiner: "Let us see who can do this the best or fastest — you or I?" (Gamstorp, 1970, 5)

The second edition, enlarged and expanded, was published in 1985.

As a person, Ingrid Gamstorp is warm and caring. I had the

pleasure of visiting her summer home on the beautiful, peaceful island of Samso in 1972. During a walk on the beach (the Scandinavian waters were much too cold for this American neurologist), she told me how, when beginning her practice, she had specifically requested that a couch be placed in her office, rather than two chairs. When I asked, "Why?" she said, "Because when I have to tell a young couple that their child has muscular dystrophy or Werdnig-Hoffmann disease or some similar fatal neurologic disease, I want the husband to be able to put his arm around his wife and comfort her, not be seated away from her."

Gamstorp published eighty-five papers in addition to her initial landmark monograph on familial periodic paralysis. These include a study on myokymia with Wohlfart (1959), some of the earliest published studies of motor and sensory nerve conduction velocities in infants and children (1963), and later studies on progressive spinal muscular atrophy (1967). In recent years her interests have expanded to include the problems faced by families with handicapped and dying children, and she has also devoted much time to the ethical problems of pediatrics.

Ingrid Gamstorp's career reflects her commitment to neurologically handicapped children and their families, her abilities as a clinician and teacher, and her skills as a gifted neuroscientist. She has served as an excellent role model for future generations of women in child neurology. She plans to retire in 1990, but her many international colleagues and friends look forward to her continuing friendship and contributions to child neurology in the years ahead.

Peggy Ferry
TUCSON, ARIZONA

REFERENCES

Gamstorp I. 1956. Adynamia Episodica Hereditaria. *Acta Ped Scand* (Suppl. 108) 45:1–126.

______. 1963. Normal Conduction Velocity of Ulnar, Median and Peroneal Nerves in Infancy, Childhood and Adolescence. *Acta Ped Scand* (Suppl.) 146:68–76.

______. 1967. Progressive Spinal Muscular Atrophy with Onset in Infancy or Early Childhood. *Acta Ped Scand* 56:408.

______. 1970. *Pediatric Neurology*. New York: Appleton-Century-Crofts.

______. 1985. *Pediatric Neurology*. 2d ed. Stoneham, MA: Butterworth.

Gamstorp, I., and G. Wohlfart. 1959. A Syndrome Characterized by Myokymia, Myotonia, Muscular Wasting and Increased Perspiration. *Acta Psych Scand* 34:181.

NEIL SIMSON GORDON

IN JUNE 1988, soon after the retirement of Neil Gordon (b. 1918) (figure 1) from practice in the National Health Service, sixty colleagues from twenty professions and thirty-three departments around Britain attended a symposium at the Royal Manchester Children's Hospital to celebrate his seventieth birthday and his career, which began as a medical student in Edinburgh in 1935. Letters and telegrams came from all over the world, indicating the extent of his reputation and the affection in which he is held. The citation accompanying the program read as follows:

His achievements in the development of paediatric neurology as a specialty are recognised world-wide. He has guided the specialty between classical neurology for children and disabled children. His clinical expertise for children with acute encephalopathies, metabolic disorders, involuntary movement disorders, language disorders, genetic disorders, epilepsies, cerebral palsies and mental retardation has been formidable but readily available. Many an unusual clinical problem has led to a comprehensive annotation in Developmental Medicine and Child Neurology. Colleagues in many departments have benefited from his support and encouragement. Development of neurophysiology services, anticonvulsant drug monitoring, insistence on high quality muscle histology and a major role in the promotion of the three child development centers in Manchester and Salford (Rodney House in 1960, Agnew Unit a few years later and Holzel Centre in the mid 70's) are examples of his foresight and hard work. His work in the Cheshire community child health

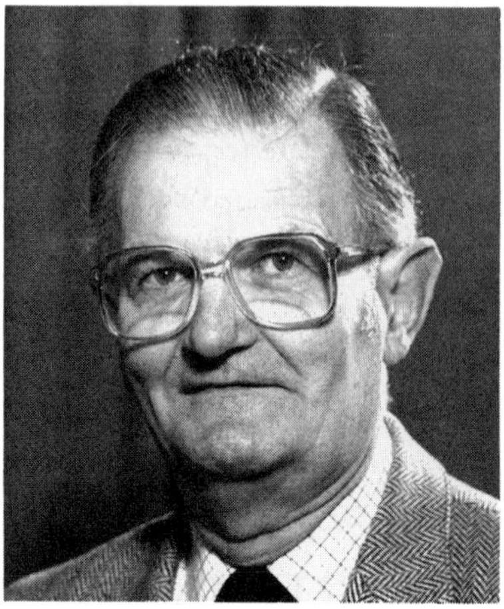

Figure 1. Neil Gordon. From Tizard, J. P. M., "James Spence Medallist, 1985: Neil Simson Gordon," *Arch Dis Child* 60(1985): 603. Courtesy of the British Medical Association.

service, since retiring from hospital paediatric neurology, has been an inspiration. Another book is planned for 1990.

The speakers and subjects reflect the range of Gordon's interests. Michael Noronha was his first senior registrar in 1969. Gordon had no junior staff for his first eleven years in Manchester, and Noronha helped develop neurophysiological and neuromuscular services and became Gordon's first consultant colleague in 1974. Like Gordon, he entered the specialty from adult neurology.

Betty Byers-Brown was a senior lecturer in speech pathology and therapy at Manchester University, where Gordon also taught. They shared their ideas about many children's clinical problems and had frequent contact through the College of Speech Therapists, for which Gordon served as an examiner for many years and of which he remains an honorary fellow. The college president, Margaret Edwards, was present at the symposium. Gordon served on the Quirk Committee on Speech Therapy Services from 1969 to 1972. In the foreword to the report from this committee, Margaret Thatcher and Keith Joseph, Secretary of State for Education and Science and Secretary of State for Social Services respectively, thanked the committee for its helpful and rigorous work but concluded "so far no decisions have been made on any of the recommendations addressed to the Government." Gordon is an enthusiastic supporter of improved in-service education for therapists.

I became his second senior registrar in 1975 and the third Manchester consultant pediatric neurologist in 1978. I came from a pediatric background, which allowed the department to open a pediatric neurology ward rather than look after patients on the pediatric ward. As a former registrar with Tom Ingram and Keith

Brown, I maintained Gordon's Edinburgh links. We have edited three books together and have acted as readers of each other's articles for many years (Gordon and McKinlay, 1986a, 1986b, 1988). When I negotiated the recognition by the British Department of Health of pediatric neurology as an independent specialty, Gordon's support in the Royal College of Physicians' neurology committee and that of Peter Tizard in the pediatric committee proved decisive.

Gordon's interest in clumsy children was stimulated by Gubbay, Ellis, Walton, and Court's 1965 article from Newcastle on developmental dyspraxia. His opinion on children with learning disorders was widely sought. He has also been involved in a prospective study of children found to be clumsy on entry to the Cheshire schools.

Martin Bax is editor of *Developmental Medicine and Child Neurology* and the *Little Club Clinics in Developmental Medicine* (formerly published by Spastics International Medical Publications, now MacKeith Press), including Gordon's book *Paediatric Neurology for the Clinician* in 1976 and many of his annotations (Gordon, 1976). Through the years, Bax and Gordon have supported and encouraged the development of pediatric neurology in England.

Ronnie MacKeith was the greatest influence on Gordon's professional career. They were involved in the biannual international meetings of the Medical, Educational and Information Unit of The Spastics Society from its inception in Oxford in 1958. From this, the British Group of Paediatric Neurologists emerged, later to become the British Paediatric Neurology Association, of which Gordon was first chairman, then president for six years. The Oxford meetings also inspired the organization of European societies for pediatric neurology, which federated in 1971. Gordon was the federation's second honorary secretary for four years and its president for two. He also became a member of the board of the International Child Neurology Association.

Stephen Brown is medical director of the David Lewis Centre, which treats people with epilepsy. For many years, Gordon visited the center to give clinical advice and involved the previous medical director in a clinic at the children's hospital in Manchester to share ideas and prevent the center from becoming isolated from mainstream services. When pupils at the center's school became ill, Gordon was always ready to admit them to the hospital for further investigation or review treatment. Half of the inpatient work of the department and a large part of Gordon's outpatient work was for children with troublesome seizures, and many families looked to him for support in difficult times, often traveling long distances for his advice.

Keith Brown was a former pupil of Gordon's, attending his marathon clinics in the 1960s, when it was not unusual for thirty-five or forty children to be seen and for the clinic to extend long into the evening. Brown went on to work with Thomas Ingram in Edinburgh and his subsequent success reflects the influence of both teachers. Brown and his colleagues in Edinburgh have kept up Ingram's innovative style, especially in the understanding of acute encephalopathies and the management of children with neural tube defects. For the symposium, Ingram wrote to say of Gordon:

His greatest achievement was to encourage adult neurologists to accept paediatric neurology as a distinct and respectable discipline — by example as well as by words. This has been of the greatest importance and only the unassuming Neil with his tact and patience could have achieved what he did.

David Taylor, Manchester's Professor of Child and Adolescent Psychiatry, also participated. The Park Hospital in Oxford influenced Gordon considerably, and he encouraged me to take an elective period there during my training. Kit Ounsted (Tom Ingram refers to him as the "Bishop" of pediatric neurology) developed the importance of biological thinking in child psychiatry, especially in understanding sex differences and children with seizure disorders. Taylor and Ounsted's creative thinking became part of Gordon's clinical practice. The opportunity to reciprocate came with the chance to support the establishment of the Manchester Chair in Child and Adolescent Psychiatry, at one time proposed to be a chair in developmental pediatrics. Taylor's appointment has transformed psychiatry in the region. His style of psychiatry is sympathetic to pediatrics and child neurology in particular; helping its establishment is typical of Neil Gordon's activity behind the scenes.

Stuart Green, senior lecturer from Birmingham, photographed the event for the archives of the British Paediatric Neurology Association. Green has inherited Gordon's voluntary clinic at Condover Hall near Shrewsbury, seventy miles south of Manchester, where Saturday morning clinics were held for some years. This was partly out of the realization of the school's need for a service and partly because of the wealth of unusual clinical problems presented by visually impaired pupils with multiple disabilities. Many special schools in the Greater Manchester area appreciated his periodic clinic visits. He created a style of service whereby pediatric neurology staff members went out to district pediatric units in the northwest of England to hold joint clinics with local colleagues. Apart from saving many families from having to travel, it fostered good professional relationships and enhanced the general understanding of the subject.

Gordon's father, Ronald Grey Gordon, was a physician in Bath, an active British Medical Association committee man, and a founding member of the Association of British Neurologists. He consulted in neurology, pediatrics, and psychotherapy and published books on child psychiatry, mental defects, paralysis in children, and the development of personality. Gordon's older brother, Ian, was a distinguished radiologist with a particular interest in pediatric radiology. He had a good reputation as a teacher and wrote a textbook on this subject. Gordon's late wife was a radiographer. They met during his second house job at the Deaconess Hospital in Edinburgh (a post I held twenty-nine yeas later). Gordon's home has a reputation for hospitality. There is an informal senior pediatric neurologists' "visiting club" that often meets there. It is not unusual to find Jean Aicardi, Bengt Hagberg, or Werner Isler staying with Gordon in Wilmslow or for Gordon to be visiting them. In either case, the conversation, with some apology on Gordon's part, is always in English.

Gordon was educated at Charterhouse School and then graduated from Edinburgh University in 1940; his first two posts were in that city. He then became a squadron medical officer attached to a mobile field hospital in North Africa, Italy, and France. This included an improbable stint as a pathologist to the Royal Air Force general hospital in Algiers. His military career lasted from 1941 to 1946, and, in the middle of this, in 1943, he received his M.D. In 1946 he became a member of the Edinburgh College of Physicians and a member of the London College the next year. Both colleges elected him to their fellowship in the 1960s. He was a registrar in the Edinburgh Royal Infirmary for two years. Between 1949 and 1954 he held a number of posts in clinical neurology at the National Hospital for Nervous Diseases, Queen's Square, London. In 1952 he spent some time as a visiting lecturer at the University of California in San Francisco. From 1952 to 1958 he assisted in the physician's clinic at Moorfields Eye Hospital, and from 1955 to 1958 he was senior registrar at St. Mary's Hospital in London.

When he moved to the northwest of England, his post was part-time adult neurologist in Preston, thirty-five miles northwest of Manchester, and part-time as the first English pediatric neurologist outside London. The latter post was to the children's hospitals of Manchester, in which he served for twenty-five years until he became a community pediatrician in Salford, Crewe, and Macclesfield in the summer of 1983.

His interest in child neurology came partly from his father, partly from Charles McNeil in Edinburgh, and also from Thomas Stapleton in London, and it was on this subject that he concentrated. He was soon able to relinquish adult neurology and went on to develop a department described by Tizard as "what must be regarded as the best staffed and organized hospital and community based child neurology service of any health region in the country" (Tizard, 1985).

Although Gordon was not a basic biological scientist, he read widely in all areas of science. It was one of his trademarks to pull an article out of his pocket for a quick read during dull moments. Because of his knowledge, good sense, and tact, he was in constant demand to give advice to colleagues all over the world. He was sent a steady stream of articles at draft stage for comment, and friends would send papers from unlikely sources when they knew he was interested in the subject. His annotations have been a reliable summary of current thinking on a wide range of interesting clinical problems.

His clinical advice has been in constant demand. When asked to see a colleague's patient, it was routine for him to see the child promptly and to keep in touch with his or her progress by frequent visits in order to keep learning. For his own patients, he sought advice readily and was resourceful in looking for ideas. He was more at ease with parents than with children, but his examination methods had a calm, purposeful, and economical style.

He encouraged parents to feel that they were helping him to understand their child. Working with him, it was impossible to avoid the addiction to clinical pediatric neurology.

He was an unenthusiastic committee man and good at keeping to the point. When he agreed to become chairman of the pediatric division at the Royal Manchester Children's Hospital, he nursed a secret ambition to abolish it as a redundant talking shop. He managed to get away with no meetings for six months, with no obvious detriment to the running of the hospital. To see him angry was a great rarity: colleagues could recall isolated instances with some awe.

Possibly his lack of malice or manipulation and optimistic faith in the good nature of others explained the limited resources made available to him until the last years of his hospital career. For nearly twenty years Booth Hall Children's Hospital denied him access to the outpatient department and obliged him to work in a tiny cubicle in the EEG department. This could seat three at a squash and a wheelchair if everyone stood up. When he made it into the outpatient department, it was on condition that his secretary ran the clinic, as the clerks and nurses were too busy with other work.

Gordon's family has always been very important to him, but as a private concern. There were difficult years for him when his daughter, then his wife, became ill and died. It was his work that kept him going, and he redoubled his efforts. For a time, he was working in Salford, Crewe, and Macclesfield, each an hours' drive from the other. In the course of dashing from one post to the other, he suffered a serious heart attack in his car. His tale of hazard warning lights, ignored by passing traffic for an hour, the wrong ambulance which arrived to collect him, with another dozen already on board, to go to the geriatric day hospital, then the correct ambulance, which had him praying for an early release as it hurtled to the coronary care unit through the tortuous Cheshire lanes, entertained worried colleagues at his bedside. He has recovered to make trips to Australia, Israel, Finland, and China.

I have seen the manuscript of his latest book handed over to his publisher today and have discussed two more for next year. He is involved in a research study on clumsy children, which should begin to bear fruit soon.

Gordon won a Hackett Fellowship to New Zealand in 1970 and the Priorsfield Fellowship to the School of Education in Birmingham, where he worked with Klaus Wedell, in 1974. In 1985 Sir Peter Tizard, president of the British Paediatric Association, presented him with the James Spence Medal (Tizard, 1985). In his address, given at a measured pace because the whereabouts of the medal had not been identified as Tizard stood up to speak, he said:

We honour you for your role in the development of paediatric neurology in Great Britain and abroad and for a lifetime of arduous, compassionate, and highly effective service to children — a record unsurpassed by any of our contemporaries — and this makes you a most fitting and distinguished recipient of our highest award. (Tizard, 1985)

Well said, well deserved.

Ian McKinlay
MANCHESTER, ENGLAND

REFERENCES

Gordon, N. S. 1976. *Paediatric Neurology for the Clinician*. Clinics in Developmental Medicine Nos. 59/60. Spastics International Medical Publications. London: Heinemann.

Gordon, N. S., and I. A. McKinlay. 1986a. *Neurologically Handicapped Children: Treatment and Management*. Oxford: Basil Blackwell.

______. 1986b. *Neurologically Sick Children: Treatment and Management*. Oxford: Basil Blackwell.

______. 1988. *Helping Clumsy Children*. Edinburgh: Churchill Livingstone.

Gubbay, S. S., et al. 1965. Clumsy Children. A Study of Apraxic and Agnosic Defects in 21 Children. *Brain* 88(2):295–312.

Tizard, J. P. M. 1985. James Spence Medallist, 1985: Neil Simson Gordon. *Arch Dis Child* 60:603–4.

JOSEPH GODWIN GREENFIELD

SAMUEL JOHNSON ONCE commented on how attractive to the Scots was the high road to London. Joseph Greenfield's father was one of those rare exceptions who left the metropolis for Edinburgh, where he was appointed professor of pathology at the university. His son, Joseph Godwin (1884–1958) (figure 1), was born in Edinburgh, where he qualified in medicine with first-class honors in 1908. Two years later he was in London, serving as house physician to the National Hospital for the Paralyzed and Epileptic in Queen's Square. There was one other resident doctor about that time, namely F. M. R. (later Sir Francis) Walshe. Two years later, Greenfield became assistant to Matthew Stewart, the distinguished professor of morbid anatomy at Leeds University.

In 1914 Greenfield was appointed pathologist to the National Hospital. With the outbreak of World War I in August of that year, Greenfield joined the Royal Army Medical Corps, serving in France with the rank of captain.

When peace came in 1918, notable changes were made in the organization of the National Hospital. Hitherto, the role of pathologist had been a temporary one held by a junior consultant whose future was to be in the practice and teaching of clinical neurology. Greenfield was the first full-time and professional pathologist.

The facilities available at that time were meager in the extreme. In the basement of the oldest part of the hospital were two rooms. A small oblong office served for Greenfield himself; he had no secretary. A larger, well-lit room was used as a work area and also housed the small but growing collection of mounted specimens. There was only one technician, but he was an exceptional individual. Before the war he had been a Yorkshire coal miner. In the war he had been batman to Greenfield, who was much impressed with his potential. When the war ended, he offered him the post of technician. This man, Anderson, proved to be a highly efficient, if not invaluable, laboratory assistant. Indeed, with Greenfield's encouragement, he actually wrote a little monograph about methods of staining specimens of nerve tissue.

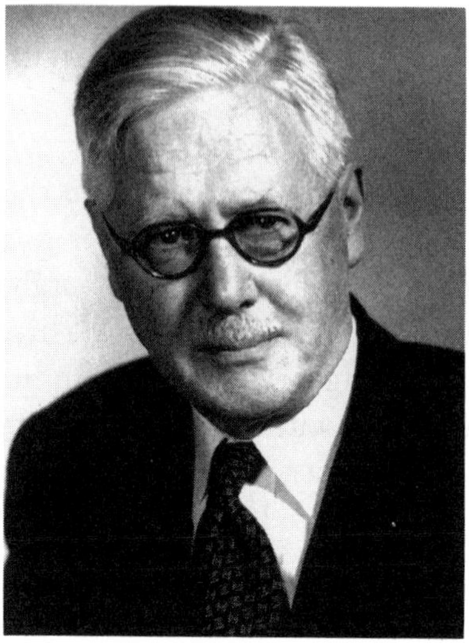

Figure 1. Joseph Godwin Greenfield (1884–1958).

If Greenfield's facilities were poor and his emolument derisory, he was rich in his access to study material. His work load was considerable, but much of it was a *terra vix incognita.* There was a considerable amount of straightforward oncology, but there was also much material where the clinical picture had been obscure in nature or rare in occurrence. For example, in my researches into the neurology of old age, I brought to him a steady supply of brains of centenarians.

It was not only the autopsy material from the National Hospital that came to him. Being one of the very few neuropathologists in the country, specimens were sent to him from all parts of England for identification, and from the United States as well.

But histological diagnosis was only one part of Greenfield's responsibilities. He set about building up a pathological museum in Queen's Square, no mean task in itself. Furthermore, he acted for many years as a biochemist, carrying out detailed examinations of the cerebrospinal fluid as well as routine blood tests. Later in his career, these duties were relegated to a full-time clinical pathologist. Microphotography was another task for which Greenfield was responsible.

As if these obligations were not enough, he carried out the duties of dean for twenty years. In his time, the medical school, although of international repute, was not officially recognized by the University of London. One consequence was that Greenfield never received the title of professor, with all the advantages and resources of an academic department, qualified assistants, and an adequate budget.

Despite his burden of work, Greenfield managed to use his opportunities well, publishing a steady output of important research work. All of it was valuable, some of it highly original. His description of the rare disease metachromatic leukodystrophy tempts us to speak of Greenfield's disease (Brain and Greenfield, 1950). This was his principal contribution to pediatric neuropathology in Great Britain.

He also published a number of standard works. In collaboration with Farquhar Buzzard (later Regius Professor of Physic at Oxford), he brought out his *Pathology of the Nervous System* in 1921. With E. A. Carmichael, he published another volume, *The Cerebrospinal Fluid* (Greenfield and Carmichael, 1925).

Greenfield was essentially an "all-round" neuropathologist, including child neuropathology. Among his considerable contributions were studies on the pathology of Parkinson's disease, diffuse sclerosis, the encephalitides, and the spinocerebellar degenerations (Greenfield, 1950, 1954).

He was deeply respected in the world of neuropathology. His colleagues at Queen's Square and, in particular, the house physicians and the postgraduate students, were devoted to him. Not only did he put at their disposal opportunities for carrying out research projects, but he was a wise mentor, advising them shrewdly upon their careers and also on personal matters. He was a loved and trusted counselor. An Irish doctor who was familiar with the neurological scene once asserted that, of the staff of the National Hospital, Greenfield was the only gentleman; all the others, he said, were too busy trying to be God.

He was not an accomplished lecturer. When illustrations were projected onto the screen, he would turn his back to the audience and continue to address his remarks to the wall. No one had the heart to tell him of this not uncommon shortcoming.

With his vast experience, Greenfield could be sternly critical of published work he considered to be unsound. But never did he display ill-feeling or rancour. With all his erudition, he remained modest and simple, a good man.

Greenfield founded the Neuropathological Club; he also served as president of both the Neurological Section of the Royal Society of Medicine and of the Association of British Neurologists. In 1955 his alma mater, the University of Edinburgh, conferred upon him an honorary Ll.D. degree.

Outside the laboratory he could relax. He was a skilled golfer and enjoyed tennis, gardening, and carpentry. In 1949 Greenfield welcomed his retirement, not because it offered leisure but for the opportunities it afforded him to record the knowledge he had accumulated but had been too busy to communicate. The Medical School of the National Hospital had become the Institute of Neurology, and Greenfield's successor was a departmental professor. Facilities were found for Greenfield to continue his work at a quieter pace.

American colleagues, too, were generous. For three successive years, he was invited to Bethesda to work in the National Institute of Neurological Disease and Blindness. Here he had the chance to document in comfort his life's work. These offers were gladly accepted, and Greenfield and his wife were enabled to enjoy the company of friendly and stimulating colleagues. He completed his magnum opus, *Neuropathology*, a tome upon which he had been working in association with William Blackwood, Joseph B. McMenemy, Adolph Meyer, and Ronald Melville Norman, in 1958.

The end, when it came, could not have been gentler. In his honor, a special party had been held at Bethesda with the twofold purpose of celebrating the appearance of *Neuropathology* in print and of bidding the Greenfields farewell on the eve of their return to England. Utterly contented, Greenfield retired to bed, promptly fell asleep, and did not wake.

Macdonald Critchley
SOMERSET, ENGLAND

REFERENCES

Brain, W. R., and J. G. Greenfield. 1950. Late Infantile Metachromatic Leuco-Encephalopathy with Primary Degeneration of the Interfascicular Oligodendroglia. *Brain* 73:291–317.

Buzzard, E. F., and J. G. Greenfield. 1921. *Pathology of the Nervous System*. London: Constable.

Greenfield, J. G. 1933. A Form of Cerebral Sclerosis in Infants Associated with Primary Degeneration of the Interfascicular Glia. *J Neur Psychopath* 13:289–302.

———. 1950. The Classification of Diffuse Demyelinating Sclerosis of the Brain on the Basis of Pathogenesis. *Folia Psych Nederl* 53:255–67.

———. 1954. *The Spinocerebellar Degenerations*. Oxford: Basil Blackwell.

Greenfield, J. G., and E. A. Carmichael. 1925. *The Cerebrospinal Fluid in Clinical Diagnosis*. London: Macmillan Co.

Greenfield, J. G., et al. 1958. *Neuropathology*. London: Arnold.

BENGT HAGBERG

BENGT ARTHUR HAGBERG (figure 1) was born on August 9, 1923, in Gothenburg, Sweden. His father was a physician, one of the first generation of radiologists in Sweden. His mother was a painter of the West-Swedish colorist school. Hagberg grew up and went to school first in Stockholm then in Boras (near Gothenburg). In 1942 he entered the University of Uppsala as a medical student and graduated in 1950. During his student years he was active in the medical students' association, chairman from 1947 to 1948, and represented Sweden at the first International Medical Students Study Group which met in England in 1948.

He married a medical student, Gudrun Wranne, in 1947. They and their five children (one architect, one teacher, two twin-son doctors, one physiotherapist) and twelve grandchildren (as of 1989) frequently spend the summer at the family's seventeenth-century fishing farm north of Gothenburg, where Hagberg's mother's family has lived for four generations.

In 1950 Hagberg began his training in pediatrics in Uppsala with Bo Vahlquist, one of the leading Scandinavian pediatricians. With Vahlquist as his tutor, Hagberg immediately started his dissertation project in pediatric hematology, "Studies on the Plasma Transport of Iron," which was presented and published in April 1953 in *Acta Paediatrica Scandinavia*.

After years of laboratory work on his thesis, Hagberg decided to leave pediatric hematology. Already, during his first months as a pediatric trainee, he had become fascinated by the numerous unsolved and challenging diagnostic and therapeutic problems in infants and children with neurological abnormalities. The field of

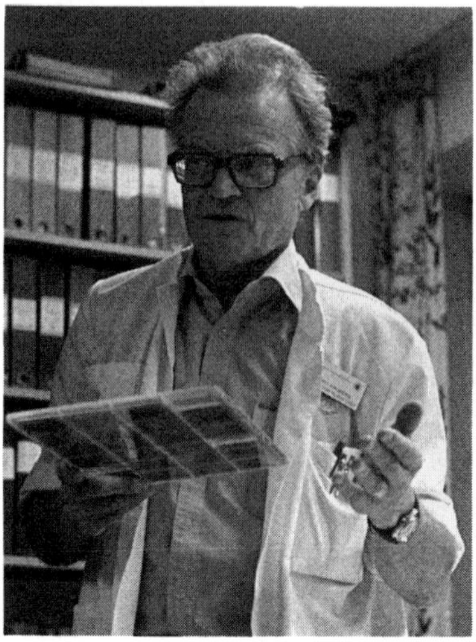

Figure 1. Bengt Hagberg.

neuropediatrics in the early 1950s was just becoming recognized as a distinct entity within pediatrics and was involving an ever-expanding sector of children, about ten times more children than the hematologic problems in the pre-oncologic era. Hagberg decided to change fields and began three years of training in adult neurology and internal medicine, especially in the area of neurology. This training was divided between the neurologic departments of Karl Ekbom in Uppsala, Tore Broman in Gothenburg, Gunnar Wohlfart in Lund, and the research-oriented internal medicine group of Jan Waldenstrom in Malmo. For a short period, Hagberg also visited Sven Brandt in Copenhagen, the only pediatric neurologist in Scandinavia at that time. He returned to Uppsala as assistant professor of pediatrics in 1956 and was lecturer in pediatrics from 1960 to 1964.

As a pediatric neurologist, Hagberg, like many of his Scandinavian colleagues, is self-taught. His original experiences were principally clinical and intensive, as he was located in the very dynamic department of pediatrics in Uppsala. In that center, pediatric subspecialization was encouraged and developed quickly. In 1964 Hagberg received a clinically oriented Swedish Medical Research Council appointment, then an associate professorship in pediatric neurology in 1967, and promotion to the first chair in pediatric neurology in the northern countries in 1969. In 1971 he was appointed professor ordinarius of pediatrics in Gothenburg, giving him yet a broader platform with better resources for pediatric subspecialization. He and his colleagues quickly developed a neuropediatric center to evaluate neurodevelopmental disorders, to manage child neurological problems, and to rehabilitate the handicapped child. Trainees from Uppsala and other parts of Sweden moved with Hagberg to the west coast of Sweden and initiated a collaboration with Ingemar Olow at the regional center at Bracke-

Ostergard, Gothenburg. Hagberg also formed a neuropediatric school, in a broad sense, as part of his administrative efforts to structure a decentralized organization in Sweden for the care of the handicapped child. Young pediatricians studied at Gothenburg for periods of improvised training in basic clinical child neurology and to learn which cases could be managed at home and which ones should be referred to the regional university centers. A large number of such "county neuropediatricians" spent a period with the Hagberg school in Uppsala or Gothenburg for clinical work, training, and also research in child neurology. This system, initiated by Hagberg, started with young, more or less "barefoot neuropediatricians," then continued with successive postgraduate training through the years. This improved competence in child neurology throughout the country. In addition, at Gothenburg, a well-functioning regional neuropediatric university center was created with four staff positions, each with a somewhat different area of interest. This was arranged because of Hagberg's administrative positions both as chairman of the Pediatric Hospital Block, which was responsible for providing child care in Gothenburg, and as prefect for the university unit of pediatrics.

Hagberg was also active in clinical research, authoring or coauthoring at least 290 papers to date, primarily in the areas of child neurology, the epidemiology of handicapping conditions, evaluation of child care, and pediatric hematology. One research area of particular importance has been in the delineation of various childhood cerebral degenerative disorders. As clinical counterpart for thirty years to Lars Svennerholm (neurochemistry) and Patrick Sourander (neuropathology), Hagberg has coauthored a series of contributions on various lysosomal diseases (Hagberg, Sourander, and Svennerholm, 1968; Ylitalo et al, 1986), neuronal ceroid lipofuscinoses (the infantile form was first described in 1968 by the team of Hagberg, Sourander, and Svennerholm) (Santavouri et al, 1973) and, later, Rett syndrome (Hagberg et al, 1983a). He also proposed clinical staging systems for late infantile metachromatic leukodystrophy (Hagberg, 1971), Krabbe's disease (Hagberg, 1984), and Rett syndrome. Together with I. Witt-Engerstrom, he has recently extensively reported on the epidemiology and natural history from infancy to middle age of Rett syndrome, including aspects of brainstem and spinal cord neurophysiology and pathology (Hagberg and Witt-Engerstrom, 1987). Hagberg has followed Rett patients since 1960, when he first observed one patient. From that time, he has collected a successive series of patients, unaware until 1982 that Andreas Rett in Vienna was pursuing the same phenomena. Together with Jean Aicardi and Ovidio Ramos in Paris and Karin Dias in Lisbon, he presented a study of a pooled series of thirty-one Swedish-French-Portuguese patients that internationally called attention to this disease, neglected since the original description by Rett in a German publication in 1966.

Among other "new" diseases described by Hagberg and coinvestigators are: malignant hyperlipemia in infancy (Hagberg et al, 1964); a Niemann-Pick simulating oligosaccharidosis (Hagberg et al, 1978); the genetic dysequilibrium syndrome (Hagberg, Sanner, and Steen, 1972); a Swedish Salla disease variant (Ylitalo et al, 1986); the recently discovered disialo-developmental deficiency (DDD) disease (Kristiansson et al, 1989); and two different familial forms of 3–methylglutaconic aciduria (Hagberg et al, 1983b).

Hagberg has also had an interest in the neuroepidemiology of cerebral palsy and infantile hydrocephalus. Organized projects were established after he moved to the western region of Sweden when his wife, Gudrun (nominated to honorary Doctor of Medicine at Gothenburg University in 1989), joined him as a competent and efficient epidemiologist and statistician. The changing panorama of cerebral palsy in Sweden was investigated in a series of papers (1975–89), using a large population-based series of cases born between 1954 and 1982. These studies were performed in collaboration also with I. Olow from Bracke-Ostergard (Hagberg, Hagberg, and Olow, 1975). Other epidemiologic investigations covered severe forms of mental deficiency (Gustavson, 1977), milder forms referring to an IQ in the 50–70 range (Hagberg et al, 1981); infantile hydrocephalus (Fernell, Hagberg, and Von Wendt, 1987); and peripheral neuropathies (Hagberg and Lyon, 1981).

Hagberg, together with Johannes Melchior from Denmark, formed The Scandinavian Neuropaediatric Society in 1963 (Melchior, 1985). The first meeting took place in Uddevalla near Hagberg's summer home. He was also one of the initiators with Melchior and Ronald MacKeith from England of the European Federation of Child Neurology Societies (Hagberg, Ingram, and MacKeith, 1985) and arranged the first conference in Kungalv, Sweden in 1973 and later served as first Secretary General (1970–77). He was also chairman of the Swedish Section of Pediatric Neurology and Rehabilitation for the Handicapped from 1975 to 1978 and has been chairman since 1977 of the Swedish Medical Research Council Committee on Medical Research in Mental Retardation and Neurological Handicaps in Children. He has been vice chairman of the Folke Bernadotte Foundation for Crippled Children since 1980 and a board member of four other foundations providing support for neuropediatric research. In addition, he is an honorary member of a number of European societies and has received many awards for his contributions to child neurology: the Lennander Award, Stockholm 1974; the Malte Award, Oslo, 1979; Ronnie MacKeith Lecturer, Honorary British Paediatric Association Lecturer, England, 1981; Finnish Paediatric Neurology Association, Helsinki, 1972 and 1983; Guest Professor Award of the University of Dundee, 1985; Oskar Medins Award, 1987; Folke Bernadotte Award, 1988; and the Segawa Price Lecturer, Japan, 1989.

Bengt Hagberg is a very active person. When one has a chance to observe him lecturing, one is immediately stimulated and curious. He is enthusiastic and so engaged that he captures an entire audience within a very short while. This, and his ability to motivate his co-workers to excellence, are the most dominant characteristics of Hagberg's personality and work, and have allowed him to make a solid contribution to contemporary child neurology.

Johannes C. Melchior
COPENHAGEN, DENMARK

REFERENCES

Fernell, E., B. Hagberg, and L. von Wendt. 1987. Epidemiology of Infantile Hydrocephalus in Sweden. II. Origin in Infants Born at Term. *Acta Paed Scand* 76(3):411–17.

Gustavson, K. H., et al. 1977. Severe Mental Retardation in a Swedish County. I. Epidemiology, Gestational Age, Birth Weight and Associated CNS Handicaps in Children Born 1959–1970. *Acta Paed Scand* 66(3):373–79.

Hagberg, B. A. 1953. The Iron-Binding Capacity of Serum in Infants and Children. *Acta Paed Scand* (Suppl.) 42:589.

______. 1971. Clinical Aspects of Globoid Cell and Metachromatic Leukodystrophies. *Birth Defects* Original Article Series 7(1):103–12.

______. 1984. Krabbe's Disease: Clinical Presentation on Neurological Variants. *Neuroped* 15(Suppl):11–15.

Hagberg, B., et al. 1964. Malignant Hyperlipemia in Infancy. *Am J Dis Child* 107:267.

Hagberg, B., et al. 1978. Neurovisceral Storage Disease Stimulating Niemann-Pick Disease. A New Form of Oligosaccharidoses? *Neuroped* 9(1):59–73.

Hagberg, B., et al. 1981. Mild Mental Retardation in Swedish School Children. I. Prevalence. *Acta Paed Scand* 70(4):441–44.

Hagberg, B., et al. 1983a. A Progressive Syndrome of Autism, Dementia, Ataxia, and Loss of Purposeful Hand Use in Girls: Rett's Syndrome: Report of 35 Cases. *Ann Neur* 14(4):471–78.

Hagberg, B., et al. 1983b. 3–Methylglutaconic Aciduria in Two Infants. *Clin Chim Acta* 134:59–67.

Hagberg, B., G. Hagberg, and I. Olow. 1975. The Changing Panorama of Cerebral Palsy in Sweden 1954–1970. I. Analysis of the General Changes. *Acta Paed Scand* 64(2):187–92.

Hagberg, B., T. T. S. Ingram, and R. MacKeith. 1985. Development of Paediatric Neurology. *Lancet* 1(653):940–42.

Hagberg, B., and G. Lyon. 1981. Pooled European Series of Hereditary Peripheral Neuropathies in Infancy and Childhood. A Correspondence Work Shop. Report of the European Federation of Child Neurology Societies (EFCNS). *Neuroped* 12(1):8–17.

Hagberg, B., G. Sanner, and M. Steen. 1972. The Dysequilibrium Syndrome in Cerebral Palsy. Clinical Aspects and Treatment. *Acta Paed Scand* (Suppl.) 226:1–63.

Hagberg, B., P. Sourander, and L. Svennerholm. 1968. Late Infantile Progressive Encephalopathy with Disturbed Poly-Unsaturated Fat Metabolism. *Acta Paed Scand* 57(6):495–99.

Hagberg, B., and I. Witt-Engerstrom. 1987. Rett Syndrome: Epidemiology and Nosology — Progress in Knowledge 1986 — A Conference Communication (Review). *Brain Dev* 9(5):451–547.

Kristiansson, B., et al. 1989. Disialotransferrin Developmental Deficiency Syndrome. *Arch Dis Child* 64:71–76.

Melchior, J. C. 1985. The Scandinavian Neuropaediatric Society. The Society's History and Present Status. *Brain Dev* 7:545–48.

Santavouri, P., et al. 1973. Infantile Type of So-called Neuronal Ceroid Lipofuscinosis I. A Clinical Study of 75 Patients. *J Neur Sci* 18:257.

Ylitalo, V., et al. 1986. Salla Disease Variants. Sialoylaciduria Encephalopathy with Increased Sialidase Activity in Two Non-Finnish Children. *Neuroped* 17(1):44–47.

THOMAS INGRAM

THOMAS THEODORE SCOTT INGRAM (b. 1927) (figure 1), known to most friends and colleagues as Tom or TTSI, was born in Carlisle, England. Both parents were medical graduates and there were seven other doctors in the family.

Ingram majored in medicine at the University of Edinburgh from 1944 through 1949, where he graduated M.B.Ch.B.and was awarded the Gunning Victoria Jubilee Prize in Child Life and Health. He became interested in pediatrics as an undergraduate and early developed an interest in child neurology under the stimulation of Richard Ellis. He took the examinations for the Diploma in Child Health and became a member of the Royal College of Physicians three years after his basic undergraduate qualification. He went on to do research on the neurological aspects of cerebral palsy. This culminated in the award by the University of Edinburgh of a Doctorate of Medicine with a Gold Medal in 1961. The following year he was elected a fellow of the Royal College of Physicians of Edinburgh.

In the early 1960s, pediatric neurology was not an established specialty and it was necessary to train in pediatrics and neurology separately and to arrange one's own program. After training in general pediatrics and neonatology at Edinburgh, Ingram became the George Guthrie Research Fellow from 1951 to 1955 in the Department of Child Life and Health and was able to pursue his studies in neurology and cerebral palsy. He subsequently became a lecturer in the pediatrics department at Edinburgh. Ingram spent the year of 1956 to 1957 with Derek Denny-Brown at the Boston City Hospital where he studied neuropathology with Paul Yakovlev at Harvard and electroencephalography with Margaret Lennox. In 1959 he was given a one-year leave of absence to attend the National Hospital for Nervous Diseases, Queen's Square, London, where he studied with Macdonald Critchley and Sir Charles Symonds. Shortly after his return, he was appointed Senior Lecturer and subsequently Reader in Pediatrics with Special Responsibility for pediatric neurology. Ingram later visited the Swedish centers of interest in pediatric neurology on a six-month study

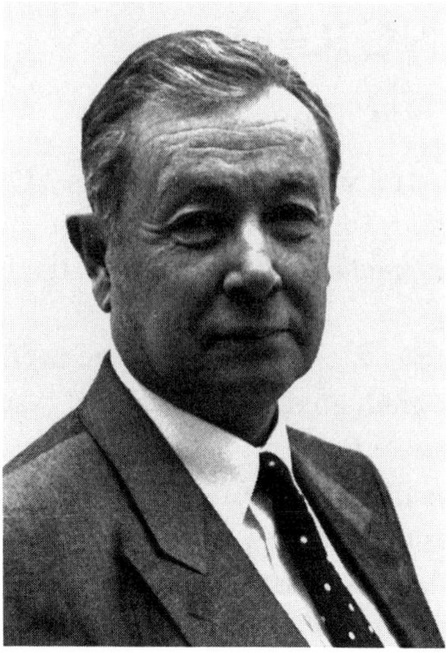

Figure 1. Thomas Ingram.

leave in 1967 and he also visited Adriano Milani Comparetti in Florence. On shorter visits, he was able to discuss common problems with Guy Tardieu in Paris, Harry Bakwin in New York, as well as with other pediatricians and neurologists interested in child neurology in Madrid, Barcelona, Heidelberg, and the Republic of Ireland.

Ingram is a member of the British Paediatric Association, a founding member of the British Paediatric Neurology Association, the Scottish Paediatric Society, the Association of British Neurologists, the Society for Research into Hydrocephalus and Spina Bifida, the Scottish Association of Mental Health, the American Academy for Cerebral Palsy, and the European Federation of Child Neurology Societies.

Many physicians have made contributions in the field of neurological disease in children since the time of Thomas Sydenham, who is often regarded as the father of child neurology in the United Kingdom. With the advent of the National Health Service in 1948, pediatrics became a much more generally available specialty to all members of the community. Specialization in child neurology followed soon afterward in the early 1950s. Three people in the United Kingdom, Paul Sandifer in London, Neil Gordon in Manchester, and Thomas Ingram in Edinburgh, initiated pediatric neurology as a separate specialty. These founding fathers were also the catalyst to formation of a pediatric neurology group in Europe. Ronald MacKeith, as a leader in the field of postgraduate medical education, linked the European group of Bengt Hagberg, Johannes Melchior, Gilles Lyon, Ingrid Gamstorp, and Jean Aicardi into what eventually became the British Paediatric Neurology Association and the European Federation of Child Neurology Societies.

Ingram is basically an academic pediatric neurologist. As Research Fellow, Lecturer, Senior Lecturer, and Reader at the University of Edinburgh, he always felt that research and scholarship were the basis of good practice. He delineated many diseases in the field of pediatric neurology with his extensive writings. His main research areas were in the field of speech and learning disorders where, with the help of the Nuffield Research Foundation, he undertook fundamental studies in higher cortical function in childhood and, with his work in cerebral palsy, he delineated cerebral palsy as a neurological disorder and defined the neurological substrate. His book, *Paediatric Aspects of Cerebral Palsy*, is a classic that highlights his scholarship and has not been bettered (Ingram, 1964).

Ingram has contributed to child neurology in three major areas. First, he was the academic of the three pediatric neurologists in the United Kingdom and stressed that pediatric neurology must be founded on scientific lines based on research and scholarship, and that it should not simply consist of "stamp collecting" of rare diseases with unpronounceable names. Secondly, he emphasized that all diseases of the brain, spinal cord, and peripheral nervous system, both acute and chronic, should be encompassed by pediatric neurology, and one should not reject mental handicaps, spina bifida, learning disorders, and cerebral palsy while collecting information on rare degenerative diseases. The important diseases to pediatric neurologists had to be those that were important to the community that he was serving. His third area of emphasis was that one should not be annihilistic about treatment in pediatric neurology. One may not be able to cure the disease but that did not mean that the condition could not be effectively managed. He pioneered the idea of working in close conjunction with orthopedic surgeons, neurosurgeons, and psychologists. However, he was most emphatic in his support of paramedical therapy and his insistence that this should have a rational scientific basis. By setting up combined cerebral palsy clinics and multidisciplinary spina bifida clinics, he showed that the study of the neurogenic bladder, the assessment of various forms of urinary diversion or catheterization, the monitoring of intracranial pressure, and early orthopedic intervention all had their place in a comprehensive management program.

Like many brilliant men, Ingram was a depressive and this meant he could not enjoy the well-deserved acclaim he received at the end of his career. He was a formidable opponent at meetings and would stand up and say in public what many were feeling privately about an unscientific presentation. He was a good teacher who was ready to impart his knowledge, not egocentric, and did not go for self-aggrandizement by keeping knowledge to himself.

Ingram was a founding editor of the journal *Neuropädiatrie*. He was also on the editorial board of *Developmental Medicine and Child Neurology* and the advisory board of the *Journal of Learning Disabilities.* His research interest centered predominantly on cerebral palsy and learning disorders. His research on cerebral palsy was incorporated in his book *Paediatric Aspects of Cerebral Palsy* (Ingram, 1964). This book was a scholarly production aimed at physicians, providing both a comprehensive historical review of the many different types of cerebral palsy with an excellent bibliography as well as a detailed analysis of Ingram's extensive clinical and epidemiological experience. He also produced a book with S. Jameson, J. Errington, and Ross Mitchell entitled *Living with Cerebral Palsy* (Ingram et al, 1964). Ingram also contributed chapters to many other books and series, such as "Spasticity in Cerebral Palsy" (Ingram, 1966). He published many scientific works as the result of specific studies, such as "The Early Manifestations and Course of Diplegia in Childhood" (Ingram, 1954a); "A Study of Cerebral Palsy in the Child Population of Edinburgh" (Ingram, 1954b); "Problems in the Classification of Cerebral Palsy in Childhood" (Ingram, 1955); and "The Long-Term Care of Patients Suffering from Cerebral Palsy" (Ingram, 1976a).

Ingram's other main area of interest was in speech, language, and learning disorders. In each area, he led a team of research workers, including audiologists, psychologists, and speech therapists, that were supported by the Medical Research Council for Research and Education and the Nuffield Foundation. He delineated several of the speech disorders seen in childhood and suggested a classification that has stood the test of time (Ingram, 1959a, 1959b, 1963, 1968, 1976b). He wrote a book with Cecil Drillien and Elsie Wilkinson, entitled *The Causes and Natural History of Cleft Lip and Palate*, which delineated the causes of speech disorders in children (Drillien, Ingram, and Wilkinson, 1966). He also published articles on behavioral and learning difficulties in brain-damaged children (Ingram, 1969a, 1969b, 1971). Among his other areas of interest were the aminoacidurias in children with chronic neurological disorders, the long-term effects of neonatal hypoglycemia on development, and studies on specific anticonvulsant drugs. With Bengt Hagberg and Ronald MacKeith, Ingram also published a paper on the importance of child neurology and the need to establish this as a separate discipline (Hagberg, Ingram, and MacKeith, 1970).

Thomas Ingram is one of the founding fathers of pediatric neurology in the United Kingdom. He is a scholar with a brilliant track record in the study of neurological diseases in childhood and an excellent teacher. He is remembered by many for his wicked sense of humor. Some may have been demolished by him. Many will be extremely grateful to him for stimulating their interest in pediatric neurology and giving them the foundation upon which the understanding of many diseases of the central nervous system in children is based.

John Keith Brown
EDINBURGH, SCOTLAND

REFERENCES

Drillien, C. M., T. T. S. Ingram, and E. M. Wilkinson. 1966. *The Causes and Natural History of Cleft Lip and Palate.* Baltimore: Williams & Wilkins Co.

Hagberg, B., T. T. S. Ingram, and R. MacKeith. 1970. Development of Paediatric Neurology. *Lancet* 1:940–42.

Ingram, T. T. S. 1954a. The Early Manifestations and Course of Diplegia in Childhood. *Arch Dis Child* 30:244.

______. 1954b. A Study of Cerebral Palsy in the Child Population of Edinburgh. *Arch Dis Child* 30:85.

______. 1955. Problems in the Classification of Cerebral Palsy in Childhood. *Brit Med J* 2:163.

______. 1959a. Specific Development Disorders of Speech in Childhood. *Brain* 82:450.

______. 1959b. A Description and Classification of the Common Disorders of Speech in Childhood. *Arch Dis Child* 34:444.

______. 1963. The Association of Speech Retardation and Educational Difficulties. *Proc Roy Soc Med* 56:199.

______. 1964. *Paediatric Aspects of Cerebral Palsy.* Edinburgh: E. & S. Livingstone, Ltd.

______. 1966. Spasticity in Cerebral palsy. *Clin Orth* 46:23–36.

______. 1968. *Speech Disorders in Childhood* (Review). *Ped Clin North Am* 15(3):611–26.

______. 1969a. The New Approach to the Early Diagnosis of Handicaps in Childhood. *Devel Med Child Neur* 11(3):279–90.

______. 1969b. *The Nature of Dyslexia.* Baltimore: Bulletin Orton Dyslexia Society.

______. 1971. Specific Learning Difficulties. A Medical Point of View. *Brit J Educ Psych* Part 1:41.

______. 1976a. The Long-Term Care of Patients Suffering from Cerebral Palsy. *J Irish Med Assoc* 67(8):205–43.

______. 1976b. Intermittent Hearing Loss in Young Children. *Devel Med Child Neur* 18:239.

Ingram, T. T. S., et al. 1964. *Living with Cerebral Palsy: A Study of School Leavers Suffering from Cerebral Palsy in Eastern Scotland.* London: The Spastics Society Medical Education and Information Unit in association with Heinemann Medical Books.

WILLIAM LENNOX

WILLIAM GORDON LENNOX (1884–1960) (figure 1) was born in Colorado Springs. His father, William Lennox, was a pioneer settler in the gold mining livery business and later had interests in mining, banking, and cattle ranching. His paternal grandfather was from Glasgow, Scotland, and was also a man of diverse interests. He was trained as a printer, farmed in Iowa, and for many years was director of schools near Colorado Springs. His mother, of English Quaker descent and an avid reader, probably stimulated Lennox's missionary bent and love of literature, including poetry. Denied admission to a theological school because of deficiencies in Greek and Latin, he realized his goal to become a missionary in China after completing his medical education at Harvard and the Massachusetts General Hospital. Married to Emma Buchtel, daughter of the chancellor of Denver University and one-time governor of Colorado, Lennox had two daughters, Mary Belle and Margaret. He moved to China with his family in 1916 and worked at the Rockefeller School and Hospital in Peking. On his return to the United States in 1920, he began a lifelong study of epilepsy, which ended in his seventy-sixth year with the publication in 1960 of a two-volume treatise entitled *Epilepsy and Related Disorders*, the summation of the advances recorded in his many original articles over a forty-year period.

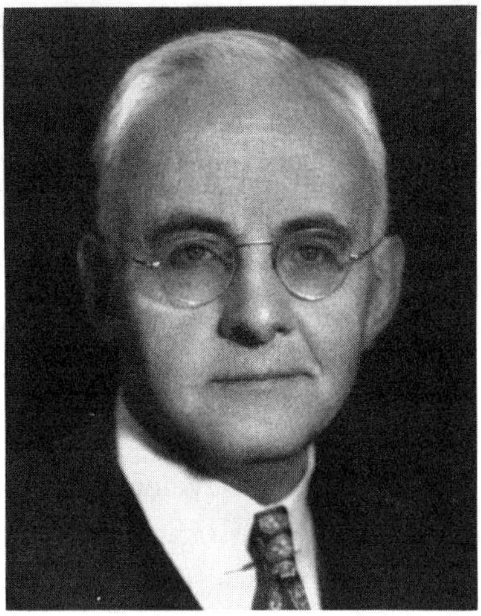

Figure 1. William Lennox (1884–1960).

Although he had no formal training in neurology, Lennox joined the Departments of Neuropathology and Neurology at Harvard Medical School and Boston City Hospital, where he worked in collaboration with Stanley Cobb. Lennox worked for more than twenty years with Cobb, and subsequently with Frederick and Erna Gibbs, first in neurology and neuropathology and later, for a short period, in psychiatry, at the Boston Psychopathic Hospital. He moved to the Children's Medical Center in Boston in 1944 to establish the Seizure Unit. Lennox considered that the problems of epilepsy and the epileptic were so diverse and complex that a group of individuals working together, each with his special training and gifts, should be able to accomplish much more than doctors of uniform training who work alone. As viewed by Cesare Lombroso (1988), the Seizure Unit was a precursor of current comprehensive epilepsy centers. It had several functions: diagnosis and treatment; training of individual doctors, psychologists, social workers, nurses, and technologists; research and publications both basic and clinical; and education of the public at large regarding epilepsy in order to remove the stigma of epilepsy and dispel the myths and misunderstandings about it.

Lennox's research into epilepsy, like the function of his Seizure Unit, was multifaceted, and his publications covered many areas.

One of his earliest articles, written in collaboration with Stanley Cobb, was "Epilepsy from the Standpoint of Physiology and Treatment" (1928). Together with Fred Gibbs and Erna Gibbs (née Leonhardt), Lennox perfected a technique of blood sampling from veins and arteries, and studied blood constituents including oxygen and carbon dioxide tensions and cerebral blood flow using a continuous recording device before, during, and after seizures (Gibbs, Gibbs, and Lennox, 1935). In these studies, Lennox usually volunteered to be the first subject before any new instrument or drug was used on patients. With Hallowell Davis and the Gibbs, Lennox helped develop the electroencephalograph machine (1935). His clinical classification of the epilepsies, petit mal, grand mal, and psychomotor, was supported by the characteristic electroencephalographic correlations. He thought of epilepsy as a variety of disorders affecting the chemistry of cerebral neurons. That petit mal could be precipitated by hyperventilation and a change in carbon dioxide tension in the blood was his discovery (Lennox and Cobb, 1928). He showed that this hyperventilation-induced response was not present to the same extent in patients with grand mal and psychomotor seizures. He knew that epilepsy was not a disease *sui generis* and investigated multiple symptomatic causes. He favored a basic biochemical mechanism responsible for an inherent tendency or predisposition to certain seizures and the associated cerebral dysrhythmia.

In his book *Science and Seizures* (1941), Lennox represented the various causes of seizures as water impounded in a reservoir. The deepest water was the fundamental cause or a hereditary predisposition and the reservoir was fed by contributory springs, for example, brain damage and emotional disorders. The dam was the seizure threshold, and the periodic overflow of the reservoir was the seizure. It is noteworthy that the latest classification of epileptic syndromes (Commission, International League Against Epilepsy, 1989) recognizes the idiopathic primary hereditary epilepsies (absence) and symptomatic epilepsies and no longer considers all epilepsies as symptomatic. Lennox would have applauded the etiologic classifications but would probably have rejected the generalized and partial pattern groupings, which, from a therapeutic standpoint, are confusing and impractical.

Of epilepsy in childhood, he wrote that seizures are predominantly a disorder of youth and not only important numerically, but also from a sociopsychological standpoint. He felt that the family doctor and pediatrician were best equipped to deal with intrafamily relationships and that the pediatrician should not resign his natural leadership in treatment to the neurologist or neurosurgeon:

Epilepsy in children differs from epilepsy in adults in several important respects: (1) Diagnosis is more difficult because of frequent borderline areas. (2) Seizures are more frequent. (3) Seizure patterns are different: Petit mal (absence attacks) are almost entirely limited to the young, whereas psychomotor (partial complex seizures) are relatively infrequent. (4) Treatment is broader in scope in that the whole family is involved. Epilepsy of childhood is more puzzling, more diversified, and treatment more rewarding. (Lennox and Lennox, 1960, 411)

However, Lennox conceded that physicians interested in epilepsy should see both children and adults, because to see one age group alone could provide a distorted view (Lennox and Lennox, 1960).

Lennox wrote papers on the significance of febrile convulsions and referred to studies by his daughter, Margaret Lennox (M. A. Lennox, 1949). He viewed the febrile convulsion as epilepsy, an "unusually pure culture of epilepsy" with a frequent hereditary transmission. By including conditions considered relatively benign under the term *epilepsy*, he hoped that such a conception would provide "a broad silver lining for the dark cloud of current thoughts about epilepsy and add force to the appellation 'Epilepsy the Hopeful Disorder'" (Lennox and Lennox , 411). Cyclic vomiting was another example of a benign disorder in childhood considered as a form of epilepsy, a subject that I investigated in his Seizure Unit (Millichap, Lombroso, and Lennox, 1955).

His vision was to have epilepsy and patients with epilepsy accepted socially and in the workplace. He aimed to unravel the basic biochemical nature of the inherited predisposition and lowered threshold to seizures, particularly in children with petit mal, but with equal emphasis he wanted to remove the stigma of the term *epilepsy*, its myths and misunderstandings, through education of physicians and the lay public. In explaining the nature of epilepsy, he often used the example of diabetes as a condition much like epilepsy, with an inherited predisposition and a chronic course often requiring lifelong treatment. He also referred to the many famous and gifted persons in history reputed to have suffered from epilepsy, including saints, world leaders, writers, artists, musicians, symphony conductors, and national sports figures.

As one of the last visiting fellows to work under his direction at the Seizure Unit, I had the opportunity to see patients who came to him from all over the world for more accurate diagnosis and improved methods of treatment. Experimentation and investigation were a mainstay of his practice. Almost all his patients would form part of a study: a trial of a new drug, an electroencephalographic study of twins or relatives, biochemical and blood-flow studies, and the investigation of psychological factors. All aspects of epilepsy were studied, and a team of secretaries was at hand to aid with the many publications produced in his Seizure Unit. He encouraged and motivated his colleagues and visiting scientists not only to investigate but to publish their findings for the better understanding of epilepsy in medicine.

Any suggestions or topic of research would receive his undivided interest and helpful comments. If not qualified to supervise a project himself, he would ask Raymond Adams, Jerome Merlis, or another colleague to become involved. My own early interest in the use of radioactive isotopes to determine changes in metabolism in the brain during convulsions in animals received his full attention, and he attempted, albeit unsuccessfully, to make arrangements for this work to be accomplished in another Harvard laboratory. When my research subsequently turned to the neuropharmacology of carbonic anhydrase inhibitors in epilepsy, Lennox helped me obtain a fellowship and subsequently a faculty research position with Louis Goodman at the University of Utah. His last words to me upon my departure were, "The discovery of the fundamental biochemical cause of epilepsy has eluded me. I want you to work toward that goal."

For his research programs, Lennox received support from the Rockefeller Foundation, the Markle Foundation, the Association for Crippled Children and Adults, the Department of Health, Education and Welfare, National Institutes of Health, and, frequently, from patients and private donors. He was honored as a recipient of the Lasker Award and by a dinner at the Harvard Club on the completion of his book, shortly before his death on July 21, 1960, three days after his seventh-sixth birthday. As Frederick A. Gibbs stated in his memoriam in 1961, "Dr. Lennox left the world as a legacy a new understanding of epilepsy and an increased acceptance of those who suffer from this disorder."

Lennox wrote four books and more than 240 medical articles on epilepsy. As a prelude to his own studies, he collected all the significant writings on epilepsy, among them the works of Galen, Thomas Willis, William Gowers, and John Hughlings Jackson. He was a dedicated physician and scientist with an understanding of epilepsy far advanced for his time. I am privileged to have had the opportunity to have known William Gordon Lennox as mentor and friend, and it is an honor to write his biography for inclusion in this book.

J. Gordon Millichap
SPRINGFIELD, ILLINOIS

REFERENCES

Cobb, S. 1961. William Gordon Lennox, M.D. Obituaries. *Arch Neur Psych* 163:463–65.

Commission on Classification and Terminology of the International League Against Epilepsy. 1989. Proposal for Revised Classification of Epilepsies and Epileptic Syndromes. *Epilepsia* 30:389–99.

Gibbs, F. A. 1961. William Gordon Lennox, 1884–1960. *Epilepsia* 2:1–8.

Gibbs, F. A., H. Davis, and W. G. Lennox. 1935. The Electroencephalogram in Epilepsy and in Conditions of Impaired Consciousness. *Arch Neur Psych* 34:1133–48.

Gibbs, F. A., E. L. Gibbs, and W. G. Lennox. 1935. Changes in Human Cerebral Blood Flow Consequent on Alterations in Blood Gases. *Am J Physiol* 111:557.

Lennox, M. A. 1949. Febrile Convulsions in Childhood: A Clinical and Electroencephalographic Study. *Am J Dis Child* 78:868–82.

Lennox, W. G. 1941. *Science and Seizures.* New York: Harper and Brothers.

Lennox, W. G., and S. Cobb. 1928. Epilepsy form the Standpoint of Physiology and Treatment. *Med* 7:105–290.

Lennox, W. G., and M. A. Lennox. 1960. *Epilepsy and Related Disorders*. Boston: Little, Brown, and Co.

Lombroso, C. T. 1988. William G. Lennox: A Remembrance. *Epilepsia* 29 (Suppl. 2):S5–S14.

Millichap, J. G., C. T. Lombroso, and W. G. Lennox. 1955. Cyclic Vomiting as a Form of Epilepsy in Childhood. *Ped* 15:705.

SAMUEL LIVINGSTON

SAMUEL LIVINGSTON (1908–1984) (figure 1) dedicated his medical career to the study of epilepsy and became one of the world's most widely recognized authorities on the subject. He reshaped methods of treatment with established drugs and actively studied new drugs as they were developed. His work on the treatment of seizures came from and was distinguished by exhaustive reviews of large groups of patients, yet the achievements that probably gave him the most satisfaction throughout his career were improvements in the social status and individual rights of epileptic patients. In essence, his primary goal was the betterment of anyone with epilepsy, and it is certainly obvious that he succeeded.

Born in Philadelphia, Livingston moved to Baltimore at age thirteen. In 1924 he graduated from City College, a prestigious Baltimore high school, and then attended Georgetown University, from which he graduated magna cum laude in 1928. During the next two years, he obtained a master's degree in chemistry at George Washington University and went on to receive his M.D. degree from Vanderbilt University in 1934. Livingston returned to Baltimore for his pediatric residency under Edwards A. Park, chairman of pediatrics at Johns Hopkins Hospital. In 1936 he entered private practice but continued to work in the epilepsy clinic at Johns Hopkins, using both positions to accumulate patient data for his many publications. He became director of the epilepsy clinic in 1946 and continued in this capacity until his retirement in 1973. Even then, his work continued fruitfully until his final illness.

As Livingston was entering practice in 1936, he married Anne Lee Pruce, and this would remain a close and mutually supportive relationship until his death. They had a daughter and son. No doubt he received great satisfaction in collaborating with his son, Herbert, a periodontist, in extensive research on phenytoin-induced gingival hyperplasia (Livingston and Livingston, 1973). Samuel and Anne Livingston regularly visited California, and in 1964 he spent much time trying to help establish the Los Angeles County

Epilepsy Society, but the going was slow. However, when he enlisted the aid of his famous nephews Stanley and Barry Livingston, who played the parts of Chip and Ernie on the television show "My Three Sons," the response was overwhelming. The situation was assessed in typical fashion by Livingston when he said, "It's not who you are but who you know."

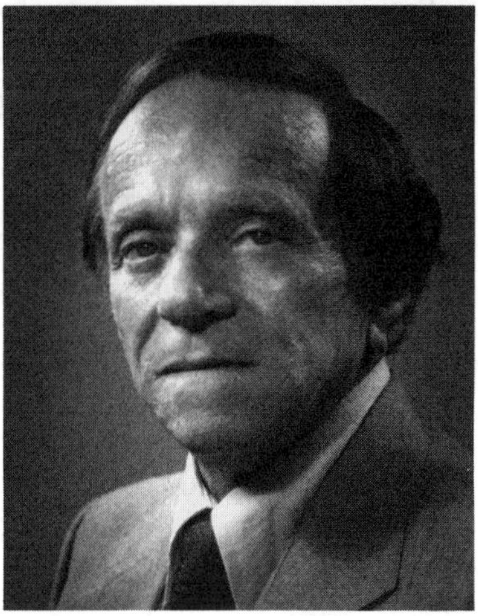

Figure 1. Samuel Livingston (1908–1984). November, 1978.

Livingston had a vast number of patients, over thirty-three thousand by his own estimate, and he used this resource to maximal advantage. He was meticulous, tenacious, and thorough in his clinical reviews. He studied virtually all the anticonvulsants, most before they were released. Perhaps his best known clinical report was the clarification of febrile seizures and why some could be managed differently from others (Livingston, Bridge, and Kajdi, 1947). Another major contribution was his initial text, "The Diagnosis and Treatment of Convulsive Disorders in Children" (Livingston, 1954). Using his clinical experience, he provided a sensible and widely appreciated way for clinicians to approach the problem of epilepsy. One of his special talents was to study a form of treatment in great detail and concisely present its advantages and disadvantages. He did this with bromides, corticosteroids, dexedrine, and the ketogenic diet (Livingston and Pearson, 1953; Klein and Livingston, 1950; Livingston, Kajdi, and Bridge, 1948). He concluded that while none of these treatments was as good as standard medications, they were potentially useful if they were used carefully and in special circumstances. His honest and unbiased stand was appreciated by the medical profession but not always by the public. When his paper on light-induced seizures (from flickering television sets) was presented (Livingston, 1952), he received numerous furious comments, mainly from parents who felt he was trying to strip them of the use of television, which had become such a good baby-sitter.

Livingston was more effective in alleviating the social and emotional problems of the epileptic patient than any other single person. Whenever he saw or heard of injustices, he began to act, sometimes locally, sometimes nationally, and occasionally, even internationally. Although he had been working with these problems throughout his career, the publication that brought this work into focus was his monograph *Living with Epileptic Seizures* (Livingston, 1963). He was concerned about the social stigma of being an epileptic, discrimination in the workplace, and the inability of epileptics to obtain life insurance. He was instrumental in getting the American Medical Association to reverse its position against contact sports for epileptics. He also proved that epileptics had better overall safety records operating motor vehicles than the general population and he fought discrimination against immigrants with epilepsy. Livingston spent much time working with the U.S. attorney general on some of these problems and would lecture anytime and anywhere as an advocate of the epileptic.

The memorials to Samuel Livingston are many. He guided the epilepsy clinic at Johns Hopkins Hospital for more than half its existence. He developed his office practice into a multidisciplinary clinic that still thrives. His personal awards from institutions and societies are far too numerous to list. His legacy includes over 350 articles, 32 chapters, 4 textbooks, teaching brochures, and films. To those of us who knew him, he was a dedicated, hard-working, pleasant man who was extremely knowledgeable about seizure disorders, especially in children.

William T. McLean, Jr.
WINSTON-SALEM, NORTH CAROLINA

REFERENCES

Klein, R., and S. Livingston. 1950. The Effect of Adrenocorticotropic Hormone in Epilepsy. *J Ped* 5:733–42.

Livingston, S. 1952. Comments on a Study of Light-Induced Epilepsy in Children. *Am J Dis Child* 83:409.

______. 1954. *The Diagnosis and Treatment of Convulsive Disorders in Children.* Springfield, IL: Charles C Thomas.

______. 1963. *Living with Epileptic Seizures*. Springfield, IL: Charles C Thomas.

Livingston, S., E. M. Bridge, and L. Kajdi. 1947. Febrile Convulsions: A Clinical Study with Special Reference to Heredity and Prognosis. *J Ped* 31:509–12.

Livingston, S., L. Kajdi, and E. M. Bridge. 1948. The Use of Benzedrine and Dexedrine Sulfate in the Treatment of Epilepsy. *J Ped* 32:490–94.

Livingston, H. L., and S. Livingston. 1973. Diphenylhydantoin Gingival Hyperplasia. *Ped Ann* 2:81–92.

Livingston, S., and P. H. Pearson. 1953. Bromides in the Treatment of Epilepsy in Children. *Am J Dis Child* 86:717–20.

CESARE LOMBROSO

CESARE LOMBROSO (figure 1) was born in 1917 in Rome, Italy, to a family that included numerous scientists and authors, many of whom had achieved worldwide fame. Perhaps most notable was his grandfather, whose name he carries and who is acknowledged internationally as the founder of criminal anthropology. Most of Lombroso's early years were spent in either Palermo or Torino, his father's home, and later in Genoa, where he received his undergraduate education.

Politics of the 1930s and 1940s, World War II, and a Lombroso family dislike of totalitarianism in any form, profoundly shaped his life. His own father was a professor of physiology in Italy until 1936, when, having refused to swear allegiance to the fascist regime, was forced to emigrate to Paris, where he worked until the Nazi invasion. Lombroso's uncle, Guglielmo Ferrero, and an aunt, Gina Lombroso, were well-known antifascist political writers who were imprisoned and exiled. Not unexpectedly, Lombroso himself was a dedicated antifascist and an active member of the clandestine Giustizia e Liberta (Justice and Liberty) movement.

After having won a trip to the United States as a result of a poetry contest, Lombroso decided to study medicine at Johns Hopkins. However, he remained a student for only one year. The war inspired him to leave medical study and become more involved in antifascist work. He served as editor of a journal advocating creation of a free Italian government in exile and actively participated in shortwave broadcasts from the United States beamed to Italy in support of the Italian resistance. After Pearl Harbor he volunteered his services to the Office of War Information. He remained active in antifascist and anticommunist organizations. During this period he met and married his wife, Rysia, who had recently arrived from Poland and was engaged in similar work against totalitarianism. They actually met at the White House, where they had been asked to attend the first World Youth Congress sponsored by Eleanor Roosevelt.

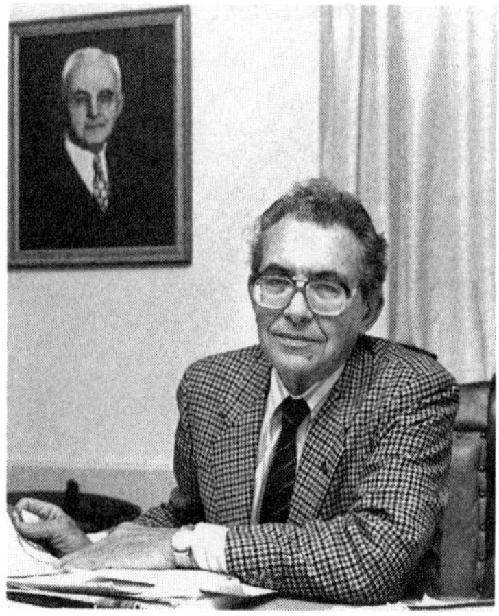

Figure 1. Cesare Lombroso in his office with a portrait of William Lennox in the background, 1987.

After the end of the war, Lombroso dropped from the political scene, returning to the study of medicine, his primary goal. He completed his medical studies in Italy at the University of Genoa in 1947. Following graduation and the M.D. degree, he worked for two years in the physiology laboratory of Arturo Bonsignore at the University of Genoa, where he obtained his Ph.D. in 1951. The attraction of clinical medicine was strong, and he undertook a residency in pediatrics under Giovanni DeToni in Genoa. He had developed special interests in brain function, and decided to emigrate to the United States. He arrived in Boston, where he took a year's fellowship with William Lennox, who had recently founded the Seizure Unit at Boston Children's Hospital, and completed his residency training in neurology and neuropathology at the Massachusetts General Hospital under Raymond Adams. He then returned to the Seizure Unit to join its staff. When Lennox retired in 1960, Lombroso was named chief of the Seizure Unit and later director of the Division of Neurophysiology, where he remained until his retirement from administrative duties in 1988. During his tenure at Children's Hospital, both the Seizure Unit and its laboratories underwent remarkable growth, not only in space and professional components, but also in scope. The excellence of the Seizure Unit training programs was recognized early, with federal grants from the Institute of Maternal and Child Health, and later from the National Institute for Neurological Disease and Stroke, allowing over a fifteen-year span for clinical and research fellowships in epilepsy. The Seizure Unit training program for technologists was among the first chosen as a national model. In the late 1960s, a laboratory for experimental research was established, which was further expanded in the 1970s, and is now engaged in several projects conducted by James Burchfield and myself with various associates.

A dedication to helping the epileptic patient from all perspectives dominated Lombroso's tenure at the Seizure Unit. He was among the first to emphasize that epilepsy was both a symptom and a disease and was most often accompanied by emotional, cognitive, social, family, financial, and other problems. He created the Family Service Team, a small group of dedicated social workers, psychologists, and psychiatrists, to assist the unit's neurologists in the management of their patients. The approach of bringing to the epileptic patient specialists from other disciplines but with experience in epilepsy, as opposed to farming epileptics out to impersonal and anonymous hospital services, became a successful and widely admired approach. Lombroso emphasized the need to follow patients over the years as they matured. He was successful in allowing the Children's Hospital to permit adults to be seen in the clinic and be admitted as inpatients when necessary. The Seizure Unit became the model upon which many other seizure units were developed, both nationally and internationally. In my many years of personal service in the unit, a month would seldom go by without visits by several other neurologists wanting to emulate Lombroso's model in their own hospitals.

Equal to his care for his patients was his dedication to training young neurologists in epileptology and electroencephalography. Lombroso took a missionary's view and intentionally chose to train neurologists from countries where their knowledge, upon return, would have the greatest impact. This gave the Seizure Unit a rich international flavor. Many graduates of the Seizure Unit fellowship training program are now the leading epileptologists in their respective countries; it is rare for Lombroso to travel internationally and not be greeted by old friends. He also refused to see training in clinical neurophysiology as separate from clinical epileptology. Although often approached for training by those wanting to profit by the unit's unique pediatric and infant electroencephalographic material, Lombroso regarded as sterile the isolated reading of clinical EEGs without fully integrating this information into the clinical practice of epileptology. Thus Lombroso's outlook, evident during the political upheavals of the 1940s, carried through in his approach to the management of his patients and the training of his fellows.

Reading EEGs while Lombroso watched could be an unsettling experience for new trainees. Fellows were encouraged to turn pages. However, if they failed to remark upon an abnormality, Lombroso would often clear his throat — a signal to stop turning pages and look more carefully. Halfway through my first year's training, and feeling quite confident in my new ability to read EEGs, I was distressed during a reading session to be interrupted every few pages by an admonishing "ahem." Only later did I discover that the interruptions were not due to my incompetence but to the Boston flu!

Lombroso's academic credentials are manifold. He is a tenured professor of neurology at Harvard Medical School, now professor emeritus; senior neurologist at Children's Hospital; principal research associate in neurosurgery at Children's Hospital; and consultant in neurology and neurophysiology at Beth Israel Hospital, Brigham and Women's Hospital, and the New England Baptist Hospital in Boston. He has served as an officer in many national and international professional societies. Among these have been the presidencies of the Eastern Association of Electroencephalographers, the American EEG Society, and the American Epilepsy Society. He is a member of the executive council of the American Academy of Neurophysiology. He has served as the chairman of Region I of the Professional Advisory Board of the Epilepsy Foundation of America. He is a fellow in a dozen American professional societies, an honorary member of six foreign ones, and has chaired committees of the International Federation of Clinical Neurophysiology and of the International League Against Epilepsy (ILAE). In 1981 he was awarded the Gold Medal of the ILAE, and a Special

Award in Clinical Neurophysiology in 1982. His curriculum vitae lists over 180 referred publications in addition to many reviews and chapters in textbooks of neurology and neurophysiology.

His research interests are largely centered on epilepsy, including several papers regarding the mechanisms of reflex myoclonus and those of perinatal hypoxia and ischemia as potential inducers of later epilepsy. Lombroso is now participating with various associates in studies to elucidate the mechanisms involved in potential epileptogenesis from perinatal hypoxia and ischemia.

His research also indicates an interest in central visual processing. He and I worked together on pattern visual-evoked potentials in human amblyopia and the role of central inhibitory factors (Lombroso, Duffy, and Robb, 1969). This work later sparked the creation of the Developmental Neurophysiology Laboratory at Children's Hospital where the inhibitory amblyopic hypotheses was confirmed in an animal model. With Ruggiero Corazza (now professor of human physiology in Modena, Italy), Lombroso and I worked on the controversial eye movement-related corollary discharge and demonstrated its physiological substratum at both cortical and subcortical levels (Corazza, Lombroso, and Duffy, 1972). Finally, Lombroso and I demonstrated the presence of an inhibitory mechanism preceding human voluntary saccades.

Lombroso's clinical contributions include one of the first descriptions of the syndrome of Sylvian seizures (Lombroso, 1967). Of note are his studies of benign infantile myoclonus (Lombroso and Fejerman, 1977), his prospective studies on West syndrome (Lombroso, 1983), and with Pincus Lerman, on the syndrome of reflex syncope — emotionally triggered vasovagal asystole, often clinically confounded with epilepsy (Lombroso and Lerman, 1967). With his associate Giuseppe Erba, he published several papers on the classification and other aspects of the myoclonic and pseudomyoclonic epileptic syndromes (Lombroso and Erba, 1982). His long experience with neonatal seizures and EEG has led to an internationally accepted classification of neonatal seizures, as well as acceptance of the value of polygraphy and organization of states as predictors of the outcome of the newborn "at risk" (Lombroso and Matsumiya, 1985). Among other contributions worth mentioning are those on primary versus secondary generalization and on the use of intravenous thiopental and diazepam to reveal poorly functioning cortical areas. There are also papers on the clinical and EEG aspects of Reye syndrome (Aoki and Lombroso, 1973), and on the clinical value of carbonic anhydrase inhibitors in the treatment of epilepsy (Lombroso and Forsythe, 1960). In 1966 he introduced the intravenous use of diazepam in the management of status epilepticus (Lombroso, 1966). Much more recently he has delineated measures for the intermittent home treatment of various paroxysmal disorders by rectal/oral administration of diazepam, after careful studies of its bioavailability. He contributed clinical observations in the syndrome of acquired aphasia in the context of brief epileptic phenomena (Landau syndrome) (Gascon et al, 1973) and proposed the pathophysiological substratum for epileptic laughter (gelastic epilepsy) by careful observations of patients with discrete lesions (Lombroso and Gascon, 1971). He recognized and collected the largest series in the United States of patients with subacute sclerosing panencephalitis and, in the late 1960s, published data obtained from direct cortical recordings that offer insights about the peculiar and distinctive EEG discharges of subacute sclerosing panencephalitis (Lombroso, 1968). With Mildred McIntyre and Paul Pritchard, he published papers on the neuropsychological profiles of right and left temporal lobe epileptic patients, outlining the diverse potential risks for psychiatric complications (Pritchard, Lombroso, and McIntyre, 1980).

With several associates, Lombroso was the first to introduce the B-mode technique of ultrasound, now further developed and adopted worldwide (Lombroso and Galicich, 1965). Classic are his papers on the controversial "14 and 6 per second positive spikes," which were proven to represent a normal developmental variant (Lombroso and Schwartz, 1966). Perhaps a latent interest in his famous grandfather's studies led to his participation with James Burchfield and me in development of the current field of computerized brain electrical activity mapping (Duffy, Burchfield, and Lombroso, 1979), especially its application to clinical epilepsy (Lombroso and Duffy, 1982).

Despite the great demands placed on his time by clinical and research activities, Lombroso remained an active member of the broad academic community. An invitation to his home often brought with it a surprise. Once I was invited for supper, along with a very interesting "visiting musician" introduced by

Lombroso as "Grommox" — or so I understood. Only weeks later, while attending a concert, did I realize I had spent the evening with the famous violinist, Arthur Grumieux. I had a similar experience with a fascinating writer named "Red" — only later to be recognized as Robert Penn Warren. Although an excellent speaker in several languages, Lombroso's English could occasionally escape full comprehension by a parochial, inattentive Yankee.

Although "retired" from his hospital duties, Lombroso continues to be actively engaged in his career-long quest to better understand and treat the epileptic patient and he remains involved in a number of clinical and experimental projects. The medical tradition of his family is continued by his three children, one a nurse, one a psychologist, and one a psychiatrist engaged in molecular biology at Yale Medical School after a fellowship at the Rockefeller Institute.

Frank H. Duffy
BOSTON, MASSACHUSETTS

REFERENCES

Aoki, Y., and C. T. Lombroso. 1973. Prognostic Value of Electroencephalography in Reye's Syndrome. *Neur* 23:333–43.

Corazza, R., C. T. Lombroso, and F. H. Duffy. 1972. Time Course of Visual Multi-Neuronal Discharges Evoked by Eye Movements in Light. *Brain Res* 38:109–16.

Duffy, F. H., J. L. Burchfield, and C. T. Lombroso. 1979. Brain Electrical Activity Mapping (BEAM): A Method for Extending the Clinical Utility of EEG and Evoked Potential Data. *Ann Neur* 5:309–21.

Gascon, G. G., et al. 1973. Language Disorders, Convulsive Disorders, and EEG Abnormalities in Children. *Arch Neur* 28:156–62.

Lombroso, C. T. 1966. Treatment of Status Epilepticus with I.V. Diazepam (Valium). *Neur* 16:629–34.

______. 1967. Sylvian Seizures and Mid-Temporal Spike Foci in Children. *Arch Neur* 17:52–59.

______. 1968. Remarks on the EEG and Movement Disorder in SSPE. *Neur* 18:69–75.

______. 1983. Infantile Spasms. In *Epilepsy: Diagnosis and Management*. 95–105. Ed. T. R. Browne and R. G. Felman. Boston: Little, Brown, and Co.

Lombroso, C. T., and F. H. Duffy. 1982. Brain Electrical Mapping in the

Epilepsies. In *Advances in Epileptology: XIIIth Epilepsy International Symposium.* Ed. H. Akimoto et al. New York: Raven Press.

Lombroso, C. T., F. H. Duffy, and R. M. Robb. 1969. Selective Suppression of Cerebral Evoked Potentials to Patterned Light in Amblyopia Ex-Anopsia. *Electroenceph Clin Neurophysiol* 27:238–47.

Lombroso, C. T., and G. Erba. 1982. Myoclonic Seizures — Considerations in Taxonomy. In *Advances in Epileptology: XIIIth Epilepsy International Symposium.* Ed. H. Akimoto et al. New York: Raven Press.

Lombroso, C. T., and N. Fejerman. 1977. Benign Myoclonus of Early Infancy. *Ann Neur* 1:138–43.

Lombroso, C. T., and I. Forsythe. 1960. A Long-Term Followup of Acetazolamide (Diamox) in the Treatment of Epilepsy. *Epilepsia* 1:493–500.

Lombroso, C. T., and J. H. Galicich. 1965. Ultrasonic B-Scanning of Brain Tumors. *Excerpta Med* 4:339–41.

Lombroso, C. T., and G. G. Gascon. 1971. Epileptic (Gelastic) Laughter. *Epilepsia* 12:63–67.

Lombroso, C. T., and P. Lerman. 1967. Breathholding Spells (Cyanotic and Pallid Infantile Syncope). *Ped* 38:563–81.

Lombroso, C. T., and Y. Matsumiya. 1985. States Profiles over Time in Normal and "At Risk" Newborns: Correlation with Long-Term Outcome. *Ped* 76:52–63.

Lombroso, C. T., and I. H. Schwartz. 1966. Ctenoids in Healthy Youth. Controlled Study of 14 and 6/sec. Positive Spiking. *Neur* 16:1152–58.

Pritchard, P. B., C. T. Lombroso, and M. McIntyre. 1980. Psychological Complications of Temporal Lobe Epilepsy. *Neur* 30:227–32.

DENISE LOUIS-BAR

DENISE BAR (b. 1914) (figure 1) was born in Liège, Belgium, but lived in Spain with her parents until the age of ten. Her early life in Spain had an important influence on her, as she explained: "The poverty, social inequalities, and severe health problems in poor children in Spain at that time were so terrible that I decided that my life would be dedicated to giving the same opportunities for all children." Her family returned to Liège when she was ten years old, later moving to Brussels (Louis-Bar, personal communication, 1989).

She graduated as an M.D. in 1939 from the Free University of Brussels and jointly obtained a degree in "éducation physique," a diploma that had recently been created in Belgium to prepare interested physicians in the supervision of sports and physical education. A few months later, she married Mr. F. Louis, a civil engineer trained at the Faculté Polytechnique of the Catholic University of Louvain, Belgium. One month after their wedding, her husband enlisted in a Belgium Army unit in the Ardennes.

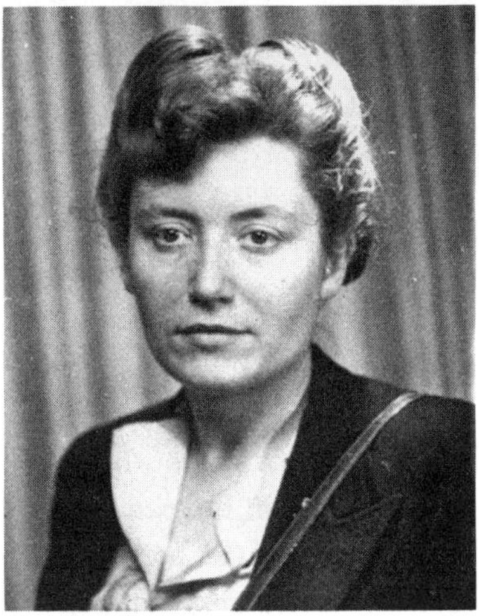

Figure 1. Denise Louis-Bar.

Louis-Bar was eager to practice general medicine immediately after graduation but changed her plans because of the difficulties in beginning a private medical practice with her husband in the army and the outbreak of World War II. She decided instead to specialize and was accepted as a "volunteer resident" in the Institute Bunge in Antwerp, Belgium. Born-Bunge was a private foundation established by Ludo van Bogaert and was primarily oriented towards clinical care and research in neurology. On October 2, 1940, at the outpatient clinic, she and van Bogaert examined a nine-year-old child displaying telangiectasias and neurological signs. Van Bogaert assigned Louis-Bar the task "to study this case in detail." The results of her study appeared in 1941 in *Confinia Neurologica* (Louis-Bar, 1941) under the title "Sur un syndrome progressif comprenant des télangiectasies capillaires cutanées et conjonctivales symétriques, à disposition naevoïde et des troubles cérébelleux." The paper was published in French but I shall quote the English summary written by the author:

The author reports the case of a 9-year-old child with a syndrome of the cerebellum with predominant ataxia-abasia together with speech disturbance and mental backwardness progressively developing since the third year of life. As regards the skin, the child shows patches of telangiectasias different from simple angioma, regularly and symmetrically arranged as also systematically ordered "café au lait" spots of fern like appearance. The double state as regards skin and nerves permits this case to be placed generally in the sphere of the phakomatoses without assigning it any particular form. The relations of this case to the Sturge-Weber-Krabbe disease are particularly discussed. (Louis-Bar, 1941)

The name of Denise Louis-Bar is now known in medicine throughout the world because of this paper that she wrote when she was twenty-seven years old.

Louis-Bar did not hear much about "her" disease until Elena Boder and her husband visited both her and Van Bogaert at the end of the 1950s. Louis-Bar does not remember whether this visit took place before or after Boder and Sedgwick published their paper about ataxia-telangiectasia in the journal *Pediatrics* (Boder and Sedgwick, 1958). This paper refers to Louis-Bar's 1941 work and to a "personal communication" of Ludo van Bogaert. Two years later, Sabine Pelc and Henri Vis suggested naming the disease "syndrome de D. Louis-Bar" (Pelc and Vis, 1960). In 1961, Stéphane Thieffry, Michel Arthuis, Jean Aicardi, and Gilles Lyon made a very significant contribution to the knowledge of this disease, noting the first description of the IgA deficiency in ataxia-telangiectasia. With the paper of Thieffry and his coworkers, the disease had entered into its modern history, well known to all pediatric neurologists (Thieffry et al, 1961).

It should be mentioned that the original description of this disorder (Syllaba and Henner, 1926), published in the *Revue neurologique* (Paris), had been omitted by all the authors quoted above. The Czech researchers L. Syllaba and Kamil Henner wrote an interesting paper about the disease entitled "Contribution à l'indépendence de l'athétose double idiopathique et congénitale. Atteinte familiale, syndrome dystrophique, signe du réseau vasculaire conjonctival, intégrité psychique." Also of interest is the fact that an Antwerp pediatrician, Alfons Lambrechts, continues to keep a complete daily record of all patients with ataxia-telangiectasia, published or not, who have come to his attention.

Until 1943, Louis-Bar pursued her training in neurology with Van Bogaert in Antwerp and in internal medicine with Professors Divry, Firket, and Roskam at the State University of Liège. She remained at Liège until 1945, serving as an instructor of pharmacology. She then accepted a position as neuropsychiatrist in the Department of Internal Medicine with Professor Lucien Brull at the State University of Liège. She left Liège in 1957 when her husband was appointed director of the Belgian Office of Study of Nuclear Energy and the family moved to Brussels.

Since 1957 Louis-Bar has oriented all her activities toward the care of severely mentally handicapped children and adults. She has founded or contributed to the foundation of twelve centers for mentally handicapped patients, mostly located in the Brussels area. Two of these centers are model institutions. One is the Entraide des Travailleuses, a day-care center for pediatric rehabilitation and an outpatient facility located in a poor area in Brussels. The other is the Centre de Réadaptation de l'Enfance à Bruxelles affiliated with the University of Louvain Medical School. Here new methods in the care of severely mentally handicapped children are tested by Marie-Claude Belpaire, with the still active participation of Louis-Bar and the help of Jean-Paul Quarre, an industrialist who, after his retirement, devoted his energies to the benefit of the associations of parents of handicapped children in Belgium and Western Europe.

We shall summarize this biographical sketch of Denise Louis-Bar in a few words. At twenty-seven years of age, she wrote one paper, known throughout the world, about a child with ataxia-telangiectasia. Since then, her inexhaustible dynamism, her devotion to mentally handicapped human beings, and her intellectual qualities have contributed to change the care of severely mentally handicapped children and adults in our country.

Philippe Evrard

Alidor Beya

Michèle Provis
BRUSSELS, BELGIUM

REFERENCES

Boder, E., and R. P. Sedgwick. 1958. Ataxia-Telangiectasia. A Familial Syndrome of Progressive Cerebellar Ataxia, Oculocutaneous Telangiectasia and Frequent Pulmonary Infection. *Ped* 21:526–54.

Louis-Bar, D. 1941. Sur un syndrome progressif comprenant des télangiectasies capillaires cutanées et conjonctivales symétriques, à disposition naevoïde et des troubles cérébelleux. *Confin Neur* 4:32–34.

______. 1989. Personal communication.

Pelc, S., and H. Vis. 1960. Ataxie familiale avec télangiectasies oculaires (Syndrome de D. Louis-Bar). *Acta Neur Psych Belg* 60:905–22.

Syllaba, L., and K. Henner. 1926. Contribution à l'étude de l'indépendance de l'athétose double idiopathique et congénitale. Atteinte familiale, syndrome dystrophique, signe du réseau vasculaire conjonctival, intégrité psychique. *Rev neur* 1:541–60.

Thieffry, S., et al. 1961. L'ataxie-télangiectasie (7 observations personnelles). *Rev neur* 105:390–405.

GILLES LYON

GILLES GILBERT CAMILLE LYON (b. 1921) (figure 1) was born in Mulhouse, a city of the Haut-Rhin, an Alsatian department in France. His father had been a lawyer and legal counselor of the French Ministry of Foreign Affairs. His mother belonged to an Alsatian family of industrialists. He attended high school in Paris.

Lyon started medical school in Paris (which includes college in continental Europe) in 1940 and two years later attempted to apply for the Externat des Hôpitaux, a rotating internship for the best young medical students, awarded on a competitive basis. However, he was prevented from applying to the Externat by the "laws of exception" promulgated by the Vichy government against those of Jewish origin. In February 1943 he crossed the Spanish border and, upon reaching England, volunteered for the Forces Françaises Libres (FFL) of General Charles de Gaulle. He spent one year at Ribbesford in the military school of the FFL. As a lieutenant, Lyon served in the Second Armoured Division (the famous "Seconde D.B." of

General Leclerc) until the Liberation and received the French War Cross.

Lyon resumed his medical training after the war. As was the custom in France for the best students, medical school was combined with an internship (internat) and afterward, a residency program (externat). Among the chiefs who had an important impact on his training and career were Raymond Garcin at the Hôpital de la Salpêtrière, Julien Marie and Robert Debre at the Hôpital des Enfants Malades, and Stéphane Thieffry at the Hôpital des Enfants Malades and later at the Hôpital des Enfants Assistés (also called the Hôpital Saint Vincent de Paul). He graduated with a doctorate in medicine and at the same time as a licensed pediatrician in 1955 from the University of Paris. It was the tradition in France to delay the official graduation as M.D. until completion of both residency and specialty training. Lyon graduated three years later than many of his high school classmates, due to his service in the army during the war. Several persons familiar with events at that time led me to understand that the postwar medical establishment did not treat former young members of the Resistance with special attention and sometimes "penalized" them by not taking into account for the age limit of the "concours," that is, the time spent in the army. His thesis was entitled "Contribution à l'étude des hémiplégies survenant au cours des premiers mois de la vie" ("Contribution on the Study of Hemiplegia Following the First Months of Life"). This early publication displayed many of the qualities of his subsequent works: a comprehensive examination of the material, deliberate in thought, original, and written in a style that was extremely concise and clear. After publication, he disdained any effort to advertise his own publication in the professional community and fully

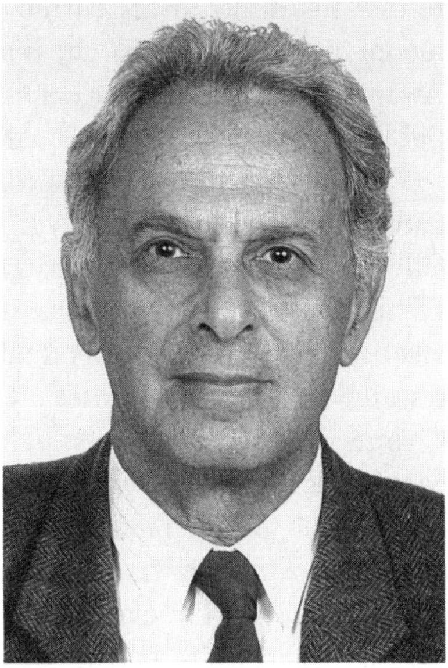

Figure 1. Gilles Lyon. Brussels, 1989.

turned his mind to his current work. The quality of this thesis, a model of clinical research, was recognized by the 1956 Thesis Award of the French National Academy of Medicine and later by publication in the international literature (Lyon, 1961).

From 1955 until 1962, Lyon completed his training in neuropathology and occupied several positions as clinical and research fellow in Paris and in Boston: 1955–57: chef de clinique (in France, clinical fellow; in the rest of Europe, associate chief of service), Hôpital des Enfants Malades, Paris; 1957–58: clinical and research fellow, Massachusetts General Hospital, Boston; 1959–62: Chargé de Recherches (research associate), Institut National de la Santé et de la Recherche Médicale (INSERM), Paris. This period was crucial for his professional development, especially his contact and neuropathology training with Raymond Adams and Edward P. Richardson, Jr. His "classmates" in the Charles Kubik Laboratory of Neuropathology at the Massachusetts General Hospital were Karl-Erik Astrom, Elliot Mancall, and Henry de F. Webster. Due to organizational problems at that time, the once-famous French school of neuropathology was in disarray, and young French scholars had to go to Adams's service at Harvard, Ludo van Bogaert's Institute at Antwerp, Belgium, or Harry Zimmerman's laboratory in New York to complete their training in this basic neurological discipline. These obligatory trips had excellent consequences and contributed to the development of a core of French scientists exposed to the international scientific community, like Lyon and his friend Jean Lapresle. This combination of clinical training in France with international research exposure was especially valuable. Research in Europe had not yet recovered from the war and was still comparatively weak, but clinical training remained excellent, especially in Paris. Recruitment of patients was unlimited and directed into a very centralized health care delivery system. In addition, the faculty, who had previously sustained difficult clinical competition (les concours) until age forty, were not pressured to publish superficial and repetitive papers but were allowed to concentrate fully on their clinical activities. Thus, the French academic system had several weaknesses but also a number of advantages.

After such a long period of preparation, Lyon was appointed pediatric neurologist, neuropathologist, and professeur agrégé at the Hôpital des Enfants Malades and the Hôpital Saint Vincent de Paul. These hospitals, which belong to the Assistance Publique de Paris, are affiliated with the University of Paris Medical School and jointly, as extramural facilities, with the Institut National de la Santé et de la Recherche Médicale. From the mid 1950s until the mid 1970s, Lyon, Jean Aicardi, Thieffry, and Michel Arthuis were associated with the same service in Paris and had almost a complete monopoly on pediatric neurology in France. This included the availability of both large numbers of children with neurological disorders and fellows interested in training, who were predominantly from French and Spanish-speaking countries. Further, both Lyon and Aicardi had excellent international contacts with child neurologists in the English-speaking countries.

During the decades following World War II, the new French pediatric establishment, founded by Robert Debre, reorganized pediatrics and made important contributions in general pediatrics, public health, genetics, metabolic disorders, social pediatrics, and several pediatric subspecialties. Pediatric neurology, after an initial period of growth in Paris under Thieffry's chairmanship, did not remain a priority. This occurred partly because pediatrics and neurology were separated by an "iron curtain," partly for local personal and organizational reasons and partly because certain powerful French pediatricians thought pediatric neurology could be indirectly covered with less disruption to the pediatric establishment by a combination of neurosurgery, genetics, metabolic diseases, and child psychiatry. As leaders of world pediatric neurology, Lyon and Aicardi found it difficult to obtain funding and space to see patients and engage in research at a time when their clinical, research, and teaching needs were dramatically increasing. More recently, however, the attitude towards pediatric neurology has improved and the importance of this field and the need for its development are better appreciated.

The Université Catholique de Louvain (UCL), with two campuses in Belgium (the Medical School in Brussels and the nonmedical faculties in Louvain-la-Neuve), is among the oldest European Universities. During the past several decades, this institution, located at the center of the European community, has enjoyed excellent support, organization, and superb academic freedom. In 1969 I was appointed to develop the Pediatric Neurology

Unit at the UCL, and by 1975 this service had expanded substantially. Transformation into an international center with new research facilities, to allow colleagues from clinical pediatric neurology and the developmental neurosciences to collaborate was proposed. At my request, Lyon was approached by the president of the university and dean of the medical school to become director and chief of service of this new center. He accepted this position, arriving in Brussels in 1976. Under his guidance, the service grew rapidly and now includes twenty-eight beds of acute pediatric neurology and eighty beds of pediatric neurology rehabilitation. With our associates, we are responsible for sections on pediatric neurology, neuroanatomy, pediatric and developmental neuropathology, pediatric neuropsychology, and metabolic disorders at the medical school and academic hospital. There are also programs in preventive medicine in child neurology, a section on developmental and fetal neuropathology, and a positron emission tomography program oriented towards pediatric neurology. A general overview of the clinical and research contributions of this center reflecting the integration of clinical pediatric neurology and neuropathology is available in a recently published textbook (Lyon and Evrard, 1987).

It is probably of interest when reading these biographies on the founders of child neurology to compare the differences in pediatric neurology in different epochs and continents. In this respect, one should mention that in most European pediatric neurology services, general care of the patient is provided by the child neurology staff. Most of us were trained in general pediatrics and keep current in order to provide care for the child, infant, and newborn. Lyon, like most child neurologists in Western Europe, has this daily responsibility. This type of organization of a pediatric neurology service is burdensome but keeps us in close contact with the patients and their parents and provides other advantages for the development of pediatric neurology. The appointment of the Frenchman Lyon as chairman in a Belgian university has been remarkably successful and is often quoted as an example to be followed at a time when the European community is officially trying to improve the circulation of academic personnel among the different universities in Western Europe.

Lyon's major research contributions relate to the prenatal encephalopathies, perinatal neuropathology, viral infections of the central nervous system, and several clinicopathological correlations. Among his 150 publications, I shall cite only a few.

Lyon was among the first to demonstrate convincingly the role played by circulatory disturbances arising in the second half of pregnancy as the origin of prenatal brain disorders (Lyon and Robain, 1967). He was the first to show that cytomegalovirus infection affects the fetal brain, particularly by creating a perfusion failure, not an arrest of neuronal migration (Marques-Dias et al, 1984). His description, with Marc Tardieu and Evrard, of the pathophysiology and management of the progressive expanding porencephalies is widely accepted (Tardieu, Evrard, and Lyon, 1981). In a seminal paper, Lyon established the existence of several "developmental microcephalies" (Robain and Lyon, 1972). With the joint efforts of Evrard, Verne S. Caviness, Olivier Robain, and Roger Williams, during the past fifteen years he has established a framework for the pathogenetic classification of prenatal malformations. More recently, Jean-François Gadisseux joined this international collaborative team. For reviews explaining the evolution of the ideas in this field, to which Lyon has been a major contributor, see Evrard, Gadisseux, and Lyon, 1982; Caviness and Williams, 1984; and Evrard et al, 1989.

In perinatal neuropathology, Lyon first described the chronic lesions of periventricular leukomalacia as early as 1959 in a paper for which he was responsible for the neuropathology (Marie, Lyon, and Bargeton, 1959). This original study has not been given sufficient recognition because it was published only in a French journal.

In neurovirology, he first described chronic rubella encephalitis (Lebon and Lyon, 1974) and the delayed type of acute measles encephalitis in immunosuppressed children (Lyon, 1972) and in immunocompetent children (Lyon, Ponsot, and Lebon, 1977). He contributed to the knowledge of chronic encephalitis in X-linked hypogammaglobulinemia (Lyon, Griscelli, and Lebon, 1972; Lyon et al, 1980). In a classic paper with Raymond Adams and Philip Dodge, he drew attention to the heterogeneous group of postviral noninflammatory acute encephalopathies of infancy (Lyon, Dodge, and Adams, 1961). Some of these patients, but not all, were retrospectively found to be affected with Reye syndrome.

Among Lyon's more general contributions, aside from his most recent textbook (Lyon and Evrard, 1987), he published with Raymond Adams *The Neurology of Hereditary Metabolic Diseases of Children* (Adams and Lyon, 1982). Alone, or with other coauthors, Lyon contributed new information on many other clinicopathological problems. He first described the in vivo diagnosis of metachromatic leukodystrophy by nerve biopsy (Thieffry and Lyon, 1959) and the importance of peripheral nerve involvement in this disease (Thieffry et al, 1964). He described a new form of sialidosis (Le Sec, Stanescu, and Lyon, 1978), and with Thieffry, Arthuis, and Aicardi first reported the IgA deficiency in ataxia-telangiectasia (Thieffry et al, 1961). He has also contributed to the description of the congenital hypomyelinating neuropathies. The characteristic ultrastructure of these disorders is now frequently referred to as the "Lyon type" of onion bulbs (Lyon, 1969; Guzzetta, Ferrière, and Lyon, 1982).

Lyon has been a pioneer and a major contributor in the field of pediatric neurology. He combines an outstanding knowledge of child neurology and neuropathology. This now rare combined competence has given him a strong and exceptional position. He is an internationally recognized authority in developmental neuropathology, the continuing importance of which is now emphasized by all concerned in the developmental neurosciences. With his powerful but liberal leadership, his influence has been effective, and he is among the creators of modern pediatric neurology in Western Europe.

Lyon was one of the founders of the Société Européenne de Neurologie Pédiatrique, a branch of the European Federation of Child Neurology Societies. He has been, and remains, an inspiring master for dozens of pediatric neurologists throughout the world, who now have great responsibilities and internationally recognized positions. In addition to his outstanding research contributions, he is well versed in literature, art, and architecture. He has an extraordinary "internationalist charm," being one of the best symbols of French medicine for American colleagues, a lost pearl for the French brain hunters, a "French pediatric neurologist drinking no wine and no Scotch" for the British, and just a Belgian pediatric neurologist for us.

Something else has made life easier and more meaningful for him; he has a marvelous and generous wife, trained first in law and afterwards in classical dance. She is a woman of culture and sophistication, and their marriage has been a source of happiness and affection for both of them.

For me, as for many other pediatric neurologists, Gilles Lyon is the best and most generous friend, always delighted to promote and eager to delegate, while remaining, for the important concerns, the most solid and final reference for his friends, colleagues, and associates.

Philippe Evrard
BRUSSELS, BELGIUM

ACKNOWLEDGMENTS

The author expresses his grateful regards to Drs. Raymond D. Adams, Jean Aicardi, Stephen Ashwal, Elizabeth C. Dooling, Barry E. Kosofsky, Jean Lapreste, Isabelle Rapin, and Henry de F. Webster, who read this manuscript and helped with insightful comments and editorial suggestions.

REFERENCES

Adams, R. D., and G. Lyon. 1982. *Neurology of Hereditary Metabolic Diseases of Children*. New York: McGraw-Hill.

Caviness, V. S., and R. Williams. 1984. Normal and Abnormal Development of the Brain. In *Advances in Clinical Neuropsychology*. Vol. 2, 1–62. Ed. R. E. Tarter and G. Goldstein. New York: Plenum.

Evrard, P., et al. 1989. Pathology of Prenatal Encephalopathies. In *Child Neurology and Developmental Disabilities,* 153–76. Ed. J. French et al. Baltimore: Paul H. Brookes.

Evrard, P., J. F. Gadisseux, and G. Lyon. 1982. Le développement prénatal du système nerveux et ses perturbations. *Prog néonat* 4:63–106.

Guzzetta, F., G. Ferrière, and G. Lyon. 1982. Congenital Hypomyelination Polyneuropathy. Pathological Findings Compared to Polyneuropathies Starting Later in Life. *Brain* 105:395–416.

Lebon, P., and G. Lyon. 1974. Non-Congenital Chronic Rubella Encephalitis. *Lancet* 2:468.

Le Sec, C., R. Stanescu, and G. Lyon. 1978. Un nouveau type de sialidose avec atteinte rénale: la néphrosialidose. Etude anatomique. *Arch fran péd* 35:830–44.

Lyon, G. 1961. First Signs and Mode of Onset of Congenital Hemiplegia. *Dev Med Child Neur* 4:33–38.

______. 1969. Ultrastructural Study of a Nerve Biopsy from a Case of Early Infantile Chronic Neuropathy. *Acta Neuropath* 13:131–42.

______. 1972. Action des immunosuppresseurs sur une encéphalite virale (rougeole): inhibition de la réaction inflammatoire. *Compt rend Acad Sci* 274D:1872–78.

Lyon, G., P. R. Dodge, and R. D. Adams. 1961. The Acute Encephalopathies of Obscure Origin in Infants. *Brain* 84:680.

Lyon, G., and P. Evrard. 1987. *Neuropédiatrie.* Paris: Masson.

Lyon, G., et al. 1980. Chronic Progressive Encephalitis in Children with X-Linked Hypogammaglobulinemia. *Neuroped* 11:57–71.

Lyon, G., C. Griscelli, and P. Lebon. 1972. Endothelial Intracisternal Tubular Inclusions in a Case of Chronic Encephalitis Associated with Immunological Deficiency. *Neuroped* 3:459–69.

Lyon, G., G. Ponsot, and P. Lebon. 1977. Acute Measles Encephalitis of the Delayed Type. *Ann Neur* 2:322–27.

Lyon, G., and O. Robain. 1967. Etude comparative des encéphalopathies circulatoires prénatales et para-natales (hydranencéphalies, porencéphalies et encéphalomalacies kystiques de la substance blanche). *Acta Neuropath* 9:79–88.

Marie, J., G. Lyon, and E. Bargeton. 1959. La sclérose cérébrale centro-lobaire (syndrome de Little). *Presse méd* 67:2286–89.

Marques-Dias, M. J., et al. 1984. Prenatal Cytomegalovirus Disease and Cerebral Microgyria. Evidence for Perfusion Failure, not Disturbance of Histogenesis, as the Major Cause of Fetal Cytomegalovirus Encephalopathy. *Neuroped* 15:18–24.

Robain, O., and G. Lyon. 1972. Les microencéphalies familiales par malformation cérébrale. Etude anatomo-clinique. *Acta Neuropath* 20:96–109.

Tardieu, M., P. Evrard, and G. Lyon. 1981. Progressive Expanding Congenital Porencephalies: A Treatable Cause of Progressive Encephalopathy. *Ped* 68:198–202.

Thieffry, S., et al. 1961. L'ataxie-télangiectasie. *Rev neur* 105:390–405.

Thieffry, S., and G. Lyon. 1959 Diagnostic d'un cas de leucodystrophie métachromatique (type Scholz) par la biopsie d'un nerf périphérique. *Rev neur* 100:425–56.

Thieffry, S., et al. 1964. L'atteinte du système nerveux périphérique dans la leucodystrophie métachromatique. *Rev neur* 110:5.

RONALD MACKEITH

UNTIL THE 1950S, individual neurologists in England such as Macdonald Critchley and Paul Sandifer had made valuable contributions to the understanding of neurological disorders in childhood, and many pediatricians were involved. However, pediatric neurology was certainly not regarded as a specialty of any kind, nor did it enter into the formal training of the neurologist. In 1958 Ronald Charles MacKeith (1908–1977) (figure 1) suggested to The Spastics Society that they should support medical education and they willingly agreed. Thus, he became the first director of the Medical, Educational and Information Unit of The Spastics Society, which since that time has organized study groups and conferences. MacKeith had the imagination to widen his scope to include almost every aspect of child neurology, both medical and nonmedical, whether or not this had a direct relevance to the child with cerebral palsy.

One of his first tasks was to organize interdisciplinary meetings biannually at Oxford and at other centers in England in the intervening years. These started in 1958 and were a great inspiration to all concerned at a time when the specialty of pediatric neurology had started to develop and exchanges of ideas were important. At each meeting guests were invited from other European countries and occasionally from the United States, Canada, and other countries (MacKeith and Bax, 1963). At the Oxford meeting in 1970, a European Federation of Child Neurology was discussed and from this developed the European Federation of Child Neurology Societies, which meets every two years in a different European country. Six European groups send members to each of these meetings, and the friendships begun in Oxford have ensured particularly close links between the various groups that have grown up together.

In 1974 it was decided that the British group of pediatric neurologists should form an autonomous group. There were twenty-seven foundation members, including MacKeith. Their first meeting was held in 1974, when MacKeith was elected secretary of the British Association for Paediatric Neurology. The association meets annually at a place of its own choosing in England and

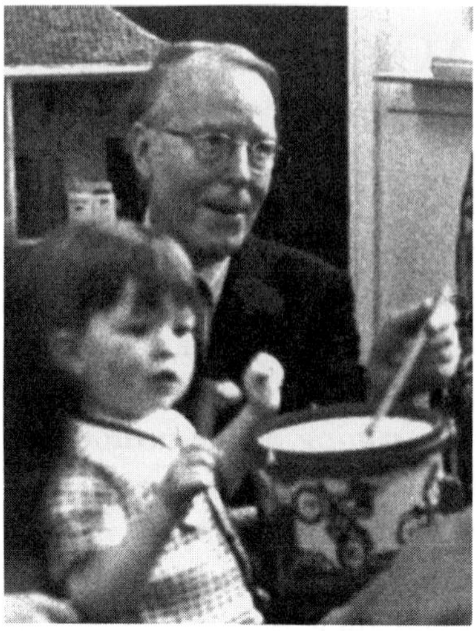

Figure 1. Ronald MacKeith (1908–1977). From Bax, M., "Ronald Charles MacKeith. A Personal Memoir," *Dev Med Child Neur* 20 (1978): 3–7.

every April at the Annual Meeting of the British Paediatric Association. The custom, founded by MacKeith, of restricting the number coming to each meeting, and always inviting a few representatives from one of the other European groups, has been maintained.

In 1977 MacKeith became the first honorary member of the British Paediatric Neurology Association. In 1978 the association founded an annual lecture in honor of Ronnie MacKeith, who died on October 30, 1977. In 1982 it was agreed that the association should award a prize, called the Ronnie MacKeith Prize, for anyone under the age of thirty-five whose published work was thought to have made a major contribution to child neurology.

Although MacKeith always maintained that he was not a pediatric neurologist, there can be no doubt that his influence was paramount in the development of pediatric neurology upon a sound foundation, and in its official recognition as a specialty in its own right with its own training and research programs in many European countries, particularly England. He wrote on numerous pediatric and neurological subjects, and pediatrics in general owes him a debt of gratitude for this (Egan, Illingworth, and MacKeith, 1969). It can be fairly said that MacKeith's interests were not in the rarities of medicine but in those common complaints that can so easily make a child's life a misery and are ignored by some practitioners. This interest is well shown by his writings on such subjects as feeding difficulties, emotional problems, and developmental disorders (MacKeith, 1968, 1971a, 1971b). He was a clinical scientist who gave remarkable attention to the details of a child's symptoms and drew conclusions from them that escaped many others. His teaching may have been unconventional at times, but when it concerned helping children in distress it was often evangelical. He was nothing less than a genius in stimulating discussion, often by making remarks that some thought were outrageous when they did not know the spirit in which they were made.

As senior editor of *Developmental Medicine and Child Neurology,* MacKeith established the journal as one of international standing and as the official journal of the American Academy for Cerebral Palsy and Developmental Medicine and the British Paediatric Neurology Association. He was also senior editor of *Clinics in Developmental Medicine*, a series of books that has covered many aspects of pediatric neurology, as well as reporting the proceedings of some of the annual meetings.

MacKeith had many interests outside medicine, in particular, the study of Samuel Johnson and the eighteenth century. His involvement with the literature of this period is well reviewed by Rousseau (1978). Martin Bax, who worked for many years with MacKeith and knew him particularly well, has recorded a number of personal memories in *Developmental Medicine and Child Neurology* (1978):

Some of them bring back to me vivid memories of this unique man. His interview with the severely mentally handicapped boy and his parents: Ronnie is leaning forward, talking, with a hand out, occasionally just touching the person sitting opposite. Dimly, through my ignorance, I become aware (and become more aware as I learn more over the years) that I am watching a brilliant display of that peculiar medical art of consultation. Until this day, I have not known what it is. Ronnie is in some way absorbing all this distress, sensing the gulf between this man and his wife, aware of all the hopes there have been for this son, and he is gently nudging them towards full reality of the situation, the need for them to accept the proffered place for their son in the local school for severely subnormal children. I sense that he is achieving something. It lasts a long time and suddenly they are gone. So too is Ronnie; he is away to some engagement for which he is probably already half an hour late. But he has quickly thrust the executive action over to the social worker who has been with us throughout. He seems to have left her with rather more than a muddle to sort out and I wonder if I should do something, but I sense suddenly that she is glad to help Ronnie, and she sends me hurrying after him with a smile and a half-joke — "Genius must be served."

His visits to assessment units and schools for handicapped children: He is all over the school; from math teaching to ophthalmological services, everything is observed. "You don't have a visiting ophthalmologist? One could easily come from. . . ." I'm not sure that the administrators who are there like all this. Their faces are gloomy ("Dr. MacKeith is always spending money"), but the headmistress does; she senses that Ronnie wants to do things for "her" children. She hasn't noticed how much he's been telling her about her job between times, but I have a feeling she won't forget the visit.

His insistence on apples for dessert: Ronnie is dining. It is always a faintly alarming process. Head waiters spend a long time finding out that they have met their match. The man at Caesar's Palace, Las Vegas, is defeated by a combination of Ronnie's adroit use of his deafness, the assumption that the waiter can't understand English, and Ronnie's vastly superior culinary knowledge. While the man at what calls itself "the best restaurant in the Mid-West" has an even worse shock when he attempts to throw out a late-arrived guest of Ronnie's because he is not wearing a jacket. Ronnie leaps up and puts his own jacket over his friend's shoulders. The waiter, who has already lost out over the missing potatoes (had they really run out?) and the absence of fresh apples ("The best restaurants always have fresh fruit") submits resignedly and comes to hang a rather greasy waiter's jacket around Ronnie's shoulders. (Bax, 1978)

John Apley comments on the link between MacKeith and the carnation:

The carnation is a badge. He [Ronnie MacKeith] once admitted to me that, in his early days, he took to wearing a carnation in his button-hole because this gave him courage and poise before an audience or when mixing with strangers. Gradually, the carnation became the badge of the Little Club, so named after Dr. W. J. Little, who studied causes of cerebral palsy a hundred years ago. Now, as a flower, or a tie or cravat, it is a badge carried by colleagues who have joined Ronnie in caring for handicapped children, for countless children in many kinds of need. He is honored and held in affection, both for the man he is and because of what he has done for them. (Apley, 1978)

The person who mattered most to MacKeith was the child, and particularly the child with a long-term handicap, which caused an obvious disadvantage to be overcome if possible; then the child's family, who so often needed advice and support; and last, the professionals. Woe betide anyone whose work could not stand up to criticism or who placed their own interests before those of the child.

MacKeith, the son of a physician, was born in 1908. He was admitted to Queen's College, Oxford, in 1926, trained at St. Mary's Hospital Medical School as an undergraduate, and completed his postgraduate training as Radcliffe Travelling Fellow at Bellevue Hospital in New York. During the war he served in the Royal Navy. After the war he was appointed to the staff of Guy's Hospital in London, where he founded a clinic for children with cerebral palsy that developed into the Newcomen Centre for Handicapped Children, one of the first such facilities in the United Kingdom to coordinate the services needed in the assessment and management of handicapped children. He showed his particular interest in community pediatrics by founding the British Community Paediatric Group, in preventive medicine by running a child health clinic at Guy's Hospital, and in child psychiatry by his appointments to the Cassel Hospital and Tavistock Clinic, leaders in this field. He also devoted a great deal of his time and energy to medical education and medical ethics. He was chairman of the Medical Association for the Prevention of War.

Among his many honors was the award in 1972 by the British Paediatric Association of the James Spence Medal for his services in pediatrics, the Rosen van Rosenstein Medal of the Swedish Pediatric Association given in 1974 for founding pediatric neurology, the Special Merit Award of the American Academy for Cerebral Palsy in 1975, and the Albrecht von Haller Medal from the University of Göttingen in 1977.

These are the bare facts of Ronnie MacKeith's career but those privileged to know him soon realized that acceptance of his ideals would ensure that pediatric neurology developed as a widely based specialty involving many disciplines.

Neil Gordon
MANCHESTER, ENGLAND

ACKNOWLEDGMENTS

I wish to acknowledge the help of Dr. Martin Bax in preparing this biography.

REFERENCES

Apley, J. 1978. Ronald Charles MacKeith. In *Care of the Handicapped Child. A Festschrift for Ronald MacKeith*, 1–9. Clinics in Developmental Medicine, No. 67. London: W. Heinemann.

Bax, M. 1978. Ronald Charles MacKeith. A Personal Memoir. *Dev Med Child Neur* 20:3–7.

Egan, D. F., R. S. Illingworth, and R. C. MacKeith. 1969. *Developmental Screening, 0–5 Years*. London: Spastics International Medical Publications/W. Heinemann.

MacKeith, R. C. 1968. Maximal Clarity on Neurodevelopmental Disorders. *Dev Med Child Neur* 10(2):143–44.

______. 1971a. A New Look at Spina Bifida Aperta. *Dev Med Child Neur* 13(3):277–78.

______. 1971b. Who Guides the Therapist? *Dev Med Child Neur* 13(1):125–26.

MacKeith, R. C., and M. Bax. 1963. *Minimal Cerebral Dysfunction; Papers from the International Study Group Held at Oxford, September 1962.* London: National Spastics Society, Medical Education and Information Unit.

Rousseau, G. S. 1978. A Non-Medical View from Across the Atlantic. In *Care of the Handicapped Child. A Festschrift for Ronald MacKeith*, 10–14. Clinics in Developmental Medicine, No. 67. London: W. Heinemann.

DONALD MATSON

DONALD DARROW MATSON (1913–1969) (figure 1) was born in Fort Hamilton, New York, the youngest of four brothers. The son of a colonel in the army, he grew up on a variety of military posts. He graduated with honors from Cornell University in 1935, excelling in sports as well as academics. During his last three years at Cornell he had a scholarship from the Telluride Foundation, which sponsored "promising young men" and supported their education.

He started medical school at Harvard in the class of 1939. As a medical student he participated in research with John Rock and Thomas Lannan, work that led to his first two publications, one on the diagnosis of infertility (Rock, Bartlett, and Matson, 1939), and the other on lung abscess (Matson, 1940). He was also influenced by one of Harvey Cushing's pupils, Franc D. Ingraham, who was the neurosurgeon at both Children's Hospital and the Peter Bent Brigham Hospital.

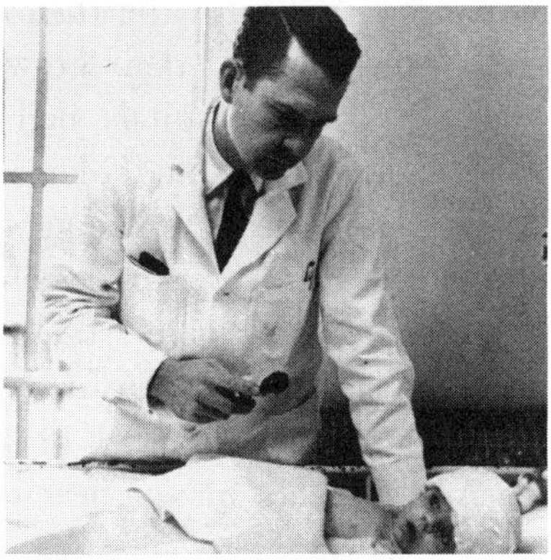

Figure 1. Donald Matson (1913–1969).

Matson took his surgical residency at the Massachusetts General Hospital, the Brigham Hospital, and the Children's Hospital. In 1943 he was called for military service. While undergoing special training in New York, he met his future wife, Dorothy Everett. They were married that year and Matson was then ordered to the European Theatre, where he started work as a surgeon with the U. S. Army, 3rd Auxiliary Surgical Group. He later became the neurosurgical consultant for the 1st Army Group under Elliot Cutler. This experience provided the basis for his first monograph, *The Treatment of Acute Craniocerebral Injuries Due to Missles,* which was published in 1948. In this monograph, operations were meticulously recorded and beautifully illustrated.

After the war, he worked for a short while with Gilbert Horrax at the Lahey Clinic and then went to Duke University Hospital under Barnes Woodall to finish his neurosurgical residency. He returned to Boston to join the staff at the Children's Hospital under Ingraham.

Cutler was beginning to rebuild the surgical department at the Peter Bent Brigham Hospital but died before this was completed. Matson's classmate and friend, Francis Moore, took over the leadership of the Brigham Surgical Services and Matson became associated with the Peter Bent Brigham Hospital for his adult practice. At this time Ingraham developed a significant essential tremor and depended more and more on Matson to do most of the surgery.

When Matson returned to the Brigham and Children's, there were no significant neurologic services. Cushing had always felt that neurosurgeons should be their own neurologists and did not tolerate neurologists in his sphere of influence. Matson encouraged and cooperated with the then developing Neurologic Services and significantly helped their growth to large academic services. Neurology in both hospitals had an excellent working relationship with Neurosurgery and Matson over the years. From 1950 until his premature death at the age of fifty-six in 1969, Donald Matson was the de facto neurosurgeon at Children's and the Peter Bent Brigham Hospital. He established a major neurosurgical training program and had an unsurpassed reputation in the field of pediatric neurosurgery. One of his early trainees, John Shillito, became his associate and, for the next two decades, they were the "Harvard neurosurgeons."

Matson's early research on cerebrospinal fluid physiology resulted from an interest in the treatment of hydrocephalus that he retained throughout his professional life. When he first returned to Boston, he worked in the surgical laboratories, publishing a number of clinical papers as well as establishing a dog model for the study of hydrocephalus (Ingraham, Alexander, and Matson, 1947a; Ingraham, Matson, and Alexander, 1948). He experimented with the use of plastics and developed a new operation for hydrocephalus that connected the ventricles to the ureter (Ingraham, Alexander, and Matson, 1947b). The ventricular-ureteral shunting procedure reported in 1949 by Matson became known as "the Matson procedure" (figure 2); at that time, it was the only alternative to the Torkelson procedure (Matson, 1949). The experience of his group led to an increasing number of neurosurgical attempts to treat hydrocephalic patients that are now routine procedures in neurosurgery.

A by-product of the procedure was removal of a kidney. This became the source of most of the early renal transplantation work done at the Brigham Hospital. Other kidneys were given to John F. Enders to use for the culturing of the polio virus, work that subsequently led to Enders receiving the Nobel Prize.

Matson always maintained a realistic attitude. In his last paper on hydrocephalus, in 1968, he noted the failure of many of his operations and the need for continued efforts and research to improve the care of these patients (Matson, 1968). For those who did not have personal contact with Matson, he is perhaps best remembered for his textbook on pediatric neurosurgery, *Neurosurgery of Infancy and Childhood.* Coauthored with Ingraham, the first edition

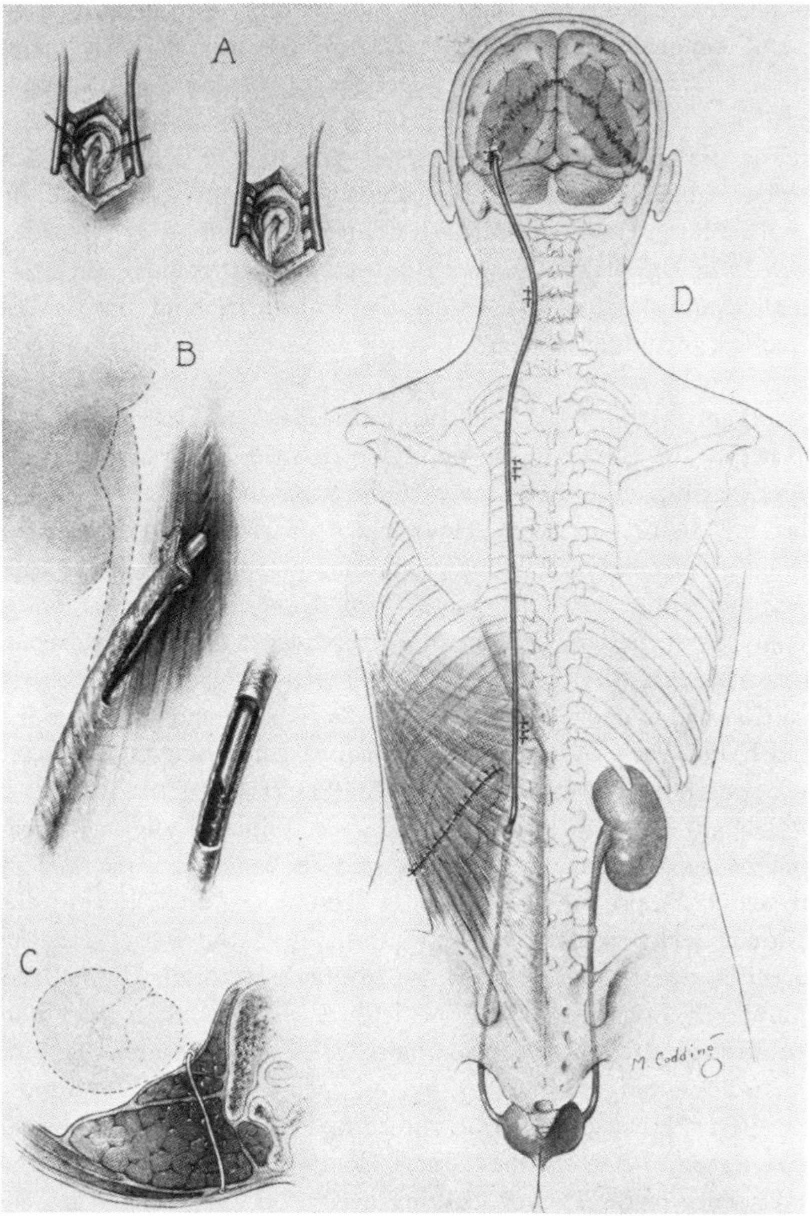

Figure 2. The Matson procedure; picture taken from his classic textbook in pediatric neurosurgery. From Ingraham and Matson, *Neurosugery of Infancy and Childhood* (Springfield, IL: Charles C Thomas, 1954).

appeared in 1954 and was 456 pages in length with numerous patient photographs and radiographs as well as many illustrations of surgical procedures. The book was divided into ten major sections: congenital anomalies, hydrocephalus, trauma, intracranial tumors, intraspinal tumors, infection, cerebrovascular disorders, epilepsy, lead encephalopathy, and pediatric neurosurgical anesthesia. Its style was clear, concise, objective, and definitive, with several tables summarizing the extensive experience of the authors at the Boston Children's Medical Center. A forerunner of this work was *Spina Bifida and Cranium Bifidum*, which Ingraham had originally published in 1943 with the collaboration of five of his trainees, including Matson.

When Ingraham retired in 1964, Matson became chief of neurosurgery at the Peter Bent Brigham Hospital. After Ingraham's death in 1965, friends and family created the Franc D. Ingraham Professorship of Neurosurgery at Harvard and, in 1968 Matson became the first recipient. However, he developed early signs of a progressive neurologic disorder in May 1968, just months after becoming professor. This disorder lasted two years and was eventually recognized as Creutzfeldt-Jakob disease. He had to give up active surgery shortly thereafter and worked mainly on the last edition of his book. Fortunately it was finished shortly before his death in 1969, thus leaving succeeding generations a landmark textbook of pediatric neurosurgery (Barlow et al, 1970).

Donald Matson was primarily a clinical and practical neurosurgeon. He was not interested in bench research but in developing procedures, training residents, and caring for patients. His advice was sought all over the world for the specific expertise he acquired at Children's Hospital. He received numerous honors and was widely recognized as a leader in neurosurgical circles. He was chairman of the American Board of Neurologic Surgery in 1965, having been its secretary for almost ten years. He also served on the editorial board of the *Journal of Neurosurgery*. One of the honors he most appreciated was the presidency of the Harvey Cushing Society in 1969. Unfortunately he was too ill to attend the meeting that year. His memory is honored by the Donald Matson Award for Excellence in Teaching, given each year by the Surgical Services of the Brigham and Women's Hospital to an outstanding teacher, and the Donald Matson Lectureship in Neurosurgery at Harvard Medical School, for which a leader in neurosurgery is invited to the university for a number of days each year (Moore, 1978).

H. Richard Tyler
BOSTON, MASSACHUSETTS

REFERENCES

Barlow, C. F., et al. 1970. Donald Darrow Matson Faculty of Medicine Memorial Minutes. In A Meeting of the Faculty of Medicine on Friday, March 13th. *Harvard Univ Gaz* 65(34): May 5.

Ingraham, F. D. 1943. *Spina Bifida and Cranium Bifidum. Papers reprinted from the New England Journal of Medicine with the Addition of a Comprehensive Bibliography*. Cambridge: The Harvard University Printing Office.

Ingraham, F. D., E. Alexander, and D. D. Matson. 1947a. Experimental Hydrocephalus. *Gen Surg* 4:164–76.

______. 1947b. Synthetic Plastic Materials in Surgery. *NEJM* 236:362–68.

Ingraham, F. D., and D. D. Matson. 1954. *Neurosurgery of Infancy and Childhood.* Springfield, IL: Charles C Thomas.

Ingraham, F. D., D. D. Matson, and E. Alexander. 1948. Studies in the Treatment of Experimental Hydrocephalus. *Gen Neuropath Exp Neur* 7:123–43.

Matson, D. D. 1940. Lung Abscess. *NEJM* 222:15–21.

______. 1948. *The Treatment of Acute Craniocerebral Injuries Due to Missles.* Springfield, IL: Charles C Thomas.

______. 1949. A New Operation for the Treatment of Communicating Hydrocephalus. *J Neurosurg* 6:238–47.

______. 1968. Hydrocephalus. In *Current Pediatric Therapy*. Ed. Sydney S. Gellis and Benjamin M. Kagan. Philadelphia: W. B. Saunders.

______. 1969. *Neurosurgery of Infancy and Childhood.* Springfield, IL: Charles C Thomas.

Moore, F. D. 1978. As We Knew Him. *Harvard Med Alum Bull* Nov./Dec., 21–27.

Rock, J., M. K. Bartlett, and D. D. Matson. 1939. The Incidence of Anovulatory Menstruation in Patients of Low Fertility. *Am J Obstet Gyn* 37:3–12.

JOHANNES MELCHIOR

CHILD NEUROLOGY'S development has varied from country to country depending on many social, historical, economic, political, and medical factors. In Denmark, although specialization did not truly develop until the early twentieth century, the field of pediatrics had taken shape somewhat earlier. The first Danish Pediatric Hospital, where construction was initiated more because of concern for the social welfare of children, opened with approximately ten beds in 1850. It was soon followed by the Queen Louises Children's Hospital in 1879 and the University Clinic of Pediatrics, Rigshospitalet, in 1910. Because of this heritage, it has been the tradition for pediatricians to assume the responsibility for the care of children with neurological disorders. It was, in fact, after World War II that neuropediatrics, or child neurology, began to develop as an independent subspecialty. Among the first of these self-trained individuals were Sven Brandt and Johannes Melchior.

Johannes Christian Melchior (figure 1) was born in 1913 in Horsens, the son of a school director and maternal grandson of a general practitioner. He began his higher education in Horsens in 1942 and studied medicine first in Aarhus and later in Copenhagen where he graduated in January 1950. That same year he married Jytte Stock, an attorney. After graduation, his first pediatric appointment was the Sundby Hospital in 1952 under Carl Friderichsen, the pediatrician well known for his description of septic shock in bacterial meningitis (Waterhouse-Friderichsen syndrome). After further clinical training in the neurology department headed by Mogens Fog, he was appointed to the University Clinic of Pediatrics, Rigshospitalet, Copenhagen and, from 1956 to 1959 to the Queen Louises Children's Hospital, Copenhagen.

In 1957 Melchior studied pediatric neuropathology and neurology at Harvard Medical School in Boston, worked with Clemens Benda at the Walter E. Fernald State School and attended teaching sessions in neurology at the Massachusetts General Hospital with Raymond Adams, Philip Dodge, and Paul Yakovlev. He received his doctor of medicine degree in 1961, based on his thesis "Pneumoencephalography in Atrophic Brain Lesions in Infancy and Childhood," from the University of Copenhagen. Several years later, in 1966, he spent three months at the Great Ormond Street Hospital in the department of clinical neurophysiology with Giuseppe Pampiglione.

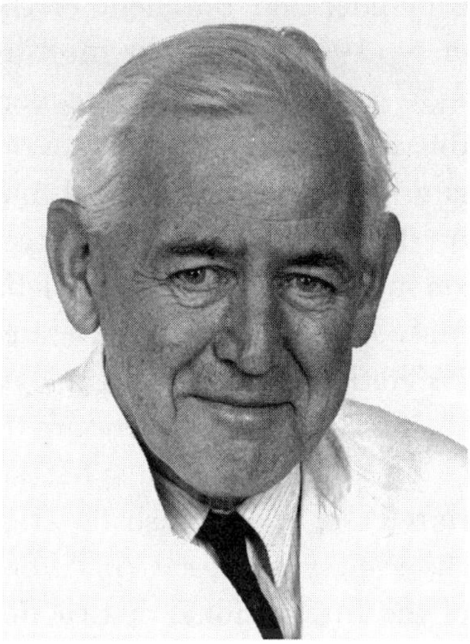

Figure 1. Johannes Melchior, 1988.

In 1964 Melchior became head of the pediatric department, Rigshospitalet, and, from 1972 to 1974, he was professor of pediatrics at the Copenhagen County Hospital, Gentofte. He then returned to the Rigshospitalet in 1974 and became chairman of the University Clinic of Pediatrics two years later, having previously been appointed professor of pediatrics at the University of Copenhagen. Despite these and other commitments, he served as chairman of the University Medical Curriculum Committee and dean of the faculty from 1975 to 1977; he was also a member of the Advisory Committee for Medical Education in the European Common Market from 1976 to 1989.

Melchior has published more than one hundred papers, including a monograph with Erna Christensen, *Cerebral Palsy: A Clinical and Neuropathological Study* (1967). He has also written a manual for medical students and a popular book for parents and their children (Melchior, 1980, 1989). His major interests in child neurology have been the progressive encephalopathies, convulsions including febrile convulsions, and cerebral palsy. In 1962 he coauthored with Holger Dyggve and Jorgen Clausen a paper entitled "Morquio-Ulrich's Disease: An Inborn Error of Metabolism?" (Dyggve, Melchior, and Clausen, 1962). This was later known as the Dyggve-Melchior-Clausen's syndrome and has been described in approximately one hundred children (Dyggve et al, 1977). These children have clinical findings of short stature, mental retardation, and skeletal abnormalities. He has also written several papers on the possible connection between immunizations, especially pertussis, and infantile spasms (Melchior, 1977).

Melchior, together with Bengt Hagberg from Gothenburg, was

a founder and president of the Scandinavian Neuropaediatric Society (1963). The first meeting organized by Bengt Hagberg was in Udevalla and was attended by twelve people from the Scandinavian countries. Now, over one hundred participants and their families enjoy these annual meetings, usually held in a remote area of the host country to foster development of collegial relations among the attendees (Melchior, 1985). Together with Ronald MacKeith, they also accelerated the development of the European Federation of Child Neurology Societies (EFCNS), which met for the first time in Gothenburg, Sweden, in 1974.

Since 1958 Melchior has also served on several different committees of the Danish Spastic Society and has been president of the society since 1976. After several years as honorary treasurer of the International Spastic Society he became an honorary member in 1984 and is also a corresponding member of the German Pediatric Society. He has been very active in the Scandinavian Pediatric Society and has served as president of this organization since 1988. Because of his numerous contributions both to pediatrics and child neurology, he was awarded the Knight of First Degree of The Order of Danneborg (Riddler af 1. grad af Dannebrogsordenen) in 1988.

Bengt Hagberg
GOTHENBURG, SWEDEN

REFERENCES

Christensen, E., and J. C. Melchior. 1967. *Cerebral Palsy: A Clinical and Neuropathological Study*. Clinics in Developmental Medicine, No. 25. London: W. Heinemann .

Dyggve, H. V., et al. 1977. The Dyggve-Melchior-Clausen (DMC) Syndrome. A 15 Year Follow-up and a Survey of the Present Clinical and Chemical Findings. *Neuropäd* 8:429–42.

Dyggve, H. V., J. C. Melchior, and J. Clausen. 1962. Morquio-Ulrich's Disease: An Inborn Error of Metabolism? *Arch Dis Child* 37:525.

Melchior, J. C. 1961. Pneumoencephalography in Atrophic Brain Lesions in Infancy and Childhood. *Acta Paed* 50 (Suppl.)(127):1–320.

______. 1977. Infantile Spasms and Early Immunization Against Whooping Cough. Danish Survey from 1970 to 1975. *Arch Dis Child* 52:134–37.

______. 1980. *Students: Paediatrisk Kompendium*. Copenhagen: FADL's Forlag.

______. 1985. The Scandinavian Neuropaediatric Society. The Society's History and Present Status. *Brain Dev* 7:545–48.

______. 1989. *Parents: Politikens Bogen om Barnet*. Copenhagen: Politikens Forlag.

RONALD MELVILLE NORMAN

RONALD MELVILLE NORMAN (1904–1968) (figure 1) was born in England's West Country on November 2, 1904. He died on August 20, 1968, of a malignant glioma. We older practitioners of pediatric neurology came to admire Norman through his magnificent chapter on malformations, birth injury/hypoxia, and heredofamilial degenerative diseases, published in the original 1958 volume of J. Godwin Greenfield's *Neuropathology*. After Greenfield's death, Norman himself edited the second edition. Current trainees in pediatric neurology learn the same material, now scattered over five chapters in the fourth edition (Adams, Corsellis, and Duchen, 1984).

Norman's academic credentials proceeded as follows: M.B., Ch.B, 1930; and M.D., 1932, from the University of Bristol; D.P.M., 1934; Member of the Royal College of Physicians in 1952; and Fellow of the Royal College of Physicians in 1961. He was lecturer in neuropathology at the University of Bristol. Norman was a founder and later president of the British Neuropathology Society and served on the editorial boards of the *Journal of Neurology, Neurosurgery, and Psychiatry*, the *Journal of Mental Science* (now the *British Journal of Psychiatry*), and *Acta Neuropathologica*.

As a young man Norman trained in psychiatry and then received several appointments. He became assistant medical director at Stoke Park Colony for Mentally Defectives in 1930, deputy superintendent of the colony in 1942, and superintendent in 1947. In 1953 he resigned his post at Stoke Park to become the full-time research neuropathologist for the Southwest Regional Hospital Board, a post that was created especially for him. His laboratory, a small converted

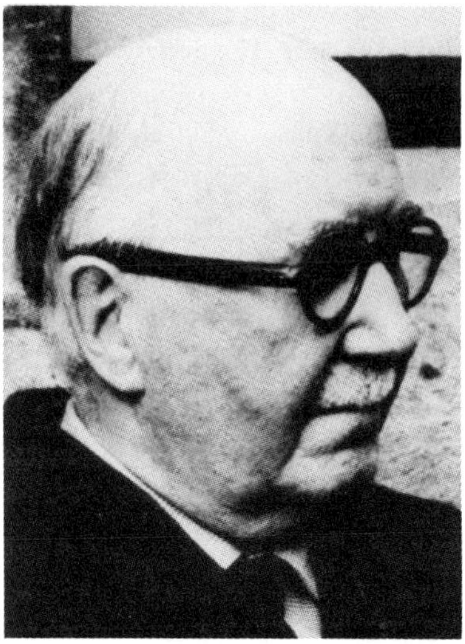

Figure 1. Ronald Melville Norman (1904–1968).

Nissan hut on the grounds of the Frenchay Hospital, Bristol, would seem primitive in this day of scintillation counters, chromatographs, computerized microscopy, and immunofluorescent staining.

Norman owed an immense debt to R. G. A. Berry, neuroanatomist (Berry, 1938) and superintendent at Stoke Park Colony, who urged him into neuropathology. Norman married Berry's daughter, Margaret. Margaret Norman, herself artistically gifted, expanded his lifelong interest in the visual arts. The couple had two sons and a daughter. Contemporaries described him as diffident and self-effacing but possessing great personal charm, erudition, wisdom, and humor.

Norman's early clinical experience with the inmates at Stoke Park Colony for Mentally Defectives sparked a lifelong interest in mental deficiency and its neuropathological substrate. In 1933 Norman published the clinical neurologic findings in five hundred mentally retarded inmates, pointing out the hard and soft signs, a classic but now little quoted paper as today's clinicians rediscover the same things. In combining clinical work and neuropathology, he was often able to study the brains of patients he had seen clinically. In this respect, Norman was typical of a long line of contemporaries, including researchers such as Paul Yakovlev and Clemens Benda, who transformed their clinical work performed at one of the large facilities for the retarded into important scientific results.

Today's neuropathologists come via departments of pathology and cannot even do a neurologic examination, much to the detriment of their ability and interest in clinicopathologic correlations. One finds the same lack of ability in today's neuroradiologists, who blanch or become bored if the clinician needs to puzzle out how a lesion, so marvelously displayed, relates to the patient's case.

Although crediting much to Greenfield, Norman was essentially self-trained. He tended to work alone, although he collaborated in his later years with the biochemist A. H. Tingey on the lipidoses and leukodystrophies, pioneering the combination of biochemistry with morphology, a synthesis that occupied much of his final decade. A self-proclaimed miniaturist, specializing in the detailed study of single brains, his insights and industry transformed him into a giant. He proclaimed that no one could adequately study more than twelve brains per year. His writings reflected his long insistence on simplicity, accuracy, and clarity of expression.

Norman adopted the whole-mount celloidin sections of the German school and frozen sections stained by the traditional methods of Franz Nissl for perikarya, Kultschitzky-Pal for myelin sheaths, Max Bielschowsky for neurons, Holzer for gliosis, and Pio del Rio Hortega for the individual silhouettes of the glia. He obviously was captivated by the beauty of these methods applied to frozen section. Anyone having seen the beauty of frozen rather than paraffin sections of the nervous system understands the tremendous aesthetic satisfaction and scientific clarity they offer, making the paraffin sections, which often pass for study of neuropathology today, seem almost useless. His publications, magnificently illustrated with his own gross and microscopic photographs, attest to his artistry. Fortunately, he was able to publish a large number of his illustrations in Greenfield's first edition because of a subsidy from the trustees of the Burden Foundation. Most of his illustrations remain in the current edition, because they cannot be surpassed.

How can we understand a person who prefers to spend a career alone in a hut, hunched over a microscope peering at slides, with caldrons of stains steaming in the background? The delightful essay of Rio Hortega, who was equally addicted to histology, explains best the dual intellectual and aesthetic satisfactions:

To wrest, by cunning stratagems of technique, a secret from nature, to penetrate to its hidden meaning, to create pure science while delighting in aesthetic contemplation is, for the histologist, something which might be compared with eagerly desired paternity. The investigator cherishes his histologic discoveries as the children of his spirit. . . . (Rio Hortega, 1949)

Over a period of thirty years Norman reported on his tripartite interests: brain malformations, perinatal and seizure-induced brain damage, and inborn errors of metabolism. Commencing with amaurotic familial idiocy (Norman, 1935; Norman and Ward, 1941), Norman contributed case studies of metachromatic leukodystrophy (Norman, 1947b; Norman, Urich, and Tingey, 1960), Gaucher disease (Norman, Urich and Lloyd, 1956), Tay-Sachs disease (Norman et al, 1959; Norman et al, 1964), Niemann-Pick disease (Oppenheimer et al, 1967; Norman, Forrester, and Tingey, 1967), Krabbe's disease (Norman, Oppenheimer, and Tingey, 1961), and maple syrup urine disease (Martin and Norman, 1967).

At the time of his studies on metachromatic leukodystrophy, some investigators suggested that the abundantly present macrophages were at fault in being unable to catabolize lipids, but he emphasized that the widespread occurrence of the metachromatic material in peripheral nerves and organs outside the central nervous system, as in Niemann-Pick and Tay-Sachs disease, meant that it could not exclusively be a macrophage or oligodendroglial disorder and suggested that it aligned with the lipidoses. He took metachromatic leukodystrophy out of the wastebasket category of Schilder's disease, arguing that

diffuse progressive metachromatic leuocencehalopathy [sic] *has pathogenetic affinity to the lipoidoses* [sic] *and that the metachromatic substance is probably formed locally in the affected organs as a result of perverted lipoid* [sic] *metabolism.* (Norman, 1947b, 243)

He emphasized that Krabbe's leukodystrophy did not show enlargement of neurons as in the lipidoses. He also noted the enlarged brains of many children with lipidoses, separating these patients with metabolic megalencephaly, who had a retrogressive course, from those with anatomic megalencephaly, who had a static course. He separated Batten's disease from Tay-Sachs disease (Greenfield, 1958) at a time when many others still linked it pathogenetically and nosologically with the lipidoses, a separation then finally and convincingly documented by the comprehensive studies of Wolfgang Zeman (Zeman, 1970). Zeman also stated that Batten's disease was the correct eponym and that neuronal ceroid lipofuscinosis was the best approximation for a systematic name.

Thus Norman's method of making detailed studies of individual brains, the sometimes decried "case-report" method, clarified and helped establish our current nosology of these conditions.

In 1945 Norman described retrograde degeneration of the nucleus medialis dorsalis and the medial one-third of the nucleus ventralis lateralis in a patient with polycystic destruction of the frontal poles and frontal granular isocortex back to area six. This paper extended to man the classical work of A. Earl Walker in 1938 on the frontal connections of the thalamus in the macaque monkey and preceded the definitive study of frontal lobe connections by Meyer, Beck, and McLardy (1946) in patients who had the Freeman-Watts prefrontal lobotomy.

The pediatric neurologists of today, so aware of the effects of hypoxia on the neonate, may have some trouble appreciating the scientific battle required to relate the perinatal events to their pathologic sequelae. Norman (1944) argued that the ulegyria of Bresler, also called atrophic sclerosis and sclerotic microgyria, resulted from destructive lesions due to perinatal vascular lesions and hypoxia and were often combined with other evidence of hypoxia, in the form of status marmoratus of the basal ganglia, thalamus, and even the corpus callosum (Norman, 1947a). He thus separated ulegyria from degenerative processes, and from the polymicrogyria of Bielschowsky, a malformation arising much earlier in the fetus rather than the consequence of perinatal hypoxic/destructive lesions.

Just as he pioneered in adding neurochemistry to neuropathological analysis, Norman was one of the early workers to describe the pathologic changes in 13–15 and 17–18 trisomy. He described heterotopic islands of granular neurons in the white matter of the cerebellum (Norman, 1966). Trisomy 17–18 differed in having milder hypoplasia of the cerebellum than trisomy 13–15 and relatively few heterotopias. Thus he helped to usher in the modern study of the neuropathology of chromosomal disorders.

Scientifically Norman was a man of his time, exploiting the best methods of the old masters, but he was far from being stuck in the past. He grasped the necessity for chemistry to shift neuropathology from static morphology and began to capitalize on another great advance of his era, the study of chromosomal errors. His publications on perinatal brain damage and heredodegenerative diseases form the basis of much that is now familiar to all pediatric neurologists, who take this information for granted, as if it had always been known.

William DeMyer
INDIANAPOLIS, INDIANA

REFERENCES

Adams, J. H., J. A. N. Corsellis, and L. W. Duchen. 1984. *Greenfield's Neuropathology*. 4th ed. New York: John Wiley.

Berry, R. G. A. 1938. *A Cerebral Atlas*. London: Oxford University Press.

Greenfield, J. G. 1958. *Neuropathology*. 1st ed. London: Edward Arnold.

Martin, J. K., and R. M. Norman. 1967. Maple Syrup Urine Disease in an Infant with Microgyria. *Dev Med Child Neur* 9:152–59.

Meyer, A., E. Beck, and T. McLardy. 1946. Prefrontal Leucotomy: A Neuroanatomical Report. *Brain* 70:18–49.

Norman, R. M. 1933. Neurological Abnormalities: Their Occurrence and Significance as Illustrated by Examination of 500 Mental Defectives. *J Neur Psychopath* 14: 97–107.

______. 1935. Case of Juvenile Amaurotic Family Iidiocy. *J Neur Psychopath* 15:219–29.

______. 1944. Atrophic Sclerosis of Cerebral Cortex Associated with Birth Injury. *Arch Dis Child* 19:111–21.

______. 1945. Thalamic Degeneration Following Bilateral Premotor Frontal Lobe Atrophy of Strumpell Type. *J Neur Neurosurg Psych* 8:52–56.

______. 1947a. Etat Marbre of Corpus Callosum Following Birth Injury. *J Neur Neurosurg Psych* 10:12–25.

______. 1947b. Diffuse Progressive Metachromatic Leucoencephalopathy: A Form of Schilder's Disease Related to Lipoidoses [sic]. *Brain* 70:234–50.

______. 1966. Neuropathological Findings in Trisomies 13–15 and 17–18 with Special Reference to the Cerebellum. *Dev Med Child Neur* 8:170–77.

Norman, R. M., R. M. Forrester, and A. H. Tingey. 1967. The Juvenile Form of Niemann-Pick's Disease. *Arch Dis Child* 42:91–96.

Norman, R. M., D. R. Oppenheimer, and A. H. Tingey. 1961. Histological and Chemical Findings in Krabbe's Leucodystrophy. *J Neur Neurosurg Psych* 24:223–32.

Norman, R. M., et al. 1964. Tay-Sachs Disease with Visceral Involvement and Its Relation to Gargoylism. *Arch Dis Child* 39:634–40.

Norman, R. M., H. Urich, O. C. Lloyd. 1956. Neuropathology of Infantile Gaucher's Disease. *J Path Bact* 72:121–31.

Norman, R. M., H. Urich, and A. H. Tingey. 1960. Metachromatic Leucoencephalopathy: A Form of Lipidosis. *Brain* 83:369–80.

Norman, R. M., et al. 1959. Tay-Sachs Disease with Visceral Involvement and Its Relationship to Niemann-Pick's Disease. *J Path Bact* 78:409–21.

Norman, R. M., and H. Ward. 1941. Congenital Form of Amaurotic Family Idiocy. *J Neur Psych* 4:175–90.

Oppenheimer, D. R., et al. 1967. Histological and Chemical Findings in Juvenile Niemann-Pick's Disease. *J Neur Sci* 5:575–88.

Rio-Hortega, P. del 1949. Art and Artifice in Histologic Science. *Texas Rep Biol Med* 7:363–90.

Urich, H., and M. G. Norman. 1987. Founders of Pediatric Pathology: Ronald Melville Norman, MD. *Perspect Ped Pathol* 9:1–3.

Zeman, W. 1970. Historical Evolution of the Nosologic Concepts of Amaurotic Familial Idiocy, 10:212–32. In *Handbook of Clinical Neurol*ology. Vol. 10, 212–32. Ed. P. J. Vinken and G. W. Bruyn. Amsterdam: North Holland.

ALBRECHT PEIPER

ALTHOUGH ALBRECHT PEIPER'S publications span forty years, little of his and his associates' investigations, commentaries, contributions in texts, and even his own book of pediatrics have been translated into English. This is regrettable because Peiper (1889–1968) (figure 1) could be considered among the first pediatric neurologists.

It was perhaps predestined that Albrecht Peiper would become a physician, a professor of pediatrics, and chairman of a pediatrics department. His father, Ernst Peiper, was both an internist and pediatrician, and was codiscoverer of neonatal tetanus and of typhoid immunization. He established the Infant and Children's Health Center in Greifswald, Germany, Albrecht Peiper's birthplace, and was himself professor of pediatrics there. Among Peiper's forebears was an ophthalmologist who described the eye findings of Sturge-Weber syndrome. On Peiper's maternal side, he was related to Max Planck, through whom he made the acquaintance of Albert Einstein.

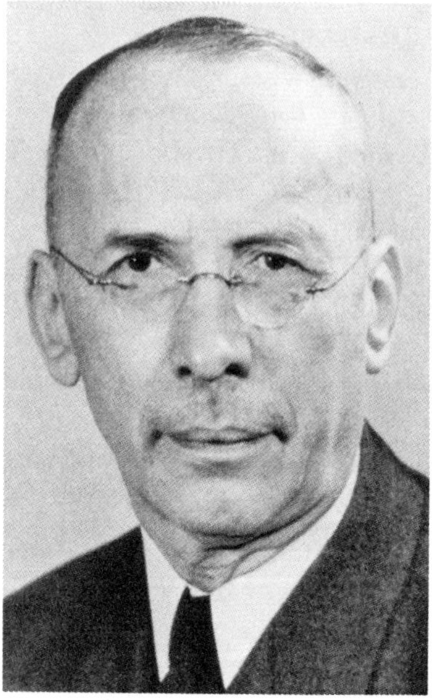

Figure 1. Albrecht Peiper (1889–1968).

Peiper began his university and medical studies in 1909, doing most of this work in Greifswald. The medical faculty was said to be quite well known, and included Ferdinand Sauerbruch, a highly respected surgeon of the time. As was common then, and like his father, Peiper began his training in internal medicine before moving on to pediatrics in Berlin in 1919 under Adalbert Czerny and others. He subsequently went on to direct the University Pediatric Clinic. From 1934 to 1943 he was director of the Pediatric Hospital in Wuppertal and in 1948 was appointed to the chair of pediatrics in Leipzig, retiring in 1958. Despite forty years of work in children's hospitals, he noted, with regret, in his book *Errinerungen eines Kinderarztes* that he was never Board-certified as a pediatrician.

Listed in the English translation of the third edition of *Cerebral Function in Infancy and Childhood* (1962) are Peiper's publications, numbering 168, most of which represent his own work. There were additional papers appearing in the German medical literature up to the year of his death. His first book on central nervous system function in infancy, *Die Hirntatigkeit des Sauglings* (*Cerebral Function in the Infant*), appeared in 1928 and was translated into Russian in 1929. The scope of Peiper's interest in the neurophysiology of the infant and child is clearly manifest in this bibliography. Even the unborn and premature infants come under his scrutiny. For example, in 1924 an article appeared entitled "Sinnesempfindungen des Kindes vor seiner Geburt" ("Sensory Perceptions of the Child Before Birth").

In 1927 in the *Archiv der Kinderheilkunde*, his was the lead article, "Über die Helligkeits-und Farbenempfindungen der Frühgeburten" ("On Light and Color Perception in Premature Infants"). Other topics about which he wrote included neonatal seizures, apneic

Figure 2. The grasp reflex in a four-week-old infant. Peiper engaged in many careful studies of infantile developmental reflexes. To emphasize his concepts of how these primitive reflexes develop in a hierarchial fashion, he frequently drew on his knowledge of the psychological functions of other species. From Peiper, *Cerebral Function in Infancy and Childhood* (New York: Consultants Bureau, 1963), 162.

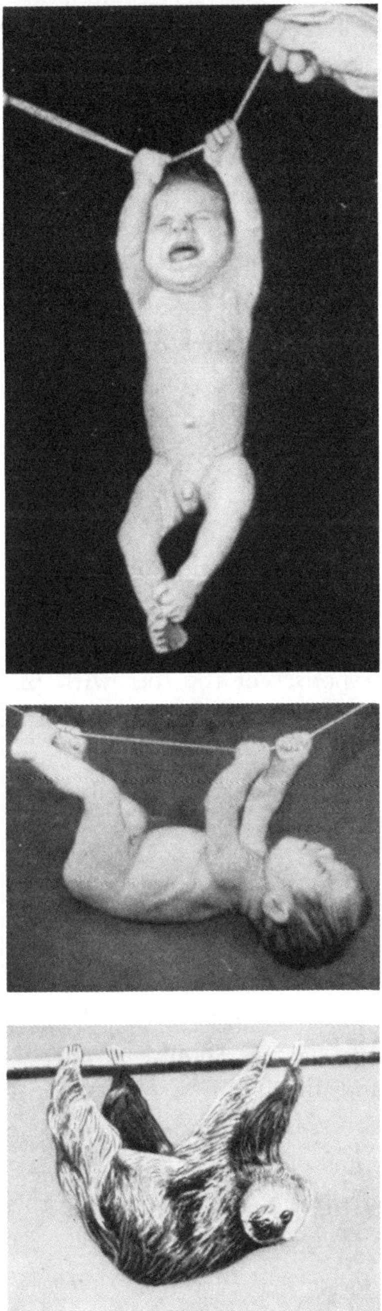

episodes, breath-holding spells, and respiratory disorders in premature infants. There are also numerous articles on various aspects of neurologic function and dysfunction in the newborn, including the acts of sucking, swallowing, and breathing, and other reflex activities (Peiper, 1963). His citations range from the ancient Greeks to modern physiologists such as Rudolf Magnus and Gijsbertus Rademaker, to animal behaviorists such as Niko Tinbergen and Konrad Lorenz, and to various psychologists.

Perhaps because of the problems of the postwar era, two editions of *Cerebral Function in Infancy and Childhood* were issued before the third was translated into English in 1963, some thirty years after the original was published. It is readily apparent that this is a work of a well-read and observant physician. Almost 800 pages in length, containing 208 figures, 16 tables, numerous quotations, and more than a thousand references, it embodies all that Peiper surveyed. One need only peruse the table of contents to appreciate the breadth and depth of this work. Among the 15 chapters are ones devoted to the development of sensory function, facial expression, reflexes of position and movement, locomotion, reflexes of clinical significance, the neurology of respiration and food intake, sleep or sleeplike states, conditioned reflexes, evolution and dissolution of cerebral function, and the child and his environment. Peiper included many photographs of infants showing different patterns of developmental reflexes with maturation. An example of this is the infantile grasp response and his comparison of this to other species (figure 2). Chapter 7, entitled "Reflexes of Clinical Significance," is just as important now as it was when it was written. For example, Peiper noted that the crossed adductor reflex is a secondary reaction to the elicitation of the patellar reflex in young infants and that either can be present alone. The chapter also contains a brief discourse on Babinski's sign. There are seven possible responses of the toes with plantar stimulation. Thus Peiper concludes from his own observations and those of others that "plantar reactions fluctuate and are inconstant at birth. . . ." He goes on to point out that the variable response of the big toe is not the result of immaturity of the pyramidal tract but due to "non-maturation of the striatum." A normal response "is possible only when the higher centers predominate permanently." Interestingly, Peiper points out that the Babinski sign is not present in newborn chimpanzees. This same chapter included a discussion of the important signs and symptoms of meningitis in children and their significance. It should be copied and given out to medical students and first year residents for the descriptive clarity of Kernig's, Brudzinski's, and Lasegue's signs and the other essential physical signs of meningitis. Perhaps the only flaw in this section is the attribution of the source of these findings to "meningitic centers."

Peiper's synthesis of an extraordinary volume of material and application to the newborn is indeed impressive, as illustrated by the following quotations taken from the last chapter, "Retrospect and Outlook":

Stimulus receptors, nerves, and the lower centers are already functioning in the newborn infant. The reflexes which can be elicited pass through the brain stem at this stage. The progressively better utilization of sensory impressions cannot generally be attributed to the improved function of the sensory organs, but rather to the progressively better evaluation of sensory impressions in the brain because of the gradual ascent of the relay station. (Peiper, 1963, 647)

In general, the development of human fetuses progresses anatomically and physiologically in the cervicocaudal direction from the brain stem to the spinal cord, and in the cervicorostral direction in the brain from the brain stem to the cerebral hemisphere. The ontogenetically younger centers break down prior to the older centers if a lack of oxygen occurs. Correspondingly, the local reflexes elicited by stimulation of the trigeminus region are the last to be extinguished in human fetuses during progressive oxygen deprivation. They are the first to be evoked in the maturing fetus. (Peiper, 1963, 648)

Extrapyramidal mass movements which are directed by the pallidum and not yet inhibited by the striatum are characteristic of the young infant. With the progressing development of the brain, these mass movements are inhibited and are gradually replaced by goal-directed voluntary individual movements; these movements are regulated by motor centers of the cerebral cortex by way of the pyramidal tracts. (Peiper, 1963, 648)

The neurological testing procedures available to us today do not yet enable us to comprehend even the young infant's entire behavior. As much as he depends on the stimuli of his environment, he nevertheless can act independently from birth. At no time is he a mere reflex creature whose behavior is completely dependent on outside stimuli. (Peiper, 1963, 652)

It is also apparent that he was concerned about the whole child, for one of the last chapters covers an array of family psychological interactions, including the mother and child, the father and children, motherless children and institutionalized children.

One year before his death, Peiper published a rather depressing review article in the *Medizinische Wochenschrift* entitled "Umgekehrte Kinderheilkunde," freely translated as "inverse" or "reverse pediatrics," paraphrased and fashioned after orthopedics in reverse, a term Peiper cites from Victor Hugo. In this article, Peiper reviewed the development of "professional beggars" and the practice of producing deformities of limbs and spine, scarring and blindness, in otherwise normal children. The roots of this form of child abuse lay in the belief that acts of goodness and mercy toward those less favored would result in a better hereafter for one's soul, though the practice existed even before the Christian era. The more the financial competition among the "professional beggars" the more widespread and grotesque the mutilations. He also commented on the practice of castration to create youthful voices for the church and court and eunuchs for the harems, and placed the government-ordered deaths of the institutionalized retarded in Germany during World War II in the framework of inverse pediatric care.

Peiper's obituary in *Monatschrift für Kinderheilkunde* in February 1969 named him one of the greatest of the German pediatricians and one of the last of the classic teachers of the time. For these attributes he was honored by numerous medical and scientific societies in Germany. A eulogy to Peiper described him as a man of heart, respectful of the work and life-style of his colleagues, perhaps reticent in the presence of strangers but easily won over by children. He was, by description, an exceptional teacher to whom many pediatricians in Germany are indebted. Undoubtedly, as we peruse his major works and texts, we will be obliged to acknowledge and posthumously honor him as a founding pediatric neurologist. Moreover, it was Albrecht Peiper, in conjunction with André-Thomas, who clearly appreciated the uniqueness of the neurology of the newborn infant. Both are to be credited with laying the foundation for that distinct area now referred to as neonatal neurology.

Jerome S. Haller
ALBANY, NEW YORK

REFERENCES

Peiper, A. 1924. Sinnesempfindungen des Kindes vor seiner Gebrut. *Mschr Kinderheilk* 29:236.

______. 1927. Über die Helligkeits und Farbenempfindungen der Frühgeburten. *Arch Kinderheilk* 80:1.

______. 1928. *Die Hirntatigkeit des Sauglings*. Berlin: J. Springer.

______. 1963. *Cerebral Function in Infancy and Childhood.* 3d ed. The International Behavioral Sciences Series. Trans. Benedict Nagler and Hilde Nagler. New York: Consultants Bureau.

______. 1967. *Errinerunge neines Kinderarztes*. Berlin: VEB Volk und Gesundheit.
______. 1967. Umgekehrte Kinderheilkunde. *Wein med Wschr* 117:895–99.
______. 1969. In Memoriam: Albrecht Peiper. *Mschr Kinderheilk* 117:2.

MEYER PERLSTEIN

IN HIS LECTURE on the parentage of child neurology at the centennial of the Hospital for Sick Children in Toronto in 1977, Sven Brandt described the pioneering contributions of pediatricians to the development of child neurology (Brandt, 1977). He mentioned two who were founders of the American Academy of Cerebral Palsy: Meyer Perlstein and Bronson Crothers.

Meyer Perlstein (1902–1969) (figure 1) was born in Chicago, the son of Moses and Rose Perlstein. His father had been commissioned by the U. S. government in the 1880s to lead Jewish settlers from the East and Midwest in covered wagons to the Dakotas. Many years later, Moses Perlstein's son Meyer helped found the Crippled Children's School in Jamestown, North Dakota, and remained as its consultant until his death (Boshes, 1970).

Perlstein attended grammar school and high school in Chicago but at the same time attended the Yeshiva, missing ordination by only three months. He attended the University of Chicago and received a B.S. in 1924 and an M.D. in 1927, when he was elected to the Alpha Omega Alpha Society. That year he published his first paper, on pygopagus twins (Perlstein, 1927). During his lifetime he published over two hundred articles on pediatric neurological topics, half of which dealt with various aspects of the etiology, diagnosis, and management of cerebral palsy, and the remainder on a variety of related topics, many of them dealing with the management of seizures with medication, in particular Gemonil and Tridione.

Perlstein interned at Cook County Hospital and subsequently attended there in pediatrics, as well as at Michael Reese Hospital, where he rose from clinic assistant in 1929 to senior attending

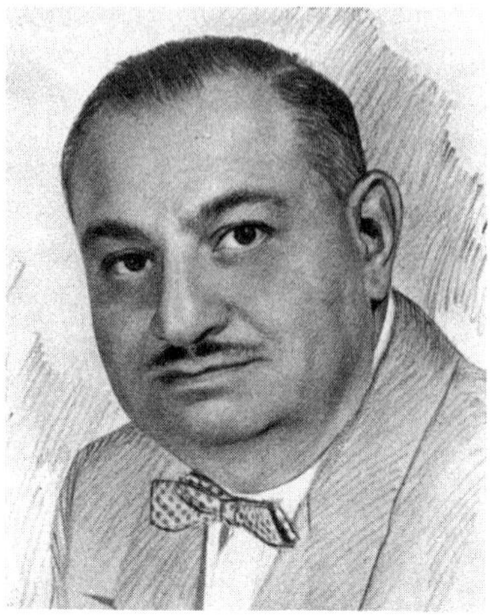

Figure 1. Meyer Perlstein (1902–1969).

physician in 1963, working closely with the pioneer pediatric neurologist Abe Levinson (Perlstein, 1956a). He trained in pediatric neurology and decided on an academic career combined with private practice. His abilities as a teacher and investigator were recognized immediately, and he progressed rapidly through the academic ranks. He was professor of pediatrics at the Cook County Postgraduate School of Medicine, associate professor of pediatrics at Northwestern University Medical School, chief of the Children's Neurology Service at Cook County Hospital, and consultant to the Department of Physical Medicine and Rehabilitation at Loyola University.

In addition to his academic appointments, he played an active role in the development of comprehensive services for the handicapped child. He was chief of the Illinois Children's Hospital School, advisor to the Cerebral Palsy Project of the National Institutes of Health, advisor on cerebral palsy to the American Public Health Association, United States representative to the World Commission on Cerebral Palsy, and member of the Scientific Council and Board of Trustees of the Brain Research Foundation. Perlstein was also a consultant on cerebral palsy to the Children's Bureau in Washington and the Armed Forces Institute and chairman of the Medical Advisory Board to the United Cerebral Palsy Association of Chicago.

Perlstein began his interest in the handicapped child in 1928, immediately upon completing his internship. He was extraordinarily active in his teaching and leadership activities. He was away from home somewhere at least once a month, speaking, holding clinics, or teaching. He made innovations in braces, for example, devising short caliper braces with removeable parts for easy repair or replacement. He introduced lighter metals for braces and taught brace makers many new methods, insisting only that, for every brace he devised, one additional be made which would go to an underprivileged handicapped child. Nor was his interest purely technical; he was always interested in the child and the family as a unit, and strove to rehabilitate the child so that he could find some place in the world (Boshes, 1970).

Perlstein initiated a cerebral palsy clinic at Michael Reese Hospital, and, because he was convinced that early and aggressive therapy would make a difference in outcome, he established the Therapeutic Day Nursery, a day school for preschool children with cerebral palsy and other motor and neuromuscular disorders, staffed by physical therapists, teachers, social workers, and others. The success of this program convinced the Chicago Board of Education to provide city-wide services for preschool children with cerebral palsy and led to the foundation of the present interdisciplinary Developmental Institute at Reese. In addition, he traveled by train to Springfield, together with Harry Barnett, an orthopedic surgeon, where they ran a cerebral palsy clinic. Barnett would then perform whatever surgery was necessary in one of the Springfield hospitals. This was a two-day project every month (Perlstein and Barnett, 1952). In addition to his extensive work on cerebral palsy, Perlstein introduced Tridione, Gemonil, and other anticonvulsants to the practicing physician (Perlstein, 1946; Perlstein, 1950).

Together with his innovative medical activities, Perlstein had many hobbies, chief among them fishing and lapidary. He collected a great variety of semi-precious stones, which he cut or engraved for his collection or for articles of jewelry. He was an expert fisherman and, with his wife, Minnie Perlstein, a professor of dermatology, he fished the rivers, lakes, and oceans of the world. Even when he went whaling off New Zealand, he remembered his medical interests and brought back the tongue of a whale to the speech department and the cochlea to the otorhinolaryngology department of Northwestern University Medical School. On another occasion, before an 8 a.m. session of a medical meeting in a seacoast town, a colleague noted that Meyer had already been deep-sea fishing that morning, caught several fish and arranged with the hotel chef to cook the catch for his friends for dinner that night. Perlstein's knowledge of literature, art, and music was profound; he could hum accurately through many a complete symphony or concert with little effort. Remarkably for one so busy, Perlstein was never angry: He had no time or place for rancor in his full life (Boshes, 1970).

Perlstein was an imposing and memorable figure, rather obese, but much more energetic than many of his slimmer colleagues. His enthusiastic teaching was enlivened by a retentive memory that never ceased to amaze his students and colleagues. His white lab coat was often crookedly buttoned, and he had a habit of polishing his eyeglasses on his necktie. For his patients, he was a charming and confident examiner. He had a very wide and enthusiastic following and was among the first to recognize the need for interdisciplinary cooperation in meeting the total needs of the neurologically impaired child. He was effective in leading discussions and had a special flair for spontaneously generating pithy and witty phrases, which he often used as capstones to terminate a discussion succinctly. Concerning the effectiveness of an experimental drug on motor behavior, he said, "Although an urgent need of this country may be a good five-cent cigar, what the medical profession needs is a good, long-acting placebo." He also noted that "a pediatrician is a doctor caring for everybody who will be, who has become, or who has been a child" (Boshes, 1970).

Perlstein was a master clinician and teacher, and the comprehensive knowledge he acquired was freely given. For twenty-two years he gave a personalized two-week course in neuromuscular diseases under the auspices of the Cook County Hospital Graduate School of Medicine. Many physicians from the United States and a number of other countries considered the course to be an important influence in redirecting their professional lives (Swinyard, 1970).

With his interest in the interdisciplinary approach to chronic neurologic afflictions of childhood, Perlstein was able to provide care to a very large number of children with cerebral palsy. In a retrospective study of his patients presented in 1965, he reported on over five thousand patients whom he had personally treated (Perlstein and Hood, 1966).

In his presidential address at the American Academy of Cerebral Palsy meeting in 1954, Perlstein noted the transformation that had occurred in the previous fifteen years from relatively few children with cerebral palsy receiving care to the plethora of new services and facilities that had been developed at that time (Perlstein,

1956b). Many of the gains in evaluation and treatment of children with cerebral palsy over the previous thirty years have been through the tireless efforts of Meyer Perlstein as a clinician, teacher, administrative leader, and humanitarian.

Charles N. Swisher
CHICAGO, ILLINOIS

ACKNOWLEDGMENTS

The personal reminiscences of Drs. Louis Boshes, Benjamin Kagan, and Irving Rozenfeld are gratefully appreciated.

REFERENCES

Boshes, L. D. 1970. Meyer A. Perlstein, 1902–1969. *Proc Inst Med Chicago* 28:35–37.

Brandt, S. 1977. The Parentage of Child Neurology. In *Topics in Child Neurology*, 3–7. Ed. M. Blaw, I. Rapin, and M. Kinsbourne. New York: Book Division of Spectrum Publications.

Perlstein, M. A. 1927. Pygopagus Twins. *Arch Path Lab Med* 3:171–92.

______. 1946. Tridione: A New Experimental Drug. *Arch Neur Psych* 55:164–65.

______. 1950. Gemonil. *Ped* 5:448–51.

______. 1956a. Obituary. Abraham Levinson. *Bull Inst Med Chicago* 21:80–82.

______. 1956b. Expanding Horizons in Cerebral Palsy. *Am J Phys Med* 55:135–43.

Perlstein, M. A., and H. E. Barnett. 1952. Nature and Recognition of Cerebral Palsy in Infancy. *JAMA* 148:1389–97.

Perlstein, M. A., and P. N. Hood. 1966. Type and Etiology of Congenital Cerebral Palsy. *Dev Med Child Neur* 8:101

Swinyard, C. 1970. Unpublished eulogy.

JOHN STOBO PRICHARD

JOHN STOBO PRICHARD (1914–1986) (figure 1), one of the pioneers of pediatric neurology in Canada, was born in Barry, Wales. Educated at Clifton Preparatory School and College and then at Cambridge, he completed his medical undergraduate training at the London Hospital.

He had a distinguished career in the British Army during World War II, serving for six years with the armored divisions on the desert, as well as in Italy, France, Holland, and Germany. He was awarded the Military Cross for bravery, as he jokingly dismissed it, "by getting mixed up with a bunch of tanks." Just before the war, Prichard married Joan Suzanne Webber, daughter of Sir Robert John Webber. Joan Prichard was also active in the war effort and was decorated for organizing and operating two hundred government-owned restaurants in Wales to insure that workers had an adequate basic diet, in spite of the heavy rationing prevalent at the time.

After the war, Prichard trained in neurology at the National Hospital, Queen's Square, and at Hammersmith Hospital. The Prichards came to Boston in 1949, into the heady atmosphere of the Massachusetts General Hospital, where Stobo worked with Robert Schwab, mainly on Parkinson disease.

In 1950 Prichard accepted a position at the Hospital for Sick Children in Toronto. After the war, the emphasis in Canada shifted from neuropsychiatry to the expanding specialty of neurology. A number of British senior registrars came over at that time to play a major role in the development of neurology in medical centers from coast to coast. Among them was Henry Dunn, who is known as the father of pediatric neurology in British Columbia. In Toronto Prichard worked with William Hawke, who at that time was associate head of neurology and head of psychiatry, social work, speech pathology and psychology at the Hospital for Sick Children, formerly the College Street Hospital. Hawke succeeded William Baracclough as head of neurology in 1952 and was the last of the neuropsychiatrists at this hospital.

Prichard threw himself into development of neurology at Sick

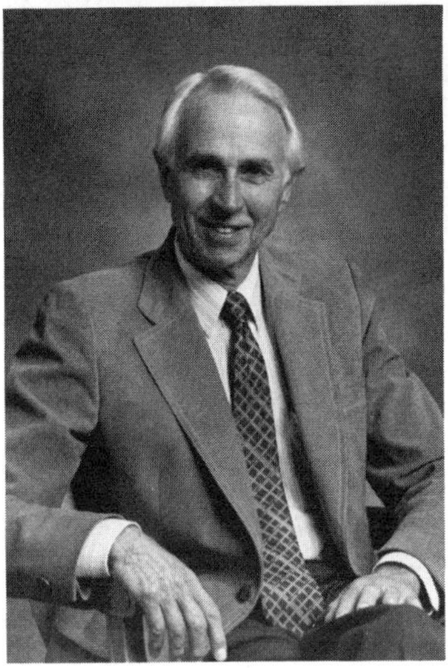

Figure 1. John Stobo Prichard (1914–1986) in 1984 when he was elected to emeritus membership of the Child Neurology Society.

Children's with characteristic enthusiasm. He found the work environment there something of a paradox: despite primitive working conditions, it was a very pleasant place. Lunch was served in a small, warm room; at that time, the staff was still an intimate family. Prichard's office was nothing more than a bedroom furnished with a few hard chairs and a simple desk. In 1951 he opened the EEG lab. A man with many skills, he did his own arteriograms, myelograms, and pneumoencephalograms.

Prichard recalled clearly the first patient he saw at the Hospital for Sick Children. A baby was brought to the hospital and testing suggested the presence of a brain tumor. When a stethoscope was held to the child's head, a loud murmur could be heard. William Keith, chief of neurosurgery at the time, performed an operation that revealed a large arteriovenous malformation, probably associated with an aneurysm of the vein of Galen.

Prichard was captivated by pediatric neurology and proceeded to attract capable and enthusiastic colleagues, such as Douglas McGreal and Edward Murphy, as well as an ever-increasing number of residents and fellows from all over the world.

Prichard succeeded Hawke as chief of neurology and, during his tenure, many important contributions originated in his department (Hawke and Prichard, 1957). Prichard himself was a pioneer in the study and treatment of epilepsy in children. His contributions in this area include publications on the significance of seizures in infancy and adulthood (Prichard, 1964, 1974), the prognostic value of the EEG in neonatal seizures (Tibbles and Prichard, 1965), breath holding spells (Gauk, Kidd, and Prichard, 1963), abdominal epilepsy (Prichard, 1958), febrile seizures (Prichard and McGreal, 1958), seizures due to toxic encephalopathies (Gordon, Prichard and Freedman, 1973), the EEG in Aicardi's syndrome (Fariello et al, 1977), and episodic coma associated with seizures (Norman, Prichard, and Harwood-Nash, 1973). His colleague, Douglas McGreal, studied the syndrome of epileptic aphasia and Simon Verret and John Steele delineated alternating hemiplegia of infancy. Prichard carefully fostered the development of neuroscience, appointing Sandy Lowden, Flavio Coceani, John Callaghan, and Cecil Pace Asciak, all brilliant neurochemists trained by Leon Wolfe at the Montreal Neurological Institute. His interest in learning disabilities led to the development of a research program that became a model for the province of Ontario. His interest in child education was reflected in a series of health books written for children in grades six through nine that were used throughout Canada as standard text books (Prichard, 1967–69).

The Provincial Ministries of Health, of Community and Social Sciences, and of Education in Ontario frequently sought Prichard's opinion and assistance in the development of programs covering matters as diverse as special education and mercury poisoning of native peoples in the North. He took on these tasks with enthusiasm, cajoling his colleagues into helping and thereby accomplishing much good that can never be uncovered in a simple reading of his curriculum vitae.

Prichard was deeply interested in fostering pediatric neurology in developing countries. He organized an exchange program with the University of the West Indies and with Thailand and was an enthusiastic participant. He and his wife traveled widely and had many friends and disciples among the pediatric neurologists of Australia, Czechoslovakia, India, Indonesia, Poland, Russia, Yugoslavia, and Japan.

Prichard was a founding member of the International Child Neurology Association and served as its first president from 1973 to 1975, when the first International Congress of Child Neurology was held in Toronto. Attended by more than 750 pediatric neurologists from around the world, the Congress gave the seal of authenticity to the specialty of pediatric neurology.

The Prichards were justifiably proud of their children. Jane is now Professor and Chairman of Sociology in the Faculty of Education at the University of British Columbia, Sarah is an associate professor of medicine and Service Chief in the Department of Medicine at the Royal Victoria Hospital at McGill University, and Robert is President Designate of the University of Toronto.

Prichard died in 1986. Douglas McGreal, his long-time friend and associate, remembers him as an excellent neurologist and clinician and, most of all, as a very warm and understanding person, attributes rather hard to find in these days of cascading, impersonal technological advances. His comments and questions at grand rounds, whatever the topic, indicated the breadth of his understanding and interest. He was a splendid teacher of both undergraduate and postgraduate students. His flair for the dramatic and his understanding of the mind of the young helped him in capturing their attention and emphasizing the important. Despite a stammer, he was an excellent orator, capable of holding a large audience enthralled through his gift for simplifying the difficult, rationalizing the detail, and utilizing his wealth of experience in solving complicated problems.

"No bubble is so iridescent or floats longer than that blown by the successful teacher" (Osler).

Fred Andermann
MONTREAL, CANADA

REFERENCES

Fariello, R. G., et al. 1977. EEG Recognition of Aicardi's Syndrome. *Arch Neur* 34(9):563–66.

Gauk, E. W., L. Kidd, and J. S. Prichard. 1963. Mechanism of Seizure Associated with Breath-Holding Spells. *NEJM* 268:1436.

Gordon, A. S., J.S. Prichard, and M. H. Freedman. 1973. Seizure Disorders and Anemia Associated with Chronic Borax Intoxication. *Can Med Assoc J* 108(6):719–21.

Hawke, W. A., and J. S. Prichard. 1957. Neurologic Disease in Infancy and Childhood. *Ped* 19:949–57.

Norman, M. G., J. S. Prichard, and D. C. Harwood-Nash. 1973. Episodic Seizures and Coma in a 14–Year-Old-Boy. *J Ped* 83:494–98.

Prichard, J. S. 1958. Abdominal Pain of Cerebral Origin in Children. *Can Med Assoc J* 78:665.

______. 1964. The Character and Significance of Epileptic Seizures in Infancy. In *Neurologic and Encephalographic Correlative Studies in Infancy,* 273–86. Ed. P. Kellaway and I. Petersen. New York: Grune and Stratton.

______. 1967–69. *Health Science and You.* Volumes 1–4. Toronto: Holt, Rinehart and Winston.

______. 1974. Convulsive Disorders in Children: Some Notes on the Diagnosis and Treatment. (Review). *Ped Clin North Am* 21(4):981–89.

Prichard, J. S., and D. A. McGreal. 1958. Febrile Convulsions. *Med Clin North Am* 42:379–87.

Tibbles, J. A. R., and J. S. Prichard. 1965. The Prognostic Value of the EEG in Neonatal Convulsions. *Ped* 35:778–86.

ANDREAS RETT

OVER THIRTY-FIVE YEARS AGO, Andreas Rett (b. 1924) (figure 1) began to work with the handicapped in Vienna. He was the first, and for many years the only, physician who cared for their problems. At that time, the handicapped were socially ostracized, and Rett lost a pediatric position because he persisted in seeing handicapped children in his clinic. Rett is now recognized as a pioneer in the care of mentally and physically handicapped children in Austria. At the time, Rett's unpopular interest led to difficulties with the medical establishment but ultimately resulted in national and international recognition of this hard-working and dedicated physician. In the words of Kathy Hunter, president of the International Rett Syndrome Association, "Andreas Rett is a charming, charismatic, loving and sensitive man. Although not highly valued in academic medicine, these characteristics are invaluable in the care of patients."

A combination of clinical acumen and lifelong dedication to the needs of brain-damaged children were the two key ingredients that resulted in the discovery of Rett syndrome in 1965. In Rett's own words,

One day in the spring of 1965, two mothers holding their children on their

laps were sitting in the waiting room. Both children were swaying and the mothers held their arms. Both children, who were treated for epileptic seizures, were well known to me. That morning I passed by them repeatedly and, incidentally, the mothers let go of their children's arms. At once, the children put their hands together and started nearly identically-looking washing movements. I asked the mothers not to stop these movements again, and was startled at the similarities. It was the same gaze, same facial expression, same weak muscles and the same stereotyped movements of their hands. Moreover, they were both females. At first, I was amazed by this enormous coincidence and thought I must have come across several other children with these symptoms. I asked my head nurse to look at these children and she immediately recalled some more names of children who behaved similarly. We invited them, placed them next to each other and found that all of them showed the same kinds of movements. Further, all patients were female. (Rett, unpublished letter to the Rett Syndrome Association, June 7, 1985)

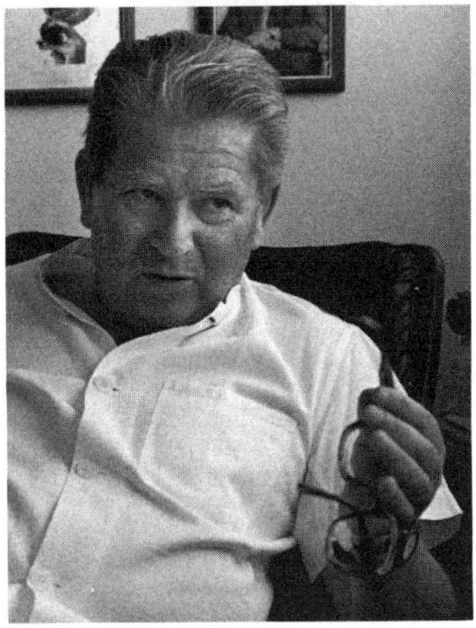

Figure 1. Andreas Rett in his office at the Ludwig Boltzmann Institute in Vienna.

The original publication of Rett's observations, which characterized the stereotyped degenerative neurological disease that now bears his name, appeared in 1966 in the Austrian medical newsletter, *Wiener Medizinische Wochenshrift* (Rett, 1966). This clinical paper, like most of Andreas Rett's publications, was not widely circulated and remained unnoticed in the English-speaking world. Realizing the limitations of publishing in the German literature alone and having become convinced that his syndrome was a discrete entity, Rett, at his own expense, prepared a film and a booklet, "A Special Kind of Atrophy," carrying it to pediatric meetings throughout Europe. The first English description of Rett syndrome appeared in the *Handbook of Clinical Neurology* (Rett, 1977) but it was Bengt Hagberg's article in the *Annals of Neurology* in 1983 that brought Rett syndrome to the attention of English-speaking neurologists (Hagberg et al, 1983). The historical significance of Rett's earlier descriptions was acknowledged in this paper.

In spite of a heavy clinical load, Rett had published 267 articles at the time of this writing. This impressive contribution to the literature is largely in German, beginning in 1951 with topics of general pediatric interest but as early as 1953 focusing on epilepsy and the diagnosis and treatment of childhood neurological conditions (Rett, 1953, 1980). In more recent years, a focus on chromosomal causes of handicapping conditions led to a number of publications on diagnosis and management of chromosomal abnormalities (Rett, 1983). Other publications have also included discussion of socially important issues such as genetic counseling (Rett, 1982).

Rett was born on January 2, 1924, in Fürth, Bavaria, and attended elementary and high school in Innsbruck. He began medical school at the University of Innsbruck, having achieved honors in the comprehensive examinations. Soon after starting medical school he was drafted into the navy but was released the next year following two injuries. In 1945 he resumed his medical studies at the University of Innsbruck and was granted his doctorate of medicine in 1949. In 1950 he moved to Vienna and began his pediatric specialist training, working as a visiting physician at the Preyersches Kinderspital, Vienna. In 1951 he studied at the University Kinderklinik in Zurich under Guido Fanconi. In 1952 he married his wife, Jutta, who is also a physician. Following neurological training with Walter Birkmayer, Rett qualified as a pediatric specialist in 1955 and soon afterward was appointed head physician of a section for developmentally retarded children in Altersheim Lainz, Austria.

Rett's contribution to the community was recognized when he received the Karl Renner Award for social services to the city of Vienna, the highest distinction awarded in Austria for social welfare activities. Following this award, his clinic became more widely known and attracted many more handicapped children:

At that time we were rather inadequately lodged in a 70–year-old building belonging to an institution for aged people with very few nurses and physicians and no water faucets in the sick bays. Within a few years, however, this clinic developed into a center for the handicapped in Austria and, sub-

sequently, we obtained more research funds, adequate staff and the first EEG machine and the first clinical psychologist in the state hospital in Austria. (Rett, personal communication)

In 1962 Rett received the Adolf Scharf Award for scientific study of the relation between early birth and brain damage. By 1965, the year of his discovery of Rett syndrome, he had produced more than 150 publications and was caring for more than five thousand handicapped patients.

In 1967 the earlier years of hard work bore fruit. Rett was awarded the Anton von Eiselsberg Award for the discovery of a brain atrophy syndrome (Rett syndrome). He was inaugurated at the University of Vienna as a university lecturer in neurology and pediatrics and was appointed director of the Ludwig Boltzmann Institute for Research on Brain Damage in Children. He was also appointed chief of the Section for Brain Damaged Children in the Austrian Pediatric Society.

Rett's focus on therapy led him to explore and publish extensively on this topic. He advocated the use of music therapy for mentally retarded individuals and found this to be helpful in treating Rett syndrome. In 1970 he became director of a school for music therapy.

Rett became an associate professor at the University of Vienna in 1973, and in 1977 became an associate member of the German Society for Child Psychiatry. A number of awards followed, including the Gold Medal of Honor from the city of Vienna in 1984 and the Ernst v. Bergmann Medal for continuing education of German physicians in 1986. Since 1983 Rett has participated in many international publications on Rett syndrome and has been an invited speaker annually at the International Symposia on Rett Syndrome, which have been held around the world. In 1989 Rett received the Distinguished Research Award from the Association of Retarded Citizens of the United States.

Open heart surgery in 1986 and a recent stroke have not quelled Andreas Rett's enthusiasm. He continues an active practice caring for pediatric neurology patients.

Richard H. Haas
SAN DIEGO, CALIFORNIA

REFERENCES

Hagberg, B., et al. 1983. A Progressive Syndrome of Autism, Dementia, Ataxia, and Loss of Purposeful Hand Use in Girls: Rett's Syndrome: Report of 35 Cases. *Ann Neur* 14(4):471–78.

Rett, A. 1953. Epileptischer Anfall und vegetatives Nervensystem. *Arztl Wschr Berlin* 49S: 1174.

______. 1966. Über ein eigenartiges hirnatrophes Syndrom bei Hyperammonaemie im Kindesalter. *Wien med Wschr* 116:723–26.

______. 1977. Cerebral Atrophy Associated with Hyperammonaemia. In *Handbook of Clinical Neurology*. Vol. 29: *Metabolic and Deficiency Diseases of the Nervous System*, 305–29. Ed. P. J. Vinken and G. W. Bruyn. Amsterdam: North Holland.

______. 1980. Das Anfallskind in Familie und Schule. *Mschr Kinderheilk* 128(5):365–69.

______. 1982. Über die Bedeutung der Humangenetik in der Behindertenbetreuung. *Wien klin Wschr* 94(12):315–17.

______. 1983. *Mongolismus — Biologische, erzieherische und soziale Aspekte. 2. ergänzte u. überarb. Aufl.* Bern: H. Huber.

DOUGLAS REYE

RALPH DOUGLAS KENNETH REYE (1912–1977) (figure 1) was born in Townsville, Queensland, Australia, the youngest of seven children of Albert and Mabel Reye (Bale, 1988). His father had emigrated from Ottendorf, Germany, to Australia in 1883. After receiving a B.S. degree from Sydney University in 1937, Reye attended St. Paul's College, Sydney University, for his medical education and obtained an M.D. degree in 1945. Less than a year after graduation he joined the staff of the Royal Alexandra Hospital for Children in Sydney as resident pathologist, where he would remain for the next thirty years (Emery, 1978). In 1941 he was appointed acting director and, in 1946, director of the Institute of Pathology, Royal Alexandra Hospital for Children, a post he retained until his retirement in 1977 (Alexander, 1978).

Between 1940 and 1977 Reye contributed at least thirty-one

publications (seventeen of these as first author) on various pathology topics about which little or no information was then available (Emery, 1978). Initially he was the only pathologist at the institute responsible for histopathology, hematology, bacteriology, and biochemistry, but as additional staff became available, Reye concentrated on histopathology, with a special interest in the nervous system. In 1951 he encountered an unusual case of cerebral edema and fatty liver, and by 1962 he had collected twenty additional cases, which, in collaboration with Graeme Morgan and James Baral, were reported in *Lancet* on October 12, 1963, under the title "Encephalopathy and Fatty Degeneration of the Viscera: An Entity in Childhood" (Reye, Morgan, and Baral, 1963).

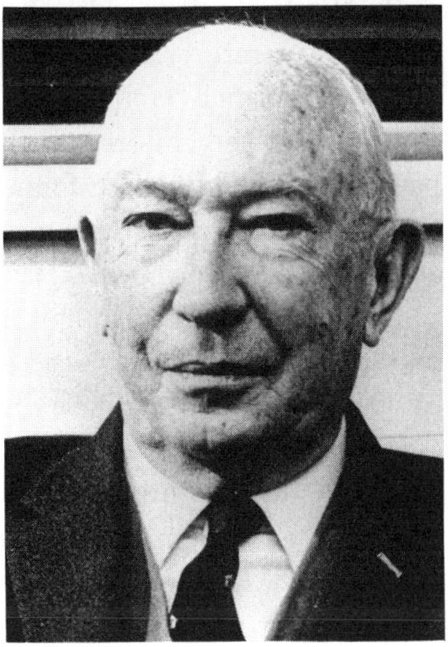

Figure 1. Douglas Reye (1912–1977).

The outstanding clinical features in Reye's cases were profoundly disturbed consciousness, fever, convulsions, vomiting, disturbed respiratory rhythm, altered muscle tone, and altered reflexes. The encephalopathy was preceded by a prodromal illness, usually manifested by cough, rhinorrhea, sore throat, or earache, and lasting from one day to three weeks. Neurologic symptoms predominated, and on admission all but two of the patients were already in stupor or coma. Nearly half of the patients had a period of delirium prior to admission, and in eight patients this was observed some time afterward. Seventeen patients had seizures, which were usually difficult to control and described as focal twitching and tetanic spasms. Twenty cases had abnormal respiratory rhythm, with hyperpnea and irregular respirations being the most common abnormalities. Sixteen patients had increased or variable tone and tendon reflexes. The plantar responses were abnormal or equivocal in half of the group. In seven patients a characteristic posture was observed with elbows flexed, legs extended, and the hands clenched (decorticate posturing). Pertinent laboratory findings included hyperammoniemia, prolonged prothrombin time, hypoglycemia, elevated transaminases, and normal cerebrospinal fluid except for hypoglycorrhachia. Seventeen of the children died, and at autopsy remarkable uniform pathologic changes were found in the form of cerebral edema and fatty changes in the liver, kidneys, and other viscera (Reye, Morgan, and Baral, 1963).

Reye regarded the changes in the liver as "degeneration," according to Virchow's classic concept that degeneration was represented by microvesicular changes, while infiltration appeared morphically as macrovesicular fatty deposits. Although Reye was aware of previous sporadic reports of cases that resembled his experience, he was certain that similar cases had not come to autopsy at the Royal Alexandra Hospital in the preceding ten years. Detailed reviews of the literature, although revealing individual reports of similar cases usually associated with varicella or chronic salicylate therapy, failed to disclose any similar outbreaks until those reported by Reye in Australia and S. E. Johnson in North Carolina (Johnson, Scurletis, and Caroll, 1963). Reye syndrome, as the disorder was soon known throughout the world, was the most common acute encephalopathy in children during the 1960s and 1970s. Electron microscopic studies of liver and brain showed morphologic abnormalities in mitochondria, and numerous investigators searched for a toxic factor that could explain the toxic changes found in brain and liver of these patients. Among those investigated experimentally and epidemiologically were ammonia, aflatoxins, short-chain fatty acids, medications including salicylates, acetaminophen, and phenothiazines — all without convincing proof (Chaves-Carballo, 1978). Other reports associated Reye syndrome with influenza B activity and with decreased ornithine transcarbamylase activity. In the early 1980s, attention once more focused on the possible relation with salicylates when case control studies from Arizona, Michigan, and Ohio reported statistically significant excess risk of Reye syndrome in association with ingestion of salicylates during antecedent varicella and respiratory illnesses. The U. S. surgeon general in 1982 advised against giving salicylates to children with influenza or chicken pox. A Public Health Service task force was then formed to design and implement a new epidemiologic study concerning the nature of the possible relationship between Reye syndrome and medications. A pilot study conducted between February and March 1984 and published in 1985 indicated that significantly more cases (93 percent) than controls (46 percent) received salicylates (Hurwitz et al, 1985).

Subsequent epidemiologic studies showed decline in the use of salicylates and in the number of reported cases of Reye syndrome. Whether these events were directly related remains controversial. Reye syndrome has become a rare disorder, and most cases seen recently are due to mitrochondrial inborn errors of metabolism. Reye syndrome, like poliomyelitis before it, helped to write an important chapter in the history of child neurology.

Reye authored four additional papers on neurological topics: Guillain-Barré syndrome (Reye, 1954), posterior fossa cysts (Schreiber and Reye, 1954), cerebrospinal fluid physiology (Reye, 1957), and subacute necrotizing encephalomyelopathy (Reye, 1960). Reye was also well-known among Australian pathologists for his description of subdermal fibrous hamartomas (Reye, 1956) and digital fibrous tumors (Reye, 1965), known by his colleagues as "Reyeoma I" and "Reyeoma II," respectively (Bale, 1988).

As the eponym appeared more frequently in the medical literature, opinion varied regarding the correct pronunciation, prompting two journal editors to request clarification (Weech, 1972; Conn, 1975). Reye replied by quoting one of his teachers in medical school, who had said: "Eye is I, so surely Reye is Rye." He thought such inquiries were "much ado about nothing."

Reye was described as "essentially shy and retiring and like many such people he gave the wrongful impression of being aloof" (Conn, 1975). A colleague comments further:

If one had any criticism of him it would be that his shyness tended to keep those registrars and residents who did not know him well, apart from him. Thus, they in turn lost the advantage of partaking of his tremendous knowledge of paediatrics, not knowing how keen he was to share his experience with them. To those who knew him well, not only was he extremely helpful in his advice but on a personal level a delightful friend with his own brand of whimsical humor. As regards hobbies, Douglas showed great interest in his garden and, in particular, had a love for tropical trees and plants. . . . He was a very keen reader and his other interest was motor cars. (Alexander, 1978)

Reye died on July 16, 1977, at age sixty-five, after a very short illness and less than twenty-four hours after his retirement as director of the Institute of Pathology.

Enrique Chaves-Carballo
NORFOLK, VIRGINIA

REFERENCES

Alexander, J. M. 1978. Obituary. Ralph Douglas Kenneth Reye. *Aust Paed J* 14:48.

Bale, P. 1988. Personal communication.

Chaves-Carballo, E. 1978. Epidemiology of Reye Syndrome. In *Neurological Epidemiology*, 231–47. Ed. R. S. Schoenberg. New York: Raven Press.

Conn, H. O. 1975. Reye or Reye, Agar or Agar, MacKay or MacKay? *Gastroent* 69:778–79.

Emery, J. L. 1978. Obituary. Ralph Douglas Kenneth Reye. *Lancet* 1:111.

Hurwitz, E. S., et al. 1985. Public Health Service Study on Reye's Syndrome and Medications. Report of the Pilot Phase. *NEJM* 313:849–57.

Johnson, G. M., T. D. Scurletis, and N. B. Carroll. 1963. A Study of Sixteen Fatal Cases of Encephalitis-like Disease in North Carolina Children. *NC Med J* 24:646.

Reye, R. D. K. 1954. The Neuropathology of the Landry-Guillain-Barré Syndrome. *Med J Aust* 2:386–88.

______. 1956. Considerations of Certain Subdermal Fibromatous Tumours of Infancy. *J Path Bact* 72:149–54.

______. 1957. Some Recent Concepts of the Physiology of the Cerebrospinal Fluid. *Med J Aust* 2:637–39.

______. 1960. Subacute Necrotizing Encephalomyelopathy. *J Path Bact* 79:165–73.

______. 1965. Recurring Digital Fibrous Tumors of Childhood. *Arch Path* 80:228–31.

Reye, R. D. K., G. Morgan, and J. Baral. 1963. Encephalopathy and Fatty Degeneration of the Viscera: A Disease Entity in Childhood. *Lancet* 2:749–52.

Schreiber, M. S., and R. D. K. Reye. 1954. Posterior Fossa Cysts Due to Congenital Atresia of the Foramina of Luschka and Magendie. *Med J Aust* 2:743–48.

Weech, A. A. 1972. Relatively Irrelevant Editorial Notation. *Am J Dis Child* 124:833.

JAMES PRESTON ROBB

FEW WOULD DENY that the man who established pediatric neurology in Quebec was James Preston Robb (figure 1). Born in 1914, the son of Joseph Doig Robb and Janie McLeod Preston, Robb took pride in a trace of Indian blood. One of his ancestors was Thayendanegea (Joseph Brant), the Mohawk chief who commanded the Iroquois forces allied with the British in the American Revolutionary War. The influence of Robb's parents lasted a lifetime; throughout his career, his father's photograph always graced his office.

Robb studied medicine at McGill University, graduating in 1939. While at the university, he played on the Canadian intercollegiate football championship team. The team skills he learned in the Molson stadium stood him in good stead years later, perhaps contributing to his outstanding abilities as captain of the rehabilitation group he created at the Montreal Children's Hospital.

Robb interned at the Montreal General Hospital and the Verdun Protestant Hospital and then joined the Royal Canadian Navy, serving overseas and then at a base in Montreal. In response to Dr. Wilder Penfield's urgent request, Robb was recommended to the Montreal Neurological Hospital. This experience sealed his fate, propelling him into a career in neurology and prompting him to return there at the end of the war. An extended tour of American pediatric neurological centers took him to Johns Hopkins, where he spent some time with Frank Ford, whose clinical skills he greatly admired, and to Boston, where he worked with Richmond Paine and Randolph Byers. He also studied neuropathology, speech pathology, and neurophysiology at the Montefiore, Massachusetts General, and Johns Hopkins Hospitals. Upon his return to Quebec, he set to work at the Montreal Children's Hospital and the Montreal Neurological Institute.

The Montreal Children's Hospital was founded by Harold Cushing. In Robb's time, it was led first by the distinguished and flamboyant Alton Goldbloom, and then by the serious and devoted Alan Ross. The Hospital's first neurological consultant was Arthur W. Young, an excellent clinician and a kind man, who began rounds so early

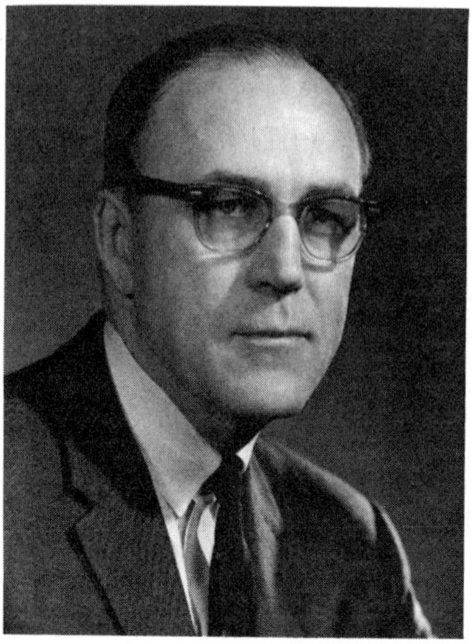

Figure 1. Preston Robb while he was neurologist-in-chief at the Montreal Neurological Institute.

in the morning that, by eight o'clock when most people started, he was gone. Young was succeeded by Francis McNaughton, who was to become McGill's first professor of neurology. A lifelong friend to Robb, McNaughton was a man of extraordinary gentleness and legendary kindness. If anyone could be called a neurologist's neurologist, it was Francis McNaughton. Upon Robb's return to Montreal, McNaughton devoted all his time to the Neurological Institute and Preston took over the work at Children's.

Initially, Robb provided consultation services only at Children's; patients who needed complex investigations or surgery were transferred to the Neurological Institute. However, in the late fifties, a resident in neurology was allotted to Children's and a true neurological service opened. Robb made rounds Monday, Wednesday, and Friday, from eight to nine. He was punctual, decisive, and his clinical judgment was phenomenal. Like many great pediatric neurologists, he obtained most of his information by watching children at play and interacting with their games. He was extraordinarily fond of children and they responded in kind, undaunted by the imposing, stern exterior known to intimidate cocky residents and obstreperous sailors alike. I joined Robb's service at the Montreal Children's Hospital in 1961. He was for me, as for generations of trainees from all over the world, a role model of rectitude and fairness. As well, he was a magnificent teacher, always nurturing independent thought and supporting initiative.

Cerebral palsy was a common problem during the years Robb was in practice. Accordingly, he developed a cerebral palsy conference staffed by a formidable team of occupational therapists, physiotherapists, speech therapists, orthopedic surgeons, social workers, psychiatrists, special education teachers, and psychologists. Robb was a magnet; he attracted the finest members of these professions to his group and they formed a dynamic, loyal team around their captain. The cerebral palsy conference at the Montreal Children's Hospital served for many years as a model for centers across Canada and abroad.

As for research, Robb did work in language localization, initially with Wilder Penfield (Robb, 1946), whom he held in high regard (Robb, 1977), and wrote about neurological complications of pregnancy, motor disability and various pediatric neurological problems (Andermann and Robb, 1972; Joubert et al, 1986). Above all, he pursued a lifelong interest in epilepsy.

In 1964, when he felt confident that he could leave the service to his junior associate without too much danger, he followed the call of his friend, Richard Masland, to the National Institutes of Health (NIH) in Bethesda. After a stint there, he travelled extensively, surveying facilities for the treatment of epilepsy across the United States and Canada. These travels culminated in a volume on the epidemiology of epilepsy entitled *Epilepsy: A Review of Basic and Clinical Research* (Robb, 1965), which was later updated (Robb, 1974). Robb pioneered the cooperative epilepsy studies launched by the NIH. Other members of the initial epilepsy study group were Dick Schmidt, Phil White, Fritz Dreyfuss, Kiffin Penry, and Herb Carp. This endeavor resulted in definitive studies on absence seizures by Dreyfuss and Penry. The centers of excellence for the treatment of epilepsy eventually created in Portland, Minneapolis, and Charlottesville, were also built on the foundation Robb helped to lay.

Returning from his travels to Montreal once more, Robb worked as director of hospitalization and chief of service at the Montreal Neurological Institute and continued his activities at the Children's Hospital. In 1970, however, he left Children's to devote all his time to the Neurological Institute, succeeding McNaughton as neurologist-in-chief and professor of neurology. His work at Children's is commemorated by an annual lectureship and research day established in his honor by his successor at the Hospital, Gordon Watters.

Robb recruited his staff wisely. George Karpati, Allan Sherwin, Andrew Eisen, Ivan Woods, Michel Aubé, Eva Andermann, and many others flourished under his guidance and support. He greatly admired the work of Julius and Kay Metrakos on the genetics of epilepsy and, in this area, he was also most supportive. Robb's own genetic counseling might today be considered somewhat brusque. When the parents of a child with an acquired problem would ask whether they should contemplate having other children, he would gruffly respond, "You shouldn't be asking me questions like this, you should be home in bed."

Robb was greatly concerned about the creation, in underdeveloped countries, of treatment facilities for epilepsy and other neurological disorders. He trained many neurologists from Africa, Asia, and South America and, toward the end of his career, served as visiting professor at the University of Nairobi. His exposure to the hurdles that must be overcome before epilepsy can be effectively treated in Third World nations, left an indelible impression. Upon his return to Canada, he wrote a practical text on the subject for paramedics and other health workers, which has since been translated into Chinese, Spanish, and Portuguese. His papers were a model of style and always to the point (Sherwin and Robb, 1972; Robb, 1975).

Robb was one of the founders of the American Academy of Neurology and of the Canadian Neurological Society. He was elected president of the latter, as well as of the American Epilepsy Society. He later received the William G. Lennox Award. He became chairman and medical advisor to many organizations, among them the YMCA Camp Board, the Canadian Rehabilitation Council for the Disabled, the US Public Health Service Advisory Committee on the Epilepsies, the Presidential Advisory Board of the Epilepsy Foundation of America, the Advisory Board of the Quebec Cerebral Palsy Association, and the Constance Lethbridge Rehabilitation Centre.

Robb was an example to his juniors in many ways, none more so than in his family life. His marriage to Mary Waller is a particularly happy one. Mary had been a head nurse at the Montreal General Hospital. Beautiful, kind, warm, and endowed with faultless social judgement, she eased her husband's heavy workload and helped generations of foreign neurological trainees and their families adapt to North American ways. They have four children, David, Christopher, Bruce, and Allison. Although Robb never seemed quite certain about the role of women in medicine, the eventual addition to the family of a physician daughter-in-law seemed to tip the scales in a favorable direction. Sociable and friendly, a droll raconteur, Robb complements his wife and is a wonderful host.

In 1982 Robb was made professor emeritus of neurology at McGill. He had always said that he did not want to be under-foot when he retired as neurologist-in-chief. True to his word, upon retirement he moved to Lyn, Ontario, near Brockville, where he embarked on a second highly successful career as chairman of the board of Joseph Robb and Company (Robco), a corporation his father founded and, at last, has time to enjoy his hobbies of tree farming and woodcarving. Always fascinated by the history of his specialty, Robb has recently completed a volume chronicling neurology at McGill.

With his colleagues, John Stobo Prichard in Toronto, and Henry Dunn in Vancouver, Preston Robb laid a solid foundation in Canada for the care of children with neurological disabilities, for the teaching of future generations, and for the study of epilepsy in North America.

During the long and satisfying years of our collaboration, I came to appreciate deeply two attitudes that set Preston Robb apart. The first was his desire to understand the cultural and emotional background of his patients, often so different from his own. This, he sensed, determined their reaction to neurological disability in themselves and their loved ones. The second was his insistence that the physician do everything possible to create an environment where patients and families were able to maintain their dignity while coping with the dreadful hurdles life placed in their path.

Fred Andermann
MONTREAL, CANADA

ACKNOWLEDGMENTS

I thank Victoria Lees for her helpful comments on this text.

REFERENCES

Andermann, F., and J. P. Robb. 1972. Absence Status. A Reappraisal Following Review of Thirty-eight Patients. *Epilepsia* 13(1):177–87.

Joubert, M., et al. 1986. Familial Agenesis of the Cerebellar Vermis. A Syndrome of Episodic Hyperpnea, Abnormal Eye Movements, Ataxia, and Retardation. *Neur* 19(9):813–25.

Robb, J. P. 1946. A Study of the Effect of Cortical Excision on Speech in Patients with Previous Cerebral Injuries. McGill University MSc thesis.

______. 1965. *Epilepsy: A Review of Basic and Clinical Research. (NINDB Monograph, No. 1).* Bethesda: National Institute of Neurological Diseases and Blindness.

______. 1974. The Epidemiology of Epilepsy. In The *Epilepsies*. Ed. O. Magnus and A. M. Lorentz de Haas. Amsterdam: North Holland Press.

______. 1975. Focal Epilepsy: The Problem, Prevalence, and Contributing Factors. In *Neurosurgical Management of the Epilepsies*. Vol. 8. *Advances in Neurology*. New York: Raven Press.

______. 1977. Wilder Penfield: His Legacy to Neurology. The Institute and Hospital. *Can Med Assoc J* 116:1368.

Sherwin, A. L., and J. P. Robb. 1972. Ethosuximide: Relation of Plasma Levels to Clinical Control (Continued). In *Antiepileptic Drugs*, 443–48. Ed. D. M. Woodbury, J. K. Penry, and R. P. Schmidt. New York: Raven Press.

DOROTHY RUSSELL

BORN IN SYDNEY, Australia, and orphaned at the age of eight, Dorothy Stuart Russell (1895–1983) (figure 1) was educated in England at the Perse School for Girls in Cambridge and at Girton College, Cambridge University, from which she graduated in 1918 with a first class degree in natural sciences. World War I determined her choice of medicine as a career, at a time when women were encouraged to join the profession. She entered the London Hospital Medical College in 1919, where she was attracted to pathology by the prestige and influence of Hubert M. Turnbull, who then occupied the chair of morbid anatomy. She was awarded the Sutton Prize in pathology and, after obtaining her medical degree in 1923, was appointed assistant in the Bernhard Baron Institute of Pathology under Turnbull. She first devoted her research efforts to a systematic study of renal disease, the results of which were published in 1929 as a special report of the Medical Research Council entitled "A Classification of Bright's Disease." This work was the basis of the thesis she submitted for her M.D. degree in 1930 and for which she was awarded the London University Medal.

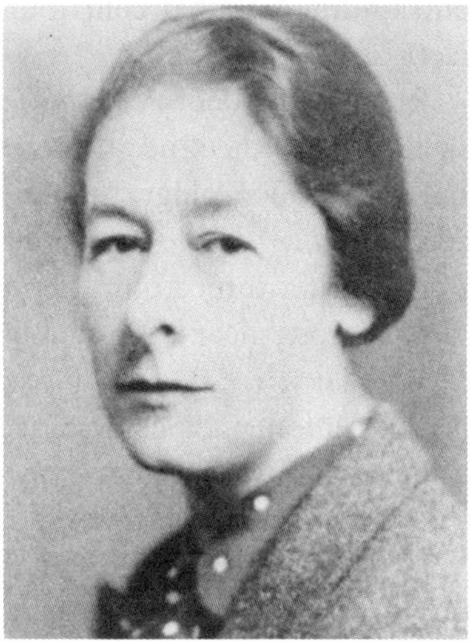

Figure 1. Dorothy Russell (1895–1983).

Her interest in neuropathology, a territory then almost unexplored in Britain, was encouraged by the distinguished neurosurgeon Hugh Cairns, who had recently returned to the London Hospital after training with Harvey Cushing at the Peter Bent Brigham Hospital in Boston. As a Rockefeller Medical Fellow, Russell first went to work with Frank Mallory in Boston in 1928 and the following year joined Wilder Penfield at the Montreal Neurological Institute. Here she rapidly gained expertise in the use and knowledge of the metallic techniques of the Spanish school and in their application to the study of the nervous system and its tumors.

She returned to the London Hospital in 1930, where she established a tradition of neuropathology that was to gain increasing renown. In 1933 she was appointed to the Scientific Staff of the Medical Research Council, still at the London Hospital. In 1939 she joined Hugh Cairns, who had been appointed Nuffield Professor of Surgery in Oxford, and one year later succeeded Pio del Rio Hortega as the neuropathologist at the Radcliffe Infirmary in Oxford. She held that position until 1944, when she was invited by Turnbull to return to the London Hospital. In 1946 she succeeded him as professor of morbid anatomy and head of the Bernhard Baron Institute of Pathology. She was appointed emeritus professor in 1960, having over the preceding three decades made a series of outstanding original contributions that encompassed almost every facet of neuropathology.

Russell was one of the pioneers of the tissue culture technique as applied to the study of cerebral tumors, and it is in the field of human neurooncology that she left her deepest mark. Among her contributions should be quoted her identification of the so-called pinealoma, a tumor more commonly seen in children, as a form of teratomatous neoplasm unrelated to the structure of the pineal gland (Russell, 1944); her recognition of the primary lymphomas of the central nervous system as a group distinct from malignant gliomas and which she termed microgliomatosis; her studies on the spread and metastases of gliomas in the cerebrospinal pathways; and the application of the wet film, or brain smear, technique for the rapid neurosurgical diagnosis of cerebral tumors. Her unparalleled experience culminated in the publication in 1959 of the book *Pathology of Tumours of the Nervous System*, a text that was widely acclaimed and that is currently in its fifth edition (Russell and Rubinstein, 1959).

Neurooncology, however, was not the only field in which she made contributions. In other papers, she wrote of the relationship of hydrocephalus to spina bifida (Russell and Donald, 1935), as well as to aneurysms of the vein of Galen (Russell and Nevin, 1940). Her monograph entitled *Observations on the Pathology of Hydrocephalus*, published in 1949 and reprinted in 1952 and 1966, is still regarded today as the most meticulous and authoritative treatise on the subject. It also constitutes her most important single contribution to child neurology. This study, which was an expansion of a series of three lectures given at the Nuffield Institute for Medical Research in Oxford in 1942, derives its value from the thoroughness with which she surveyed the morbid anatomy of hydrocephalus. She found no grounds for retaining the word *idiopathic* in connection with the etiology of the condition. On the contrary, she felt that, in every case, some form of obstruction could be demonstrated in the cerebrospinal pathway. Thus, congenital hydrocephalus was usually due to a malformation that involved the aqueduct or was associated with an Arnold-Chiari malformation, the latter being almost always accompanied by spina bifida. She emphasized the need for distinguishing aqueductal atresia, which classically consisted in a forking of the channel from gliosis, which, in most cases, seems to have been the result of a low-grade inflammatory process. She found evidence that a widespread disturbance of the ependyma and of the subependymal glia was demonstrable in the last instance and concluded that the obstructive effects of hydrocephalus were manifested in the aqueduct solely on account of its small size.

From a historical perspective, Dorothy Russell's monograph on hydrocephalus also provides worthwhile reading. The following extract testifies to her succinct and accurate expression, her ability to ferret out obscure information, and her delight in tracing the historical origins of the disorder.

The clinical observation of hydrocephalus, with its striking cranial deformity, is doubtless as old as medicine itself. But, in the brief historical notes that follow, no attempt will be made to trace records into ancient times since, on the authority of Morgagni (1761), it appears that the physicians of earlier periods had somewhat vague ideas as to where in the brain and its integuments the fluid accumulated. It was most generally supposed that the fluid lay external to the brain. Vesalius (1514–64), iconoclastic in this as in other matters, appears to have given the first clear account of internal hydrocephalus. The relevant passage, from Chapter V of Book I of the Opera Omnia (1725), for the translation of which I am indebted to Mrs. Isobel Henderson of Somerville College, Oxford, is as follows:

Galen declared that this shape (of skull) can, indeed, be conceived as existing in another world, but cannot exist in nature. Nevertheless, a boy may be seen to-day in Venice, deformed in many of his parts and quite insane, with a head of this shape. And, in fact, a beggar who goes about at Bologna has a head which is square, but a little broader than it is long. Besides, at Genoa there was a small boy who was carried round from door to door by a beggar-woman, and was soon afterwards exhibited by play-actors in the most noble province of Brabant in Belgium: and his head bulged out on both sides and was bigger than two men's heads. Now I think that boy suffered from a disease like that which I observed at Augsburg in a two-year-old girl whose head had grown in seven months, more or less, to such a size that I never saw any man's head which was not surpassed by it in bulk. This disease was what the ancients called hydrocephalus, from the water which is stored in the head and gradually collects. In this girl's case, however, the water had not collected between the skull and its outer surrounding membrane, or the skin (where the doctors' books teach that water is deposited in other cases), but in the cavity of the brain itself, and actually in the right and left ventricles of the brain. The cavity and breadth of these had so increased — and the brain itself was so distended — that they contained about nine pounds of water, or three Augsburg wine-measures (so help me God). Moreover, just as the brain in the crown of the head was of an almost membrane-like thinness, and formed in a manner of speaking one continuous body with its own thin membrane, so also the skull was quite membranous — but, at the same time, its bony seat was still of the size of the girl's skull before her head began to grow abnormally. The manner of this was much the same as that which we perceive in new-born children, in the structure of the frontal bone and the bones of the head, which are normally contiguous with each other, but in quite small children are observed to have a considerable gap, with a stretch of membrane. The cerebellum, nevertheless, and the entire base of the brain, were in their natural state; and so were the extensions of the nerves. And I found no water in any other places but in the ventricles of the brain, which were enlarged to the extent that I have stated; and the girl had the full use of all her senses up to her death. I inspected her a few days before her death, and then, whenever her head was moved by the persons attending, and was somewhat raised, however slightly at once a severe cough troubled the girl, with difficult respiration, an extraordinary redness of the whole face, a suffusion of blood, and a flow of tears. The condition of the rest of her body was moderate; her joints, though loose and weak, were not slack; there was no marked emaciation, nor any watery swelling in the limbs, nor signs of epilepsy or any kind of convulsion. The liver, which was examined soon after death, appeared rather pale, and a good deal harder and more shrunken than a natural liver would otherwise be; the spleen, however, was extremely large and conspicuously soft, just as if it had for some time past been performing the functions of the liver. Indeed I, with the doctors who were present, found nothing more surprising than the fact that such a great force of water had been accumulated for so long in the ventricles of the brain without more extensive symptoms. (Russell, 1949, 2)

Other areas of descriptive neuropathology in which Russell was a pioneer include the pathology of radiation changes in the brain; neurotoxicology, in which she threw light on the pathogenesis of cerebellar atrophy following organic mercury poisoning; the experimental production of cerebral abscesses and their response to chemotherapy and antibiotics; the pathology of subacute sclerosing panencephalitis; and the nosological relationship between acute hemorrhagic leukoencephalitis and disseminated encephalomyelitis. All these publications, which were models of clarity and accuracy and are listed in a recent memorial, can still be read with profit today (Rubinstein, 1984b).

Russell played a major role in the foundation and growth of British neuropathology, and her achievements contributed greatly to the advancement of the position of women in British medicine. She was the first woman to become head of a department of pathology in a London medical school or, indeed, anywhere in the Western world, and she was the first woman member of the Medical Research Club. Numerous honors recognized her accomplishments. She also wielded a profound influence as a teacher. One of her main sources of pride was that so many of those whom she had attracted to her department subsequently came to occupy chairs in pathology, neuropathology, or medicine.

Dorothy Russell was a woman of stately dignity. Few knew her really well, and many were awe-struck by the ascendancy of her personality, in which a penetrating intellect, uncompromising honesty, and gravity of demeanor were combined with a felicity and clarity of expression, both verbal and written, that were almost legendary. At the London Hospital she was known as "The Lady," a description that sums up the mixture of affection and respect in which she was held. Her somewhat reserved public persona concealed a sensitive and receptive nature and, in particular, a warm sympathy for her junior colleagues, whom she not only protected and encouraged in their academic careers but in whose personal problems she was genuinely concerned.

She was fortunate, after her retirement in 1960, to enjoy many years of personal happiness in Westcott, near Dorking, Surrey, maintaining a vigorous interest in her field, helping and counseling colleagues and friends, while her scientific contributions continued to be widely quoted. In the surroundings of her simple but comfortable house, with its lofty view of the Surrey hills, she was able to pursue her long-standing interests in gardening and botany. Numerous friends visited her. She loved music and made the regular yearly pilgrimage to the opera in Glyndebourne. She long maintained a spirit of indomitable energy, which made her willing to undertake travels to Puerto Rico, Yucatan, and Ethiopia in her late seventies. Her mind stayed active and its acuity unimpaired till almost the very end. She died in 1983 at the age of eighty-eight, following a massive cerebrovascular accident (Bailey, 1984). She left an imposing body of scientific work that continues to stand the test of time, a model to others in its intellectual standards, and the memory of a scholar and teacher whose influence and example have immeasurably enriched those who knew her. For those in the field of child neurology, her legacy in the studies of tumors, hydrocephalus, and other developmental malformations remains of exceptional clarity and clinical significance.

Lucien J. Rubinstein
CHARLOTTESVILLE, VIRGINIA

REFERENCES

Bailey, O. T. 1984. In Memoriam: Dorothy S. Russell, Sc.D., M.A., M.D., F.R.C.P. (1895–1983). *J Neuropath Exp Neur* 43:546–48.

Rubinstein, L. J. 1984a. Obituary. Dorothy Stuart Russell: 27 June 1895–October 1983. *J Path* 142:iii-iv, 3.

______. 1984b. Obituary. Dorothy Stuart Russell, 1895–1983. *Neuropath Appl Neurobiol* 10:314–20.

Russell, D. S. 1944. The Pinealoma: Its Relationship to Teratoma. *J Path Bact* 56:145–50.

______. 1949. *Observations on the Pathology of Hydrocephalus*. London: His Majesty's Stationery Office.

Russell, D. S., and C. Donald. 1935. The Mechanism of Internal Hydrocephalus in Spina Bifida. *Brain* 58:203–15.

Russell, D. S., and S. Nevin. 1940. Aneurysm of the Great Vein of Galen Causing Internal Hydrocephalus: Report of Two Cases. *J Path Bact* 51:375–83.

Russell, D. S., and L. J. Rubinstein. 1959. *Pathology of Tumours of the Nervous System*. London: Edward Arnold.

PAUL SANDIFER

PAUL HARMER SANDIFER (1908–1964) (figure 1) was the son of a London general practitioner, Henry Stephen Sandifer. After doing well at Mill Hill School in North London, where he excelled in athletics and was captain of the rugby football team, he took up medicine at the Middlesex Hospital Medical School of the University of London after reading law for a short time. Sandifer qualified in 1934 and served at the Middlesex Hospital as house physician to neurologist Douglas MacAlpine and Sir Alan Moncrieff in the Department of Pediatrics, appointments that were to guide his later career. After further residency posts at the Brompton Hospital in London, he was appointed casualty medical officer at the Middlesex Hospital in 1936. By then he had obtained, by examination, membership in the Royal College of Physicians. A year later he obtained the diploma of psychologic medicine following a residency post at Maudesley Hospital. With this impressive clinical start, he went to the well-known National Hospital at Queen's Square in London, first as a house physician and later as senior resident medical officer (Obituary, 1965) .

During the war years he was appointed neurologist to a sector of the emergency medical service and then joined the Royal Air Force as a neuropsychiatrist, rising to the rank of wing commander. After the war was over, he continued his connection with the RAF as a civilian consultant until 1951. In 1946 he was appointed assistant physician to the Maida Vale Hospital for Nervous Disorders and also to the Royal National Orthopedic Hospital. Two years later he was also appointed neurologist to the Mount Vernon Hospital and Radium Institute. In addition to these important posts, he served from 1948 to 1955 as neurologist to the Oxford Regional Hospital Board. It was at the Maida Vale Hospital for Nervous Disorders that he met Wyllie McKissock, the distinguished neurosurgeon who praised his intellect and his rare quality of enhancing the lives of others. His case sheets, it is reported, betrayed his initial legal training by their precise wording.

Sandifer was appointed in 1953 to the newly created post of

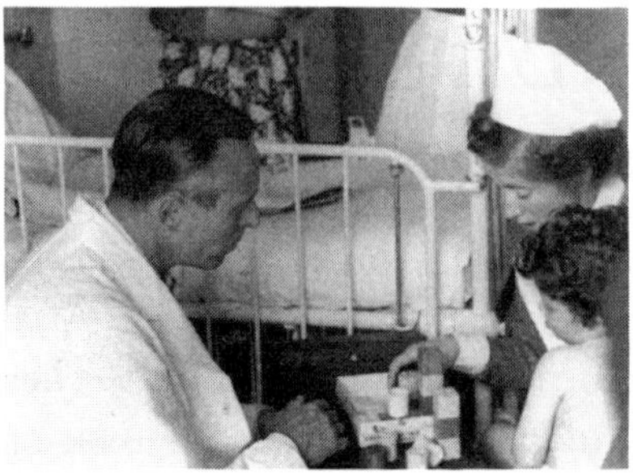

Figure 1. Paul Sandifer (1908–1964).

pediatric neurologist at the Hospital for Sick Children in Great Ormond Street, the premier children's hospital in England (Pampiglione, 1965). Here he again linked up with Moncrieff, professor of child health and one of the great pediatricians, who pioneered social pediatrics in its widest terms and supported the philosophy of the "whole child," meaning the child as an entity and not the subject of just one discipline. Sandifer was the obvious choice for this new and challenging post, which brought him to the peak of his professional career through his enthusiasm and dedication. His previous training under Moncrieff proved invaluable, for he gained a significant ability to understand the sick child and command its trust and affection. A remote successor to Frederick Batten at Great Ormond Street and William Gifford Wyllie, Sandifer spent many hours of service at the hospitals to which he was appointed, particularly ministering to the needs of children and young adults. The 1950s saw a realignment in the clinical practice of medicine with new techniques and therapies, the consequent development of new departments, and an increase in specialization. It was therefore not surprising that a physician of Sandifer's outstanding ability, and working in an area of medicine given more than a fair share of difficult clinical problems, should not then have time for much research or indeed for contributions to the literature. The clinical demands were great, and the hospital's status and reputation ensured a constant supply of difficult cases and second opinion referrals for consultation. He was elected a fellow of the Royal College of Physicians in 1950, which, in itself, was a form of approval of his clinical ability and distinction.

His many hours of hospital service, particularly at Great Ormond Street, involved an exhaustive but gentle study of his patients, followed by the writing of the most conscientious and detailed case reports and correspondence. Sandifer was held in great esteem and affection by his patients and their parents as well as by his colleagues. His ward rounds were always well attended and his demonstrations were meticulous. He was a most popular teacher. His magnetic manner of teaching was coupled with an informality in terminology that veered away from the many polysyllabic words that afflicted much descriptive neurological jargon, and he kept up an unusual enthusiasm without ever becoming too assertive or repetitive. He was possessed of elegance and a youthful charm and a gentleness with both patients and staff. Honest in his opinions and readily acknowledging the fact if anything defeated him, he had no hesitation in seeking the aid of a senior colleague whenever necessary.

Sandifer was a pioneer of British pediatric neurology and made a significant contribution to the specialty. He started a special clinic, which he named E.K.D. (Epileptic and Kindred Disorders) so as to avoid the public use of the terms *seizures* or *epileptic clinic*.

For years he was intrigued by the diverse and progressive cerebral syndromes of infancy and early childhood, including subacute sclerosing panencephalitis and the interactions of immunizations and encephalitis (Sandifer, 1963). He recognized a pseudo-dystonic movement disorder in infants and recognized that it was not a primary neurological disorder but was due to reflux esophagitis, a condition now usually known as the Sandifer syndrome (Kinsbourne, 1964). He also differentiated the so-called "dancing eye syndrome" from other acquired ataxic syndromes and was the first to show that treatment with ACTH was beneficial (Kinsbourne, 1962).

His principle interest was an attempt to unravel the mystery of such "untidy" syndromes as the "floppy infant" and "spastic" child (Sandifer, 1953, 1961). He firmly held that the diplegias of childhood were essentially problems of pediatric neurology. The establishment at the Hospital for Sick Children in 1958 of the first Cerebral Palsy Centre in Britain was the work of Sandifer, who recognized the lack of treatment facilities for children with that condition.

Sandifer had been preparing a book of pediatric neurology as well as a paper on metachromatic leukodystrophy when his untimely death intervened. However, his keenness on documenting and filming all the extraordinary cases that were referred to him resulted in a monumental photographic library, which is a record of his work.

His interests outside medicine were wide and varied. He was skilled in drawing and sketching, and he occasionally painted. He was very fond of music and ballet, was an excellent cook, and knew much about good food and wine. Old furniture, indoor plants, photography, travel and an interest in sports cars (he had a Lagonda) convey the talents of a man who had a sense of humor, a dislike of pomposity, a great sympathy for the sick, especially children and adolescents, and a genuine sincerity. He was an approachable person but always remained a shy man.

His devotion to his work and his clinical drive stretched him considerably. A serious illness some years before his death, which he bore stoically knowing that at any moment it could return to end his life, eventually took its toll, on December 29, 1964, of a great neurologist in his prime who still had much to offer from his unrecorded wealth of experience. His monument stands within the Hospital for Sick Children. Perhaps Macdonald Critchley's comments about Sandifer sum up his contribution to child neurology in England most succinctly:

Sandifer's greatest hour, in his professional sense, was when he was appointed to the coveted and important post of neurological physician to the Hospital for Sick Children, Great Ormond Street. This achievement led to his appearance on the scene as the premier paediatric neurologist — a remote successor of Frederick Batten. His practice among the manifold and obscure nervous disorders of childhood was pioneering indeed, and to this work he brought him many talents — vision, zeal, sagacity, and clinical discernment. (Critchley, 1965, 131)

Posthumously, a monograph entitled *Neurology in Orthopedics* was published for Sandifer. In addition, a unit bearing his name opened in March 1970, and a thriving pediatric neurological department at the Hospital for Sick Children is now headed by John Wilson and Edward Brett.

Gordon Piller
LONDON, ENGLAND

REFERENCES

Critchley, M. 1965. P. H. Sandifer, F.R.C.P., D.P.M.. *Brit Med J* 1:131.

Kinsbourne, M. 1962. Myoclonic Encephalopathy of Infancy. *J Neur Neurosurg Psych* 25:271–76.

______. 1964. Hiatus Hernia with Contortions of the Neck. *Lancet* 1:1058.

Munk's Roll. 1968. *Lives of the Fellows of the Royal Colleges of Physicians of London*, 364. London: The College of Physicians

Obituary. 1965. Paul Harmer Sandifer, F.R.C.P, D.P.M. *Lancet* 1:113.

Pampiglione, G. 1965. Obituary. Paul Harmer Sandifer, F.R.C.P., D.P.M. *Dev Med Child Neur* 7:93–94.

Sandifer, P. H. 1953. Incidence of Infantile Cerebral Palsy. *Proc Roy Soc Med* 46:632.

______. 1961. Critical Evaluation of Treatment of Cerebral Palsy. *Proc Roy Soc Med* 54:143–46.

______. 1963. Immunization and Encephalitis. *Dev Med Child Neur* 5:395–97.

______. 1967. *Neurology in Orthopaedics*. London: Butterworth and Co.

PETER TIZARD

SIR JOHN PETER MILLS TIZARD (figure 1) was one of the outstanding British pediatricians of his day. He would not have claimed to be a pediatric neurologist, but neurology was one of two special interests; the other was neonatal medicine. Nevertheless, he made some original contributions to pediatric neurology and through his considerable talents for organization and leadership, his eager and infectious spirit of inquiry, and a genuine concern and compassion for his patients and their families, he had an important influence on its development in Britain.

Tizard was born in London in 1916, the eldest son of Henry Thomas and Kathleen Eleanor Tizard. His father, later Sir Henry, was a scientist of distinction and a fellow of the Royal Society. Both his father and his equally intelligent mother imbued their son with a love of English literature. He was educated at Rugby School, Oxford University, and the Middlesex Hospital Medical

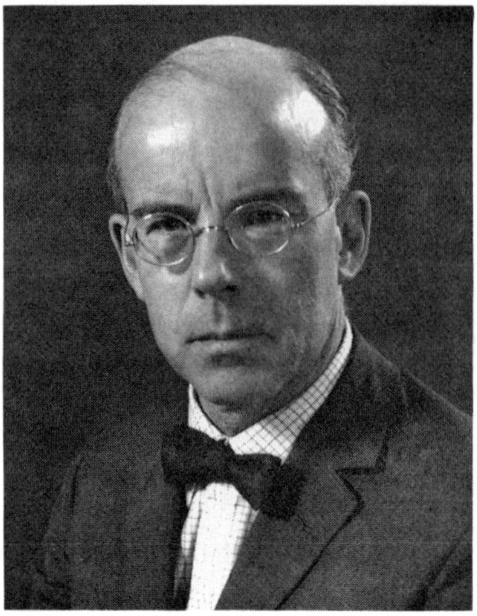

Figure 1. John Peter Mills Tizard.

School, qualifying M.A., B.M., and B.Ch. in 1941. He served in the Royal Army Medical Corps for the remaining years of World War II, after which he began his pediatric training at the Hospital for Sick Children, Great Ormond Street, London. Then, as indeed now, most pediatrics in the United Kingdom was undertaken by general (family) practitioners. Moreover, at the time Tizard embarked on his pediatric training, there were only a few dozen pediatric consultants in the country, almost all attached to teaching hospitals. Pediatric specialists were rarities, and there was only one pediatric neurologist, William Gifford Wyllie. It was during the next five years, as assistant director of the Pediatric Unit at St. Mary's Hospital Medical School in London, that his interest in pediatric neurology developed, where he came to know and be profoundly influenced by Donald Winnicott (Tizard, 1981). As a young doctor, Tizard was one of few to realize, long before others, the older man's supreme contributions as a pediatrician and child analyst. Perhaps it was this association that fostered Tizard's concern for the emotional well-being of his patients (Tizard et al, 1959). He later served as secretary to a subcommittee of the British Paediatric Association on the Welfare of Children in Hospital (British Paediatric Association, 1959). The dean of the Medical School at St. Mary's, Denis Brinton, himself a neurologist of distinction, encouraged Tizard to apply for a Nuffield Foundation Medical Fellowship to study pediatric neurology. This he did successfully. The period of the fellowship, from 1951 through 1952, was divided between the National Hospital for Nervous Diseases, Queen's Square, in London, and the Children's Hospital Medical Center in Boston, Massachusetts.

In 1954 Tizard was appointed reader at the Institute of Child Health in London, and ten years later he was appointed professor of pediatrics at the Institute and also at the Royal Postgraduate

Medical School, with special responsibilities for neonatal medicine. Support from the Nuffield Foundation enabled him to set up the Nuffield Neonatal Research Unit at Hammersmith Hospital, which he directed until his appointment as first professor of pediatrics at Oxford in 1972. He stayed there until his retirement in 1982, when the title of professor emeritus was conferred upon him by the university.

The year of his Nuffield Fellowship, divided between London and Boston, was to see the beginnings of his two personal contributions to pediatric neurology. His first was to show, for the first time, the presence of disturbances of peripheral sensation in hemiplegic children (Tizard and Crothers, 1952; Tizard, 1953; Tizard, Paine, and Crothers, 1954). During his work in Boston, he found that approximately half of over one hundred such patients had some degree of impairment of discriminatory sensation on the affected side, including most often, total or partial astereognosis. The extent of the impairment was usually greater when the hemiplegia had been acquired in the prenatal period. Homonymous hemianopia was also present in a quarter of them — not surprisingly, almost all of whom had peripheral sensory deficits. While there was close correlation with shortening of the affected limb, the presence or absence of sensory impairment or hemianopia showed no correlation with the degree of motor disability or muscular underdevelopment, mental status, seizure activity, or age of onset in postnatally acquired hemiplegia. The possibility of sensory disturbances had previously been largely ignored in pediatric texts, and earlier scrutiny of the patients examined by Tizard failed to detect their presence. He showed that testing was feasible at a much earlier age than had hitherto been thought possible (Tizard, 1955, 1960). This was an important piece of work, for the sensory impairment could constitute a limiting factor for expected results from physiotherapy or orthopedic surgery. It was doubtless achieved because of Tizard's empathy with his young patients. It was always delightful as well as instructive to watch him conduct a revealing examination of the central nervous system in an initially apprehensive or reluctant child. He later took pains to explain to therapists that the learning of skilled voluntary movement depended on the ability to store memories of previous movements made correctly and incorrectly and that the child with peripheral defects might be unable to accomplish this. Training had to comprise visual attention to the movement (Tizard, 1960). Countless families have been grateful to him for his clear and careful explanation of the meaning of their children's disability.

Tizard's second contribution arose in consequence of his training in electroencephalograpy with W. A. Cobb at Queen's Square. Tizard was later to be the first in Britain, with his research assistant, Ruth Harris, to study the electroencephalogram (EEG) in the newborn infant (Harris and Tizard, 1957, 1960; Harris et al, 1957). This work attempted to analyze for the first time the significance of the abnormal EEG in terms of clinical state and progress in babies who developed seizures in the neonatal period. Six abnormalities not seen in the records of normal newborn infants were described. These were rhythmic slow waves, persistent focal sharp waves, spikes, repeated stereotyped sharp waves or wave complexes, gross asymmetry, and a low amplitude background. Although abnormal EEGs were invariably accompanied by abnormal clinical states, the reverse did not hold true. Interseizure EEGs were normal in 15 percent of the infants studied, and clinical abnormalities suggesting a cerebral disorder without seizures were not always accompanied by abnormal EEG findings. The work confirmed a previous suggestion that neonatal seizures appeared to be of focal cerebral origin; the spread of abnormal discharges was characteristically unaccompanied by bilateral synchrony. The clinical associations suggested previous anoxia to be the cause of focal hemispheric brain damage. The other major group of seizures seen were those associated with acute anoxia and characterized by flattening of the record. Neither clinical nor electroencephalographic findings in the original illness appeared to bear any definite relationship to eventual prognosis, but bilateral interseizure abnormalities tended to have a poor prognosis in terms of neurological outcome. Over twenty years later Janet Eyre, working under his supervision at Oxford, was to make a further contribution in this field in seriously ill infants. Continuous recording and rapid analysis of the EEG allowed recognition of seizure activity in infants who were paralyzed by muscle relaxants to allow more effective artificial ventilation (Eyre, Oozeer, and Wilkinson, 1983a). This technique made it possible to relate the total duration of electroencephalographic seizure activity with eventual outcome (Eyre,

Oozeer, and Wilkinson, 1983b). Tizard's interest in seizures extended to older children, and he contributed, with other neurologists, to a collection of cases of self-induced epilepsy (Andermann, 1962).

Tizard's most important contributions to pediatric neurology were undoubtedly organizational, educational, and inspirational. He was a founding member of the British Paediatric Neurology Association in 1975 and became its second chairman, following Neil Gordon, for the years 1979–82. He was convener of a British Paediatric Association/British Paediatric Neurology Association working party and prepared the detailed recommendations for neurological services for children in the United Kingdom (British Paediatric Association, 1983).

As director of the first neonatal research unit in the country, he spearheaded the technological revolution in neonatal medicine that started in the 1960s. At a time when his contemporaries were obsessed with the neonatal respiratory disorders of preterm infants, he was one of the first to recognize the importance of studying the developing nervous system (Robinson and Tizard, 1966).

Tizard also attracted a large number of able young doctors to work with him at Hammersmith and later at Oxford. They were given help, encouragement, and every opportunity to develop their talents. Thus, Roger Robinson, working in the Hammersmith unit, conducted one of the earliest studies of the assessment of gestational age in newborn infants by neurological examination (Robinson, 1966). David Baum undertook the important task of measuring changes in retinal vessel diameter, which occurred in preterm infants when levels of arterial oxygenation were altered between measured limits. This work confirmed for the first time in newborns observations previously made in adults and experimental animals, showing that raising the arterial oxygen tension led to a constriction of retinal blood vessels. More important, it showed that absence of extreme vasospasm was not an indication that the oxygen tension was within safe limits and that ophthalmoscopy could not be used as an alternative to direct measurement of the latter in infants at risk for retinopathy of prematurity (Baum and Bulpitt, 1970; Baum and Tizard, 1970). At Oxford, Richard Cooke used venous occlusion plethysmography in one of the earliest efforts to demonstrate apparent cerebral blood flow in the newborn infant (Cooke, Rolfe, and Howat, 1979).

Peter Tizard was elected a member of the Association of British Neurologists in 1969. He was elected a member of the British Paediatric Association in 1953 (honorary, 1989), served as its president from 1982 to 1985, and was awarded its highest honor, the James Spence Medal, in 1986. He was also president of the Paediatric Section of the Royal Society of Medicine, to which, as a young doctor in training, he presented cases of diastematomyelia and of an unusual brachial plexus palsy (Tizard, 1957). He was a founding member and later president (1975–78) of the Neonatal Society. He was an excellent ambassador for British pediatrics in general, and for pediatric neurology and neonatology in particular. He was a founding member of the European Society for Paediatric Research and served as its president from 1971 to 1972. Tizard was a corresponding member of four foreign pediatric societies and honorary member of six. He received the honor of knighthood in 1982. He wrote elegantly and clearly, contributing seven chapters on pediatric neurology to Gaisford and Lightwood's three-volume treatise, *Paediatrics for the Practitioner* (Tizard, 1955). He also wrote chapters on disorders of the nervous system and on mental defects for *Paterson's Sick Children* (Tizard, 1956). He contributed to the first four editions of Walton's *Disorders of Voluntary Muscle* (Tizard, 1964, 1969, 1974; Gardner-Medwin and Tizard, 1981). He spoke eloquently and wittily, his lectures spiced with quotations from his favorite authors. He was consequently much in demand as a lecturer at home and abroad. His Croonian Lecture to the Royal College of Physicians in London was entitled "Cerebral Palsies: Treatment and Prevention" (Tizard, 1980). His views on successively fashionable systems of therapy resembled those of his deeply admired teacher, Bronson Crothers; however, from his knowledge of perinatal medicine, he held out realistic hope of a reduced incidence of these disorders.

Pamela A. Davies
LONDON, ENGLAND

REFERENCES

Andermann, K., et al. 1962. Self-Induced Epilepsy: A Collection of Self-Induced Epilepsy Cases Compared with Some Other Photoconvulsive Cases. *Arch Neur* 6:49–65.

Baum, J. D., and C. J. Bulpitt. 1970. Retinal Vasoconstriction in Premature Infants with Increased Arterial Oxygen Tension. *Arch Dis Child* 45:350–53.

Baum, J. D., and J. P. M. Tizard. 1970. Retrolental Fibroplasia: Management of Oxygen Therapy. *Brit Med Bull* 26:171–74.

British Paediatric Association. 1959. The Welfare of Children in Hospital. *Brit Med J* 1:166–69.

______. 1983. *Neurological Services for Children in the United Kingdom. Report of a BPA/BPNA Working Party*. London: British Paediatric Association.

Cooke, R. W. I., P. Rolfe, and P. Howat. 1979. Apparent Cerebral Blood Flow in Newborns with Respiratory Disease. *Dev Med Child Neur* 21:154–60.

Crothers, B. and R. Paine. 1988. *The Natural History of Cerebral Palsy*. Oxford and Philadelphia: Blackwell Scientific Publications Ltd. / J. B. Lippincott.

Eyre, J. A., R. C. Oozeer, and A. R. Wilkinson. 1983a. Continuous Electroencephalographic Recording to Detect Seizures in Paralyzed Newborn Babies. *Brit Med J* 286:1017–18.

______. 1983b. Diagnosis of Neonatal Seizures by Continuous Recording and Rapid Analysis of the Electroencephalogram. *Arch Dis Child* 58:785–90.

Gardner-Medwin, D., and J. P. M. Tizard. 1981. Neuromuscular Disorders in Infancy and Early Childhood. In *Disorders of Voluntary Muscle*, 625–65. Ed. Sir J. Walton. 4th ed. Edinburgh: Churchill Livingstone.

Harris, R. F., and J. P. M. Tizard. 1957. Electroencephalograpy in the Normal and Abnormal Newborn. *Arch Dis Child* 32:364–65.

______. 1960. The Electroencephalogram in Neonatal Convulsions. *J Ped* 57:501–20.

Harris, R. F., et al. 1957. Electroencephalography in the Newborn. *Electroen Clin Neurophys* 9:372.

Robinson, R. J. 1966. Assessment of Gestational Age by Neurological Examination. *Arch Dis Child* 41:437–47.

Robinson, R. J., and J. P. M. Tizard. 1966. The Central Nervous System in the New-Born. *Brit Med Bull* 22:49–55.

Tizard, J. P. M. 1953. The Future of Infantile Hemiplegics. *Proc Roy Soc Med* 46:637–40.

______. 1955. Chapter 1: General Comments on Examination and Clinical Signs; Chapter 2: Infections of the Nervous System; Chapter 3: Intracranial Vascular Lesions; Chapter 4: Degenerative Diseases of the Nervous System; Chapter 5: Cerebral Palsy; Chapter 6: Epilepsy and Convulsions; and Chapter 7: Diseases of Muscle. In *Paediatrics for the Practitioner*. Vol. 3. Ed. W. Gaisford and R. Lightwood. London: Butterworth.

______. 1956. Disorders of the Nervous System; Mental Defect. In *Paterson's Sick Children*, 323–87, 388–402. Ed. R. Lightwood. London: Cassell.

______. 1957. Diastematomyelia. Brachial plexus Palsy Associated with Soft Tissue Atrophy in the Scapular Region. *Proc Roy Soc Med* 50:330.

______. 1960. Sensory, Auditory and Speech Defects in Cerebral Palsy: Sensory Defects. *Cerebral Palsy Bull* 2:40–41.

______. 1964. Neuromuscular Disorders in Infancy, 369–88. In *Disorders of Voluntary Muscle*, 369–88. Ed. J. N. Walton. London: J. & A. Churchill.

______. 1969. Neuromuscular Disorders in Infancy, 579–605. In *Disorders of Voluntary Muscle*, 579–605. Ed. J. N. Walton. 2d ed. London: J. & A. Churchill.

______. 1974. Neuromuscular Disorders in Infancy and Early Childhood. In *Disorders of Voluntary Muscle*, 693–725. Ed. J. N. Walton. 3d ed. Edinburgh: Churchill Livingstone.

______. 1980. Cerebral Palsies: Treatment and Prevention. The Croonian Lecture 1978. *J Roy Coll Phys London* 14:72–80.

______. 1981. Donald Winnicott: The President's View of a Past President. Presidential Address to the Section on Paediatrics, Royal Society of Medicine. *J Roy Soc Med* 74:267–74.

Tizard, J. P. M., and B. Crothers. 1952. Sensory Disturbances in Hemiplegia in Childhood. *Trans Am Neur Assoc* 77:227–29.

Tizard, J. P. M., R. S. Paine, and B. Crothers. 1954. Disturbances of Sensation in Children with Hemiplegia. *JAMA* 155:628–32.

Tizard, J. P. M., et al. 1959. The Role of the Paediatrician in Mental Illness. *Lancet* 2:193–95.

LUDO VAN BOGAERT

LUDO VAN BOGAERT (1897–1989) (figure 1) was born into an old Flemish family in Antwerp, Belgium, the city where he made important contributions to child neurology during a long career and where he died. Antwerp, with its large harbor and flourishing businesses, has been a cosmopolitan center for centuries, but until recently it had no university. Van Bogaert's father was a successful practitioner who provided a model for a caring, dedicated clinician. Graduating from high school in 1914, Van Bogaert fled occupied Belgium to start his medical studies at the University of Utrecht (Institut Bunge, 1962). A prodigious learner, he completed the first two years of study by age eighteen. He then joined the Belgian

Army as a volunteer, but in September 1918 suffered a spinal concussion secondary to a fractured vertebra and was discharged.

The following year he resumed his medical studies at the Free University of Brussels, graduating summa cum laude in 1922. While a medical student, Van Bogaert conducted neuroanatomical research in Albert Dustin's laboratory. In September 1922 he began his neurological training under Pierre Marie in Paris and worked in the laboratory of nutrition and metabolism with Marcel Labbe. Ivan Bertrand, his first mentor in neuropathology, introduced him to the cytological methods of the German school of neuropathology. During this time, Van Bogaert became acquainted with many of the leading French neurologists, starting both lifelong friendships and mutual collaborations. Van Bogaert returned to Antwerp in 1923 as a voluntary assistant in internal medicine at St. Elizabeth Hospital. This was the beginning of an extensive, well-rounded clinical experience. He was appointed staff physician at Stuivenberg Hospital, where he started a small pathology laboratory and in 1925 successfully defended his doctoral thesis on amyotrophic lateral sclerosis at the Free University of Brussels. This made him eligible for a professorship, which, however, was never offered under acceptable conditions to a fiercely independent man. During the next few years, Van Bogaert visited Cornelius Winkler in Utrecht, Bernard Brouwer in Amsterdam, S. Kinnier Wilson in London, Constantin von Economo in Vienna, Alfons Jakob in Hamburg, Constantin von Monakow in Zurich, and Walther Spielmeyer and Willibald Scholz in Munich. His busy life was extremely productive, resulting in the publication of seventeen papers in 1924 and thirty in 1925. Van Bogaert continued at the same pace for the next forty years. Although some of these papers were short notes,

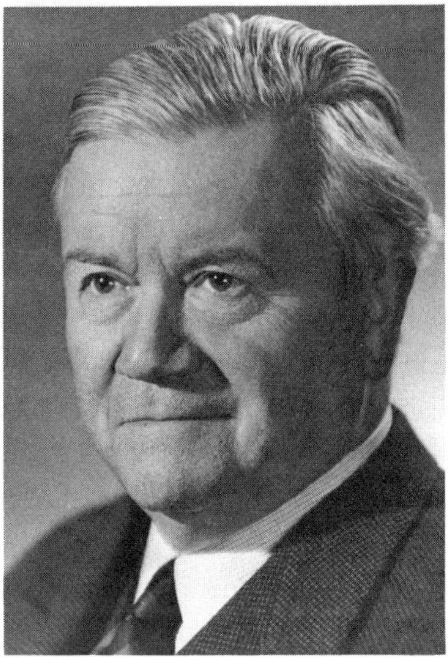

Figure 1. Ludo van Bogaert (1897–1989). Photograph taken at age sixty-five.

many others were elaborate reviews; Van Bogaert was the single or first author on the majority of them. The range of topics was astounding, covering the whole field of neurology, with special emphasis on infectious processes, demyelinating disorders, and inherited metabolic and neurodegenerative diseases.

His clinical base for the next decade remained the Department of Internal Medicine in the Stuivenberg Hospital. His expertise in child neurology was quickly recognized, and he became a valued consultant and collaborator. Pediatrics was not yet widely established in Belgium as a specialty outside of the universities. Neurology fared even worse: there was only one department of neurology, at the University of Louvain. In 1933 Edouard Bunge, a businessman, financed the establishment of a private institute, the Institut Bunge, for medical and surgical research. Van Bogaert was offered the opportunity to organize the clinical services and, more important, to open the institute's pathology laboratory, which, under his direction, became famous.

Hans Joachim Scherer, a student of Spielmeyer and a political refugee from Germany, joined the institute in 1934 to organize the laboratory. Joseph Radermecker became the first clinical assistant. Neurologists and neuropathologists were encouraged to visit or train in the privately funded institute, and by 1936 the first volume of collected reprints from the Institut Bunge was issued. Van Bogaert's works, based on his investigations at the institute, were extensively cited in S. Kinnier Wilson's *Neurology* (1940).

In 1925 Van Bogaert founded a Belgian group made up of neurologists, neurosurgeons, otorhinolaryngolists, and ophthalmologists who meet annually, fostering mutual interaction, collaboration, and publication. The success of this undertaking is illustrated by the seven hundred-page book on intracranial aneurysms and angiomatoses published at its twenty-fifth anniversary meeting (Groupement Belge, 1951).

World War II reduced the productivity of the institute until 1946. However, the clinical records and laboratory collections survived heavy bombing, and clinical work and monthly meetings continued almost without interruption during the war. In 1946 new laboratories in electroencephalography, electromyography, biochemistry, and histochemistry were opened, scientific activity rebounded, and trainees began to arrive from all over Europe and from North and South America.

The quality, breadth, and influence of organized scientific meetings continued to increase. Some were on a small scale, such as the 1955 Symposium on Cerebral Lipidoses (Van Bogaert, Cumings, and Lowenthal, 1957), which gathered together many scientists who later formed the International Society for Neurochemistry. Others were large international gatherings as the epoch-making First Congress of Neurological Sciences, at which more then three thousand participants met in Brussels in 1957 and agreed to form the World Federation of Neurology. Van Bogaert was elected the new organization's first president, capping thirty years of efforts to foster the interaction of neurology with the increasingly isolated old and new subspecialties. Multiple research groups were created, pediatric neurology being one of them. Thereafter, Van Bogaert received national and international recognition with honorary doctorates and election to more than fifty medical academies and scientific societies.

Van Bogaert's contributions resulted from the unique combination, in a single mind, of meticulous clinical skills learned from the traditional French school of neurology and the equally meticulous pathological skills learned from the great German neuropathologists. Charcot, of course, had been the pioneer in such an endeavor, but the pathology laboratory of the nineteenth century was rather elementary and did not require much personal involvement. The proliferation of eponymic syndromes whose distinctive clinical signs could be correlated with equally distinctive pathological features that resulted from a facile dogmatism has not weathered medical progress, especially in biochemistry, although the logical attractiveness of such concepts has always remained popular in textbooks. Van Bogaert's works demonstrate the weakness and limitations of clinical investigations not corroborated by autopsies. They are like a tapestry where all the facts are registered and organized. This was his great strength; he presented data in their diversity, never attempting to force them into shaky theories. The sheer number and variety of Van Bogaert's publications defy summaries or even brief outlines. Only an arbitrary selection of his publications more pertinent to child neurology will be mentioned.

The outbreaks of encephalitis that occurred throughout the

world from 1916 on attracted a great deal of interest regarding their etiology, clinical manifestations, pathology, and sequelae. In the 1920s interest in primary encephalitis kindled investigations into the neurologic complications of childhood diseases and immunizations. Van Bogaert published on these themes in 1924. In 1933 he focused his attention on subacute leukoencephalitis (Barré and Van Bogaert, 1933). The clinical delineation of subacute sclerosing panencephalitis (SSPE) was firmly made in 1945. His classic paper described the distinctive presentation in a child of progressive dementia, followed by myoclonus and variable dyskinesia, ending in death after a terminal phase of extrapyramidal hypertonia (Van Bogaert, 1945). The wealth of documents accumulated at the Institut Bunge on SSPE was the basis for François Lhermitte's thesis, "Les leucoencéphalites" (1950).

A 1937 monograph elegantly described two cousins with a condition subsequently labeled by others as cerebrotendinous xanthomatosis. Cholestanol was later identified as the abnormal metabolite (Menkes and Philippart, 1968), and this finding was confirmed in a cousin of the original case (Philippart and Van Bogaert, 1969). Van Bogaert recognized three clinical phases: progressive cognitive and behavioral difficulties during the second decade with juvenile onset cataracts, ataxia and spasticity during the third decade, and finally bulbar palsy. The second patient died at age fifty-five without any tendinous xanthoma. Van Bogaert had wisely used "generalized" instead of "tendinous" in his original title, an example of his innate ability to avoid mistaking striking for constant features in the diagnosis of an uncommon disorder. The need to use chemistry to supplement classic clinicopathological studies was acknowledged by the participation of a Viennese chemist, Emile Epstein, as coinvestigator (Van Bogaert, Scherer, and Epstein, 1937).

In 1939 van Bogaert reported on a new disorder, which he distinguished from Tay-Sachs disease. The autopsy showed an enlarged spongy brain with cavitation under the gray matter and dense diffuse gliosis with abnormally large glial cells (Van Bogaert, 1939). The material entrusted to Epstein for chemical studies was lost during World War II, delaying final publication (Van Bogaert and Bertrand, 1949). Additional cases were published under the title "Familial Spongy Degeneration of the Brain" (Van Bogaert, 1962a)

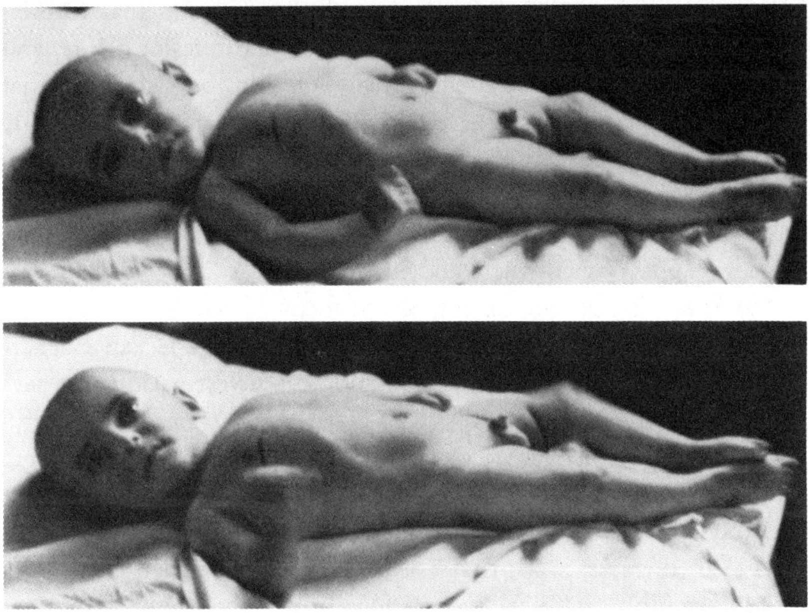

Figure 2. Van Bogaert's first patient with "spongy degeneration of the brain," seen in 1937 and presented in 1939. However, photographs of the child and histopathology were not reported until later. These figures show the posture of the child and involuntary movements of the right upper and left lower limbs. From Van Bogaert and Bertrand, *Spongy Degeneration of the Brain in Infancy* (Amsterdam: North Holland, 1967), 5.

and a classic monograph in collaboration with Ivan Bertrand was issued in 1967 (figure 2) (Van Bogaert and Bertrand, 1967). Canavan had previously published an example of this condition as a case of Schilder's encephalitis, recognizing neither its distinctive character nor the large fibrillary astrocytes (Canavan, 1931). This disorder has generally been labeled Canavan's disease in the English literature, despite the anecdotal character of Canavan's isolated report.

In 1962 Van Bogaert was invited to lecture on inborn metabolic disorders of the nervous system at the University of Liège. The lysosomal storage disorders had not yet been recognized. This overview may now appear to be mostly of historical interest, but this work documented how a lucid mind groped through a wide variety of poorly understood facts (Van Bogaert, 1962b).

Most of Van Bogaert's works were published in French. A first-rate polyglot, he knew that the subtlety of his thought could not be properly conveyed in his secondary languages, and that translation was actually not necessary for foreign colleagues of his generation. A more serious hindrance than language was the fact that many invaluable articles were in publications that were not easily available. As an example I shall cite only the remarkable chapters on neurocutaneous diseases in *Traité de médecine*, infantile cerebral sclerosis, multisystemic diseases, and extrapyramidal diseases (Van Bogaert, 1949, Van Bogaert and Nyssen, 1949).

Inherited diseases are an important focus of pediatric neurology. Starting with a paper on Friedreich's disease in 1924, Van Bogaert undertook careful clinical and pathological investigations on several generations whenever possible. He seemed to have read everything, conveying a treasure of facts in a succinct and lucid fashion, always buttressed by his own experience, which clearly but unobtrusively guided his selection. His lecture on systemic nervous diseases (Van Bogaert, 1948) is a remarkable essay, in which he stressed the uncertainty of clinical observations in the absence of pathological studies. Further, he acknowledged the limitations of pathology and predicted that chemistry would provide the key to many of these scientific enigmas. In this essay, the underlying philosophy of his work, its aims, and methods can be clearly appreciated, providing rare insights into a mind not given to explaining itself.

Van Bogaert's personality defies sketches. He was the kind of person one meets only once in a lifetime. He was elemental like the sea, powerful and illusory. People and facts were taken and understood as they were. The intimate feelings of this master diplomat remained carefully hidden behind his open and kind manner. His activities were prodigious but under complete control. There was never any sense of inner or outer pressure. He never gave orders or proffered opinions. Everything and everyone fell into place, and the work was completed. As one would expect from a man whose scientific tool was the microscope, he was a visual person. Inconspicuous details of a patient's examination were grasped within minutes and sorted out against his well-furnished memory. Even the most humble, inarticulate patient was treated with compassion and provided with warm, reasonable reassurance. Patients understandably become attached to him for the rest of their lives.

No ivory tower hermit, he was eminently sociable. His extraordinarily busy professional life did not preclude innumerable extracurricular activities. The range of his cultural and other interests was vast and varied, encompassing painting, literature, and precious books, to cite but a few. He was a brilliant conversationalist, equally able to captivate the attention of colleagues, young assistants, or people of social renown and importance.

Van Bogaert started his career when scientific nationalism and chauvinism were at their peak. He had a powerful influence in erasing artificial frontiers, helping to bring into existence a world community of neurology and fostering its growth from a somewhat narrow clinical specialty into the diversified neurological sciences we know today. He was conscious of the growing need for subspecialization, but he saw the danger of losing the laboriously acquired unity of the mother discipline unless the different subspecialists could regularly meet together. This will remain the challenge facing the next generation.

Michel Philippart
LOS ANGELES, CALIFORNIA

REFERENCES

Barré, J. A., and L. van Bogaert. 1933. Contribution à la dissociation anatomique et clinique des leucoencéphalites subaigues. Le type concentrique de Balo. *Rev neur* 1:547–78.

Canavan, N. M. 1931. Schilder's Encephalitis Periaxialis Diffusa. Report of a Case in a Child Aged Sixteen and One-Half Months. *Arch Neur* 25:229–308.

Groupement Belge d'études oto-neuro-ophtalmologiques et neuro-chirurgicales. 1951. *Livre jubilaire*. Bruxelles: Les Editions *Acta Neurologica et Psychiatrica Belgica*.

Lhermitte, F. 1950. *Les leucoencéphalites*. Paris: Editions Médicales Flammarion.

Menkes, J. M., and M. Philippart. 1968. Cholestanol Storage in the Nervous Ssystem of Two Patients with Cerebrotendinous Xanthomatosis. *Trans Am Neur Assoc* 93:66–69.

Philippart, M., and L. van Bogaert. 1969. Cholestanolosis. (Cerebrotendinous Xanthomatosis). A Follow-up Study on the Original Family. *Arch Neur* 21:603–10.

Institut Bunge. 1962. *Livre jubilaire: Hommage au Docteur Ludo van Bogaert* (includes bibliography up to 1961). Vol. 15, 24. Bruxelles: Les Editions *Acta Medica Belgica*.

Van Bogaert, L. 1924. Encéphalite léthargique avec syndrome respiratoire et hépatique. *J belge neur* 24:1–12.

______. 1924. Maladie de Friedreich et scoliose éssentielle tardive héréditaire. *Arch int méd exp* 1:75–95.

______. 1939. Idiotie avec amaurose chez un enfant d'Israelites polonais en dehors de la maladie de Tay-Sachs. *J belge neur* 39:470–71.

______. 1945. Une leucoencéphalite sclérosante subaigue. *J neur neurosurg psych* 8:101–20.

______. 1948. Maladies nerveuses systematisées et problèmes de l'hérédité. *Acta neur psych belg* 48:308–29.

______. 1949. Les dysplasies à tendance blastomateuse; les scléroses cérébrales; les maladies systematisées. In *Traité de Médecine*. Vol. 16, 117–41, 142–218. Paris: Masson.

______. 1962a. Familial Spongy Degeneration of the Brain. *Acta Neur Psych Scand* 39:617–26.

______. 1962b. *Maladies nerveuses génétiques d'ordre métabolique*. Liège: Revue médicale de Liège.

Van Bogaert, L., and I. Bertrand. 1949. Sur une idiotie familiale avec dégénérescence spongieuse du névraxe. *Acta Neur Belg* 49:572.

Van Bogaert, L., and I. Bertrand. 1967. *Spongy Degeneration of the Brain in Infancy*. Amsterdam: North Holland.

Van Bogaert, L., J. N. Cumings, and A. Lowenthal. 1957. *Cerebral Lipidosis: A Symposium*. Oxford: Basil Blackwell.

Van Bogaert, L., and R. Nyssen. 1949. Les maladies extrapyramidales. In *Traité de Médecine*. Vol. 16, 219–80. Paris: Masson.

Van Bogaert, L., H. J. Scherer, and E. Epstein. 1937. *Une forme cérébrale de la cholestérinose géneralisée*. Paris: Masson.

Wilson, S. A. K. 1940. *Neurology*. London: Arnold.

JOHN WALTON

LORD JOHN NICHOLAS WALTON (figure 1) was born on September 16, 1922, in Rowlands Gill in County Durham, the son of a headmaster. With the exception of military service in the Royal Army Medical Corps and periods of training and research in London and Boston in the early 1950s, he remained in the north of

England until 1983 when he accepted an invitation to become the Warden of Green College, Oxford.

A man of immense intellectual energy, a fluent and gifted teacher, a born organizer and leader of men, hospitable, charismatic, urbane, ambitious and hugely efficient, Walton has made major contributions as a physician, teacher, director of research, medical administrator, and politician, and is currently one of the most distinguished medical men of his generation. As a student, he admired the personality and achievements of Sir William Osler and, nearly half a century later in 1989, he took up residence in Osler's Oxford house the "Open Arms" at 13 Norham Gardens, part of which he and his wife have been restoring in Osler's memory. There is much to compare in the two men, especially their charm and capacity for hard work, but if there was deliberate emulation, it stopped short of imitating Osler's mischievous sense of humor or his passion for bibliography, and Walton's military background and his proficiency and passion for cricket and golf had no counterpart in Osler's life.

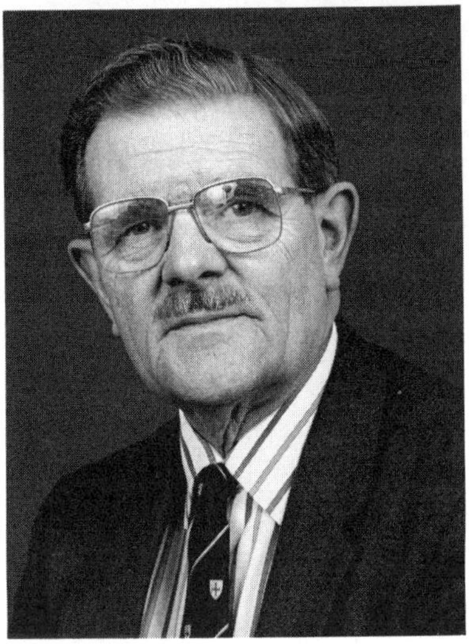

Figure 1. John Walton.

Walton's major medical interest for thirty-eight years has been in neuromuscular disease, particularly muscular dystrophy, but he deliberately and successfully maintained the widest possible knowledge of neurology and his approach has always been to practice neurology as inseparable from medicine as a whole. Before he was a professor, he used the title "Physician in Neurology" on his correspondence, rather than "Neurologist."

Walton entered Durham University Medical School at King's College, Newcastle upon Tyne, in 1941 and qualified with first-class honors and with distinctions in all subjects in 1945, a feat not repeated for nearly twenty years. His interest in medical politics was evident early. He was president of the Medical Students' Representative Council and treasurer of the British Medical Students' Association. After qualifying, he was house physician to Frederick John Nattrass (the professor of medicine whose major interest was neurology) and, later, to Sir James Spence (the first professor of child health in England), both deeply impressive individuals whose influence was lasting. Nattrass later kindled Walton's interest in muscular dystrophy and Spence very nearly persuaded him to take up pediatrics. Together, they originated Walton's contributions to pediatric neurology. In 1947 he joined the Royal Army Medical Corps for two years, serving ultimately as Second in Command on the Hospital Ship *Oxfordshire*, and later on the *El Nil*. He continued to serve in the Territorial Army for twenty years, eventually retiring in 1970 with the rank of colonel.

Walton returned to Newcastle in 1949 as medical registrar to Alan Gordon Ogilvie and Henry Miller at the Royal Victoria Infirmary and there began a remarkable neurological relationship that continued until Miller's death in 1976. Both men were destined to become neurologists of international renown: Miller was flamboyant, brilliantly intuitive, and had a devastating wit; Walton was methodical, organized, exceedingly well informed and, to Miller's irritation, frequently right. As Miller's registrar, Walton's interest shifted away from pediatrics and into neurology. Miller later established the first university Department of Neurology at the Royal Victoria Infirmary with Walton as its first assistant from 1956 to 1958. Walton wrote his M. D. thesis on subarachnoid hemorrhage in 1952 and later expanded it into a book (Walton, 1956a). He worked with Raymond Adams for a year at the Massachusetts General Hospital as Nuffield Foundation Fellow (1953–54), where he collaborated on their book on polymyositis (Walton and Adams, 1958). He spent periods of three months and later, a year, at the National Hospital for Nervous Diseases, Queen's Square, working with Edward Arnold Carmichael and doing an important study on amyotonia congenita. He developed an interest in clinical electrophysiology, both EEG and automatic frequency analysis of the EMG, and made his first major study of the muscular dystrophies with Nattrass. Even during this busy period, he found time to be chairman of the Registrar's Group of the British Medical Association (1952–53 and 1954–55) and a member of the standing committee of members of the Royal College of Physicians.

In 1958 John Walton was appointed consultant neurologist at

Newcastle General Hospital and, with the neurosurgeon George Frederick Rowbotham, created the Regional Neurological Centre in 1962, the first of its kind in Britain. Walton persuaded the Health Authority to devote nearly one third of the space on the neurological floor to research laboratories. Over the next twenty years, this research space was greatly expanded as Walton recruited an increasingly large team of research scientists and physicians to work on the neuromuscular diseases. The two neurology departments flourished in a friendly competitive spirit under their rival directors. Miller's research interest in demyelination and Walton's in muscle never conflicted and each attracted visitors, researchers, and a high caliber of staff. The two teams met unfailingly for an hour on Friday mornings, alternately in each unit, to see interesting or difficult cases; anyone's opinion might be sought, starting with one of the most junior visitors and finishing with an analysis by the boss of the visiting team before the results of the investigations and the answer, or lack of one, were revealed. This tradition remains one of the trademarks of Newcastle neurology to this day.

In 1968 Walton was appointed Professor of Neurology and, from 1971 to 1981, he succeeded Miller as Dean of Medicine at the University of Newcastle. During this period, he was the driving force behind the planning and funding of a major new building for the medical school. He was created a Knight Bachelor in 1979 and was elevated to the Peerage with the title of Lord Walton of Detchant in 1989. He has been elected an honorary member of many neurology societies throughout the world and of the British Paediatric Association. He has served as chairman of the Research Committee of the World Federation of Neurology since 1977, as its president since 1989, and successively as president of the British Medical Association (1980–82), the General Medical Council (1982–89), the Royal Society of Medicine (1984–86), and the Association of British Neurologists (1987–88), and as a member of the Council of the Royal College of Physicians (1979–88).

Walton's major contributions to neurology have been of three kinds: his teaching and inspiration of a generation of neurologists, his building of a research team that has made important contributions to knowledge of neuromuscular disease, and his writings. Far more than most neurologists of his day, he studied and wrote about the neurological disorders of childhood, particularly Duchenne muscular dystrophy and the congenital myopathies. In 1972 he was instrumental, together with Henry Miller and Donald Court, in persuading the Newcastle Health Authority to create the first consultant appointment in the United Kingdom outside London specifically devoted to pediatric neurology.

His contribution to the study of the floppy infant, or children with myotonia congenita (which, as he wrote in 1956, "for more than half a century . . . have come to be regarded as valid explanations rather than tentative labels") was to review the literature exhaustively and analyze a series of 109 cases in London, Newcastle, and Boston, examining 50 of them personally (Walton, 1956b). He brought order to a muddled subject and created a nosological framework that remains valid today. Walton recognized that some floppy infants suffered from systemic illness or disorders of the central nervous system and that the largest category of severe neuromuscular causes was spinal muscular atrophy. Most of the remaining 17 cases he classified as cases of benign congenital hypotonia with or without complete recovery. In the latter group, with the limited techniques for studying muscle biopsy material that were available at the time, he found unconvincing evidence of myopathy, although he later recognized that such cases were, in fact, suffering from benign congenital myopathies. Indeed, it was in the same year (1956) that Milton Shy and Kenneth R. Magee in the United States described central core disease, the first to be discovered of many specific genetic entities causing such myopathies. Walton's term *benign congenital hypotonia*, used to describe floppy infants without identifiable etiological factors or pathological changes on investigation who tended to improve with time, has remained controversial. Today, those children who completely recover tend to be viewed from a different point of view, although perhaps with no clearer insight, as suffering from specific delay in motor development.

The work on which Walton's early reputation was founded was his paper, written with Nattrass and published in *Brain* in 1954, "On the Classification, Natural History and Treatment of the Myopathies," which was a major review of the muscular dystrophies and myotonias based on 105 cases that they observed. A comprehensive genetic survey of the same cases was published in the *Annals of Human Genetics* in 1955 (Walton, Race, and Phillip,

1955) with a supplement the following year (Walton, 1956c). The three-fold importance of this study was that it established a clear and consistent classification of the muscular dystrophies based on firm genetic and clinical grounds, proposed a category of "limb-girdle" muscular dystrophy, and aroused a lasting medical interest in the United Kingdom in the muscular dystrophies. In their classification, Walton and Nattrass decided that the milder forms of X-linked muscular dystrophy, which they discussed in some detail, were so precisely similar in their pattern of muscle involvement of classic Duchenne cases that they should be included in that category. They thus missed being the first to describe the Becker type that had previously been separated by P. E. Becker and F. Keiner in 1955 and, in fact, it was not until 1968 that Walton was persuaded to accept Becker muscular dystrophy as a separate disorder. Recent events, including the recognition that the genes for both were located at the same site on the X chromosome (Xp21) and that variable dystrophin abnormalities were to be found in both, have returned us virtually to the nosological position Walton adopted in his definition of the disorder in 1954. Walton included a few girls in his Duchenne category, as Duchenne himself and Gowers had done before him. Some of them may have suffered from other disorders, but one girl with Turner syndrome and Duchenne muscular dystrophy (Walton, 1956c) was a seminal case. She was the first example in the literature in which a clear reason for the manifestation of X-linked muscular dystrophy in a female was discovered, and the precursor of the cases reported from the 1970s onward in which 46XY females were found to have X/autosomal translocations with breaks at the Xp21 site. These cases were the first to provide evidence of the localization of the Duchenne gene from which all the subsequent advances in our knowledge of the molecular biology of the disease have developed.

The introduction of limb-girdle muscular dystrophy as a nosological entity, rather than as a provisional term for a mixed group of cases as Stevenson had used it in 1953, was less successful. Subsequent experience showed that patients with spinal muscular atrophy and the scapulohumeral and Emery-Dreifuss types of muscular dystrophy had probably been included, possibly together with other disorders, and the delineation of these and especially of other autosomal recessive myopathies of adolescence and adult life might have proceeded more quickly if the concept of limb-girdle muscular dystrophy had never been introduced. Nevertheless, the attractive clarity of the classification of Walton and Nattrass and the gifted advocacy both of this and a wider research interest in the myopathies that Walton achieved in his writings and spell-binding lectures over the subsequent three decades were major contributing factors to the worldwide development of knowledge about these disorders during this period.

The Muscular Dystrophy Group of Great Britain, and later of Northern Ireland, had its origin in 1955 in an organization of parents of disabled children and achieved independence in 1959. Nattrass and Walton were, from the beginning, its principal medical protagonists. Nattrass died in 1979 and Walton has continued as chairman of the Group. Nattrass's and Walton's insistence on the highest standards of scientific appraisal of applications for research grants ensured that much would always be achieved, even with quite modest funding; in addition, both men were held in such affection and respect because of their transparent devotion to the task of finding the cause and care of muscular dystrophy, that they inspired generations of members of the Group to feats of fund raising that became the envy of other British medical charities.

A more direct contribution to the facilitation of research into the neuromuscular diseases was Walton's direction of the muscular dystrophy research laboratories at Newcastle General Hospital from 1963 until 1983. A constant succession of notable researchers from many parts of the world who worked there during this period included Ronald J. Pennington, Keith Ross, Alan McComas, John Pearce, Arthur Rose, Konstanty Mrozek, Adrian Upton, David Barwick, Albert Aguayo, Walter Bradley, Peter Hudgson, Frank Mastaglia, A. K. Susheela, Paul Larson, Malcolm Campbell, Ram Ayyar, Frans Jennekens, John Pearn, Michael Cullen, John Fulthorpe, Clarke Slater, John Harris, Margaret Johnson, and many others. Research was on a broad front involving, from the beginning, biochemistry, neurophysiology, and clinical and experimental histology, and was soon followed by histochemistry, tissue culture techniques, and a strong interest in experimental pharmacology. Walton's publications include numerous books, 30 or more chapters in books, and 187 published papers; of these, 163 have been on neuromuscular disorders, 78 reporting the results of research on neuromuscular diseases with his collaborators. A selection of these publications, particularly relating to pediatric neurology or to basic science include the following: his book *Disorders of Voluntary Muscle* (1964), which is now in its fifth edition; benign congenital myopathy with myasthenic features (Walton, Geschwind, and Simpson, 1956); the limp child (Walton, 1957); polymyositis (Rose and Walton, 1966; Currie and Walton, 1971); benign spinal muscular atrophy (Gardner-Medwin, Hudgson, and Walton, 1967); juvenile onset spinal muscular atrophy (Mastaglia and Walton, 1971); subacute and chronic spinal muscular atrophy in childhood (Pearn et al, 1978); nemaline myopathy (Fulthorpe et al, 1969); myotubular myopathy (Campbell, Rebeiz, and Walton, 1969); mitochondrial myopathies (Mechler et al, 1986); and studies on muscle fiber size during normal development (Aherne et al, 1971).

Another quite separate contribution to pediatric neurology was Walton's work on clumsy children. He collaborated first with two pediatricians, Errington Ellis and Donald Court. The latter was Sir James Spence's successor to the Chair of Child Health in Newcastle, and later worked with Sonny Gubbay. Walton's chief contribution to the neurological analysis of this previously, and subsequently ill-defined, but often severely handicapped group of children was to apply strict criteria for the diagnosis of apraxia or agnosia in individual children once pyramidal, sensory, or cerebellar disorders had been identified or excluded (Walton, Ellis, and Court, 1962; Gubbay et al, 1965). The emphasis in these papers on the undoubted value of a relatively low performance score on the Wechsler Intelligence Scale for Children in drawing attention to such children may have led unwittingly to the dependence in subsequent studies by other workers on psychological tests, but it was the demonstration of the value of detailed neurological examination of cognitive function that was Walton's crucial contribution to this field.

Walton's contributions to pediatric neurology and to neurology as a whole have been important and far reaching. They have been those of a codifier, teacher, catalyst, and organizer, rather than a discoverer of new disorders or new principles. He made no major new discovery about muscular dystrophy, yet without him, muscular dystrophy research since 1950 would certainly have been less successful. Like Osler, he has made his most lasting impression on his patients as a superb physician and on his students as a superb teacher and writer.

David Gardner-Medwin
NEWCASTLE, ENGLAND

REFERENCES

Aherne, W., et al. 1971. Muscle Fibre Size in Normal Infants, Children and Adolescents: An Autopsy Study. *J Neur Sci* 14:171.

Campbell, M. J., J. J. Rebeiz, and J. N. Walton. 1969. Myotubular Centronuclear or Pericentronuclear Myopathy? *J Neur Sci* 8:425.

Currie, S., and J. N. Walton. 1971. Immunosuppressive Therapy in Polymyositis. *J Neur Neurosurg Psych* 34:447.

Fulthorpe, J. J., et al. 1969. Nemaline Myopathy: A Histological and Ultrastructural Study of Skeletal Muscle from a Case Presenting with Infantile Hypotonia. *Neur* 19:735.

Gardner-Medwin, D., P. Hudgson, and J. N. Walton. 1967. Benign Spinal Muscular Atrophy Arising in Childhood and Adolescence. *J Neur Sci* 5:121.

Gubbay, S. S., et al. 1965. Clumsy Children: A Study of Apraxic and Agnosic Defects in 21 Children. *Brain* 88:295.

Mastaglia, F. L., and J. N. Walton. 1971. Histological and Histochemical Changes in Skeletal Muscle from Cases of Chronic Juvenile and Early Adult Spinal Muscular Atrophy (the Kugelberg-Welander Syndrome). *J Neur Sci* 12:15.

Mechler, F., et al. 1986. Mitochondrial Myopathies. A Clinico-Pathological Study of Cases with and without Extra-Ocular Muscle Involvement. *Aust NZ J Med* 16:185.

Pearn, J., et al. 1978. A Genetic Study of Subacute and Chronic Spinal Muscular Atrophy in Childhood: A Nosological Analysis of 124 Index Patients. *J Neur Sci* 37:227.

Rose, A. L., and J. N. Walton. 1966. Polymyositis: A Survey of 89 cases with Particular Reference to Treatment and Prognosis. *Brain* 89:747.

Walton, J. N. 1956a. *Subarachnoid Haemorrhage*. Edinburgh: Livingstone.

______. 1956b. "Amyotonia congenita": A Follow-up Study. *Lancet* 1:1023.

______. 1956c. The Inheritance of Muscular Dystrophy: Further Observations. *Ann Hum Genet* 21:40.

______. 1957. The Limp Child. *J Neur Neurosurg Psych* 20:144.

______. 1964. *Disorders of Voluntary Muscle*. Edinburgh: Churchill Livingstone.

Walton, J. N., and R. D. Adams. 1958. *Polymyositis*. Edinburgh: Livingstone.

Walton, J. N., E. Ellis, and S. D. M. Court. 1962. Clumsy Children: A Study of Developmental Apraxia and Agnosia. *Brain* 85:603.

Walton, J. N., N. Geschwind, and J. A. Simpson. 1956. Benign Congenital Myopathy with Myasthenic Features. *J Neur Neurosurg Psych* 19:224.

Walton, J. N., and F. J. Nattrass. 1954. On the Classification, Natural History and Treatment of the Myopathies. *Brain* 77:169.

Walton, J. N., R. R. Race, and U. Phillip. 1955. On the Inheritance of Muscular Dystrophy. *Ann Hum Genet* 20:1.

WILLIAM WYLLIE

WILLIAM GIFFORD WYLLIE (1889–1969) (figure 1) was born in Edinburgh and was educated at Edinburgh Academy and Edinburgh University. He graduated M.D., Ch.B. in 1913 and was appointed house physician (intern) at the Royal Edinburgh Infirmary. In 1914 he joined the Royal Navy as a surgeon lieutenant and served mainly in the Mediterranean. After demobilization in 1918, he moved to London to continue his medical career, as many good Scots have done, and became resident medical officer at the National Hospital for Nervous Diseases, Queen's Square, from 1919 to 1922.

Wyllie's training and specialization in pediatric neurology began in 1922 with his appointment as registrar (resident) and pathologist at the Hospital for Sick Children, Great Ormond Street, and his election to the staff as honorary consulting pediatrician in 1925. Great Ormond Street Hospital had been without a neurologist since Frederick Batten died in 1918, and with four years of previous training in neurology, Wyllie was groomed for the position.

Wyllie was the first fully qualified pediatric neurologist in Great Britain and was trained in both neurology and pediatrics. He was a pioneer in the specialty, but combined his neurologic practice and interests with general pediatrics. The first issue of the *Archives of Disease in Childhood* opened with a paper on hepatic cirrhosis by Wyllie and F. J. Poynton (1926). He also wrote on the

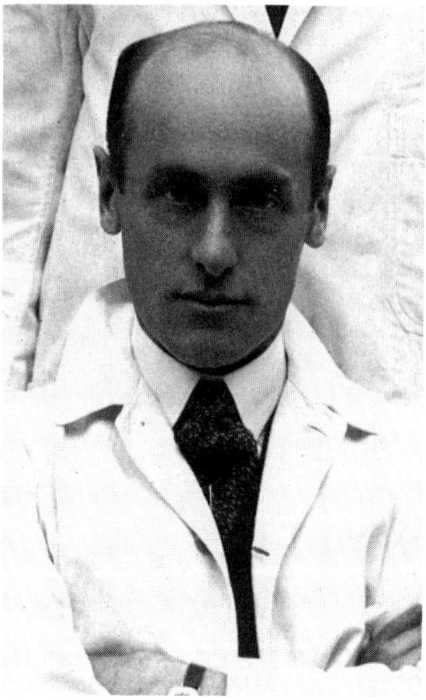

Figure 1. William Wyilie (1889–1969).

periodic syndromes, such as cyclical vomiting, idiopathic pulmonary hemosiderosis, and bronchiectasis, among other pediatric subjects. He coauthored a book entitled *Recent Advances in Diseases of Children* (Pearson and Wyllie, 1935) and taught pediatrics and neurology to postgraduate fellows and students. He was president of the Paediatric Section of the Royal Society of Medicine and was offered the chair of the British Paediatric Association.

His special interests in pediatric neurology were many, and he contributed chapters on the nervous system in Archibald Garrod, Batten, and Hugh Thursfield's *Diseases of Children* and Sir Leonard Parsons and Seymour Balings's *Diseases of Infancy and Childhood.* He elucidated the condition of encephalitis following infectious diseases (1934), the pathology of Pink disease (1944), and the pathology of hemiplegia in childhood (1948), and was one of the first to recognize neonatal myasthenia gravis (1946). Children with psychiatric problems were of special concern, and he started one of the earliest child guidance clinics in London (Wyllie, 1926).

In addition to his appointment to the staff of Great Ormond Street, he was physician to the Children's Department of the Westminster Hospital, and for twenty years (1925–45) consultant physician to the Maida Vale Hospital for Nervous Diseases. During World War II, he was a member of the Emergency Medical Service. When the Institute of Child Health in the University of London was created, he became its first dean and was responsible for the planning of postgraduate teaching at the Hospital for Sick Children. He was a member of the Board of Governors of the hospital from 1948 until he retired in 1951.

As one of his last house physicians, appointed in 1950, I was privileged to have begun my training in pediatric neurology under Wyllie. His gentleness with children and quiet manner, and his sympathetic and sensible approach to his patients and their parents made him an ideal children's physician. As a mentor and chief, he was very much a gentleman — reserved, dignified, courteous, and perfectly tailored, but his manner was sometimes austere and at first intimidating to a young house physician. His ward rounds, conducted with the very able assistance of Janet Booth, were punctual, orderly, disciplined, and never hurried. All test results and X rays were expected to be on hand and available for his inspection. Case reports for presentation at his postgraduate teaching rounds had to be prepared with care and delivered succinctly and clearly. He reviewed one of my earliest manuscripts for publication and returned it to me with the comment, "Millichap, I suggest you read Robert Louis Stevenson and then rewrite it." He believed in lucid, short sentences without unnecessary adjectives or repetitious phrases.

Visitors to Wyllie's ward rounds were many, both national and international. I have clear and pleasant memories of presenting cases to David Clark when he was on sabbatical from Frank Ford's service at Johns Hopkins in Baltimore. Wyllie knew the literature and was ready to take advantage of new and promising treatments developed at home or abroad. He motivated my interest in epilepsy and anticonvulsants and drew my attention to the work of William Lennox in Boston. In fact, while serving as Wyllie's house physician, I had occasion to write a letter of referral to Lennox about the medications available in Britain for a child with a refractory petit mal seizure disorder. Wyllie's counsel in dealing with difficult patients was wise. He never hesitated to refer a patient when he thought superior treatment might be available elsewhere, particularly if the parent made the slightest suggestion of dissatisfaction with his management of the case.

In addition to medicine, Wyllie was a connoisseur of the good things of life — literature, travel, paintings, fishing, gardening, and, not least, food and wine. As a guest for dinner at his bachelor's apartment toward completion of my appointment, I was introduced to the cheese soufflé prepared by his Scottish housekeeper, to vintage champagne, and to VSOP Cognac. I remember little more of that night, except that my appreciation and understanding of Wyllie had changed from the intimidating and austere to a genial, witty host with a sense of fun, dry humor, and excellent conversation.

Wyllie retired early at sixty-two, lived in the country, and took up bird watching and gardening as hobbies. At sixty-seven, he became interested in fishing and moved to Strathtay in Scotland, where he lived for many years with a companion, a poodle named Kim. At seventy-eight, while standing in the river, he had a heart attack, which put an end to fishing but not to reading the lesson in church or greeting occasional and well-chosen friends from London or Edinburgh. He later moved to a flat in Edinburgh, where he died on October 24, 1969, at the age of eighty. Characteristically, he instructed the executor of his will that there was to be no memorial service. If alive today, he would have declined the inclusion of his biography, which would have been a serious and unfortunate omission from this book.

J. Gordon Millichap
SPRINGFIELD, ILLINOIS

REFERENCES

Munk's Roll. 1982. *Lives of the Fellows of the Royal College of Physicians of London.* Ed. G. Wolstenholme. Oxford and Washington, D.C.: IRL Press.

Obituary. 1969. *Brit Med J* 4:372.

Obituary. 1969. *Lancet* 2:1016.

Pearson, W. J., and W. G. Wyllie. 1935. *Recent Advances in Disease of Children.* London: Churchill.

Wyllie. W. G. 1926. Treatment of Hysterical Disorders in Children. *Lancet* 1:301–2.

______. 1934. Encephalitis. *Brit Med J* 2:241–43.

______. 1944. Signs, Symptoms and Treatment of Pink Disease. *Med Press* 212:212–13.

______. 1946. Myasthenia Gravis (2 Cases). *Proc Roy Soc Med* 39:591–93.

______. 1948. Acute Infantile Hemiplegia; President's Address. *Proc Roy Soc Med* 41:459–66.

Wyllie, W. G., and F. J. Poynton. 1926. Hepatic Cirrhosis in Children; Biliary Forms. *Arch Dis Child* 1:1–20.

PAUL YAKOVLEV

PAUL YAKOVLEV (1894–1983) (figure 1) was a friendly, outspoken man. Although he was never directly responsible for training neurology residents, he exerted a profound influence on those trained in Boston for over three decades.

Yakovlev was born in Touretz, Russia, on December 28, 1894. His father and grandfather were military officers, and his mother was from the "upper class." His parents died when he was young, and he was raised by an aunt. Yakovlev went to the Military Medical Academy of St. Petersburg in 1914 and here was exposed to Vladimer Bekhterev, Ivan Pavlov, Paul Fleschig, and Alexander Maximow. After receiving his medical diploma in 1919, he quickly escaped from Russia by crossing the Gulf of Finland in the middle of winter. In Finland he worked as a dockhand until he could arrange for a visa. Making his way to Paris via England, he worked with Pierre Marie at the Salpêtrière and Joseph Babinski at the Hôpital de la Pitié. He received his M.D. from the University of Paris in 1925. On the advice of Maximow, who was now at the University of Chicago, Yakovlev came to America. He went into practice in Rhode Island for the first six months, but found this arrangement unsatisfactory. He then met Stanley Cobb at the neurological unit of the Boston City Hospital and was hired to survey foreign literature for a book being prepared by Cobb and William Lennox (Kemper, 1984). He also worked in the Neurological Outpatient Clinic. This early period of his life, as well as his other contributions, noted specifically in this paper, were described in some detail in an excellent biographical sketch by Kemper (1984).

Yakovlev obtained his first stable medical position at the Monson State Hospital for Epileptics in Massachusetts. He often said that he regarded the work there with patients as his "vocation" and the study of their brains when they died as his "avocation." While at Monson he wrote on epilepsy and some of the syndromes he saw there (Yakovlev, 1937). He had a meager pathological laboratory, but one in which he could develop his ideas and neuroanatomical and neuropathological expertise. He subsequently became director of

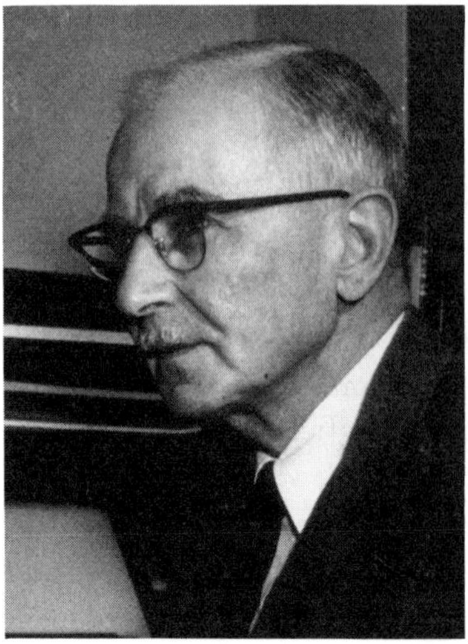

Figure 1. Paul Yakovlev (1894–1983).

laboratories at the Metropolitan State Hospital, where he started his famous anatomy of the brain classes that physicians who were preparing for the new Board examinations in neurology and psychiatry found helpful. These lectures were subsequently published (Yakovlev, 1942). In 1938 he moved across the street and became clinical director of the Fernald State School. He finally received significant laboratory space, built a giant microtome, and began his collection of abnormal and normal brain material. Many of his best articles were written while at Fernald, including the articles on schizencephalies and paraplegia with hydrocephalus, as well as several conceptual papers on the embryology of the brain (Yakovlev and Wadsworth, 1946; Yakovlev, 1947). His book with Harold Solomon concerning military psychiatry was written at this time, (Yakovlev and Solomon, 1944). In 1947 he went to Yale, subsequently returning to Harvard in 1951.

In these and subsequent years, Yakovlev made a liaison with Derek Denny-Brown's service at the neurologic unit at Boston City Hospital. He had always had professional relationships with neurologists in this area, first with Cobb and Lennox, and through Lennox he obtained his position in the institutions where he could initiate his studies of epileptics. He would "visit" for one month each year on Denny-Brown's service, and it was here that neurologic residents first encountered this unique neurologist — their only exposure to "continental neurology." Yakovlev introduced them to approaches and examination techniques quite foreign to those of the English school, which they had traditionally used for the previous eleven months. His monthly visit was one of the most stimulating of the year and always unpredictable. His ways of looking at patients, his examinations, and his discussions always opened up grand vistas and new literature for the residents. As his resident, I recall taking Parkinsonian patients to the swimming pool to study their motility in swimming (as opposed to walking) to see if some of his bedside predictions were correct. To settle questions that he raised during rounds, I tested certain types of ataxia by having patients walk on seesaws at the local playground to see if ataxia was a problem of faulty recognition of the spatial orientation of the floor. At the end of the week, interesting patients were presented to "the Professor" (Denny-Brown), but he rarely encouraged discussion from the members of his staff at these conferences. He felt that most people were coming to hear him discuss patients; however, Yakovlev was someone who Denny-Brown encouraged to speak, as he obviously found this man as fascinating as the residents did. Few people were able to steal the limelight from the Professor, and clearly Yakovlev was one who could. An original thinker, he dealt in generalizations that tied together his vast knowledge of anatomical, embryological, and comparative anatomy. These expositions, expressed in enthusiastic language with a slight Russian accent, captivated all. He was primarily interested in organization and development of the brain with respect to clinical neurology.

In later years, after his return to Harvard, he was curator of the Warren Anatomical Museum at the Medical School, and had a huge neuropathological laboratory at the Medical School. By 1957 Yakovlev had ascended the academic ladder and was a clinical professor of neuropathology. He continued to amass neuropathologic specimens, studied by serial sections of the whole brain. He also published works dealing with mental retardation, epilepsy, frontal leukotomy, and arrhinencephaly (Yakovlev, 1952, 1954, 1959). He had a special interest in the anatomy of the limbic cortex, corpus callosum, and thalamus, which resulted in a number of classic studies with his collaborators Simon Locke, Jan Angevine, and Pasko Rakic (Yakovlev, Locke, and Angevine, 1966; Rakic and Yakovlev 1967; Yakovlev, 1969). He and his collaborators published two classic anatomical atlases at this time, one of the sagittal sections of the brain and one of the cerebellum (Yakovlev and Singer, 1954; Angevine, Mancall, and Yakovlev, 1962). He also published a number of articles dealing with the development and myelination of the brain (Yakovlev, 1962).

On his retirement, Yakovlev took his glass slides with him to the Fernald State School and to his home in Brookline. When one visited him at home, he would say that he lived on a huge glass mountain. He was particularly concerned about what would happen to this collection and was reluctant to see it in any place without some guarantee of its future stability. In 1974 the collection was relocated to the Armed Forces Institute of Pathology in Washington, D.C. It had now reached the monumental size of 250,000 slides collected over forty-two years, based on nine hundred specimens. He spent his last years in Washington, enjoying the permanent installation of his great collection, satisfied to see that his life's work would be the base for future advances in neurologic knowledge. This national treasure provided, and will continue to provide, investigative material of enduring value.

Yakovlev was a man who was liked by everyone. He always seemed to be interested in the activities and families of his colleagues; he loved to discuss neurology, anatomy, politics, theater, or to just "talk" with charming enthusiasm. He was always sought out at receptions and had a devoted group of colleagues and followers who delighted in his company. In his later years, Yakovlev was secure in the respect shown him by almost all his neurologic colleagues and became one of the "grand old men" of his profession. More than anything else, he enjoyed his professional contact with young residents, physicians, and neurological investigators, and was a constant figure near the front row at the national meetings.

Yakovlev received many honors in his life, most notably the presidency of the American Association of Neuropathologists in 1951, the Max Weinstein Award for Outstanding Scientific Achievements in Cerebral Palsy in 1955, officer of the American Neurologic Associations in 1958, and, more recently, in 1979, he was the recipient of the Hower Award from the Child Neurology Society for his outstanding contribution to developmental neuropathology.

H. Richard Tyler
BOSTON, MASSACHUSETTS

REFERENCES

Angevine, J. B., E. Mancall, and P. I. Yakovlev. 1962. *The Human Cerebellum: An Atlas and Topography in Serial Sections*. Boston: Little, Brown, and Co..

Kemper, T. 1984. Paul Ivan Yakovlev. *Arch Neur* 41:536–40.

Rakic, P., and P. I. Yakovlev. 1967. Development of Corpus Collosum and Cavum Septi in Man. *J Comp Neur* 132:45–72.

Yakovlev, P. I. 1937. Neurologic Mechanisms Concerned in Epileptic Seizures. *Arch Neur Psych* 37:523–54.

______. 1942. *Collected Lectures of the Seventh Post Graduate Seminar in Neurology and Psychiatry*. Waltham, MA: Metropolitan State Hospital.

______. 1947. Paraplegia of Hydrocephalics. *Am J Ment Def* 51:561–76.

______. 1952. Patterns of Neuronal Assemblies and Anatomical Substratum of Seizures. *Epilepsia* 1:51–68.

______. 1954. Paraplegia in Flexion of Cerebral Origin. *J Neuropath Exp Neur* 13:267–96.

______. 1959. Pathoarchitectonic Studies of Cerebral Malformations: III, Arrhinecephalies. *J Neuropath Exp Neur* 18:22–55.

______. 1962. Morphological Criteria of Growth and Maturation of the Nervous System in Man. *Res Pub Assoc Research Nerv Ment Dis* 39:3–46.

______. 1969. Development of the Nuclei of the Dorsal Thalamus and of the Cerebral Cortex. In *Modern Neurology*, 15–53. Ed. S. Locke. Boston: Little, Brown, and Co.

Yakovlev, P. I., S. Locke, and J. B. Angevine. 1966. The Limbus of the Cerebral Hemisphere, Limbic of the Thalamus and Cingulum Bundles. In *The Thalamus*, 77–79. Ed. D. P. Purpura and M. D. Yahr. New York: Columbia University Press.

Yakovlev, P. I., and M. Singer. 1954. *Human Brain in Sagittal Section*. Springfield, IL: Charles C Thomas.

Yakovlev, P. I., and H. G. Solomon. 1944. *Manual of Military Psychiatry*. Philadelphia: W. B. Saunders.

Yakovlev, P. I., and R. G. Wadsworth. 1946. Schizencephalies: A Study of the Congenital Clefts in the Cerebral Mantle. *J Neuropath Exp Neur* 5:116–30, 169–206.

NAME INDEX

NOTE: Page numbers in **boldface type** indicate chapters of founders.

SUBJECT INDEX

CREDITS

CHAPTER I

UNDERWOOD:
Figure 1 from J. R. Paul, *A History of Poliomyelitis.* New Haven: Yale University Press, 1971.

WHYTT:
Figure 1 courtesy of the National Library of Medicine.

CHAPTER 2

CHEYNE:
Figure 1 courtesy of the History and Special Collections Division, Louise M. Darling Biomedical Library, University of California, Los Angeles.

CLARKE:
Figure 1 courtesy of the National Library of Medicine.

GERHARD:
Figure 1 courtesy of the National Library of Medicine.

HEINE:
Figure 1 courtesy of Yale University School of Medicine.

ITARD:
Figure 2 courtesy of Jeremy Norman & Co., Inc.

MAUTHNER:
Figure 1 courtesy of Dr. H. Gadner of the Saint Anna's Childrens Hospital, Vienna. Figure 2 courtesy of Dr. Stephen Ashwal.

TIEDEMANN:
Figure 1 courtesy of the Louise M. Darling Biomedical Library, UCLA.

WEST:
Figure 1 by permission of The Hospital for Sick Children, Great Ormond Street, London.

CHAPTER 3

BOURNEVILLE:
Figure 1 courtesy of the Louise M. Darling Biomedical Library, UCLA.

CHARCOT:
Figures 1, 2a, and 2b courtesy of the Louise M. Darling Biomedical Library, UCLA.

COPEMAN:
Figure 1 courtesy of Dr. Anthony Batty Shaw and the Norfolk and Norwich Hospital.

DEJERINE:
Figures 1 and 2 courtesy of the National Library of Medicine.

DEJERINE-KLUMPKE:
Figure 1 courtesy of the National Library of Medicine.

DOWN:
Figure 1 by permission of Little Brown and Company. From *Mongolism*, CIBA Foundation Study Group, No. 25. Boston: Little, Brown and Company, 1967.

DUCHENNE:
Figure 1 by permission of the Library of the National Academy of Medicine, Paris.

ERB:
Figure 1 by permission of the American Medical Association. *Archives of Neurology and Psychiatry* 7:250–51. Copyright 1922, American Medical Association.

FREUD:
Figure 1 courtesy of the Louise M. Darling Biomedical Library, UCLA.

FRIEDREICH:
Figure 1 courtesy of Dr. Erich Kuhn, Heidelburg and Dr. Dieter Schjeffner, Berlin.

GAUCHER:
Figure 1 by permission of the Wellcome Institute Library, London.

GILLES DE LA TOURETTE:
Figure 1 courtesy of the National Library of Medicine.

GOWERS:
Figure 1 is from Macdonald Critchley, *Sir William Gowers, 1845–1915: A Biographical Appreciation*. London: Heinemann, 1949.

HUGHLINGS JACKSON:
Figure 1 courtesy of the Louise M. Darling Biomedical Library, UCLA.

Figures 2a–2c courtesy of the National Hospital Library, Queen's Square, London.

LITTLE:
Figures 1 and 2 courtesy of Wellcome Institute Library, London. Figure 3 courtesy of the Louise M. Darling Biomedical Library, UCLA.

MACEWEN:
Figure 1 courtesy of the National Library of Medicine.

MARIE:
Figure 1 by permission of the *Revue neurologique.*

OPPENHEIM:
Figure 1 courtesy of J. Ulbricht, Universitätsbibliothek der Freien Universität, Berlin.

OSLER:
Figure 1 courtesy of the National Library of Medicine.

QUINCKE:
Figure 1 courtesy of the National Library of Medicine.

SOLTMANN:
Figure 1 by permission of Institut für Geschichte der Medizin der Universität Wien.

STURGES:
Figure 1 courtesy of M. P. Coomer, Deputy Secretary, Charing Cross and Westminister Medical School.

THOMSEN:
Figure 1 is based on information from E. Thomasen, *Myotonia: Thomsen's disease (Myotonia congentia), Paramyotonia, and Dystrophia Myotonica: A Clinical and Heredobiologic Investigation.* Cophenhagen: Egnar Munsgaard, 1948; and K. Nissen, "Beiträge zur

Kenntnis der Thomsenchen Krankheit (Myotonia congenita) mit Besonderer Berücksichtigung des hereditären momentes und seinen Beziehungen zu den Mendelschen Vererbungsregeln," *Zeit Klin Med* 97 (1923):58–93.

UNVERRICHT:
Figure 1 courtesy of the Francis A. Countway Library of Medicine, Boston.

VON RECKLINGHAUSEN:
Figure 1 courtesy of the National Library of Medicine.

WERDNIG:
Figures 1 and 2 courtesy of the Institut für Geschichte der Medizin der Universität Wien.

CHAPTER 4

BAILEY:
Figure 1 courtesy of the National Library of Medicine.

BALÓ:
Figure 1 courtesy of Ilona Banga, M.D.

BRUNS:
Figure 1 by permission of Georg Thieme Verlag.

CANAVAN:
Figure 1 courtesy of the National Library of Medicine.

COLLIER:
Figure 1 courtesy of the Photography Department, National Hospital, Queen's Square, London. Figures 2a and 2b courtesy of the National Library of Medicine.

CROTHERS:
Figure 1 by permission of the C. V. Mosby Company. Figure 2 by permission of Williams & Wilkins.

CROUZON:
Figure 1 courtesy of the National Library of Medicine.

CUSHING:
Figure 1 by permission of the Yale Medical Historical Library, New Haven, Connecticut.

DANDY:
Figure 1 courtesy of the National Library of Medicine.

FÖLLING:
Figure 1 from Lyman, Frank L. *Phenylketonuria* (1963). Courtesy of Charles C Thomas, Publisher, Springfield, Illinois.

HALLERVORDEN:
Figure 1 by permission of Springer-Verlag, Heidelberg.

HUNT:
Figure 1 courtesy of the National Library of Medicine.

HUNTER:
Figure 1 courtesy of Dr. Allan R. Ronald, University of Manitoba.

HURLER:
Figure 1 courtesy of Dr. H. R. Wiedemann.

LAFORA:
Figure 1 courtesy of the New York Academy of Medicine Library.

ORTON:
Figure 1 by permission of the Orton Dyslexia Society.

RACHFORD:
Figure 2 From a private collection of the Condon School.

SACHS:
Figure 1 is from Stumpf, David, "The Founding of Pediatric Neurology in America," *Bull NY Acad Med* 57(1981): 804-16.

SCHILDER:
Figure 1 courtesy of Warren Marks and Ilsa von Braukitch.

SPIELMEYER:
Figure 1 courtesy of the National Library of Medicine.

TREDGOLD:
Figure 1 courtesy of Dr. Stephen Lock, editor of the *British Medical Journal*.

VOGT:
Figure 1 courtesy of Dr. Wiesner, Vogt-Institut, Bad Soden.

CHAPTER 5

ADAMS:
Figure 1 courtesy of Dr. Raymond Adams.

AICARDI:
Figure 1 courtesy of Dr. Jean Aicardi.

ALPERS:
Figure 1 by Bachrach.

ANDRÉ-THOMAS:
Figure 1 courtesy of Dr. Saint-Anne Dargassies.

BRANDT:
Figure 1 courtesy of Rigshospitalet, Denmark.

BYERS:
Figure 1 courtesy of the family of Dr. Randolph Byers.

CARTER:
Figure 1 courtesy of Dr. Sidney Carter.

CLARK:
Figure 1 courtesy of Dr. David Clark

COURVILLE:
Figure 1 from his work *Birth and Brain Damage*, published by his wife posthumously.

CRITCHLEY:
Figure 1 courtesy of the Department of Medical Illustration, Institute of Neurology, the National Hospital, Queen's Square, London.

DODGE:
Figures 1 and 2 courtesy of Dr. Philip Dodge.

DUBOWITZ:
Figure 1 courtesy of Dr. Victor Dubowitz.

FORD:
Figure 1: Courtesy of the Johns Hopkins Medical Institutions, the Alan Mason Chesney Medical Archives.

FUKUYAMA:
Figure 1 courtesy of Dr. Yukio Fukuyama.

GAMSTORP:
Figure 1 courtesy of Dr. Ingrid Gamstorp.

HAGBERG:
Figure 1 courtesy of Dr. Bengt Hagberg.

INGRAM:
Figure 1 courtesy of the Royal Hospital for Sick Children, Edinburgh.

LENNOX:
Figure 1 courtesy of Dr. J. Gordon Millichap.

LIVINGSTON:
Figure 1 courtesy of Mrs. Anne Livingston and Dr. Irving Pruce.

LOMBROSO:
Figure 1 courtesy of Dr. Cesare Lombroso.

LOUIS-BAR:
Figure 1 courtesy of Dr. Philippe Evrard.

LYON:
Figure 1 courtesy of Dr. Gilles Lyon.

MATSON:
Figure 1 courtesy of Dr. John Shillito, Department of Neurosurgery, Children's Hospital Medical Center, Boston.

MELCHIOR:
Figure 1 courtesy of Dr. Johannes Melchior.

NORMAN:
Figure 1 reproduced by permission from H. Urich and M. G. Norman.

PEIPER:
Figure 1 courtesy of the National Library of Medicine.

PERLSTEIN:
Figure 1 courtesy of Dr. Louis Boshes.

PRICHARD:
Figure 1 courtesy of the family of Dr. John Prichard.

RETT:
Figure 1 courtesy of the Rett Syndrome Foundation.

REYE:
Figure 1 courtesy of Dr. Corrie Reye.

ROBB:
Figure 1 courtesy of Dr. Fred Andermann.

RUSSELL:
Figure 1 reproduced with the permission of the Controller of Her Majesty's Stationery Office.

SANDIFER:
Figure 1 courtesy of the Museum and Archives Service, the Hospital for Sick Children, London.

TIZARD:
Figure 1 courtesy of Sir Peter Tizard.

WALTON:
Figure 1 courtesy of Lord John Walton.

WYLLIE:
Figure 1 courtesy of The Hospital for Sick Children.

NORMAN
PUBLISHING ®

Collaborators on the production of *The Founders of Child Neurology:*

Desktop Publishing Inc., Linotronic Output
Elinor Lindheimer, Indexer
Jill Lustig, Project Manager
Seventeenth Street Studios, Designer
Martha Nicholson Steele, Editor
Technical Publications, Electronic Page Composition
Thomson-Shore, Inc., Printer and Binder

The text type is Garamond #3, from Adobe Systems.